OBSTETRICS AND GYNECOLOGY

Second Edition

CHARLES R. B. BECKMANN, M. D., M.H.P.E.
Professor and Associate Chairman in the Department of Obstetrics
and Gynecology
Professor in the Department of Community and Family Medicine
University of Missouri — Kansas City, School of Medicine
Kansas City, Missouri

FRANK W. LING, M.D.
Faculty Professor and Chairman
Department of Obstetrics and Gynecology
University of Tennessee College of Medicine
Memphis, Tennessee

BARBARA M. BARZANSKY, Ph.D., M.H.P.E.
Assistant Director, Division of Undergraduate Medical Education
The American Medical Association
Chicago, Illinois

G. WILLIAM BATES, M.D.
Professor of Obstetrics and Gynecology
University of South Carolina
Vice President, Medical Education
Greenville Hospital System
Greenville, South Carolina

WILLIAM N. P. HERBERT, M.D.
Professor and Director
Division of Maternal and Fetal Medicine
Department of Obstetrics and Gynecology
Duke University School of Medicine
Durham, North Carolina

DOUGLAS W. LAUBE, M.D., M.Ed.
Professor and Chairman
Department of Obstetrics and Gynecology
University of Wisconsin Medical School
Madison, Wisconsin

ROGER P. SMITH, M.D.
Professor and Director
Section of General Obstetrics and Gynecology
Department of Obstetrics and Gynecology
Medical College of Georgia
Augusta, Georgia

OBSTETRICS AND GYNECOLOGY

SECOND EDITION

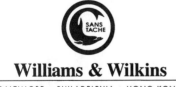

Williams & Wilkins

BALTIMORE • PHILADELPHIA • HONG KONG
LONDON • MUNICH • SYDNEY • TOKYO

A WAVERLY COMPANY

Editor: Patricia A. Coryell
Managing Editor: Linda S. Napora
Copy Editor: Candace B. Levy
Designer: Dan Pfisterer
Illustration Planner: Ray Lowman
Production Coordinator: Anne G. Seitz

Copyright © 1995
Williams & Wilkins
428 East Preston Street
Baltimore, Maryland 21202, USA

Accurate indications, adverse reactions, and dosage schedules for drugs are provided in this book, but it is possible that they may change. The reader is urged to review the package information data of the manufacturers of the medications mentioned.

Printed in the United States of America

First Edition 1992

ISBN 0-683-00503-0

95 96
1 2 3 4 5 6 7 8 9 10

FOREWORD

Most second editions are usually just updates and reorganization of the first. Such is not the case with the second edition of this unique and excellent textbook, *Obstetrics and Gynecology*. In addition to updating with current information where indicated, the new edition includes summary information tables, more illustrations, a well organized self-evaluation section, and a valuable discussion on primary care for the obstetrician-gynecologist.

As in the first edition, the material, based on APGO Educational Objectives, is presented in a concise and readable fashion and supplies more important information than outline-type review books. This edition will fulfill the needs of all medical students. Its organization and content make it a valuable resource for residents and practitioners as well, particularly when reviewing for examinations.

The authors, all involved in the first edition, are to be congratulated on maintaining their original concept and achieving their objective of a textbook for learning. I enthusiastically recommend this new edition and am confident that it will secure its position as the standard text for all obstetric and gynecologic clerkships.

MARTIN L. STONE, M.D.
PROFESSOR AND CHAIRMAN (EMERITUS)
SUNY AT STONY BROOK, NEW YORK

PREFACE

Obstetrics and Gynecology, 2nd edition, is written specifically for medical students taking their clerkship in obstetrics and gynecology. The goals of the book are to provide the basic information about obstetrics and gynecology that all medical school graduates should possess, to provide the specific information that medical students need to complete an obstetrics and gynecology clerkship successfully, and the information medical students need to pass national standardized examinations in this content area. This book also is designed to provide the basic information needed by other physicians whose primary care responsibilities include the care of women, such as internists, family medicine physicians, and pediatricians. Nurse midwives, nurse practitioners, and nurses will find the content specifically suitable for their needs as well.

Obstetrics and Gynecology, 2nd edition, is unique in two important ways:

1. This textbook was written by seven professional medical educators. Six are experienced obstetrician-gynecologists who have expertise and interest in education, including additional degrees in education, experience as clerkship and residency directors, and involvement in the preparation of national standardized examinations and issues of primary care for women. The seventh author is a professional educator and anatomist with extensive experience in curriculum development and evaluation. With the exception of special sections and one chapter that was written by four contributors, the entire book was written, reviewed, and revised by these seven individuals.
2. This textbook was designed to facilitate learning and self-evaluation. To do this, the book is based on the "Instructional Objectives for a Clinical Curriculum in Obstetrics and Gynecology" of the Association of Professors of Gynecology and Obstetrics, 6th edition. These national standards are used to organize most OB-GYN clerkships in the United States and Canada, and they are used as a guideline in the development of national standardized examinations. They contain objectives that cover basic information that any health care provider engaged in the primary care of women should know. A summary of these objectives is provided in the book as well as a comprehensive "APGO Objectives Index" which will facilitate access to the objectives. This APGO objectives index will provide students with a fast method of studying a particular topic across all the chapters of the book.

Each chapter has a section devoted to case studies, and at the end of the book, there is an extensive self-evaluation section that contain questions organized by chapter. The use of these tools will help learners gauge their progress and focus their efforts with maximum efficiency. The use of these special facets of the book is discussed in the introductory section, "How to Use This Book."

Medical school textbooks often contain large amounts of information more useful to residents and practicing physicians than to medical students. In contrast, *Obstetrics and Gynecology*, 2nd edition, focuses specifically on the basic information needed for the primary obstetric and gynecologic care of women, the same information medical students need during the 6- to 8-week OB-GYN clerkship. *Obstetrics and Gynecology*, 2nd edition, written by professional educators according to sound educational principles, accomplishes this goal. The concise and easy-to-read chapters, correlated with national learning objectives and the self-evaluation sections for measuring progress fulfill our intention: to provide the fundamental information about obstetrics and gynecology required for the basic care of women.

ACKNOWLEDGMENTS

We extend our appreciation to Pat Coryell, Tim Satterfield, Linda Napora, Anne Seitz, Dan Pfisterer, Ray Lowman, and Candace Levy and all the staff at Williams & Wilkins for their seemingly tireless help and encouragement during the arduous preparation of *Obstetrics and Gynecology*, 2nd edition. Likewise, we appreciate the innovative educational art provided by Joyce Lavery, which adds so much to the usefulness of the book. We also extend thanks to Judy Klingbeil for her coordination of the manuscript chapters and figures and to our secretaries for their good-spirited efforts as we produced revision after revision of each chapter. Finally, we again extend a special thanks to Carol-Lynn Brown, our first editor at Williams & Wilkins, for her foresight and support in the early development of the first edition of this book, and our best wishes in her new career in medicine.

CONTRIBUTORS

BARBARA F. SHARF, Ph.D. *(contributor, chapter 1)*
Associate Professor of Health Communication and Medical Education
Department of Medical Education
University of Illinois College of Medicine
Chicago, Illinois

DANIEL L. CLARKE-PEARSON, M.D. *(contributor, chapter 1)*
Professor and Director, Division of Gynecologic Oncology
Department of Obstetrics and Gynecology
Duke Medical Center
Durham, North Carolina

LEE P. SHULMAN, M.D. *(contributor, Reproductive Genetics in chapter 3)*
Associate Professor of Obstetrics and Gynecology
Director, Division of Reproductive Genetics
Department of Obstetrics and Gynecology
University of Tennessee College of Medicine
Memphis, Tennessee

JOANNA M. CAIN, M.D. *(Author, chapter 47)*
Associate Professor of Obstetrics and Gynecology
Division of Gynecologic Oncology
University of Washington
Seattle, Washington

HOW TO USE THIS BOOK

Obstetrics and Gynecology, 2nd edition, is specifically written to help the medical student learn the basics of obstetrics-gynecology. It is useful in studying during the clerkship and in reviewing for clerkship written and oral examinations as well as for standardized national examinations. The following suggestions will make the use of the book most efficient.

Indexes

There are two indexes in this book. One is a traditional subject index giving the page references for specific topics. The other is an APGO objectives index based on the 6th edition of the objectives of the Association of Professors of Gynecology and Obstetrics (APGO). Each APGO objective has been condensed, and the pages where content relating to that objective can be found are listed. It would be useful for you to review these objectives at the start of the clerkship to get an idea of the basic content that you will be expected to master during the clerkship. The "APGO Objectives Index" will also be useful when it is time to study for national standardized examinations.

To Study a Topic for the First Time

Each chapter covers a general topic and most of the chapters are directly related to one of the APGO objectives. Locate the appropriate objective summary and read it carefully. Then read the chapter and attempt to answer the study questions in the Case Studies and the questions for each chapter at the end of the book. The questions are to help you assess whether you have learned the chapter's main points. Based on your answers, you may choose to go back and reread the relevant portion(s) of the chapter.

Many chapters contain references to content contained in other parts of the book. Sometimes this information is required for you to understand the topic that you are studying. In this case, you should read these additional pages. For example, terms in the book are defined only once in any detail. You will need to find the definition of important terms related to the topic by using the "Subject Index". To ensure that you have read all the information about a topic, consult both the "Subject Index" and the "APGO Objectives Index" and read the cited pages.

After you have studied a chapter and completed the study questions, go back and reread the APGO objective. Make sure that you know the information asked for in the objective.

To Review for Examinations after the Clerkship

For the review, you may want to study units or sections as a whole. Begin by attempting to answer the study questions for each chapter again and reviewing the case studies and their commentary. If you answer the questions correctly, you should briefly reread the chapter to stimulate your memory. If you cannot answer the study questions, read the chapter carefully, along with related content that is contained elsewhere in the book.

APGO OBJECTIVES, 6th EDITION (condensed)

The following is a condensation of the *Medical Student Educational Objectives*, 6th Edition of the Association of Professors of Gynecology and Obstetrics (APGO). The numbers correspond to the numbers of the APGO objectives.

The student should be able to:

Unit 1: Approach to the Patient

1. HISTORY
   Take a thorough obstetric-gynecologic history, utilizing appropriate communication skills, and transmit the results in written and oral form.
2. EXAMINATION
   a. Perform a thorough obstetric-gynecologic examination (breasts, abdomen, pelvis), utilizing appropriate communication skills and attention to patient comfort and modesty, and transmit the results in written and oral form.
   b. Explain breast and external genital self-examination to the patient.
3. PAP SMEAR AND CULTURES
   Obtain and properly handle specimens for a Pap smear and microbiologic cultures to detect sexually transmitted diseases and explain the purpose of these tests to the patient.
4. DIAGNOSIS AND MANAGEMENT PLAN
   Based on the results of the patient history and physical examination, generate a problem list, identify likely diagnoses, and develop a management plan (laboratory and diagnostic studies, patient education plan and plans for continuing care and treatment).

Unit 2: Obstetrics

SECTION A: NORMAL OBSTETRICS

5. Maternal-Fetal Physiology
   Explain the maternal physiologic changes associated with pregnancy and the physiology of the placenta and fetus.
6. Preconception and Antepartum Care
   a. Describe the conditions warranting special attention in preconceptional care and counseling and explain the nature of this care.
   b. Explain the initial and ongoing elements of antepartum care, including methods to diagnose pregnancy and establish gestational age; determination of obstetric risk status;

techniques to assess fetal growth, maturity, and well-being; and appropriate diagnostic studies.

c. Perform a physical examination on an obstetric patient and develop a problem list and management plan based on the initial assessment and ongoing evaluation.

d. Answer commonly asked patient questions concerning pregnancy, labor, and delivery.

7. INTRAPARTUM CARE

Describe the stages and mechanisms of labor, including the differences between false and true labor; the initial and ongoing assessment of the fetus and the laboring patient; the management of normal labor and delivery, including the indications for operative delivery; and the immediate postpartum care of the mother.

8. IMMEDIATE CARE OF THE NEWBORN

Explain the assessment and immediate postpartum care of the newborn, including situations requiring immediate intervention.

9. POSTPARTUM CARE

Explain normal postpartum care and the appropriate counseling of the postpartum patient. Explain the normal physiologic changes in the postpartum period.

SECTION B: ABNORMAL OBSTETRICS

10. ECTOPIC PREGNANCY

Describe the diagnosis and management of ectopic pregnancy, including risk factors, symptoms/physical findings, diagnostic procedures, and treatment options.

11. SPONTANEOUS ABORTION

Explain the diagnosis and management of the causes of first-trimester bleeding, including incomplete, threatened, and missed abortion as well as the potential complications of spontaneous and septic abortion.

12. MEDICAL AND SURGICAL CONDITIONS IN PREGNANCY

Describe the diagnosis and management of the common medical and surgical complications in the pregnant patient, including their effects on the pregnancy and the effects of pregnancy on the condition, including anemia, diabetes, urinary tract disease, infectious disease (herpes, rubella, streptococcus, hepatitis B, HIV), cardiac disease, asthma, substance abuse, and acute abdominal symptoms.

13. PREECLAMPSIA-ECLAMPSIA SYNDROME

Define pregnancy-induced hypertension, preeclampsia, and eclampsia and describe the pathophysiology, diagnosis, management, and potential maternal and fetal complications of these conditions.

14. D ISOIMMUNIZATION

Describe the circumstances leading to Rh isoimmunization and the techniques used to determine its presence in the mother, the methods used to assess the severity of disease in the fetus and newborn, and the appropriate use of immuno-globulin prophylaxis.

15. MULTIFETAL GESTATION
Describe the mechanism of twinning and the altered physiology associated with multifetal gestation. Describe the diagnosis and the antepartum, intrapartum, and postpartum management of multifetal gestation.

16. FETAL DEATH
Describe the diagnosis and management of fetal death, including methods to determine the cause, the potential maternal complications (including disseminated intravascular coagulation), and the emotional consequences.

17. ABNORMAL LABOR
   a. Describe the causes, labor patterns, evaluation, and management of abnormal labor, fetopelvic disproportion, and abnormal fetal presentations.
   b. Describe the indications and contraindications for oxytocin administration and vaginal birth after cesarean section.
   c. Describe the maternal and fetal complications resulting from abnormal labor.

18. THIRD TRIMESTER BLEEDING
Describe the approach to the patient with third-trimester bleeding, including the methods to differentiate among the causes (such as placenta previa and abruptio placentae), the maternal and fetal complications, and the management of shock secondary to bleeding.

19. PRETERM LABOR
Describe the predisposing factors and causes of preterm labor and preterm delivery and the approach to the patient with premature contractions, including the principles of tocolysis.

20. PREMATURE RUPTURE OF MEMBRANES
Describe the diagnosis and management of premature rupture of the membranes, including the indications and methods for expectant management versus immediate delivery and the methods used to monitor maternal and fetal status during expectant management.

21. INTRAPARTUM FETAL DISTRESS
Explain the techniques for intrapartum electronic and biochemical fetal monitoring. Describe normal, abnormal, and reassuring fetal heart rate patterns and the approach to management when there is an abnormal or nonreassuring fetal heart rate pattern, including auscultation, electronic fetal monitoring, and fetal scalp sampling.

22. POSTPARTUM HEMORRHAGE
Describe the likely causes and predisposing factors of postpartum hemorrhage and the approach to its diagnosis and management, including identification of lacerations and the use of contractile agents.

23. POSTPARTUM INFECTION

Describe the risk factors associated with postpartum infection, the possible causes and the means to distinguish among them, and the approach to the management of a patient with fever and presumed postpartum infection. Describe the use of prophylactic antibiotics to prevent postpartum infection.

24. ANXIETY AND DEPRESSION

Describe the factors commonly associated with and symptoms of postpartum anxiety, depression, and psychosis in normal and high-risk pregnancy and the management of these situations.

25. MORTALITY

Define the common causes of and describe the formula for calculating the rate of maternal death, fetal death, neonatal death, and perinatal death.

26. POSTTERM PREGNANCY

Define and describe postterm pregnancy and its associated risks and complications. Explain the methods used in antepartum monitoring and management of the fetus.

27. FETAL GROWTH ABNORMALITIES

Define macrosomia and intrauterine growth retardation and for each, describe the associated risk factors, recognized causes, methods used in diagnosis and management, and associated maternal and fetal abnormalities.

SECTION C: PROCEDURES

28. OBSTETRICAL PROCEDURES

Define, supply the indications and contraindications for, and list the risks of the following procedures: ultrasonography, episiotomy, cesarean delivery, forceps delivery, induction and augmentation of labor, vacuum-assisted delivery, breech delivery, antepartum fetal assessment, amniocentesis and cordocentesis, chorionic villus sampling, newborn circumcision, vaginal birth after cesarean delivery, spontaneous vaginal delivery, and fetal monitoring.

Unit 3: Gynecology

SECTION A: GYNECOLOGY

29. CONTRACEPTION

Describe the mechanism of action, degree of effectiveness, advantages and disadvantages, contraindications, financial considerations, and potential complications for each commonly utilized method of contraception.

30. STERILIZATION

Describe the advantages and disadvantages, contraindications, failure rates, reversibility, financial considerations, and potential complications for each commonly used method of male and female sterilization.

31. VULVAR AND VAGINAL DISEASE

    Describe the physiologic or infectious causes, history/physical findings, methods of diagnosis and management of physiologic changes in normal vaginal discharge, infectious and atrophic vaginitis and vulvitis, dermatologic conditions of the vulva, and Bartholin's gland disease.

32. SEXUALLY TRANSMITTED DISEASES

    Describe the causative agent, method of transmission, symptoms/physical findings, and methods of diagnosis/screening and management for gonorrhea, *chlamydia*, herpes, syphilis, condyloma acuminatum (HPV) and HIV infection.

33. SALPINGITIS

    Describe the anatomical location, causes, symptoms/physical findings, methods of diagnosis, and possible sequelae of acute and chronic salpingitis. Discuss the relationship of salpingitis to tuboovarian abscess, chronic salpingitis, ectopic pregnancy, and infertility.

34. PELVIC RELAXATION

    Discuss the predisposing factors, anatomy, pathophysiology, and diagnosis of pelvic relaxation and urinary incontinence, including discussion of cystocele, rectocele, and vaginal and uterine prolapse.

35. ENDOMETRIOSIS AND ADENOMYOSIS

    Compare and contrast the pathogenesis, diagnosis, and treatment of endometriosis and adenomyosis. Explain the differences between endometriosis and adenomyosis.

36. CHRONIC PELVIC PAIN

    Define chronic pelvic pain and discuss the diagnosis, pathophysiology, and management of the heterogeneous group of disorders causing it.

SECTION B: BREASTS

37. DISORDERS OF THE BREAST

    a. Describe the indications for and timing of breast self-examination, physical examination of the breast, and mammography.

    b. Describe the diagnostic approach to a woman with a breast mass, nipple discharge, or breast pain.

    c. Explain the history/physical findings associated with intraductal papilloma, fibrocystic changes in the breast, fibroadenoma, breast carcinoma, and mastitis.

SECTION C: PROCEDURES

38. GYNECOLOGIC PROCEDURES

    a. Define and describe the indications and contraindications for and the risks of the following gynecologic procedures: colpscopy and cervical biopsy, cone biopsy, cyrotherapy, culdocentesis, dilation and curettage, electrosurgical excision of cervix, endometrial biopsy, hysterectomy, hysterosalpingography, hysteroscopy, laparoscopy, laser vaporization, mam-

mography, needle aspiration of breast mass, pelvic ultrasonography, pregnancy termination, vulvar biopsy.
  b. Explain each of the above procedures in language under-
     standable to the patient.

Unit 4: Reproductive Endocrinology, Infertility, and Related Topics

39. PUBERTY
    a. Describe the physiologic and psychologic events associ-
       ated with normal puberty and the approximate ages at
       which these occur.
    b. Explain the causes, characteristics, diagnostic approach to,
       and counseling issues about abnormal puberty.
    c. Define true precocious puberty, pseudoprecocious pu-
       berty, and delayed puberty.

40. AMENORRHEA
    a. Define primary amenorrhea, secondary amenorrhea, and
       oligomenorrhea.
    b. Describe the physical, endocrinologic, and psychologic
       causes of amenorrhea and the diagnostic approach to the
       patient with this problem.

41. HIRSUTISM AND VIRILIZATION
    a. Define hirsutism, defeminization, and virilization.
    b. Describe the causes of hirsutism and virilization and the
       diagnostic approach to the patient with these problems.

42. NORMAL AND ABNORMAL UTERINE BLEEDING
    a. Define and discuss the physiology/pathophysiology of
       normal menstruation, abnormal uterine bleeding and dys-
       functional uterine bleeding.
    b. Describe the causes of abnormal uterine bleeding and the
       diagnostic approach to the patient with this problem.

43. DYSMENORRHEA
    Define primary and secondary dysmenorrhea and describe
    the causes and approach to the evaluation and management
    of each.

44. CLIMACTERIC
    a. Describe the physiologic changes in the hypothalmic-pi-
       tuitary-ovarian axis related to the climacteric and meno-
       pause and the associated physical, emotional, and sexual
       symptoms/physical findings.
    b. Describe the indications, contraindications, risks and ben-
       efits, and method of hormone-replacement therapy.

45. INFERTILITY
    a. Define infertility.
    b. Describe the causes of infertility and the diagnostic meth-
       ods used to evaluate the presence of each.

46. PREMENSTRUAL SYNDROME
    a. Describe the premenstrual syndrome and its possible
       causes.

b. Describe the diagnostic and therapeutic options for symptomatic patients with premenstrual syndrome.

Unit 5: NEOPLASIA

47. GESTATIONAL TROPHOBLASTIC DISEASE
    a. List symptoms/physical findings commonly found in patients with gestational trophoblastic disease.
    b. Describe the diagnostic methods used to confirm this condition and the management and follow-up of patients.

48. VULVAR NEOPLASMS
    a. Define the risk factors for vulvar neoplasia.
    b. Describe the diagnostic approach and management of the patient with vulvar symptoms.

49. CERVICAL DISEASE AND NEOPLASIA
    a. Describe the risk factors, symptoms, and physical findings characteristic of cervicitis and cervical neoplasia.
    b. Describe the management of a patient with an abnormal Pap smear.
    c. Explain the common course of cervical neoplastic disease, including the histologic categories of cervical neoplasia and the FIGO staging to cervical cancer.

50. UTERINE LEIOMYOMAS
    Describe the symptoms/physical findings characteristic of uterine leiomyomas; the diagnostic methods employed to confirm the condition; and the management options, including indications for surgical intervention.

51. ENDOMETRIAL CARCINOMA
    a. Describe the approach to the patient with postmenopausal bleeding.
    b. Describe the risk factors and the symptoms/physical findings characteristic of endometrial carcinoma, the methods used in diagnosis and staging of the disease, and the typical disease course.

52. OVARIAN NEOPLASMS
    a. Describe how specific factors (such as patient age, characteristics of the mass) affect the approach to the patient with an adnexal mass.
    b. Describe the symptoms/physical findings, methods used in diagnosis and staging, and histologic systems used for classification of functional and benign ovarian neoplasia and ovarian carcinoma.

Unit 6: Human Sexuality

53. SEXUALITY
    a. Explain the phases of the female sexual response and the physiologic basis of each.
    b. Describe the influences on sexuality at various stages in the female life cycle, including menarche, initiation of sexual activity, pregnancy, postpartum, and menopause.

  c. List and answer commonly asked questions about sexual function.
  d. Describe common examples of sexual dysfunction and their preliminary assessment and identify those problems that require referral.
54. MODES OF SEXUAL EXPRESSION
  Define heterosexual, homosexual, bisexual, transsexual, and transvestite.
55. PHYSICIAN SEXUALITY
  a. Demonstrate empathetic and nonjudgmental behaviors in interactions with patients.
  b. Demonstrate awareness of the influence of the physician's own sexuality on his/her interactions with patients.
  c. Describe the behavioral patterns of seductive patients.
56. SEXUAL ASSAULT AND DOMESTIC VIOLENCE
  a. Define domestic violence and the rape trauma syndrome.
  b. Describe the management of suspected cases of sexual assault in children and adults.

Unit 7: Professional Behavior, Ethics, and Legal Issues

57. PERSONAL INTERACTION AND COMMUNICATION SKILLS
  a. Establish rapport and work dependably with patients.
  b. Work cooperatively and dependably with other members of the health care team.
  c. Recognize personal limitations.
58. LEGAL ISSUES IN OBSTETRICS AND GYNECOLOGY
  a. Demonstrate a knowledge of the elements of informed consent: right to refuse care, outcomes, options, capacity to choose, and surrogate decision makers.
  b. Describe the following legal obligations to protect patient interests: advance directives for health care, confidentiality, abandonment, contractual nature of medical benefits, fraud.
59. ETHICS IN OBSTETRICS AND GYNECOLOGY
  a. Describe approaches to the definition of ethical problems and the bases of ethical conflict in maternal/fetal medicine.
  b. Describe how the concept of justice applies to access to care in obstetrics and gynecology.
  c. Describe the ethical issues raised by termination of pregnancy and reproductive technology.

Unit 8: Preventive Care and Health Maintenance

60. PREVENTIVE CARE
  a. Describe the indications for and appropriate intervals between the following screening procedures that are part of routine health surveillance: Pap smear, mammogram, blood pressure monitoring, and blood lipid profiles.

b. Describe the appropriate patient education associated with the following: contraception, STD prevention, diet, exercise, stress management, smoking, and immunization.

c. Describe the costs/benefits of routine health surveillance.

CONTENTS

SECTION I: APPROACH TO THE PATIENT: PREVENTIVE CARE AND HEALTH MAINTENANCE

SECTION II: OBSTETRICS

SECTION III: GYNECOLOGY

SECTION IV: REPRODUCTIVE ENDOCRINOLOGY AND INFERTILITY

SECTION V: NEOPLASIA

SECTION VI: ETHICS

chapter 1

HEALTH CARE FOR WOMEN:
Obstetrics and Gynecology as Specialty and Primary-Preventive Health Care

While obstetrician-gynecologists provide specialty care for women, they also serve as the primary care physician for over one-half of women in the United States. As "specialists," they provide obstetric and gynecologic care. As primary care physicians for women, obstetrician-gynecologists assume responsibility for primary-preventive health care, where the annual gynecologic examinations are enhanced to become periodic health examinations timed and tailored to address the important causes of morbidity and mortality in each age group of women.

To be successful with these diverse but important responsibilities, the obstetrician-gynecologist must understand the wide range of issues encompassed by the primary-preventive health care responsibility as well as the specialty of obstetrics and gynecology, must be able to establish a good professional relationship with patients, and must be able to perform an excellent women's health evaluation (history and physical examination).

THE SPECIALIST AND PRIMARY-PREVENTIVE HEALTH CARE ROLES OF THE OBSTETRICIAN-GYNECOLOGIST

Obstetrics was originally a separate branch of medicine and gynecology, a division of surgery. Obstetrics and gynecology merged into a single specialty as knowledge of the pathophysiology of the female reproductive tract led to a natural integration of the two areas of medicine that were so clearly interrelated. In the United States,

obstetrics is now somewhat indistinctly divided into general obstetrics (dealing with uncomplicated pregnancy) and maternal-fetal medicine (dealing with complicated, or high-risk, pregnancy) as well as reproductive genetics. Likewise, gynecology now includes general gynecology (dealing with nonmalignant disorders of the reproductive tract and associated organ systems), urogynecology, gynecologic infectious disease, gynecologic oncology, and reproductive endocrinology-infertility.

Obstetrician-gynecologists have traditionally dealt with diseases of the reproductive tract and pregnancy. However, many obstetrician-gynecologists have also assumed responsibility for the overall health of women, including treatment of some nongynecologic problems and coordinating their care by appropriate diagnosis and referral to other physicians and specialists.

To facilitate the primary-preventive health care responsibility, the Task Force on Primary and Preventive Health Care of the American College of Obstetricians and Gynecologists (1993) published *The Obstetrician-Gynecologist and Primary-Preventive Health Care*, which contains guidelines for this care. By means of screening testing, counseling, behavioral intervention, and/or consultation, the obstetrician-gynecologist is able to address the major causes of morbidity (Table 1.1) and mortality (Table 1.2) for women in each of the major age groups. Recommendations for screening testing (Table 1.3) are associated with high-risk situations and conditions; recommendations for immunization (Table 1.4) complete the tasks.

1

Table 1.1.
Leading Causes of Morbidity in Women in the United States

Cause of Morbidity	Age 12–18	19–39	40–64	>65
HEENT[a] conditions	+	+	+	+
URI[b]	+	+	+	+
Infection (viral, parasites, bacterial)	+	+		
Sexual abuse	+			
Accidental injury	+	+		+
Digestive tract conditions	+			
Acute urinary conditions	+	+		
Osteoporosis/arthritis			+	+
Hypertension			+	+
Orthopaedic conditions			+	
Heart disease			+	+
Hearing and vision impairments			+	+
Urinary incontinence				+

[a] Head, ears, eyes, nose, and throat.
[b] Upper respiratory infection.

Table 1.2.
Leading Causes of Death in Women in the United States

Cause of Death	Age 12–18	19–39	40–64	>65
Motor vehicle accidents	+	+		
Homicide	+	+		
Suicide	+			
Leukemia	+			
Cardiovascular disease		+	+	+
Coronary artery disease		+	+	+
AIDS		+		
Breast cancer		+	+	+
Uterine cancer		+		
Lung cancer			+	+
Cerebrovascular accident			+	+
Colorectal cancer			+	+
Obstructive lung disease		+	+	+
Ovarian cancer		+		
Pneumonia/influenza				+
Accidents				+

ESTABLISHING A PROFESSIONAL RELATIONSHIP: LISTENING AND RESPONDING

Starting with the first interaction between physician and patient and continuing in each subsequent visit, the physician strives to establish and develop a professional relationship of mutual trust and respect with the patient. The physician gathers the historical and physical information needed for the patient's care, makes differential and presumptive diagnoses, identifies issues involving health maintenance and disease prevention, and formulates a management plan in cooperation with the patient. At the same time, the patient usually decides if the physician is knowledgeable and trustworthy and whether she will accept and follow the regimens and recommendations that are made.

The process begins with an appropriate greeting, which deserves special attention because of the importance of initial impressions. A handshake is commonly used. Surnames should generally be used. First names are more appropriate for friendship relationships, whereas the patient-physician relationship, while friendly, is professional. "What brought you to the office today?" or "How may I help you today?" are neutral opening questions that allow the patient to frame a response that includes her problems, concerns, and/or reasons for the visit.

Attentive, thoughtful listening is essential for accurate patient evaluation. Sometimes issues are uncomfortably personal. Letting the patient know that your interest is not personal, but instead reflects your desire to learn what you need to know to help, often facilitates these difficult communications. When faced with a negative, perhaps hostile, response, the physician may use such a comment to resolve the conflict and reestablish a positive interaction. Ignoring a negative response usually dooms the professional relationship. Furthermore, a highly emotional response may be the first indication of an unstated problem that requires attention.

HEALTH EVALUATION: HISTORY, PHYSICAL EXAMINATION, AND COMPREHENSIVE HEALTH PLANNING

History

Chief Complaint

The chief complaint is the reason for the patient's visit. This may be expressed and recorded as a quote or as a paraphrased statement, although care must be taken in the latter case to avoid obscuring the pa-

Table 1.3.
Recommended Screening Testing and Health Care Interventions for Women

Risk Factor/Condition	Screening Test Recommendation or Intervention
Cervical dysplasia/cancer (high risk: immunosuppression, AIDS, multiple STDs or sexual partners, smokers)	Pap annually from onset of sexual activity or age 18; physician and patient discretion after three consecutive normal Paps after age 19
Skin cancer (high risk: extensive sun exposure, family/personal history of skin cancer, suspicious lesions)	Physical examination; counseling about sun exposure; consultation for suspicious lesions
Anemia (high risk: Caribbean, Latin American, Asian, Mediterranean, or African descent or history of menorrhagia)	Hemogram/sickle cell preparation; hemoglobin electrophoresis
Hypercholesterolemia, coronary artery disease (high risk: elevated cholesterol; patient or sibling with cholesterol 240 mg/DL or higher; sibling, parent, or grandparent with coronary artery disease, esp. at age 55 or under; smoking; diabetes mellitus)	Cholesterol/lipid profile every 5 years from age 19, every 3 to 4 years from age 65
Breast cancer (high risk: first-degree relative with breast cancer, esp. if diagnosed premenopausally)	Screening mammography every other year from age 40, every year from age 50; yearly physician breast examination; self-breast examination instruction
Lung cancer, coronary artery disease	Counseling about smoking
Colorectal cancer	Sigmoidoscopy every 3 to 5 years after age 40; fecal occult blood test at physician discretion
Thyroid disease/risk for autoimmune disease (high risk: family history of thyroid disease, autoimmune disease)	Thyroid-stimulating hormone (TSH) every 3 to 5 years after age 65
Tuberculosis (TB) (high risk: patients with AIDS, who are immunosuppressed, or have close contact with those with TB; alcoholics and drug users; inmates of residential care facilities and prisons)	TB skin testing
Sexually transmitted diseases	As indicated by history/physical examination: cultures for gonorrhea and chlamydia; RPR/VDRL; hepatitis; HIV
Diabetes mellitus (high risk: family history of diabetes; obesity; personal history of gestational diabetes mellitus)	Fasting blood glucose as indicated
Osteoporosis	Diet and exercise counseling combined with menopausal hormone-replacement therapy and calcium supplementation

tient's true meaning with medical jargon. Establishing the chronology of a problem carefully is important because chronological organization of symptoms may suggest a specific disorder. Issues of health maintenance and disease prevention may come directly from the stated chief complaint or may be derived from other history or specific questions about high-risk situations.

Menstrual History

Menstrual history begins with *menarche*, the age at which menses began. The basic menstrual history should then include the duration of bleeding, the interval between the first day of menstrual flow and the first day of the next menstrual flow, the frequency of menses, and the *last menstrual period (LMP)*, dated from the first day of the last normal period. Episodes of bleeding that are "light but on time" should be noted as such, as they may have diagnostic significance. Estimation of the amount of menstrual flow can be made by asking whether the patient uses pads or tampons, how many are used during the heavy days of her flow, and whether they are soaked or just soiled when they are changed. It is normal for women to pass clots during menstruation, but they should not nor-

Table 1.4.
Immunization Recommendations

Immunization	Recommendations
Tetanus-diphtheria booster	Once between ages 14 and 16
Influenza vaccine	Every 10 years from age 19 to 64 for residents of chronic care facilities; persons with chronic cardiopulmonary disorders; and persons with metabolic diseases such as diabetes mellitus, hemoglobinopathies, immunosuppression, or renal dysfunction; annually for women 65 years old
Pneumococcal vaccine	Every 10 years from age 19 to 64 for women with medical conditions that increase the risk of pneumococcal infection, e.g., chronic cardiac or pulmonary disease, sickle-cell disease, nephrotic syndrome, Hodgkin's disease, asplenia, diabetes mellitus, alcoholism, cirrhosis, multiple myeloma, renal disease, or other immunosuppression
Measles, mumps, rubella (MMR)	Rubella titer vaccine for women of childbearing age lacking evidence of immunity; a second measles immunization, preferably as MMR, for all women unable to show proof of immunity
Hepatitis B vaccine	Intravenous drug users; current recipients of blood products; persons in health-related jobs with exposure to blood or blood products; household and sexual contacts of hepatitis B virus carriers; prostitutes; persons with a history of sexual activity with multiple partners in the previous 6 months

mally be larger than the size of a dime. Asking the size of clots relative to coins is useful, because it provides patient and clinician with a standard reference. Specific inquiry should be made about irregular or intermenstrual bleeding or spotting and contact bleeding (postcoital or postdouching bleeding or spotting). Such abnormal bleeding must be correlated with information about contraceptive method, infections, concurrent gynecologic problems, and sexual practices.

The menstrual history may include perimenstrual symptoms (molimina) such as anxiety, fluid retention, nervousness, mood fluctuations, food cravings, variations in sexual feelings, and difficulty sleeping. Any medications used during this time should be noted. Crampy pain during the menses is common. It is abnormal when it interferes with daily activities or when it requires more analgesia than provided by plain aspirin, acetaminophen, or ibuprofen. Inquiry about duration, quality, radiation of the pain to areas outside the pelvis, and association with body position or daily activities completes the pain history.

The term *menopause* refers to the cessation of menses. The *climacteric* is the time of transition when ovarian function begins to wane. The climacteric history often begins with increasing menstrual irregularity and varying or decreased flow, associated with hot flashes, nervousness, mood changes, and decreased vaginal lubrication. The physician should ask the patient whether she

has had or is undergoing *hormonal therapy* (estrogen replacement with or without progestin and/or other hormonal treatment) as well as other medical treatment such as psychoactive medications. A history of medical (radiation or chemotherapy) or surgical oophorectomy should be taken. *Postmenopausal bleeding* is abnormal; it is usually defined as bleeding 6 months after cessation of menses. It is an important historical fact that should be documented or stated as a pertinent negative because of its association with genital malignancy, especially endometrial carcinoma.

Obstetric History

Obstetric history includes the number of pregnancies (*gravidity*) and outcomes of each (*parity*). The following abbreviation may be used:

gravida (G) a Para (P) b c d e
where
a number of pregnancies
b number of term pregnancies ($\geq$37 weeks)
c number of preterm pregnancies (viability through 36 weeks)
d number of abortions (spontaneous or induced) and ectopic pregnancies
e number of living children

Specific information about each item should be included. For term and preterm deliveries, determine the outcome, any complications, and mode of delivery. For abortions and ectopic pregnancies,

Table 1.5.
Obstetric Definitions

Gravida	A woman who is or has been pregnant
Primigravida	A woman who is in or who has experienced her first pregnancy
Multigravida	A woman who has been pregnant more than once
Nulligravida	A woman who has never been and is not now pregnant
Primipara	A woman who has delivered one pregnancy (regardless of the number of fetuses) that progressed beyond the gestational age of an abortion
Multipara	A woman who has delivered two or more pregnancies that progressed beyond the gestational age of an abortion
Nullipara	A woman who has never had a pregnancy progress beyond the gestational age of an abortion
Parturient	A woman currently in labor
Puerpera	A woman who has just recently given birth

determine any known causes, medical therapy and/or surgical procedure(s) done, complications, and feelings about these events. Some obstetric terms are defined in Table 1.5.

Gynecologic History

The gynecologic history includes information about any *gynecologic disease and/or treatment* the patient has had, including the diagnosis or as much as the patient can remember about her illness, the medical and/or surgical treatment, and the results. Questions about previous gynecologic surgery should include what surgery, reason for the surgery, when and where and by whom the surgery was performed, the results as the patient understands them and whether they agree with her expectations for the surgery, and the emotional and physical effects of the surgery.

Information about *infectious and sexually transmitted disease* (STD) should be obtained. Information about vaginitis should include frequency, duration, treatment, and effect of treatment. Vaginal discharge should be characterized by color, odor, consistency, quantity, association with rectal or urethral discharge, associated symptoms such as pain or pruritus, relationship to medication such as antibiotics and exogenous steroids, and relationship to exacerbations of diseases such as diabetes. Localized lesions or ulcerations should be characterized by date of recognition, location, growth, associated symptoms (pain, pruritus, bleeding, discharge), similar nonperineal lesions, treatment, and results of treatment. Pelvic inflammatory disease (PID) is a frequently encountered history. PID is classically characterized by fever, chills, abdominopelvic pain, and an appropriate response to oral or parenteral

antibiotic therapy. PID is often confused with vaginitis, which may be differentiated by the different history of vaginal discharge, characterized by local symptoms such as pruritus or irritation and treatment with topical medications. The patient should be asked specifically about a history of sexually transmitted and infectious disease such as gonorrhea, herpes, chlamydia, warts (condyloma), hepatitis, AIDS, and syphilis as well as the the use of intrauterine devices (IUDs) since these have been associated with PID. Finally, patients should be asked about behaviors that are high risk for the acquisition of HIV or hepatitis, including parenteral drug use, sexual relationships with drug users or bisexuals, transfusion before approximately 1980, and prostitution or promiscuity.

A history about *breast disease and breast cancer* should include previous known breast disease or cancer; previous breast biopsy; previous mammography or other imaging study; family history of breast cancer; and appreciation by the patient of a mass, discharge, or painful area. Correlation with the patient's age, menstrual status, and hormonal therapy should be made.

If a patient has a history of *infertility*, questions concerning both partners should cover previous diseases or surgery that may affect fertility, previous fertility (previous children with the same or other partners), duration of time that pregnancy has been attempted, and a history of sexual practices.

Finally, *diethylstilbestrol (DES)* use by the patient's mother during her pregnancy should be noted, since it may be associated with infertility problems and/or vaginal carcinoma in the daughter. A personal hygiene history should address the use of douching and vaginal "feminine sprays," deodorants, or self-medications. A history of gastrointestinal and urinary disorders completes the gynecologic history.

Sexual and Contraceptive History

Taking a *sexual history* will be facilitated by behaviors, attitudes, and direct statements by the physician that project a nonjudgmental manner of acceptance and respect for the patient's lifestyle. The initial questions are often the most difficult. A good opening question is, "Please tell me about your sexual partner or partners." This question is gender neutral, leaves the issue of number of partners open, and also gives the patient considerable latitude for response. In the final analysis, however, these questions must be individualized to each patient. If faced with an untoward emotional response, the physician should address the situation directly, assuring the patient that no disrespect or judgment was meant or implied and that the goal is solely to provide good health care. Data to be elicited should include age at first intercourse, the patient's present sexual partner(s) (including gender), types of sexual practices, and the patient's level of satisfaction with her sex life. Finally, questions regarding *child and/or adult sexual abuse and assault* should be asked. The patient may be asked, "Have you ever been touched against your will, either as a child or an adult?"

A patient's *contraceptive history* should include the contraceptive method currently used, when it was begun, any problems or complications, and the patient's and her partner's satisfaction with the method. Previous contraceptive methods should also be noted as well as the reasons they were discontinued. The history concludes with inquiry about the patient's future conceptive or contraceptive plans (Table 1.6).

Physical Examination

Breast Examination

The breast examination by a physician remains the most cost-effective and reliable means of early detection of breast cancer when combined with appropriately

Table 1.6.
The OB-GYN History and Physical Examination: Generalized Report Format

I. History
  A. Chief complaint
  B. Menstrual history
    1. Last menstrual period; previous menstrual period
    2. Menarche
    3. Usual menstrual duration; interval between first days of menstrual periods
    4. Menstrual flow
    5. Abnormal menses
    6. Pain
  C. Menopause
    1. Climacteric symptoms, if any
    2. Perimenopausal and postmenopausal history
    3. Postmenopausal bleeding
  D. Obstetric history
    1. Gravidity and parity
    2. Obstetric complications
  E. Gynecologic history
    1. Gynecologic diseases and treatment, including surgery and medical treatment
    2. Sexually transmitted diseases
      a. Vaginitis, vulvitis
      b. Local lesions
      c. Pelvic inflammatory disease
    3. Breast disease (history, biopsy information, any family history of breast carcinoma)
    4. Infertility
    5. DES exposure
    6. Personal hygiene
    7. Gastrointestinal and genitourinary review of systems
  F. Sexual history (activity, problems, satisfaction)
  G. Sexual assault and abuse, adult and child
  H. Contraceptive history
    1. Present contraception
    2. Past contraception
    3. Conception plans
II. Physical examination
  A. Height, weight, and blood pressure
  B. Breast examination
  C. Examination of the abdomen, back, and lymphatics
  D. Pelvic examination
    1. Vulva
    2. Clitoris
    3. BUS (Bartholin's, urethral, Skene's glands)
    4. Vagina
    5. Cervix
    6. Uterus
    7. Adnexa
    8. Rectovaginal examination (guaiac determination, if needed)

scheduled mammography. It should be combined with patient education, including teaching the technique of the breast self-examination.

The results of the breast examination may be expressed by description or diagram or both, usually with reference to the quadrants and tail region of the breast or by allusion to the breast as a clock face with the nipple at the center (Fig. 1.1). Development of the female breast as described in Tanner's sex maturity ratings is used in the description of the breast examination (Fig. 1.2).

How to Do the Breast Examination

The breasts are first examined by *inspection*. Inspection begins with the patient's arms at her sides and then with her hands pressed against her hips and/or with her arms raised over her head. If the patient's breasts are especially large and pendulous, leaning forward so that the breasts hang free of the chest may facilitate inspection. The patient's breasts are observed before and after these maneuvers, which alter the relations of the supportive fascia of the breast tissue as the arms move. Tumors often distort the relationships of these tissues, causing disruption of the shape, contour, or symmetry of the breast or position of the nipple. Some asymmetry of the breasts is common, but marked differences or recent changes deserve further evaluation.

Discolorations and/or ulcerations of the skin of the breast or areola/nipple, or edema of the lymphatics, causing a leathery puckered appearance of the skin

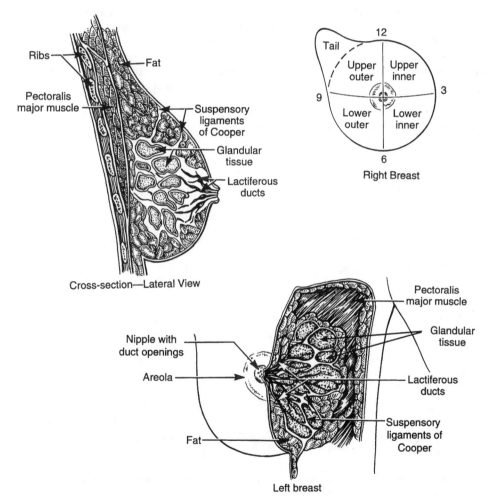

Figure 1.1. Clinical anatomy and associated examination schema of the breast.

(like an orange skin, hence called peau d'orange) are abnormal. A clear or milky breast discharge (galactorrhea) requires evaluation. Bloody discharge from the breast is abnormal; it usually does not represent carcinoma but rather inflammation of a breast structure. Pus usually indicates infection, although an underlying tumor may be encountered.

Palpation follows inspection, first with the patient's arms at her sides and then with the arms raised over her head. This is usually done in the supine position, although sometimes use of the sitting position with the patient's arm resting on the examiner's shoulder or over her head for examination of the most lateral aspects of the axilla is helpful. Palpation should be done with slow, careful maneuvers using the flat of the fingers and not the tips. The fingers are moved up and down in a wavelike motion, moving the tissues under them back and forth. By so doing breast masses are moved so that they may be more easily felt. A spiral or radial pattern is described over each breast to uniformly cover all of the breast tissue, including that of the axillary tail. If masses are found, their size, shape, consistency (soft, hard, firm, cys-

tic), and mobility as well as their position should be determined. Women with large breasts may demonstrate a firm ridge of tissue found transversely along the lower edge of the breast. This is the inframammary ridge and is a normal finding. The examination is concluded with gentle pressure inward and then upward at the sides of the areola — a gentle "squeezing" action to express fluid. If fluid is expressed, it should be sent for culture and sensitivity and cytopathology if indicated by its character and the clinical situation (Fig. 1.3).

Pelvic Examination

Despite advances in ultrasonography and other imaging technologies, the pelvic examination (inspection and palpation of the external genitalia, the speculum examination with Pap smear and culturing, and the vaginal and rectovaginal bimanual examinations) remains a mainstay of clinical obstetrics and gynecology. The results of the pelvic examination may be expressed by description or diagram or both.

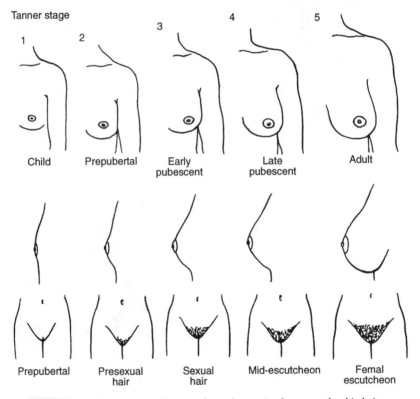

Figure 1.2.   Tanner's classification of sexual maturity: breasts and pubic hair.

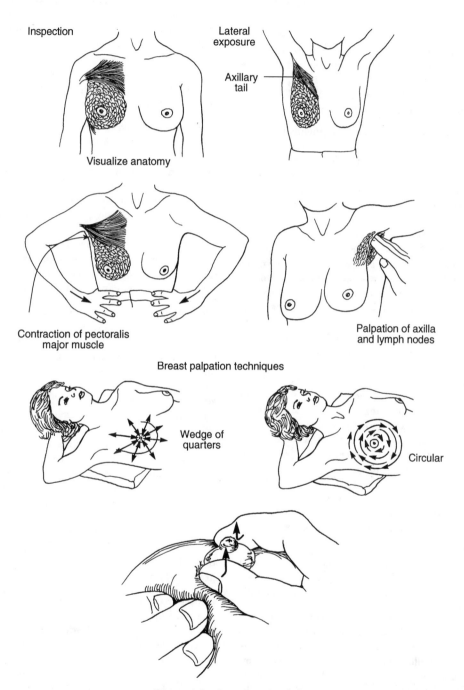

Figure 1.3. Breast examination.

How to Do the Pelvic Examination

Preparation for the pelvic examination begins with the patient emptying her bladder and donning an examination gown. An assistant should usually be present for the pelvic examination to assist in the preparation of specimens and act as a chaperon. It is important to thoroughly explain everything that is going to happen to a patient before it happens. The cardinal rule is "TALK BEFORE YOU TOUCH," as an unexpected touch is disconcerting.

Abdominal and especially pelvic examinations require relaxation of the muscles. An abrupt or stern command, such as "Relax now; I'm not going to hurt you," may raise the patient's fears, whereas a phrase such as "Try to relax as much as you can, although I know that it's a lot easier for me to say than for you to do" sends two messages: (a) that the patient needs to relax and (b) that you recognize that it is difficult, both of which demonstrate patience and understanding. A phrase such as "Let me know if anything is uncomfortable, and I will stop and then we will try to do it differently" tells the patient that there might be discomfort but that she has control and can stop the examination if discomfort occurs. If any maneuvers require deep palpation or may cause discomfort, the patient should be told what to expect before such maneuvers are done. Few positions leave a woman with such a feeling of helplessness as the lithotomy position; returning a degree of control to her is most helpful. Using the word we also demonstrates that the examination is a cooperative effort, further empowering the patient and facilitating care. Techniques that help the patient to relax include encouraging the patient to breathe in and out gently and regularly rather than holding her breath and helping the patient to identify specific muscle groups (such as the abdominal muscle groups or the perineal muscle groups) that need to be relaxed.

The patient is asked to sit at the edge of the examination table and an opened, draping sheet is placed over the patient's knees. If a patient requests that a drape not be used, the request should be honored.

Positioning the patient for examination begins with the elevation of the head of the examining table to about 30° from horizontal. This serves three purposes: (a) it allows eye contact and facilitates communication between physician and patient; (b) it relaxes the abdominal wall muscle groups, making the examination much easier; and (c) it allows the clinician to observe the patient for responses to the examination, which may provide valuable information, e.g., wincing as evidence of pain on examination. The physician and/or an assistant should help the patient assume the lithotomy position. The patient should be asked to lie back, place her heels in the stirrups, and then slide down to the end of the table until her buttocks are flush with the edge of the table. After the patient is in the lithotomy position, the drape is adjusted so that it does not obscure the clinician's view of the perineum or obscure eye contact between patient and physician.

The physician should sit at the foot of the examining table with the examination lamp adjusted to shine on the perineum. The lamp is optimally positioned in front of the physician's chest a few inches or so below the level of the chin, just at the level of the perineum but at about an arm's length distance from it, allowing the examination maneuvers. The physician should glove both hands. This protects the patient's modesty and sense of privacy and also protects the clinician from sexually transmitted disease. After contact with the patient, there should be minimal contact with equipment such as the lamp.

The pelvic examination begins with the inspection and examination of the external genitalia. The physician begins by firmly placing the back of his hand on the patient's inner thigh, progressing to both hands touching the external genitalia, and thereafter to a sequential inspection and palpation of the external genitalia. Initial touching of the inner thigh begins the examination in a "personal and sensitive" area, although not as sensitive as the perineum. Throughout the pelvic examination, the examiner should make use of the bilateral symmetry of the body. Dissymmetry shows that one side is different from the other, perhaps because of disease, which then requires an explanation. All maneuvers should be performed gently yet with a firmness that is comfortable. Deliberate speed is important but do not be abrupt; neither linger beyond the time needed to do the task nor move too quickly, failing to gain the needed information.

Inspection should include the mons pubis, labia majora and labia minora, perineum, and perianal area. Inspection continues as palpation is performed in an orderly sequence, starting with the clitoral hood, which may be pulled back to inspect the glans proper. The labia are spread laterally to allow inspection of the introitus and outer vagina. The urethral meatus and the areas of the urethra and Skene's glands should be inspected. After forewarning the patient about the possible sensation of having to uri-nate, the forefinger is placed an inch or so into the vagina to gently milk the urethra. A culture should be taken of any discharge from the urethral opening. The forefinger is then rotated posteriorly to palpate the area of the Bartholin's glands between that fin-ger and the thumb. The patient is then asked to bear down slightly as if she were going to have a bowel movement while the vaginal walls are inspected for cystocele or rectocele. Just as with the breast exami-nation, women at different ages will demonstrate different stages of development of the genitals and associated hair, as seen in Tanner's classification (see Fig. 1.2).

The next step is the speculum examination. The parts of the speculum are seen in Figure 1.4. There are two types of specula in common use for the ex-amination of adults. The Pederson speculum has flat and narrow blades that barely curve on the sides. The Pederson works well for most nulliparous women and postmenopausal women with atrophic, narrowed vaginas. The Graves speculum has blades that are wider, higher, and curved on the sides and is more appropriate for most parous women. Its wider, curved blades keep the looser vaginal walls on the multiparous women separated for visualization. A Pederson with extra narrow blades may be used for visualizing the cervix in pubertal girls.

First, the speculum is examined to be sure it is clean and in proper working order. If not already warm, the speculum should be warmed, because insertion of a cold speculum is unacceptable.

Speculum insertion and visualization of the vagina and cervix are performed in a stepwise manner (Fig. 1.5). Moistening the speculum with warm water may help with insertion. Lubricants should not be used routinely as they interfere with cytologic and micro-biologic specimens. Situations that require their use are encountered infrequently; examples include some prepubertal girls, some postmenopausal women, and patients with irritation or lesions of the vagina mak-ing manipulative examination uncomfortable.

Most physicians find the control of pressure and movement of the speculum facilitated by holding the speculum with the dominant hand. The speculum is held by the handle with the blades completely closed. The first two fingers of the opposite hand are placed on the perineum laterally and just below the introitus and pressure is applied downward and slightly inward until the introitus is opened slightly.

If the patient is sufficiently relaxed, this downward pressure on the perineum results in an open introi-tus into which the speculum may be easily inserted. The speculum is initially inserted in a horizontal plane with the width of the blades perpendicular to the vertical axis of the introitus. The speculum is then inclined at approximately a 45° angle from hor-izontal; the angle is adjusted as the speculum is in-serted so that the speculum slides into the vagina with minimal resistance. Inserting the speculum in a more vertical plane and then rotating the speculum is another method of introduction that is widely used. If the patient is not relaxed, posterior pressure from a finger inserted in the vagina will sometimes relax the perineal musculature.

As the speculum is inserted, a slight continuous downward pressure is exerted so that distention of the perineum is used to create space into which the speculum may advance. Taking advantage of the dis-tensibility of the perineum and vagina posterior to the introitus is a crucial concept for the efficient and comfortable manipulation of the speculum (and later for the bimanual and rectovaginal) examination. Pressure superiorly causes pain in the sensitive area of the urethra and clitoris. The speculum is inserted as far as it will go, which in most women means in-sertion of the entire speculum length. The speculum is then opened in a smooth deliberate fashion. With slight tilting of the speculum, the cervix will slide into view between the blades of the speculum. The speculum is then locked into the open position using the thumb screw. Failure to find the cervix most commonly results from not having the speculum in-serted far enough. Keeping the speculum fully in-serted while opening the speculum does not result in discomfort.

When the speculum is locked into position, it will usually stay in place without being held. For most patients, the speculum is opened sufficiently by use of the upper thumb screw. In some cases, however, more space is required. This may be obtained by gently expanding the vertical distance between the speculum blades by use of the screw on the handle of the speculum.

With the speculum in place, the cervix and the deep lateral vaginal vault may be inspected. The Pap smear, "wet prep," and/or cultures may be taken at this time.

Before obtaining the Pap smear, the patient should be told that she may feel a slight "scraping" sensa-

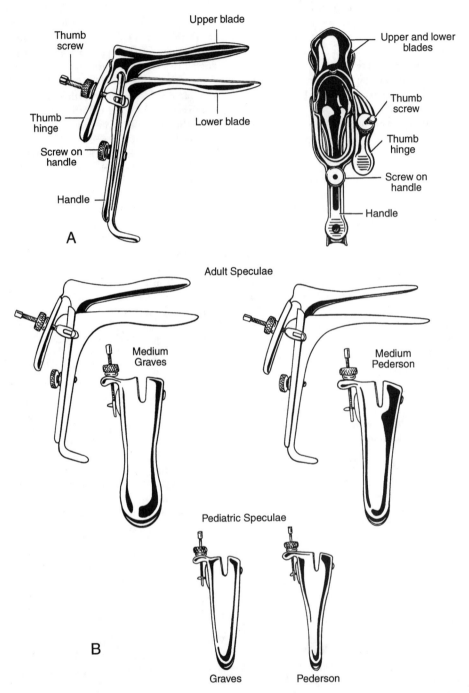

Figure 1.4.   The vaginal speculum. **A,** Parts of the vaginal speculum. **B,** Types of vaginal speculae.

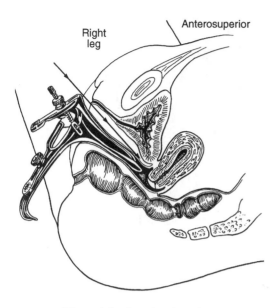

Figure 1.5. Speculum insertion.

tion but no pain. Specimens are collected to fully evaluate the transformation zone where cervical intraepithelial neoplasia is more likely to be encountered. Both an endocervical sample and an exocervical sample are obtained using appropriate sampling devices. The material is thinly smeared on a slide, avoiding large accumulations of mucus and other material. Thick accumulations of material cannot be accurately evaluated. *Immediate fixation* is important to avoid air drying artifacts, which compromise cytopathologic evaluation. Slides left in air longer than 10 sec demonstrate a very high incidence of such artifacts (Fig. 1.6).

When specimen collection is completed, it is time for speculum withdrawal and inspection of the vaginal walls. After telling the patient that the speculum is to be removed and that she should not tighten her vaginal muscles upon movement of the speculum, the blades of the speculum are opened very slightly by putting pressure on the thumb hinge and the thumb screw is completely loosened. Opening the speculum blades slightly farther before starting to withdraw the speculum avoids pinching the cervix between the blades. The speculum is withdrawn about 1 inch before pressure on the thumb hinge is slowly released. The speculum is withdrawn slowly enough to allow inspection of the vaginal walls. As the end of the speculum blades approaches the introitus, there should be no pressure on the thumb hinge, otherwise the ante-

rior blade can flip up, hitting the sensitive vaginal, urethral, and clitoral tissues.

The *bimanual examination* uses both hands (the "vaginal" hand and the "abdominal" hand) to entrap and palpate the pelvic organs. The bimanual examination begins by exerting gentle pressure on the abdomen about halfway between the umbilicus and the pubic hair line with the abdominal hand, while at the same time inserting one finger of the vaginal hand into the vagina to about 2 inches and gently pushing downward, distending the vaginal canal. The patient is asked to feel the muscles being pushed on and to relax them as much as possible. Then two fingers are inserted into the vagina until they rest at the limit of the vaginal vault in the posterior fornix behind and below the cervix. A great deal of space may be created by posterior distention of the perineum.

During the bimanual examination, the pelvic structures are "caught" and palpated between the abdominal and vaginal hands. Whether to use the dominant hand as the abdominal or vaginal hand is a question of personal preference. The most common error in this part of the pelvic examination is failure to make effective use of the abdominal hand. Pressure should be applied with the flat of the fingers, not the tips, starting midway between the umbilicus and the hairline, moving downward in conjunction with upward movements of the vaginal hand. The bimanual examination continues with the circumferential examination of the cervix for its size, shape, position, mobility, and the presence or absence of tenderness or mass lesions. Cervical position is often related to uterine position. A posterior cervix is often associated with an anteverted or midposition uterus, whereas an anterior cervix is often associated with a retroverted uterus. Sharp flexion of the uterus, however, may alter these relationships.

Bimanual examination of the uterus is accomplished by lifting the uterus up toward the abdominal fingers so that it may be palpated between the vaginal and abdominal hands. The uterus is evaluated for its size, shape, consistency, configuration, and mobility as well as masses or tenderness and for position (anteversion, midposition, retroversion, anteflexion, or retroflexion). The technique varies somewhat with the position of the uterus. Examination of the anterior and midposition uterus is facilitated with the vaginal fingers lateral and deep to the cervix in the posterior fornix. The uterus is gently lifted upward to the abdominal fingers and a gentle side-to-side "searching" motion of the vaginal fingers is combined with steady

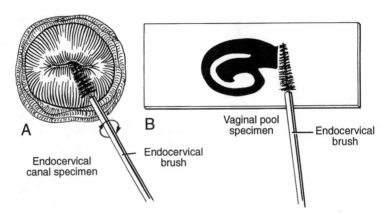

Figure 1.6. Pap smear. **A,** Obtaining endocervical portion of Pap smear. **B,** Strong specimen before fixation within 10 sec.

pressure and palpation by the abdominal hand to determine the characteristics of the uterus (Fig. 1.7). Examination of the retroverted uterus is more difficult. In some cases the vaginal fingers may be slowly pushed below or at the level of the uterine fundus, after which gentle pressure exerted inward and upward will cause the uterus to antevert or at least move "upward," somewhat facilitating palpation. Then palpation is accomplished as in the normally anteverted uterus. If this cannot be done, a waving motion with the vaginal fingers in the posterior fornix must be combined with an extensive rectovaginal examination to assess the retroverted uterus.

Bimanual examination of the adnexa to assess the ovaries, fallopian tubes, and support structures begins by placing the vaginal fingers to the side of the cervix deep in the lateral fornix. The abdominal hand is moved to the same side just inside the flare of the sacral arch and above the pubic hairline. Pressure is then applied downward and toward the symphysis with the abdominal hand while at the same time lifting upward with the vaginal fingers. The same movements of the fingers of both hands used to assess the uterus are used to assess the adnexal structures, which are brought between the fingers by these maneuvers to evaluate their size, shape, consistency, configuration, mobility, and tenderness as well as to palpate for masses. Special care must be taken when examining the ovaries, which are sensitive such that excessive pressure or sudden movements causes a deep visceral pain. It is important to note that the ovaries are palpable in normal menstrual women about one-half of the time, whereas palpation of ovaries in postmenopausal women implies the possibility of ovarian pathology requiring further evaluation.

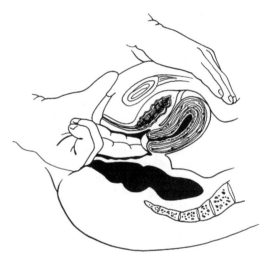

Figure 1.7. Bimanual examination of the uterus and adnexa.

The rectovaginal examination is an integral part of the complete pelvic examination on initial and annual examination as well as at interval examinations whenever clinically indicated. Full evaluation of the posterior aspect of the pelvic structures and of the support structures is possible only by this method in many patients. As patients may have had bad experiences with this part of the pelvic examination, a careful explanation of the value of the examination and reassurance that the examination will be gently done is helpful.

The rectovaginal examination is begun by changing the glove on the vaginal hand and using a liberal supply of lubricant. The examination may be comfortably performed if the natural inclination of the rectal canal is followed: upward at a 45° angle for about

1 to 2 cm, then downward (Fig. 1.8). This is accomplished by positioning the fingers of the vaginal hand as for the bimanual examination except that the index finger is also flexed. The second finger is then gently inserted through the rectal opening and inserted to the "bend" where the angle turns downward. The index (vaginal) finger is inserted into the vagina, and both fingers are inserted until the vaginal finger rests in the posterior fornix below the cervix and the rectal finger rests as far as it can go into the rectal canal. Asking the patient to bear down as the rectal finger is inserted is not necessary and may add to the tension for the patient. Palpation of the pelvic structures is then accomplished as in their vaginal palpation. The uterosacral ligaments are also palpated to determine if they are symmetrical, smooth, and nontender (as normally) or if they are nodular, slack, or thickened. The rectal canal is evaluated as are the integrity and function of the rectal sphincter. After palpation is complete, the fingers are rapidly but steadily removed in a reversal of the sequence of movements used on insertion. Care should be taken to avoid contamination of the vagina with fecal matter. A guaiac determination is made from fecal material collected on the rectal finger.

At the conclusion of the pelvic examination, the patient is asked to move back up on the table and thereafter to sit up. It is both good manners and helpful to offer a hand to the patient when she sits up. Discussion of the findings and recommendations for further care should be done after the patient has had a chance to clean herself, go to the washroom if needed, and dress.

Comprehensive Health Planning and Patient Management

Obstetrician-gynecologists are involved with their patients in two broad kinds of health care activities: (*a*) activities to promote good health and prevent disease and (*b*) management plans to address specific disease states or medical conditions. In both cases, the issues may fall within the scope of the obstetrician-gynecologist's practice or may require consultation or referral. Thus the obstetrician-gynecologist will facilitate the health screening discussed earlier in this chapter, caring for identified problems (e.g., counseling about smoking cessation) or referral/consultation (e.g., referral for evaluation of guaiac-positive stools). At times, the obstetrician-gynecologist will pro-

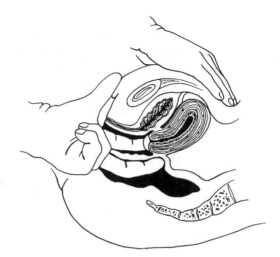

Figure 1.8. Rectovaginal examination.

vide care and at other times will serve as the coordinator/facilitator of care, the primary care responsibility. When a specific problem is identified, the classic schema of diagnosis and treatment facilitates care is followed. The five tasks are discussed below.

1. FORMULATION OF DIFFERENTIAL DIAGNOSIS

The differential diagnosis is a list of conditions whose characteristics may correspond to one or more of the historical, physical examination, and/or laboratory findings. This list should be inclusive of all entities that reasonably may fit the information at hand, not exhaustive of all that in theory could fit the situation. The purpose of a differential diagnosis is to avoid failure to consider unusual or rare conditions and to provide a list for reconsideration should the presumptive diagnosis prove to be in error.

2. SELECTION OF LABORATORY TESTING

Only those laboratory tests that are sufficient and necessary to select among the elements of the differential diagnosis and confirm the presumptive diagnosis should be obtained. Each test should be valid (validity is the closeness with which the measurements reflect the true value) and reliable (reliability is the property of a test to reproducibly identify the testable goal when present) and should not impose risks for the patient disproportionate to the severity of the malady under evaluation or be more costly than justifiable for the same reason. As a general policy, the minimum number of tests needed to confirm the presumptive diagnosis and allow management to begin should be obtained.

3. FORMULATION OF A PRESUMPTIVE DIAGNOSIS

That diagnosis that best fits the information at hand is chosen as the presumptive diagnosis. At times this will clearly be the correct diagnosis; other times the correctness of the selection may be very much in doubt. In addition, a patient may often have more than one problem.

4. DEVELOPMENT OF A MANAGEMENT PLAN

The management selected should be an effective treatment for the presumptive diagnosis and the benefits and risks of the proposed therapy should outweigh the risk of no treatment. In some cases, there will be only one management that fits these requirements; in other cases several management alternatives may exist.

Whether there are one or more possible managements, an informed consent for treatment must be made by the patient before treatment. Informed consent is an educational process wherein the physician explains the diagnosis; the natural course of the process if untreated (i.e., risk of no treatment); and the management(s) available, including the risks, benefits, and anticipated results of each. The patient and physician should discuss this information until both are satisfied with their understandings of the situation. The patient then consents to treatment, which is begun. In the case of a surgical procedure, participation in a research protocol, and/or other situations, a written "consent form" is completed to document that this process has occurred.

5. FOLLOW-UP MANAGEMENT

During and after treatment, the patient's clinical course should be followed to ascertain if the de-

sired outcome is being or has been achieved. If not, the presumptive diagnosis may be in error, the management plan or its execution may be faulty, or both. Reconsideration of the diagnosis and management is made and a new or revised diagnosis/management plan instituted. This process is iterated until the desired outcome is achieved.

CASE STUDIES

Case 1A

A 68-year-old G4 P4004 comes to your office for her annual examination. She has been in good health except for some constipation, which she treats with Milk of Magnesia. She has been on hormone replacement therapy — Premarin 1.25 mg q.d. and Provera 2.5 mg q.d. — since menopause, about 15 years ago. She is widowed and lives in a retirement community in an efficiency apartment.

On physical examination her blood pressure, pulse, and weight are normal as is her general physical examination, including her breasts, chest, and abdomen. You note that her vulva and vagina are normal, although the latter is somewhat atrophic. Her uterus and cervix are surgically absent, and on questioning you learn that "they took my uterus out a long time ago because of tumors." Her rectovaginal examination is negative; her guaiac, positive.

Question Case 1A

Appropriate diagnostic studies include

A. Hemogram
B. Pap smear of vaginal vault
C. Coagulation profile
D. Sigmoidoscopy
E. Ultrasound of the pelvis

Answer: A, B, D

A hemogram in an elderly patient is always a useful measure of health but especially where there is the possibility of blood loss. A yearly Pap smear is also a routine screening test. Sigmoidoscopy is indicated because of the positive guaiac test. There is no history of a bleeding disorder warranting coagulation evaluation, and without physical findings or symptoms, ultrasound of the pelvis is likewise unnecessary.

Case 1B

An 18-year-old white G4 P1031 presents with a complaint of vaginal discharge for 3 weeks, which has not responded to an over-the-counter vaginal douche.

Question Case 1B

While all the components of a new patient evaluation are important, the history so far makes which of the following lines of questioning especially pertinent?

A. Sexual history
B. Obstetric history
C. Contraceptive history
D. STD history
E. Social history

Answer: All

Questions about contraception and sexual practice are obvious, including the outcome of her four pregnancies. The complaint of vaginal discharge combined with multiparity at 18 years renders questions about frequency and number of partners and STDs pertinent. Her social situation, given her age and having a living child, is also important for the evaluation of her well-being as well as that of her child.

chapter 2

OBSTETRIC AND GYNECOLOGIC PROCEDURES

Any physician who cares for women must be familiar with some of the procedures common in obstetric and gynecologic practice. Whether the physician performs the procedure or not, he or she should understand the indications, contraindications, risks, benefits, and the appropriate language needed to inform the patient about her diagnoses and therapeutic options.

OBSTETRIC PROCEDURES

Amniocentesis

Amniocentesis is the withdrawal of fluid from the amniotic sac to obtain fluid and cells for a variety of tests (Fig. 2.1). Biochemical studies can identify the presence of fetal physiologic markers (e.g., deficiency of hexosaminidase A or Tay-Sachs disease) or the presence of substances indicating fetal abnormalities (e.g., α-fetoprotein in neural tube defects or bilirubin in Rh incompatibility). Tissue culture of fetal cells allows genetic evaluation of the fetus.

In more advanced gestations, fluid obtained through amniocentesis is used to assess the degree of fetal lung maturity. This indication of fetal lung readiness is extremely valuable in the management of premature labor or the timing of delivery for patients with medical complications. Fluid obtained at amniocentesis may also be cultured and stained to evaluate for intrauterine infection, i.e., chorioamnionitis.

Amniocentesis is associated with a 0.5% risk of fetal loss because of bleeding, infection, preterm labor, or fetal injury. To reduce this risk, the procedure is usually performed using ultrasonographic guidance.

Chorionic Villus Sampling

In chorionic villus sampling (CVS), a small cannula is passed through the cervix to aspirate villus cells for genetic analysis of an early gestation (Fig. 2.2). Cells may also be acquired via transabdominal aspiration. The cells that are obtained are cultured for genetic studies.

Because chorionic villus sampling carries about a 0.5% risk of fetal loss, it is usually reserved for patients with a >0.5% chance of an abnormality, e.g., those over the age of 35 or with a history of genetic abnormalities. Bleeding or infections are infrequent complications.

Compared with amniocentesis, chorionic villus sampling can be performed earlier in pregnancy with a more rapid availability of results. This allows for an earlier decision regarding possible pregnancy termination in the case of significant fetal abnormality. Isolated reports of an association of CVS with limb reduction defects should be noted, but as yet an association has not been confirmed.

Periumbilical Artery Blood Sampling

The physician uses real-time ultrasonographic guidance for periumbilical artery blood sampling (PUBS). The umbilical artery is sampled using a needle introduced transabdominally. Various analyses may be performed on the fetal blood sample obtained, including fetal blood gas and metabolic evaluation, fetal hemogram and blood chemistries, and fetal genetics studies. The risks of this procedure are the same as those of amnioncentesis plus an approximately 1% risk to the fetus from bleeding at the umbilical puncture site. This procedure is also referred to as *cordocentesis*.

Forceps Delivery and Vacuum Extraction

Vaginal delivery may be assisted with obstetric forceps or a vacuum extractor. These methods augment the expulsive forces during the second

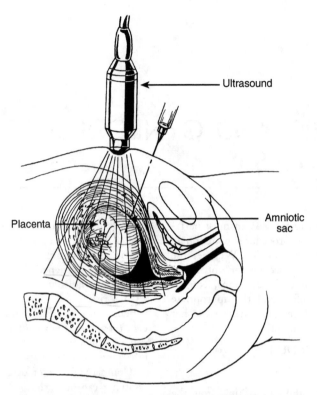

Figure 2.1. Amniocentesis with ultrasound guidance. Cross-section of uterus and fetus with the needle in a pocket of amniotic fluid.

stage of labor as well as direct these forces in an optimal manner.

Obstetric forceps are designed either to provide traction to augment and/or direct the expulsive forces of the second stage of labor or to facilitate the rotation of the fetal head (Figs. 2.3 and 2.4). Each type is applied to the fetal head and is classified as low (or outlet), mid, or high, based on the level of descent of the fetal head (station) at the time the forceps are applied. In general, low or outlet forceps describe application when the fetal scalp is visible at the introitus; midforceps, when the head is engaged but above the pelvic outlet or in those cases in which a forceps rotation of the head is performed; and high forceps, when the presenting part is above zero station.

Although virtually any forceps may be used in a low forceps delivery, some specific types of forceps are often chosen for midforceps deliveries. The Kjelland's (Kielland) forceps are especially suited for midforceps deliveries involving rotation of the fetal head.

Because of the risk of injury to fetus and mother, it is inappropriate to use high forceps. In-

stead, delivery should be accomplished by cesarean section. Piper's forceps are specially designed to facilitate the delivery of the "after-coming head" in vaginal breech deliveries (Fig. 2.5).

Forceps may cause injury to either the fetus or mother unless applied carefully and used judiciously. Transient bruising over the zygomatic arch is common and is generally of little consequence. More dangerous are lacerations of the birth canal or cervix, which may result from excessive force or improper manipulation of the forceps during delivery.

The vacuum extractor is a suction cup-like device that is applied to the fetal scalp (Fig. 2.6). Traction is then used to aid maternal expulsive efforts and expedite delivery. Although damage to maternal structures is less likely with the use of the vacuum extractor than with forceps, hematomas or abrasions of the fetal scalp can occur.

Cesarean Delivery

Cesarean delivery (or cesarean section) is the delivery of the fetus through an abdominal incision.

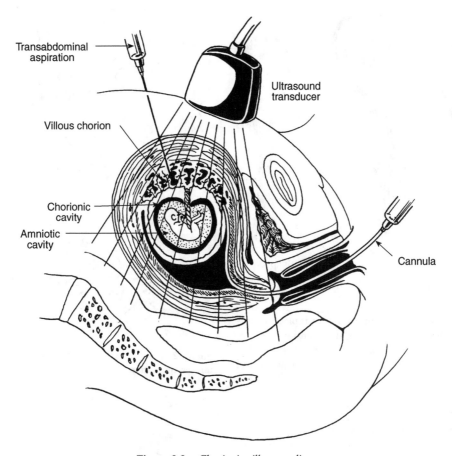

Figure 2.2. Chorionic villus sampling.

This route may be chosen when rapid delivery is required and vaginal delivery is not imminent (e.g., nonreassuring fetal status — "fetal distress" — or abruptio placentae), when vaginal delivery is not advisable (e.g., placenta previa, fetal anomalies, or malpresentation), or when vaginal delivery cannot be accomplished by the normal forces of labor (e.g., cephalopelvic disproportion, macrosomia, or uterine dysfunction). Cesarean deliveries are classified as *lower uterine segment* (transverse or vertical) when the incision is in the lower uterine segment or *classical* when the incision is in the upper, contractile portion of the uterus (Fig. 2.8). Patients with lower uterine segment cesarean deliveries may be candidates for future vaginal delivery (vaginal birth after cesarean; VBAC), if careful maternal and fetal monitoring are available as well as staff and facilities for emergency cesarean section. Patients with classical incisions are at greater risk of rupture of the uterine scar before or during labor and are generally not allowed to labor in subsequent pregnancies.

Circumcision

Circumcision of the newborn (the removal of the foreskin from the penis) has been practiced for centuries as social custom and for religious and health reasons. Controversy continues over the health value of this surgical procedure. It has been argued that circumcision represents mutilation, reduces penile sensitivity, and carries a greater risk of operative complications (surgical damage, bleeding, and infection) than is warranted by its benefits. Proponents point to improved hygiene and a reduced incidence of penile cancer.

GYNECOLOGIC PROCEDURES

Imaging

The ability to image various parts and organs of the body has dramatically enhanced our diagnostic

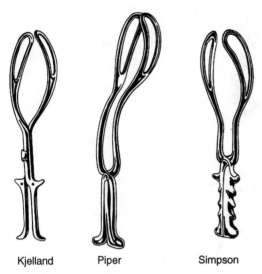

Kjelland   Piper   Simpson

Figure 2.3. Obstetric forceps.

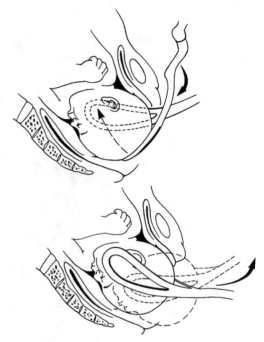

capabilities. These methods do not replace a careful and thoughtful history and physical evaluation. The effective use of these modalities requires that the physician be familiar with the benefits and limitations of each.

Figure 2.4. Correct biparietal, bimalar, cephalic forceps application.

Ultrasonography

Ultrasonography is based on the use of high-frequency sound reflections to identify different body tissues and structures. The term *sonography* literally means "sound writing" and is often described as using sound waves to make a picture. Very short bursts of low-energy sound waves are sent into the body. When these waves encounter the interface between two tissues that transmit sound differently, some of the sound energy is reflected back toward the sound source (Fig. 2.8). The returning sound waves are detected and the distance from the sensor is deduced using the elapsed time from transmission to reception. This information is displayed graphically as a cross-sectional view of the structure encountered by the beam.

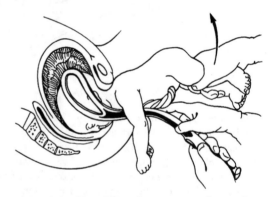

Figure 2.5. Use of Piper forceps on an after-coming head.

Since ultrasonography uses low-energy sound waves, it is safe for use in pregnancy. Its reliance on subtle tissue differences limits the ability to distinguish some tissues. It is also affected by interference from substances such as bowel gas. Despite these limitations, ultrasonography is very good at distinguishing solid from cystic structures and for fetal assessments. In obstetrics, measurement of fetal anatomy to allow estimation of fetal

age and weight is often carried out. Detailed evaluations of fetal structures such as heart, brain, spinal column, and kidneys can be performed. Fetal gender may frequently be determined as well.

In gynecology, ultrasonography may be used to distinguish the character of pelvic masses (solid versus cystic) or to provide accurate measurement of tumors such as fibroids. These applications often have little impact on clinical management or decision making and provide only a false sense of precision. Because of cost and limited return, ultrasonography should be used only to evaluate pelvic masses when an adequate examination is not possible (e.g., extreme obesity) or when the information gathered will alter patient management. Routine ultrasonography to confirm findings on pelvic examination is not warranted.

Improved resolution for imaging intrauterine and adnexal structures may be obtained by placing the ultrasound transducer inside the vagina. The higher frequencies of sound used for transvaginal imaging allow enhanced details to be seen but limit the depth of penetration of the sound. Therefore, transvaginal ultrasound is especially useful for conditions located near the apex of the vagina, e.g., early gestations and possible ectopic pregnancies, and for ovarian follicle monitoring during assisted reproduction.

Doppler ultrasound is a form of ultrasonography that uses changes in the frequency of the reflected

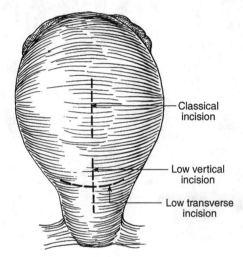

Figure 2.7. Uterine incisions used for cesarean delivery.

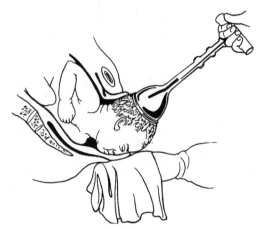

Figure 2.6. Vacuum extractor applied to head.

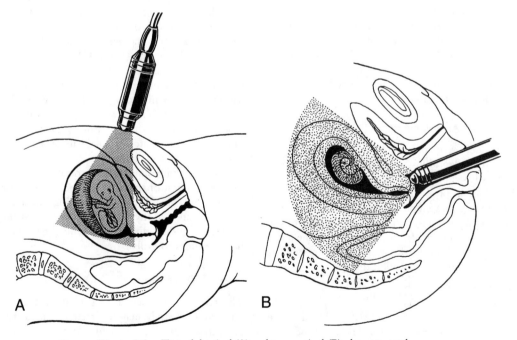

Figure 2.8. Transabdominal (**A**) and transvaginal (**B**) ultrasonography.

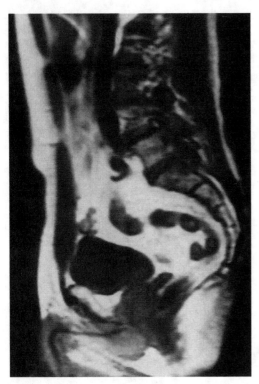

Figure 2.9. Computed axial tomography (CT) of the pelvis.

sound to infer motion of the reflecting surface. This can be useful in detecting cardiac motion or assessing blood flow. A growing application of Doppler ultrasound has been the evaluation of blood flow patterns in the umbilical vessels, because changes in these patterns may be an indication of fetal stress.

Computed Axial Tomography

Computed axial tomography (CT scanning) uses computer algorithms to construct cross-sectional images based on x-ray information (Fig. 2.9). This technique involves slightly greater radiation exposure than a conventional single-exposure x-ray but provides significantly more information. With the use of contrast agents, this modality can help the physician evaluate pelvic masses, look for signs of adenopathy, or plan radiation therapy.

Magnetic Resonance Imaging

Magnetic resonance imaging (MRI) is based on the magnetic characteristics of various atoms and molecules in the body. Because of the variations in

chemical composition of body tissues (especially the content of hydrogen, sodium, fluoride, or phosphorus), MRI offers exceptional images of many soft tissues. The relatively longer time needed to form images and MRI's somewhat experimental nature make this modality exciting in its possibilities but limited in direct clinical application in obstetrics and gynecology.

Mammography

The need to develop an effective screening method for breast cancer has prompted the evaluation of many imaging technologies such as thermography (based on skin temperature patterns), ultrasonography, transillumination by light, and x-ray. It has been the latter (mammography) that has proven to be the most effective for screening and evaluation of recognized abnormalities (Fig. 2.10). In mammography, breast tissue is compressed against an imaging plate, and a small amount of radiation is used to form the image. Improved films, imaging screens, and xerographic technologies have led to better images with the lower radiation exposures, usually less than 0.5 rad per image set.

Hysterosalpingography

For hysterosalpingography, contrast material is introduced through the cervix into the uterine cavity and fallopian tubes and x-rays are taken at specific intervals to reveal the progression of the dye through the uterus, fallopian tubes, and into the abdominopelvic cavity (Fig. 2.11). This technique is useful for assessment of the size, shape, and configuration of the uterine cavity as part of the evaluation for infertility or genital anomalies. The contrast material will flow through the fallopian tubes and spill into the peritoneal cavity, which can be a good indicator of tubal patency and allow examination of tubal anatomy.

Hysterosalpingography is associated with the risk of infection of the uterus or pelvis as well as bleeding or pain. With the increasing availability of and reliance on hysteroscopy and laparoscopy, the role of hysterosalpingography in clinical practice continues to evolve.

Genital Tract Biopsy

The removal of tissue from genital tract lesions for histologic study may be safely obtained from the vulva, vagina, cervix, and endometrial cavity. Usually performed in the office, most of these

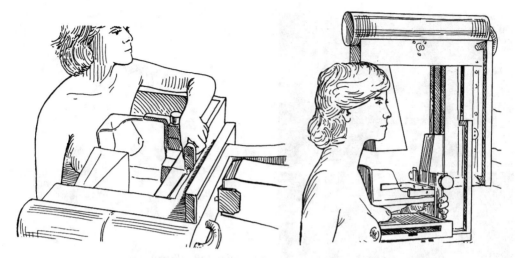

Figure 2.10. Technique of screening mammography.

procedures require little or no anesthetics and are associated with minimal risk.

Vulvar biopsies are generally accomplished with the use of a local anesthetic. Tissue may be removed by circumscribing the biopsy specimen with a Keyes biopsy instrument (a sharp hollow punch), elevating the tissue, and cutting across the base or by simple excision with a scalpel (Fig. 2.12). Local pressure or the use of styptics such as Monsel's solution (ferric subsulfate) is usually adequate for hemostasis; sutures are seldom required.

Biopsy of *vaginal* lesions is generally carried out using either the pinch technique for lesions low in the canal or a biopsy forceps. The biopsy forceps is also used for cervical biopsy. Local anesthesia is usually not required for vaginal or cervical biopsies.

An *endometrial* biopsy may be obtained in several ways. A small hollow tube may be passed through the cervix and tissue fragments aspirated using the suction pressure generated by removal of the stylet (Fig. 2.13). Larger, more rigid cannula may be used to aspirate or even curette the endometrium. This sharp curettage may require slightly greater cervical dilation, producing more discomfort and may warrant use of a paracervical anesthetic block.

Colposcopy

A colposcope is a fixed stereomicroscope with an internal light source used to facilitate detailed evaluation of the surface of the cervix, vagina, and vulva when malignancy is suspected based on history, physical examination, or cytologic report. It is used to make directed biopsies of suspicious areas and is an improvement over random biopsies in the face of abnormal cytologic reports. Colposcopy may be performed in the office — almost always without the need for analgesia or anesthesia — and has minimal morbidity.

Cryotherapy

Cryotherapy is the term used to describe tissue destruction by freezing. Liquid carbon dioxide or nitrogen is run through a metal probe that is placed on the tissue to be treated, allowing freezing of the tissue. Cryotherapy is most frequently used to treat dysplastic changes and benign lesions such as condyloma (Fig. 2.14). The formation of ice crystals within the cells of the treated tissue leads to tissue destruction and subsequent slough. As a result, patients who have had cryotherapy of the cervix can be expected to have a watery discharge for several weeks as the tissue sloughs and healing occurs. Cryotherapy is inexpensive and generally effective, but it is less precise than other tissue destruction procedures such as laser ablation.

Laser Vaporization

Energy from intense beams of light may be transferred to tissue to produce a therapeutic effect. This effect may vary from "sunburn" to explosive vaporization of the tissue. Light from laser (light amplification by stimulated emission of radiation)

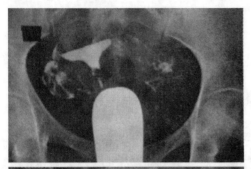

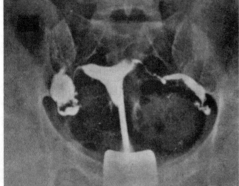

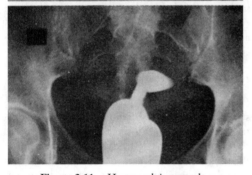

Figure 2.11. Hysterosalpingography.

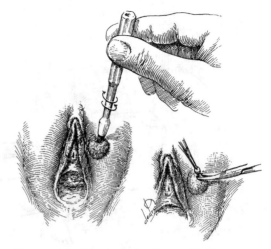

Figure 2.12. Biopsy of vulvar lesion with Keyes punch.

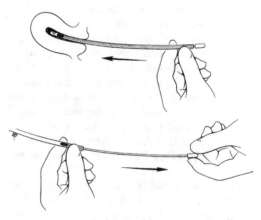

Figure 2.13. Endometrial biopsy using Pipelle.

sources is used because of its coherence (allowing the beam to be manipulated) and the purity of wavelength (decreasing extraneous effects and interactions). The interaction of the light and tissue depends on the wavelength of light and the *power density*, or intensity, of the beam.

One of the most common lasers used in gynecology is the infrared laser. The infrared energy emitted by this device is readily absorbed by the water molecules in tissue. This results in efficient energy transfer and relatively shallow depth of penetration. These two characteristics allow for precise control and selective tissue destruction. Laser therapy may be used to remove tissue by vaporization or to act as a "light knife" to excise tissues. The

precise control possible with this technique makes its use for cervical and vulvar lesions attractive. Laser may also be used for operative laparoscopic procedures and endometrial ablation.

Dilation and Curettage

The *dilation* of dilation and curettage (D&C) refers to opening the cervix to allow access to the endometrial cavity. This is usually done by gently using a series of graduated dilators to stretch the cervical opening. Because stretching of the cervix is painful, D&C is usually performed under a local (paracervical) or general anesthetic in an operating room. *Curettage* is a scraping of the uterine lining.

For the purpose of obtaining a representative sample of the uterine cavity, i.e., endometrial biopsy, D&C is supplanted by more easily accomplished office endometrial biopsy techniques, such as the Novak or Pipelle endometrial biopsy technique, or by biopsy under direct hysteroscopic visualization. Removal of polyps and other tumors may be accomplished by D&C, although direct removal under hysteroscopic visualization is sometimes chosen.

Hysteroscopy

Improved optics have led to the availability of small endoscopes that allow a direct view of the endocervix and endometrial cavity (Fig. 2.15). These endoscopes may be used for diagnosis (such as the evaluation of bleeding or congenital malformations, the staging of cancer, or the location of missing intrauterine devices) or for therapy (such as polypectomy, myomectomy, endometrial abla-

tion, and removal of a uterine septum). Usually done as an outpatient procedure under local or general anesthesia, hysteroscopy shares most of the same problems and complications found in dilation and curettage. Fluid may be used to distend the uterine cavity to improve visualization or the endometrium may be directly visualized (contact hysteroscopy). *Limited by Fluid Overload Monitor I/O*

Pregnancy Termination

Pregnancy termination refers to the planned interruption of a pregnancy before viability and is often referred to as induced abortion. It is generally accomplished surgically through dilation of the cervix and evacuation of the uterine contents (sometimes called D&E). Removal of the products of conception in the first and early second trimester uses either a suction or a sharp curette (suction and curet-

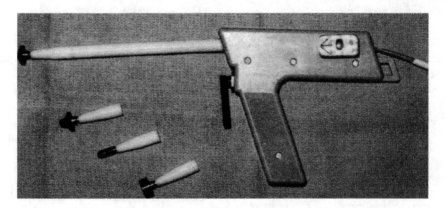

Figure 2.14. Cryosurgical equipment.

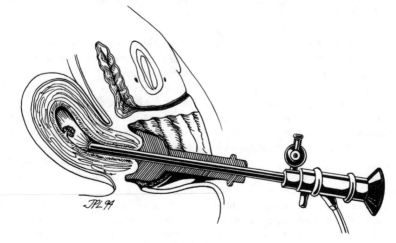

Figure 2.15. Hysteroscopy.

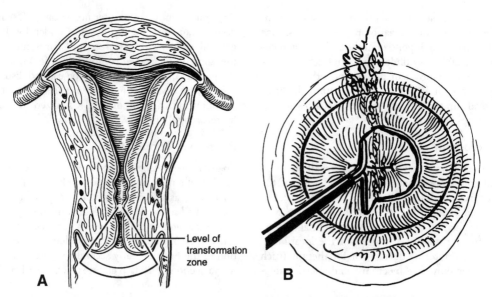

Figure 2.16. Conization of the cervix. **A**, Cold knife technique. **B**, LLETZ technique.

tage; S&C). Suction curettes are often preferred because they are less likely to cause uterine damage such as endometrial scarring or perforation.

In the second trimester, destructive grasping forceps may be used to remove the pregnancy through a dilated cervix (D&E). Alternatively, medical induction of labor can be performed. In the rarest of instances, an advanced pregnancy may be terminated by surgical removal, the hysterotomy (an operation similar to cesarean section, although incision through a relatively avascular lower uterine segment may not be possible).

Cervical Conization

Conization is a surgical procedure performed for either diagnostic or therapeutic purposes in which a cone-shaped sample of tissue, encompassing the entire cervical transformation zone and extending up the endocervical canal, is removed from the cervix (Fig. 2.16). Conization is required for the definitive evaluation of patients with abnormal Pap smears for whom adequate colposcopic examinations are impossible or are inconsistent with Pap smear data.

Conization may be performed using a variety of techniques, including sharp dissection (cold knife cone), laser excision, and electrocautery (large loop excision of the transformation zone; LLETZ). An early complication of conization is excessive bleeding, which can occur 5 to 10 days after surgery. Cervical stenosis or incompetence is an infrequent complication.

Laparoscopy

Laparoscopy (or pelviscopy) involves inspection and manipulation of tissue within the abdominal cavity using endoscopic instruments. The laparoscope is inserted into the abdominal cavity, usually through a periumbilical incision. To facilitate viewing and to decrease the chance of bowel injury, the abdominal cavity is distended with either carbon dioxide or nitrous oxide gas. Additional incisions in the lower abdomen may be made to allow supplementary instruments to be placed into the abdominal cavity for surgical or other manipulations (Fig. 2.17). A probe or other device is often inserted into the uterine cavity to facilitate uterine manipulations.

Laparoscopy is used for diagnostic or therapeutic purposes. Laparoscopic inspection of the pelvis can be invaluable in the diagnosis of pelvic pain, infertility, congenital abnormalities, or small pelvic masses. Operative laparoscopy may be used to perform lysis of adhesions, treat endometriosis, or carry out surgical sterilizations and other gynecologic procedures.

Because laparoscopy involves the penetration of the abdominal cavity, it is considered major surgery. Even though it is usually done on an outpatient basis under local or general anesthe-

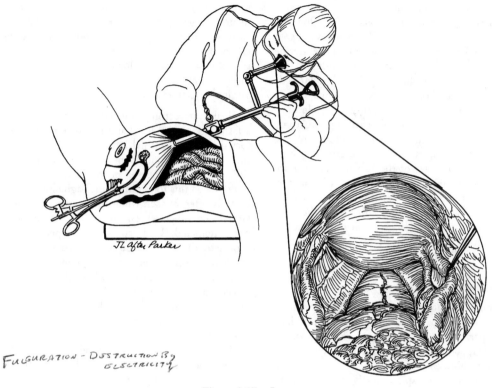

FULGURATION - DESTRUCTION By ELECTRICITY

Figure 2.17. Laparoscopy.

sia, the surgical nature of the procedure must be recognized. Serious complications from injury to the bowel or great vessels can occur. Intraperitoneal bleeding or injuries such as unappreciated damage to bowel during fulguration or laser also pose a risk. Anesthetic complications are possible, as are infections and bleeding at the incision site.

Hysterectomy

Hysterectomy, the removal of the uterus, is still one of the most common surgical procedures performed. In the United States, approximately 500,000 hysterectomies are performed each year. Removing the uterus may be indicated for patients with benign or malignant changes in the uterine wall or cavity, abnormalities of the cervix, or menstrual disturbances that do not respond to more conservative therapy. Hysterectomy essentially eliminates the posibility of pregnancy, causes cessation of menses, and removes the risk of cervical disease. Despite these apparent advantages, hysterectomy is sufficiently

expensive, time-consuming, and risky that it cannot be recommended for the sole purpose of sterilization.

In discussing hysterectomy with patients, it is important to recognize the correct use and common misuse of terms associated with the procedure. When physicians use the term *total* hysterectomy, they are referring to the removal of all of the uterus. The term does not indicate removal of the ovaries (oophorectomy) or fallopian tubes (salpingectomy). These distinctions are important and should be emphasized when taking the patient's history and providing preoperative counseling. A *subtotal*, or *supracervical*, hysterectomy is one in which the body of the uterus is removed near the level of the internal cervical os, leaving the cervix in place. A *radical* hysterectomy is a cancer surgery procedure in which the uterus is removed with very wide margins of surrounding tissues.

Removal of the uterus may be accomplished by entering the abdominal cavity from above (abdominal hysterectomy) or by extracting the uterus through the vagina (vaginal hysterectomy). Each has advantages and disadvantages that must be evaluated for each patient. With either approach, certain steps must be accomplished to allow the safe removal of the uterus. The blood supply to the uterus is interrupted by ligation of the uterine arteries and the anastomotic connections to the vaginal and ovarian blood supplies. The latter is ligated at the level of the uteroovarian ligament (if the ovaries are to be preserved) or at the level of the infundibulopelvic ligament (if oophorectomy is planned). The supporting structures of the uterus (the round, cardinal, and uterosacral ligaments and the leaves of the broad ligament) are severed. The sequence of these steps is dictated by the route of surgery chosen (fundus to cervix for the abdominal route; cervix to fundus for the vaginal route) and the local exigencies mandated by the pathology encountered (e.g., distortion of anatomy by fibroids).

Abdominal Hysterectomy

Removal of the uterus through an abdominal incision allows the surgeon maximal exposure and latitude in performing the procedure. This approach is used when substantial pathology is anticipated (as with large fibroids or pelvic scarring), when wide margins or further exploration is required (as in cancer surgery), when additional abdominal procedures are contemplated (such as bladder suspension), or when surgery is done at the time of cesarean delivery. Abdominal hysterectomies generally involve longer operating times, because of the time spent making and repairing the abdominal wall incision. This route also is associated with a greater rate of morbidity and a longer hospital stay.

Vaginal Hysterectomy

Vaginal hysterectomy is generally associated with a faster recovery period and less patient discomfort than an abdominal hysterectomy. Offsetting this is the higher incidence of fever and infection, although the use of prophylactic antibiotics has reduced this to a minimum. Vaginal hysterectomy is often chosen when the uterus is not enlarged and other adnexal or pelvic pathology is not anticipated. This procedure is especially appropriate for patients who require repair of a cystocele, rectocele, or enterocele. Vaginal hysterectomy is typically avoided when the uterus is larger than 10 to 12 weeks' size, movement of the pelvic organs is restricted by scarring or endometriosis, or further abdominal exploration is required.

The role of laparoscopic-assisted vaginal hysterectomy (LAVH) — in which some of the initial stages of hysterectomy are done with laparoscopic instrumentation, but the uterus is ultimately removed transvaginally — remains to be fully identified.

chapter 3

EMBRYOLOGY, ANATOMY, AND REPRODUCTIVE GENETICS

A knowledge of the embryology of the female reproductive system is helpful in understanding both normal anatomy and the structural anomalies that can sometimes occur. Although this chapter concentrates on development in the female, comparisons with the development of the male reproductive system are made for illustration.

EMBRYOLOGY

The genital system develops from embryonic intermediate mesoderm. With the folding of the embryo, the intermediate mesoderm comes to lie as two longitudinal rods on either side of the primitive aorta. In the trunk region, the rods are called nephrogenic cords (Fig. 3.1*A*). There is a dorsal outgrowth of each nephrogenic cord, which bulges into the celomic cavity. These bulges, called the *urogenital ridges,* are covered with celomic epithelium. The urogenital ridges give rise to elements of both the urinary and the reproductive systems (Fig. 3.1*B*).

In general, the elements of the reproductive system pass through an undifferentiated stage in the early embryo. That is, development is identical in the male and female. Later, sex-specific differentiation occurs.

Development of the Ovary

Genetic sex, determined at fertilization, depends on whether the X-bearing oocyte is fertilized by an X- or Y-bearing sperm. However, early in development, the gonads are undifferentiated, i.e., the sex of the embryo cannot be determined from the appearance of the gonad.

The gonads begin to develop during the 5th week, when a portion of the urogenital ridge on the medial side of the mesonephric kidney thickens to form the *gonadal ridge.* The celomic epithelium divides to form finger-like bands of cells (the *primary sex cords*), which project into the underlying mesodermal mesenchyme of the gonadal ridge. In the female, it is the cortical area that predominates in the mature gonad, and it is this cortical tissue that contains the follicles. This growth results in the creation of a cortex and a medulla in the indifferent (undifferentiated) gonad.

During the 4th week, the *primordial germ cells* (which will eventually give rise to the gametes) can be identified in the yolk sac. As the embryo folds, some of the yolk sac is incorporated into the embryo. During the 6th week, the primordial germ cells migrate into the mesenchyme of the gonadal ridge, where they become associated with the primary sex cords. In the female, the primordial germ cells become oogonia, which divide by mitosis during fetal life. No oogonia form after birth.

If a Y chromosome is present, the tunica albuginea of the testis will begin to form in the mesenchymal tissue of the medulla during the 8th week. This is the first indication of the sex of the embryo. In the absence of a Y chromosome, the undifferentiated gonad will develop into an ovary, which will be identifiable by about the 10th week of development. In the ovary, the primary sex cords degenerate, and secondary sex cords (cortical cords) appear and extend from the surface epithelium into the underlying mesenchyme. The *oogonia* are incorporated into them, and at about 16 weeks of development, the cortical cords organize into *primordial follicles.* Each follicle eventually consists of an oogonium, derived from a primary germ cell, surrounded by a single layer of squamous follicular cells, derived from the cortical cords. *Follicular maturation* begins when the oogonia enter the first

31

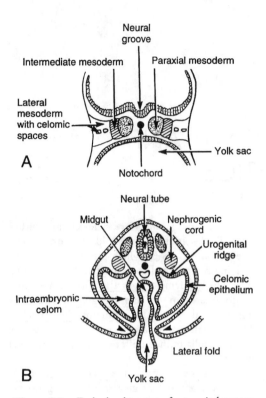

Figure 3.1. Early development of urogenital system.

stage of meiotic division (at which point they are called oocytes). Oocyte development is then arrested until puberty, when one or more follicles are stimulated to continue development each month (see Chapters 34 and 35).

Development of the Genital Ducts

In both the male and female, two pairs of ducts initially develop, the mesonephric (wolffian) and the paramesonephric (müllerian). As with the gonad, there is an indifferent (undifferentiated) stage in ductal development. During this stage, both sets of ducts are present in both the male and the female.

In the male, the *mesonephric ducts*, which drain the embryonic mesonephric kidneys, eventually form the *epididymis, ductus deferens*, and *ejaculatory ducts*. In the female, the mesonephric ducts almost completely disappear.

In the female, it is the *paramesonephric* ducts (or müllerian) that persist to form major parts of the reproductive tract (the *fallopian tubes, uterus*, and *parts of the vagina*). The paramesonephric ducts start to develop early in the 6th week, beginning

as invaginations of the celomic epithelium in the vicinity of the mesonephric kidneys (Fig. 3.2*A*). For each duct, the invagination fuses to form a tube. The cranial end of each duct opens into the celomic (future peritoneal) cavity. The ducts grow caudally, and the caudal segments fuse at about the 8th week of development into the Y-shaped *uterovaginal primordium* or *canal* (Fig. 3.2*B*). The cranial (unfused) portion of each duct becomes a fallopian tube, and the fused portions become the uterus and parts of the vagina. This differentiation does not depend on the presence of ovaries.

When the two paramesonephric ducts fuse, two peritoneal folds are brought together. This creates the broad ligaments of the uterus (Fig. 3.2*C*).

Development of the Vagina

Between weeks 5 and 7, the *primitive cloaca*, a pouch-like enlargement of the caudal end of the hindgut, is divided into the *urogenital sinus* (ventral) and the *anorectal canal* (dorsal). The contact of the caudally growing uterovaginal primordium with the urogenital sinus results in the formation of a solid mass of cells called the vaginal plate. The vaginal plate extends from the urogenital sinus into the caudal end of the uterovaginal primordium. The central cells of the vaginal plate disappear, forming the lumen of the vagina. The peripheral cells of the plate persist as the vaginal epithelium. In addition to contributing to the vagina, the urogenital sinus also gives rise to the *epithelium of the urinary bladder*, the *urethra*, the *greater vestibular glands*, and the *hymen*.

Development of the External Genitalia

The external genitalia also pass through an indifferent stage. Early in the 4th week, the *genital tubercle*, or phallus, develops at the cranial end of the cloacal membrane. Soon after, labioscrotal swellings and urogenital folds appear at either side of the cloacal membrane (Fig. 3.3*A*). The genital tubercle enlarges in both the male and the female (Fig. 3.3*B*).

The division of the cloaca by the urorectal septum divides the cloacal membrane into the dorsal anal membrane and the ventral urogenital membrane. At about week 7, these membranes rupture.

At about 9 weeks, distinguishing sexual characteristics begin to appear, but the external genital organs are not fully formed until week 12. In the absence of androgens, the external genitalia are feminized (Fig. 3.3*C*). The phallus develops into

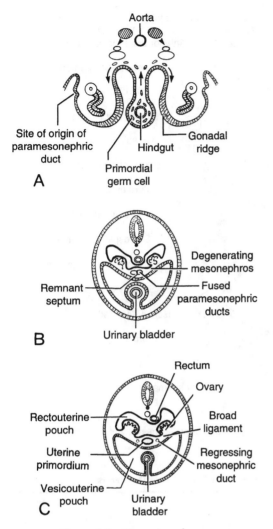

Figure 3.2. Formation of uterus.

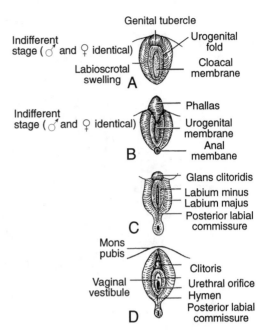

Figure 3.3. Development of the external genitalia.

the relatively small *clitoris*. The unfused urogenital folds form the *labia minora* and the labioscrotal swellings become the *labia majora* (Fig. 3.3D).

ANATOMY

This section first describes the normal anatomy of the female reproductive system. Anomalies, arising from defects in development, will then be discussed.

Bony Pelvis

The bony pelvis is composed of the paired *innominate bones* and the sacrum. The innominate bones are joined anteriorly to form the symphysis pubis, and each is articulated posteriorly with the sacrum through the sacroiliac joint (Fig. 3.4).

The innominate bones are composed of three portions — the *ilium*, the *ischium*, and the *pubis* — which become fused during adolescence. The three parts come together to contribute to the acetabulum. The sacrum is composed of five or six sacral vertebrae, which are fused in adulthood. The sacrum articulates with the coccyx inferiorly and with the fifth lumbar vertebra superiorly.

The pelvis is divided into the pelvis major (*false pelvis*) and the pelvis minor (*true pelvis*), which are separated by the linea terminalis. The false pelvis, whose main function is to support the pregnant uterus, is bounded by the lumbar vertebrae posteriorly, an iliac fossa bilaterally, and the abdominal wall anteriorly.

The true pelvis is formed by the sacrum and coccyx posteriorly and by the ischium and pubis laterally and anteriorly. Concern arises when its dimensions are inadequate to permit passage of the fetus.

There are *four pelvic planes*: the *pelvic inlet*, the *plane of the greatest diameter*, the *plane of least diameter* (midplane), and the *pelvic outlet*. The pelvic inlet is bounded posteriorly by the promontory and alae of the sacrum, laterally by the linea terminalis, and anteriorly by the superior surface of the

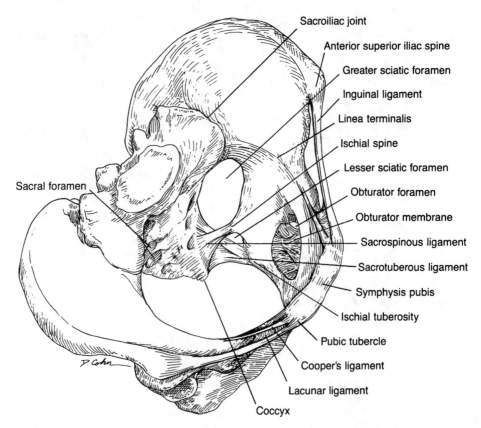

Figure 3.4. View of the pelvis from above, showing bones, joints, ligaments, and foramina.

pubic bones. Thus the plane of the inlet separates the false pelvis and the true pelvis. The plane of the greatest diameter is bounded by the junction of the second and third sacral vertebrae posteriorly, the upper part of the obturator foramina laterally, and the midpoint of the pubis anteriorly. The plane of least diameter (the midplane) extends from the lower border of the pubis anteriorly to the lower sacrum at the level of the ischial spines. This plane is most important clinically, because arrest of fetal descent occurs most frequently at this point. The plane of the outlet is irregular, consisting of two intersecting triangles. It is bounded posteriorly by the tip of the sacrum, laterally by the ischial tuberosities and the sacrotuberous ligaments, and anteriorly by the lower border of the symphysis. There are certain key diameters of the pelvis that are important in assessing the space available during fetal descent (Fig. 3.5, Table 3.1).

The female pelvis is classified into four basic types, according to the scheme of Caldwell and Moloy

Table 3.1.
Length of Pelvic Plane Diameters

Pelvic Plane	Diameter	Average Length (cm)
Inlet	True conjugate	10.5–11.5
	Obstetric conjugate	10.0–11.0
	Diagonal conjugate	12.5
	Transverse diameter	13.5
	Oblique diameter	12.5
Greatest diameter	Anterior-posterior	12.75
	Transverse	12.5
Midplane	Anterior-posterior	11.5–12.0
	Bispinous	10.0
Outlet	Anterior-posterior	11.5
	Bituberous	8.0–11.0

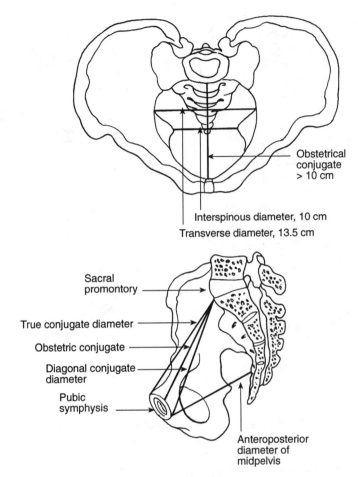

Figure 3.5. Pelvic diameters.

(Fig. 3.6). The most common type is the *gynecoid,* occurring in about 40 to 50% of women. In this type, the inlet is rounded, the side walls are straight, the sacrum is well curved, and the sacrosciatic notch is adequate. In general, this gives the pelvis a cylindrical shape, which has adequate space along its length. The *platypelloid* pelvis occurs in only about 2 to 5% of women. There is an oval inlet, the sacrum is normal, the side walls are straight, the sacrosciatic notch is narrower, and the interspinous and intertuberous diameters are increased compared with the other pelvic types. Any individual may be of a pure or mixed pelvic type. The *android* pelvis occurs in about 30% of all women but in only 10 to 15% of African-American women. There is a wedge-shaped inlet, the side walls converge, the sacrum is inclined forward, and the sacrosciatic notch is narrow. This pelvic type has limited space at the inlet, and the funnel shape results in even less space below. Fetal descent may be arrested at the midpelvis. The *anthropoid* type occurs in about 20% of all women and in about 40% of black women. The inlet is oval, long, and narrow; the side walls are straight (do not converge); the sacrum is long and narrow; and the sacrosciatic notch is wide. Both the interspinous and intertuberous diameters are somewhat smaller than in the gynecoid pelvis.

Vulva and Perineum

The vulva contains the labia majora, labia minora, mons pubis, clitoris, vestibule, and ducts of glands that open into the vestibule (Fig. 3.7). The labia majora are folds of skin with underlying adipose tissue; they are fused anteriorly with the mons pubis and posteriorly with the perineum. The skin of

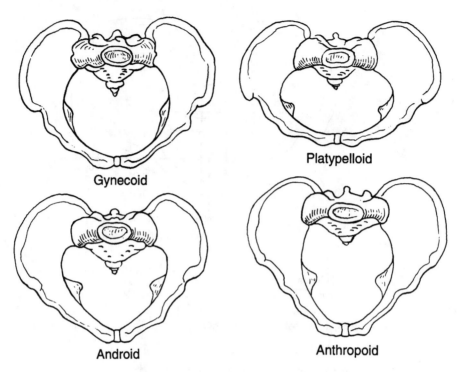

Figure 3.6. Caldwell-Moloy pelvic types.

the labia majora contains hair follicles and sebaceous and sweat glands. The labia minora are narrow skin folds, which lie inside the labia majora. The labia minora merge anteriorly with the prepuce and frenulum of the clitoris and posteriorly with the labia majora and the perineum. The labia minora contain sebaceous and sweat glands but no hair follicles, and there is no underlying adipose tissue. The clitoris, which is located anterior to the labia minora, is the embryologic homolog of the penis. It consists of two crura (corresponding to the corpora cavernosa in the male) and the glans, which is found superior to the point of fusion of the crura. On the ventral surface of the glans is the *frenulum*, the fused junction of the labia minora. The *vestibule* lies between the labia minora and is bounded anteriorly by the clitoris and posteriorly by the perineum. The urethra and the vagina open into the vestibule in the midline. The ducts of *Skene's (paraurethral) glands* and *Bartholin's glands* also empty into the vestibule.

The *muscles of the vulva* (superior transverse perineal, bulbocavernosus, and ischiocavernosus) lie superficial to the fascia of the urogenital diaphragm (Fig. 3.8). The vulva rests on the triangular-shaped urogenital diaphragm, which lies in the anterior part of the pelvis between the ischiopubic rami. The urogenital diaphragm surrounds and supports the urethra and the vagina.

Vagina

The vagina is a muscular tube that extends from the vestibule to the uterus (Figs. 3.9 and 3.10). The long axis of the vagina is approximately parallel to the lower portion of the sacrum. The uterine cervix projects into the upper portion of the vagina. Therefore, the anterior vaginal wall is about 2 cm shorter than the posterior wall. The area around the cervix, the fornix, is divided into four regions: the *anterior fornix*, two *lateral fornices*, and the *posterior fornix*. The posterior fornix is in close proximity to the peritoneum that forms the floor of the posterior pelvic cul-de-sac (pouch of Douglas). This allows access to the peritoneal cavity from the vagina, e.g., during culdocentesis.

At its lower end, the vagina traverses the urogenital diaphragm and is then surrounded by the two bulbocavernosus muscles. These act as a sphincter. The *hymen*, a fold of mucosal-covered connective tissue, somewhat obscures the external

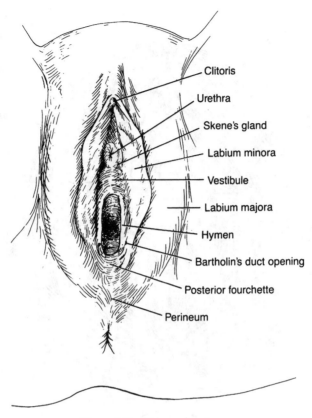

- Clitoris
- Urethra
- Skene's gland
- Labium minora
- Vestibule
- Labium majora
- Hymen
- Bartholin's duct opening
- Posterior fourchette
- Perineum

Figure 3.7. Vulva and perineum.

vaginal orifice in the child. The hymen is fragmented into irregular remnants with sexual activity and childbearing.

The major *blood supply* to the vagina is from the vaginal artery, a branch of the hypogastric artery. The veins follow the path of the arteries.

The *vaginal wall* consists of a mucous membrane and an external muscular layer. The lumen is lined by a stratified squamous epithelium. Beneath this is a submucosal layer of connective tissue, which contains a rich supply of veins and lymphatics. Submucosal rugae throw the lumen of the vagina into the characteristic H shape in the young; these folds become less prominent with age. The muscular wall has three layers of smooth muscle. The vaginal wall is extremely distensible, especially under hormonal influences during childbirth.

Uterus

The uterus is covered on each side by the two layers of the broad ligament, and it lies between the rectum and the bladder (Figs. 3.9 and 3.10).

The close relationship with structures in the broad ligament, especially the uterine arteries and veins and the ureters, has important implications during surgery. The two major portions of the uterus are the *cervix* and the body (*corpus*), which are separated by a narrower isthmus. Before puberty, the length of the cervix and the body are approximately equal; after puberty, the ratio of the body to the cervix is between 2:1 and 3:1. The part of the body where the two uterine (fallopian) tubes enter is called the *cornu*. The part of the corpus above the cornu is termed the *fundus*. In the nonparous adult, the uterus is about 7 to 8 cm long and 4 to 5 cm wide at the widest part. The cervix is relatively cylindrical in shape and is 2 to 3 cm long. The corpus is generally pear shaped, with the anterior surface being flat and the posterior surface, convex. In cross section, the lumen of the corpus is triangular.

The normal position of the uterus is variable. The angle between the long axis of the corpus and the cervix varies from *anteflexion* to *retroflexion*,

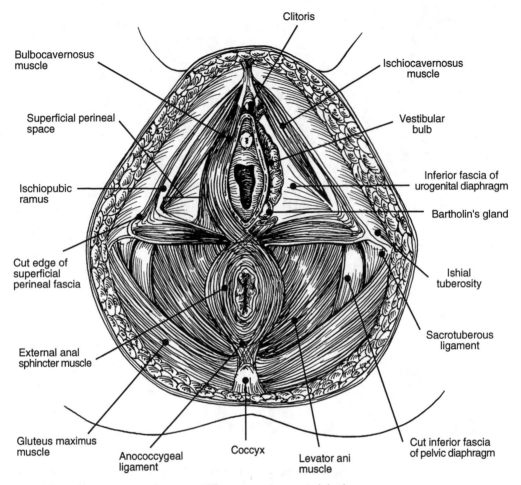

Figure 3.8. Perineum and urogenital diaphragm.

and the angle between the cervix and the vagina varies from *anteversion* to *retroversion*. Unless caused by underlying pathology, these variations are normal. The uterus is supported by the following ligaments: *uterosacral, cardinal, round,* and *broad.* The *blood supply* to the uterus comes primarily from the uterine arteries and also from the ovarian arteries, whereas the venous plexus drains through the uterine vein.

The cervix joins the vagina at an angle between 45 and 90°. The opening to the vagina, the external os, is round to oval in nonparous women but is a transverse slit after childbirth. The portion of the cervix that projects into the vagina is covered with stratified squamous epithelium, which resembles the vaginal epithelium. The squamous epithelium changes to a simple columnar epithelium in

the *transition* (transformation) *zone.* This zone is found at about the level of the external cervical os, although it is found higher in the endocervical canal in postmenopausal women. The importance of this zone in the process of neoplastic transformation is discussed in Chapter 42.

There are *three basic layers in the wall of the uterine body* (Fig. 3.11). The inner mucosa (the endometrium) consists of the simple columnar epithelium with underlying connective tissue. The changes in the structure of this layer that occur during the normal menstrual cycle are described in Chapter 44. Beneath the mucosa is a thick muscular layer (the myometrium), covered by a peritoneal serosa. The muscle layer is continuous with the muscular walls of the vagina and the fallopian tubes.

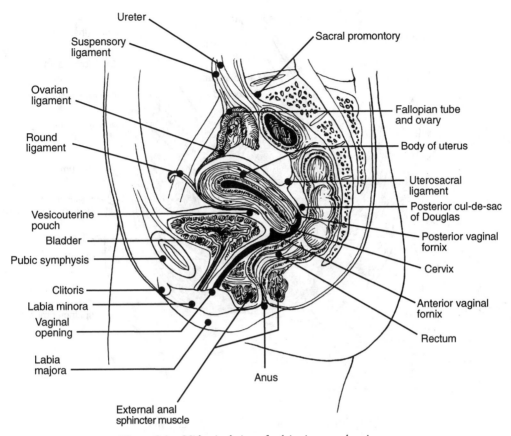

Figure 3.9. Midsagittal view of pelvic viscera and perineum.

Fallopian Tubes

The fallopian tubes (the oviducts) average about 7 to 14 cm in length. Each tube can be divided into three portions: a narrow and straight isthmus, which adjoins the opening into the uterus; the ampulla, or central portion; and the infundibulum, which is fringed by the finger-shaped fimbriae. These surround the ovary and help to collect the oocyte at the time of ovulation. The fallopian tubes are supplied by the ovarian and uterine arteries. The epithelial lining of the fallopian tube is ciliated columnar. The cilia beat toward the uterus, assisting in oocyte transport.

Ovaries

Each ovary is about 3 to 5 cm long, 2 to 3 cm wide, and 1 to 3 cm thick in the menstrual years. The size decreases by about two-thirds after menopause, when follicular development ceases. The ovary is attached to the broad ligament by the mesovarium,

to the uterus by the ovarian ligament, and to the side of the pelvis by the suspensory ligament of the ovary (infundibulopelvic ligament), which is the lateral margin of the broad ligament (Figs. 3.10 and 3.11). The outer ovarian cortex consists of follicles embedded in a connective tissue stroma. The connective tissue medulla contains smooth muscle fibers, blood vessels, nerves, and lymphatics.

The ovaries are mainly supplied by the ovarian arteries, which are direct branches of the abdominal aorta, but there also is a blood supply from the uterine artery, a branch of the hypogastric artery (internal iliac artery) (Fig. 3.12). Venous return via the right ovarian vein is directly into the inferior vena cava, and from the left ovary into the left renal vein.

Anomalies of the Female Reproductive System

Anatomic anomalies arise from defects during embryologic development, and all occur very in-

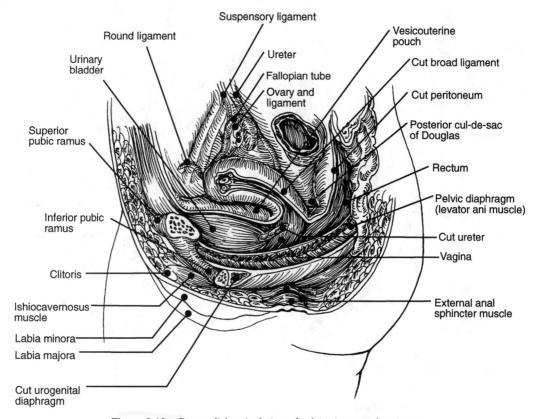

Figure 3.10. Paramedial sagittal view of pelvic viscera and perineum.

frequently. Absence of the ovary is rare and usually associated with óther genital tract anomalies. Ectopic ovarian tissue may occur, as supernumerary ovaries or as accessory ovarian tissue. In general, various kinds of uterine and vaginal malformations can arise from incomplete fusion of the paramesonephric ducts, incomplete development of one or both paramesonephric ducts, or incomplete canalization of the vaginal plate.

Absence of the uterus occurs when the paramesonephric ducts degenerate. This condition is associated with vaginal anomalies (such as absence of the vagina), because vaginal development is stimulated by the developing uterovaginal primordium. A double uterus (uterus didelphys) occurs when the inferior parts of the paramesonephric ducts do not fuse; this condition may be associated with a double or a single vagina. A bicornuate uterus results when lack of fusion is limited to the superior portion of the uterine body. If one of the paramesonephric ducts is poorly developed and fusion with the other duct does not occur, the result is a bicornuate

uterus with a rudimentary horn. This horn may or may not communicate with the uterine cavity.

Absence of the vagina occurs when the vaginal plate does not develop. It is usually coupled with the absence of the uterus. If the vaginal plate does not canalize, the result is vaginal atresia. Imperforate hymen is a minor example of this.

REPRODUCTIVE GENETICS

Genetics has become an integral part of obstetric care. Obstetricians must identify women at increased risk for fetal abnormalities and offer appropriate genetic screening and testing to patients based on their personal, family, and medical histories. This section reviews current indications and techniques of genetic screening and testing applicable to the pregnant patient.

Genetic Counseling

Genetic counseling serves two important functions: (*a*) to obtain information from the patient to properly assess her risk for developing disease and

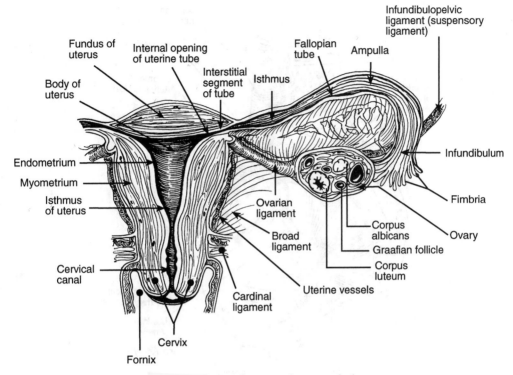

Figure 3.11. Frontal section of uterus and adnexa.

for being delivered of an infant with congenital abnormalities and (*b*) to provide information to the patient regarding appropriate screening or diagnostic tests. Data forms, questionnaires, pedigree construction, and patient interviews are all effective methods for obtaining information concerning personal and family medical history, parental exposure to potentially harmful substances, and other issues that may impact risk assessment. No single method or combination thereof is universally effective in obtaining all appropriate patient information. The specific methods used to gather information depend on the type of information required and the physician-patient relationship.

Genetic counseling should never be used to coerce a patient to undergo or forego certain tests or pregnancy management decisions. Information should be obtained and provided in a nondirective fashion so that the counselor acts in a completely objective manner, never interjecting personal opinions into the counseling session. Patients may then arrive at reproductive decisions based on their own values, ethics, and desires as well as

written and verbal information provided by the counselor. In addition to decisions concerning genetic screening or testing, counselors must be able to review alternative reproductive options (e.g., pregnancy termination, permanent sterilization, selective pregnancy reduction, and donor insemination) with their patients in an empathetic yet nondirective manner.

Chromosome Abnormalities

In the United States, the most common indication for invasive prenatal diagnostic testing is increased risk for fetal chromosome abnormalities (Table 3.2). Chromosome abnormalities also play an important role in spontaneous abortion and infertility; at least 50 to 60% of first-trimester spontaneous abortions, 5% of stillbirths, and 2 to 3% of couples experiencing multiple miscarriage or infertility will be found to have a structural or numerical chromosome alteration. Overall, 0.6% of all liveborn infants have a chromosome abnormality.

Couples who desire chromosome analysis because of a history of multiple miscarriage or infertility are evaluated by cytogenetic analysis of cul-

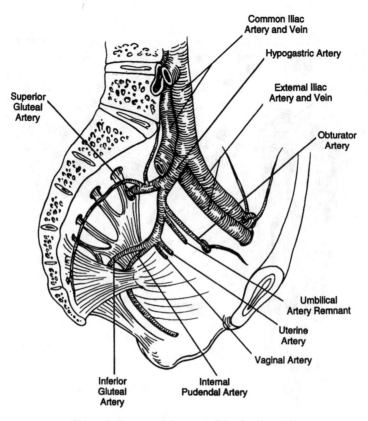

Figure 3.12.   Arterial system of the female pelvis.

tured lymphocytes obtained from their peripheral blood (Fig. 3.13). Determination of fetal chromosome complement, however, is not as simple or safe, because obtaining fetal cells involves invasive procedures that increase fetal morbidity and mortality. Fetal chromosome analysis, either of continuing pregnancies or of spontaneous or induced abortions, is currently performed on cells obtained from amniotic fluid, placenta (chorionic villi), or fetal tissue. The procedures used to obtain these specimens are described later in this section.

Indications for Prenatal Cytogenetic Analysis

Advanced Maternal Age

The most common indication for invasive prenatal diagnosis is advanced maternal age. The incidence of Down syndrome among newborns is approximately 1:800; however, the incidence of Down syndrome among newborns delivered to 35-year-old women is 1:385, and the incidence

among 45-year-old women is 1:33. Down syndrome is not the only chromosome abnormality that increases in frequency with advanced maternal age; other autosomal trisomies and some sex chromosome polysomies increase in incidence as parturients get older (Table 3.2).

In the United States, it was standard obstetric practice to offer all women 35 years old or older at their estimated day of delivery invasive prenatal diagnostic testing to detect fetal chromosome abnormalities. Recently, the Committee on Obstetric Practice of the American College of Obstetricians and Gynecologists reviewed this practice with reference to Down syndrome. They noted that only 5 to 8% of pregnancies occur in women over 35 years of age but that 20% of Down syndrome babies are born to women in this age group. Thus 80% of Down syndrome babies are born to women under 35 years of age, often to women who in addition have no identified risk of Down syndrome. The committee now recommends that serum screening testing be offered to all women between the 15th

Table 3.2.
Common Cytogenetic Abnormalities

Chromosome Abnormality	Live-Birth Incidence	Characteristics
Trisomy 21 (Down syndrome)	1:800	Moderate to severe mental retardation; characteristic facies; cardiac abnormalities; increased incidence of respiratory infections and leukemia; only 2% live beyond 50 years
Trisomy 18 (Edwards syndrome)	1:8,000	Severe mental retardation; multiple organic abnormalities; less than 10% survive 1 year
Trisomy 13 (Patau syndrome)	1:20,000	Severe mental retardation; neurologic, ophthalmologic, and organic abnormalities; less than 5% survive 3 years
Trisomy 16	0	Lethal anomaly occurs frequently in first-trimester spontaneous abortions; no infants are known to have trisomy 16
45,X (Turner syndrome)	1:10,000	Occurs frequently in first-trimester spontaneous abortions; associated primarily with unique somatic features; patients are not mentally retarded, although IQ of affected individuals is lower than sibs
47,XXX; 47,XYY; 47,XYY; 47,XXY (Klinefelter syndrome)	each approximately 1:900	Minimal somatic abnormalities; individuals with Klinefelter syndrome are characterized by a tall, eunuchoid habitus and small testes. 47,XXX and 47,XYY individuals do not usually exhibit somatic abnormalities, but 47,XYY individuals may be tall and may exhibit social pathology
del(5p) (cri du chat (syndrome)	1:20,000	Severe mental retardation; microcephaly; distinctive facial features; characteristic "cat's cry" sound

and 18th week of gestation. Such testing is voluntary and should be preceded by counseling about the nature of the screening tests and their predictive value and limitations as well as comparison with diagnostic cytogenetic tests. In addition, the committee suggests that serum testing — single marker maternal serum α-fetoprotein (MSAFP) or triple marker MSAFP plus human chorionic gonadotropin (hCG) plus unconjugated estriol (uE3) — should not be recommended for routine Down syndrome screening as an equivalent alternative to prenatal cytogenetic diagnosis. Some women over 35 years of age may choose this less invasive serum screening testing as opposed to the more invasive cytogenetic diagnostic procedures after complete counseling about the risks and benefits of both. Finally, the committee does not recommend ultrasonography as a screening test in any age group because of lack of sensitivity and issues of cost.

The incidence of fetal chromosome abnormalities is higher at midtrimester (e.g., 16th week ges-

tation) than at term, because many chromosomally abnormal fetuses will be aborted spontaneously after the 16th gestational week. It is, therefore, important to use consistently either midtrimester or live-born data when counseling patients concerning risks for fetal chromosome abnormalities.

Parental Chromosome Abnormality

Although an *unbalanced* parental chromosome complement is a rare occurrence, a *balanced* parental chromosome rearrangement is not uncommon. Approximately 4% of Down syndrome children are the result of an unbalanced robertsonian translocation (see below) between chromosome 21 and either chromosome 13, 14, 15, 21, or 22. Although 60% of these unbalanced translocations are the result of a de novo (i.e., new) rearrangement, the other 40% are the result of an unbalanced gamete inherited from a parent with a balanced chromosome rearrangement (Fig. 3.14).

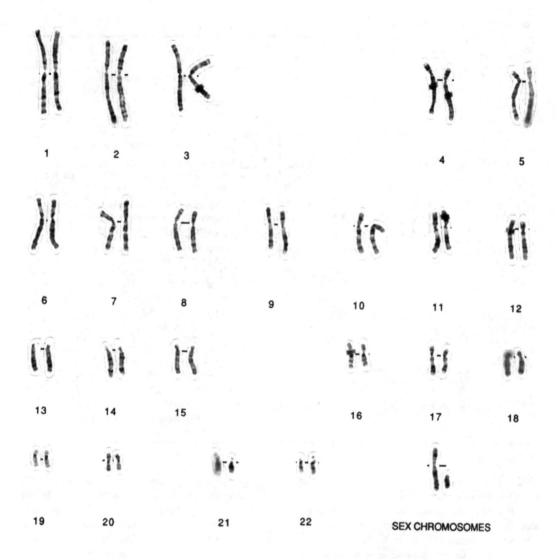

Figure 3.13. Normal (46,XY) metaphase spread of a cultured lymphocyte obtained from peripheral blood.

Three types of parental chromosome rearrangements that can result in chromosomally abnormal offspring are robertsonian translocations, reciprocal translocations, and inversions. Robertsonian translocations involve the two groups of acrocentric chromosomes, namely the D group (chromosomes 13, 14, and 15) and the G group (chromosomes 21 and 22); it is this type of balanced parental translocation that most frequently results in Down syndrome in offspring. The theoretical risk for a parent who has a balanced robertsonian translocation involving chromo-

some 21 to have a child with Down syndrome is 33%. However, the actual risk for Down syndrome in offspring depends on which parent has the translocation and which chromosomes are involved. For example, if the mother carries a balanced robertsonian translocation involving chromosomes 14 and 21 (45,XX,−14,−21,+t(14q; 21q)), the risk is approximately 10%, whereas if the father carries the same translocation, the risk is 1% or less. In addition, if the balanced translocation involves two number 21 chromosomes, the risk for Down syndrome in live borns is

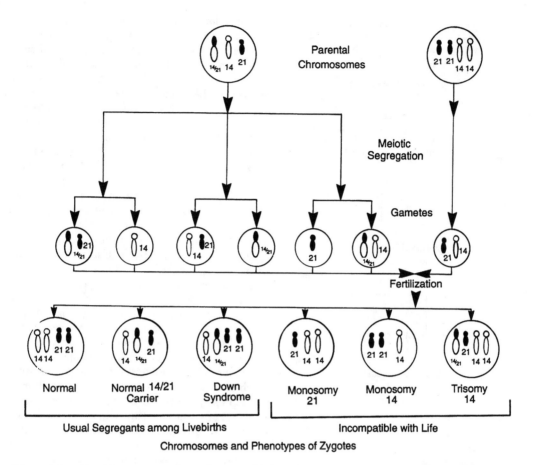

Figure 3.14. Possible gametic products of a parental balanced translocation. Although theoretical risk for abnormal live borns is 33%, the empiric risk is frequently lower.

100%, irrespective of which parent carries the translocation.

Balanced reciprocal translocations may involve any chromosome and are the result of a reciprocal "trade" of material between two or more chromosomes. This results in a rearranged complement characterized by the same amount of genetic material found in a "normal" complement. Similar to robertsonian translocations, empiric risk for newborn chromosome abnormality is less than the theoretical risk (33%). However, unlike robertsonian translocations, empiric risk of newborn chromosome abnormalities is approximately 11%, irrespective of which parent carries the translocation or which chromosomes are involved.

Detection of a parental inversion resulting in fetal or newborn chromosome abnormalities is

rare, despite the relatively common occurrence of certain specific inversions (e.g., inv9(p11q13)) in the population. Such commonly occurring inversions do not apparently place couples at increased risk for chromosome abnormalities in offspring. Empiric data for unique inversions that result in chromosomally unbalanced progeny are unavailable; theoretical risks depend on whether the centromere is involved and the size of the inverted portion.

Screening Tests

In addition to the aforementioned indications, results from noninvasive screening techniques such as ultrasonography and maternal serum screening for Down syndrome (including measurement of maternal serum levels of α-fetoprotein (AFP), hCG, and/or uE3) may prompt a woman to con-

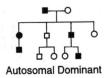

Autosomal Dominant

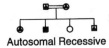

Autosomal Recessive

X-linked Dominant

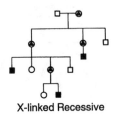

X-linked Recessive

□   Males
○   Females
■●   Affected
▫⊙   Unaffected but heterozygous
═   Consanguineous

Figure 3.15. Patterns of familial transmission expected for autosomal dominant, autosomal recessive, X-linked recessive, and X-linked dominant inheritance.

sider invasive prenatal diagnostic testing. A thorough discussion of the particular protocol used to detect women at increased risk for Down syndrome or other chromosome abnormalities should be undertaken, as results may significantly alter pregnancy management.

Mendelian Disorders

Mendelian disorders result from mutations of specific genes. Expression of a disease or trait may result from expression of a single gene at a specific genetic locus on an autosomal chromosome (auto-

somal dominant) or may require expression of two genes at an autosomal locus (autosomal recessive) (Fig. 3.15). In addition, those genes located on the X chromosome that result in specific disorders or traits are known as *X-linked*; X-linked conditions may also be dominant or recessive. Because males have only one X chromosome, those males possessing a single recessive X-linked gene will express that condition, even though they have only a single copy of that gene (hemizygosity) (Fig. 3.15). Expression of the same condition in females would require two copies of the recessive gene.

A plethora of Mendelian disorders and traits have been described, and a description of them is beyond the scope of this section. Many Mendelian disorders occur more frequently in certain groups (e.g., sickle-cell disease in blacks, cystic fibrosis in whites, Tay-Sachs disease in Ashkenazic Jews, β-thalassemia in southern Europeans and α-thalassemia in Asians) and usually have frequencies of less than 1:1000 in the at-risk group. Although screening for some Mendelian disorders is now available (e.g., sickle cell-disease, Tay-Sachs disease, thalassemia) or is being developed (e.g., cystic fibrosis), couples found to be at risk for having children affected with most Mendelian disorders are usually discovered as a result of previously affected offspring or relatives. In addition, advanced paternal age (usually 50 years old or older) has been demonstrated to increase risk for Mendelian disorders characterized by gene mutations (*new mutations*) associated with autosomal dominant conditions such as Marfan's syndrome and achondroplasia. Counseling thus plays a critical role in determining risk for a couple having a child with a specific Mendelian disorder. Information that better defines a couple's risk for affected offspring includes family history — specifically in regard to Mendelian disorders or similar conditions — and the race, religion, or national origin of relatives. This information helps reassess risk and permits couples to further delineate their risk or, in appropriate situations, to undergo invasive prenatal testing.

Prenatal detection of many Mendelian disorders is now possible as result of recent advances in molecular biology. DNA base (adenine, guanine, cytosine, and thymine) sequences of specific lengths that are associated with, but not necessarily included within, a gene locus are called restriction fragment length polymorphisms (RFLPs). RFLPs are formed by the cleavage of the genome by restriction enzymes that cut the genome at known specific sequences. RFLPs are not genes but rather are sequences physically close to the actual genes; the number and constitution of RFLPs differ among individuals. The association of certain RFLPs with specific Mendelian disorders has permitted us to prenatally diagnose Mendelian disorders, albeit using a nonabsolute mathematical algorithm determining the *linkage*, or proximity, of a specific RFLP to a specific gene. The sensitivity of RFLP analysis depends on the proximity of the RFLP to the gene, i.e., the closer the RFLP to the gene in question, the more sensitive the analysis. It is, therefore, important to recognize the presence of a RFLP does not always indicate presence of a mutant gene, and conversely, absence of the same does not always indicate a disease-free state. More recently, direct detection of specific gene mutations, detection of abnormal proteins associated with specific diseases, and gene sequencing have permitted us to directly diagnose certain Mendelian disorders (e.g., sickle-cell disease) without the inherent inaccuracies of RFLP analysis.

Despite advances in molecular biology that have identified an increasing number of RFLPs, actual mutations, and normal and *wild-type* genes, certain disorders elude characterization by classical Mendelian paradigms. One such advancement is polymerase chain reaction (PCR). This technique permits the identification, delineation, and amplification of small DNA sequences. Using PCR, a new group of genetic disorders has recently been described; namely, disorders resulting from a markedly increased number of specific trinucleotide repeats within a given gene. Fragile X syndrome and Huntington disease are two such disorders. Fragile X syndrome, a relatively common cause of developmental delay in males, is caused by inactivation of the FMR1 gene by an increase in the numbers of CGG (cytosine-guanine-guanine) repeats within the gene. On the other hand, Huntington disease is caused by gene activation, resulting from an increased number of CAG (cytosine-adenine-guanine) repeats within the Huntington disease gene located on chromosome 4. Our increasing experience with sequencing the human genome will no doubt delineate new mechanisms of gene function and novel modes of heritability.

Irrespective of the specific DNA analytic method used, all DNA tests require recovery of DNA; this is accomplished by obtaining nucleated cells. For DNA analysis of newborns, children,

and adults, nucleated cells are easily recoverable from peripheral blood samples. However, prenatal DNA analyses require fetal nucleated cells; obtaining fetal cells is currently performed by chorionic villus sampling (CVS), amniocentesis, or percutaneous umbilical blood sampling (PUBS). As sequences of more genes are delineated, diagnosis of Mendelian disorders heretofore undetectable will be possible.

Polygenic/Multifactorial Disorders

Certain relatively common disorders result in a 2 to 5% recurrence risk if first-degree relatives (parents, siblings, and/or children) are affected. Such recurrence risks suggest a polygenic/multifactorial etiology in which undetermined genes and environmental stimuli are involved in disease expression. Many of these disorders are manifest by anatomical abnormalities. Some examples include cardiac anomalies, such as ventricular and atrial septal defects and hypoplastic left heart syndrome; gastrointestinal anomalies, including omphalocele, small bowel atresia, and diaphragmatic hernia; and urologic anomalies, including renal agenesis and ureteropelvic junction obstruction.

A group of polygenic/multifactorial disorders frequently encountered by the obstetrician-gynecologist is neural tube defects, comprised of cranial (anencephaly and encephalocele) and spinal (spina bifida) fusion abnormalities that occur relatively frequently in the United Kingdom and United States. Neural tube defects occur in approximately 1 in 1500 births in the United States; however, in certain regions of the country, neural tube defects occur more frequently (1 in 750 live births), and in some parts of the UK, the rate may be as high as 1 in 300 live births. Fetal neural tube defects are prenatally diagnosed by ultrasonography and α-fetoprotein and acetylcholinesterase assays of amniotic fluid obtained by amniocentesis. However, approximately 85% of newborns with neural tube defects are born to women with no family or medication history that would have indicated their being at increased risk, which would have resulted in their being offered amniocentesis.

Fortunately, a maternal blood test is now available to screen low-risk women for fetal neural tube defects. MSAFP screening measures the maternal serum level of α-fetoprotein, a fetal protein markedly elevated in the amniotic fluid and maternal serum in most women carrying fetuses with open neural tube defects. However, as with most screening tests, many women found to have elevated

MSAFP levels are not carrying an affected fetus. Accordingly, physicians and health care professionals who provide MSAFP screening must inform their patients of possible false-positive and false-negative results as well as availability of further diagnostic testing if screening results are abnormal.

Invasive Prenatal Diagnostic Procedures

Amniocentesis has been used for prenatal diagnosis for almost 20 years. The procedure involves removing, usually under concurrent ultrasonographic guidance, 20 to 40 mL of amniotic fluid. Traditionally, amniocentesis is performed between 15 and 20 weeks gestation. Cytogenetic and DNA analyses of amniotic fluid specimens require culture of amniotic fluid cells, as most cells obtained from amniocentesis are not in metaphase and the number of viable cells is relatively small. Direct analysis of the amniotic fluid supernatant (amniotic fluid liquor) is possible for α-fetoprotein and acetylcholinesterase assays; such analyses permit detection of fetal neural tube defects and other fetal structural defects (e.g., omphalocele and gastroschisis). In addition, some centers have begun to perform amniocentesis before 15 weeks gestation; however, the safety and accuracy of early amniocentesis are still undetermined.

Chorionic villus sampling was developed to provide early prenatal diagnosis. CVS is usually done between 9 and 12 weeks gestation and is performed by transcervical or transabdominal aspiration of chorionic villi (immature placenta) under concurrent ultrasonographic guidance. Recent multicenter trials have demonstrated CVS to have similar safety and accuracy to that of traditional (i.e., performed at or after 15 weeks gestation) amniocentesis. A benefit of CVS is direct, and therefore rapid, cytogenetic and DNA analyses, because cytotrophoblasts obtained from first-trimester placentas are more likely to be in metaphase than amniotic fluid cells. However, disorders that require analysis of amniotic fluid liquor, such as neural tube defects, are not amenable to prenatal diagnosis by CVS. Concern regarding a possible association of CVS with terminal fetal limb defects is currently being addressed. However, data from a World Health Organization (WHO) study reviewing more than 100,000 procedures indicate no significant increased risk of fetal limb defects if CVS is performed by experienced personnel after 9 weeks of gestation.

Percutaneous umbilical blood sampling is usually performed after 20 weeks of gestation and is used to obtain fetal blood for blood component analyses (e.g., hematocrit, Rh status, and platelet count) as well as cytogenetic and DNA analyses. One major benefit of PUBS is the ability to obtain rapid (in 18 to 24 hr) fetal karyotypes. However, the safety of PUBS remains undetermined; accordingly, PUBS should not be used when amniocentesis or CVS can obtain similar diagnostic results in a timely fashion.

Other prenatal diagnostic procedures include fetal skin sampling, fetal tissue (muscle, liver) biopsy, and fetoscopy. These procedures are used only for the diagnosis of rare disorders not amenable to diagnosis by less invasive methods.

Teratogenesis

Teratogenesis is the development of fetal defects as a result of maternal exposure to specific compounds (agents) in the environment. Potential teratogenetic agents range from viruses and bacteria to heavy metals and organic compounds. Some agents are obviously teratogenetic (e.g., isotretinoin), whereas other agents are not as consistent in their embryotoxic affect. Determination of teratogenicity of a specific agent is frequently difficult, and counseling women exposed to a particular agent is invariably incomplete. Many agents will be teratogenetic in some species but not in others, e.g., cortisol ingestion increases the risk of cleft palate in mice but not in humans. In addition, some agents may be teratogenetic only at certain doses, at certain stages of embryonic or fetal development, in combination with other specific agents, or in specific groups or populations more susceptible to the agent's embryotoxic effects than other groups or populations. Despite the inherent difficulty in arriving at an accurate risk assessment, a thorough review of maternal drug ingestion and environmental toxin exposure is essential to estimate a woman's risk for fetal malformation and should be a part of the initial antenatal assessment, along with family and medical-surgical history.

Future Trends

The ultimate prenatal diagnostic test would have high sensitivity and specificity but would not increase maternal or fetal morbidity and mortality. To this end, several centers are currently attempting to identify and isolate fetal cells in maternal circulation. If fetal cells can be isolated from maternal blood, and if these cells can be analyzed for cytogenetic and Mendelian disorders, a noninvasive method for prenatal screening — and possibly diagnosis — would be possible. Even if fetal cells can be consistently isolated from maternal blood, the clinical application of this technology is years away; however, initial results are promising.

Ethics

Our increasing ability to detect fetal abnormalities by ultrasonography and invasive prenatal diagnostic techniques has permitted couples to make pregnancy management decisions in cases in which fetal abnormalities are detected. However, our ability to detect fetal sex and other nonlethal characteristics creates a great ethical dilemma: To what extent should prenatal diagnostic techniques be used to prenatally identify fetal characteristics, and which characteristics, traits, or disorders are appropriate for prenatal diagnosis. Accordingly, new applications of current prenatal diagnostic techniques and development of new prenatal diagnostic modalities should be undertaken only with due consideration of the ethical, moral, and social ramifications of such new applications and/or technologies.

CASE STUDIES

Case 3A

A 24-year-old G1 P0, accompanied by her 27-year-old husband, presents with a history of 8 weeks of amenorrhea and the onset, earlier in the day, of cramping and bleeding. Clinical examination reveals an incomplete abortion and a suction and curettage is performed without incident. At the parents' request, the tissue is sent for genetic evaluation. She is Rh+ and in good health. Each has a negative family history of congenital anomalies and inherited disease and negative personal medical histories. Her physical examination is entirely normal.

On her first office visit 1 week after the miscarriage, her course has been unremarkable, her physical examination is normal, and she feels well, although depressed. The couple questions what the significance of the miscarriage will be for future pregnancies.

Questions Case 3A

Your answer will include which of the following:

A. The likelihood of the next or subsequent pregnancies carrying to term is less than 35%
B. The likelihood of this pregnancy demonstrating a genetic disorder is less than 5%
C. The likelihood of their being able to conceive is reduced by 67% compared with couples who have had no miscarriage
D. All of the above
E. None of the above

Answer: E

Absent identified risk factors, the chances of conceiving and carrying the next pregnancy to term are not reduced. Provided the tissue obtained at suction and curettage is viable enough to permit culturing, the chances of a genetic anomalies are about 50%.

Three weeks later a genetic report is received indicating trisomy 16. You inform the patient and her husband of this information and suggest

A. They consider adoption
B. They consider sterilization of one or both partners and adoption
C. The continue with their plans to have another pregnancy in about six months
D. All of the above
E. None of the above

Answer: C

Trisomy 16 is associated with lethal outcomes in the first trimester. Your previous advice about future pregnancy remains valid.

chapter 4

MATERNAL-FETAL PHYSIOLOGY

There are many normal physiologic changes in pregnancy. Some mimic the signs, symptoms, or laboratory findings of disease in the nonpregnant patient yet are normal in pregnancy. Therefore, knowledge of normal maternal physiology will help avoid unnecessary diagnostic or therapeutic interventions.

MATERNAL PHYSIOLOGY

Gastrointestinal Changes (Table 4.1)

One of the earliest symptoms of pregnancy is *nausea* and *vomiting*, or "morning sickness." Morning sickness typically begins between 4 and 8 weeks of gestational age and abates by the middle of the second trimester, usually by 14 to 16 weeks. Although the exact etiology of this nausea is unknown, it appears related to elevated levels of progesterone, human chorionic gonadotropin (hCG), and relaxation of the smooth muscle of the stomach. There are usually no significant nutritional deficits or weight loss associated with this distressing but transient symptom complex. Treatment consists primarily of reassurance, frequent small meals, and inclusion of bland foods as well as avoidance of those foods found to exacerbate the nausea and vomiting.

If the symptoms persist beyond the middle of the second trimester or if there is an associated weight loss, ketonemia, and electrolyte imbalance at any time, the diagnosis of *hyperemesis gravidarum* should be considered. Patients with this severe variety of nausea and vomiting in pregnancy must be hospitalized to receive parenteral fluid and electrolyte replacement. Environmental stressors and/or other psychological underpinning are common in these patients, and evaluation should attempt to assess these factors and reduce them, if possible.

Despite the gastrointestinal upset seen in early pregnancy, many patients report *dietary cravings* during pregnancy. Some may be the result of the patient's perception that a particular food may help with nausea and heartburn. *Pica* is an especially intense craving for such things as ice, laundry starch, or clay. Other patients develop dietary aversions during pregnancy. *Ptyalism* is perceived by the patient to be the excessive production of saliva but probably represents the inability of a nauseated patient to swallow the normal amounts of saliva that are produced.

In general, there is decreased gastrointestinal motility during pregnancy because of increasing levels of progesterone. As a result, gastric emptying time is prolonged and there is decreased esophageal tone and incompetence of the esophageal-stomach sphincter, leading to gastric reflux and heartburn, common complaints in pregnancy.

Gallbladder function is also delayed in pregnancy, with the subsequent cholestasis resulting in an increased tendency to form gallstones. Elevated liver enzymes and lowered serum protein levels are seen with resultant signs of spider angioma and palmar erythema, which are commonly found in association with liver disease. Alkaline phosphatase may be elevated as much as twofold during pregnancy. Serum cholesterol levels are increased during pregnancy while serum albumin decreases.

Anatomic changes of the GI system associated with pregnancy include hyperemia and softening of the gums. A highly vascular swelling may occur, the *epulis of pregnancy*. This typically regresses after pregnancy. *Hemorrhoids* are common in pregnancy and are caused by both constipation and elevated venous pressures. The treatment for hemorrhoids during pregnancy is generally reassurance and topical medication for symptomatic relief; surgery is reserved for intractable cases.

Table 4.1.
Key Gastrointestinal Changes in Pregnancy

Appetite	Usually increases, sometimes with unusual cravings (pica)
Gastric reflux	Results from cardiac sphincter relaxation and anatomic displacement
Gastric motility	Decreases
Intestinal transit time	Slower
Liver	Does not change functionally
Gallbladder	Dilates
Bile composition	Does not change

Pulmonary Changes

Pregnancy-related changes of the respiratory systems are the result of both anatomic and functional changes (Table 4.2). Mucosal hyperemia results in marked nasal stuffiness and an increased amount of nasal secretions. Patients often complain of allergy-like symptoms or chronic colds. Anatomically, there are also pregnancy-induced accommodations for the enlarging uterus. The subcostal angle increases from approximately 68 to 103°, the chest circumference increases up to 7 cm and the chest diameter increases 1 to 2 cm. There is increased diaphragmatic excursion and the diaphragm is elevated approximately 4 cm.

Pulmonary functions are altered in pregnancy. There is a 30 to 40% increase in tidal volume. Inspiratory capacity increases approximately 5%, with respiratory rate, vital capacity, and inspiratory reserve remaining the same as in the nonpregnant state. The functional residual capacity, expiratory volume, and residual volume are all decreased by approximately 20%. The total lung capacity is also decreased by 5% with a resulting increase in minute ventilation of 30 to 40%. Arterial blood gases reflect this change in pulmonary function in the following ways: oxygen (P_{O_2}) is increased, carbon dioxide (P_{CO_2}) is decreased, and serum bicarbonate is reduced. In summary, there is a mild respiratory alkalosis, with the patient being aware of dyspnea, hyperventilation, and a relative decrease in exercise tolerance.

Cardiovascular Changes

The dramatic changes in the maternal cardiovascular system during pregnancy improve oxygenation and flow of nutrition to the fetus (Table 4.3).

Cardiac output increases up to 50% as a result of an increase in both heart rate and stroke volume. Particularly late in pregnancy, however, cardiac output may be decreased, depending on maternal position. In the supine position, the inferior vena cava is compressed by the enlarged uterus, resulting in decreased venous return to the heart with decreased cardiac output. Although most women do not become overtly hypotensive when lying supine, some may have symptoms that include dizziness, light-headedness, and syncope. This is often termed the *inferior vena cava syndrome*.

Because of the smooth muscle relaxing effect of increased levels of progesterone during pregnancy, *peripheral vascular resistance* is decreased. There is a decrease in arterial blood pressure during the first

Table 4.2.
Key Pulmonary Changes in Pregnancy

Increases	Does Not Change	Decreases
Oxygen requirement	Arterial pH	Carbon dioxide pressure
Oxygen pressure		Expiratory reserve volume
Tidal volume		Residual volume
Inspiratory capacity		Total lung capacity
Vital capacity		P_{CO_2}
Minute volume		Serum bicarbonate
P_{O_2}		

Table 4.3.
Key Cardiovascular Changes in Pregnancy

Increases	Decreases
Cardiac output	Systemic vascular resistance
Stroke volume	Pulmonary vascular resistance
Heart rate	Colloid osmotic pressure
Left ventricular stroke work index	
Mean arterial pressure (slight)	
Blood flow Uterus Kidney Breasts Skin Brain	

Table 4.4.
Key Hematologic and Biochemical Changes in Pregnancy

Increases	Does Not Change	Decreases
Plasma volume		Hemoglobin concentration
Total erythrocyte volume		Hematocrit
Mean cell volume		
Total iron-binding capacity		Serum iron
Erythrocyte sedimentation rate		
Alkaline phosphatase	Amylase	Total protein
	Lactic acid dehydrogenase (LDH)	Albumin
	Glutamic oxaloacetic transaminase (GOT)	Osmolality
	Glutamic pyruvic transaminase (GPT)	

24 weeks of pregnancy with a gradual rise returning to nonpregnant levels by term. Blood pressures higher than the nonpregnant values for a particular patient should be considered abnormal.

Because the cardiovascular system is in a hyperdynamic state, normal physical findings on *cardiovascular examination* during pregnancy include an increased second heart sound split with inspiration, distended neck veins, and low-grade systolic ejection murmurs. Most normal pregnant women will have an S_3 gallop, or third heart sound, after midpregnancy. Systolic ejection murmurs are believed to be caused by a normal increased blood flow across the aortic and pulmonic valves. Diastolic murmurs should not be considered normal findings in pregnancy.

Anatomically, the heart is displaced upward and to the left. Because the diaphragms are elevated and because the heart is in a more horizontal position, chest x-rays might appear to demonstrate cardiomegaly when no such abnormality exists.

During the course of *labor*, cardiac output increases approximately 40% above that in late pregnancy. Much of this is a result of pain and apprehension, as these findings are significantly reduced when a patient has an epidural anesthetic administered. Mean arterial blood pressure rises approximately 10 mm Hg during each contraction, unless adequate analgesia is provided. Immediately postpartum, because the obstruction to venous return is released and because extracellular fluid is quickly mobilized, cardiac output increases 10 to 20%.

Hematologic Changes

Maternal *plasma volume* begins to increase as early as the 6th week of pregnancy and reaches maxi-

mum at approximately 30 to 34 weeks, after which it is stable. The mean increase in plasma volume is approximately 50%; there is a greater increase in patients with multiple gestation. Similarly, larger babies are associated with a greater increase of maternal plasma volume, whereas a pregnancy complicated by intrauterine growth retardation is often associated with a less-than-normal increase in blood volume.

Red cell mass begins to increase later in pregnancy and increases to a lesser degree than does plasma volume. As a result, there is a "physiologic" anemia caused by dilution of approximately 15% compared with nonpregnancy levels. Whereas erythrocyte volume increases by approximately 18% without iron supplementation, it can increase up to 30% when iron supplements are used. After 30 to 34 weeks, the hematocrit (Hct) may increase somewhat, as erythrocyte volume continues to increase while plasma volume is stable (Table 4.4).

White blood cell (WBC) counts also rise as pregnancy advances. This progressive increase may reach 20,000/mL during the late third trimester. During labor, the WBC count may further rise to 30,000/mL, with a return to nonpregnant levels during the puerperium. The increase in the WBC count is caused primarily by an increased number of granulocytes. Platelet counts during pregnancy may decline slightly but remain within the normal range of those of nonpregnant patients.

Pregnancy is considered a hypercoaguable state with an increased risk of *venous thromboembolism* both during pregnancy and the puerperium. The risk of thromboembolism is approximately 2 times normal during pregnancy and rises to 5.5 times nor-

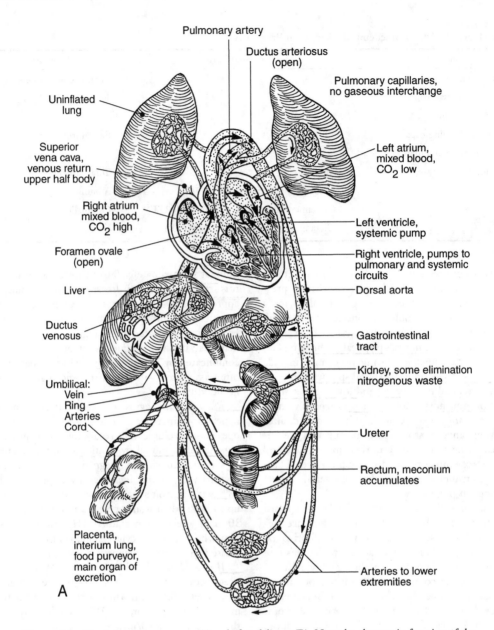

Figure 4.1. Fetal circulation at term (**A**) and after delivery (**B**). Note the changes in function of the ductus venosus, foramen ovale, and ductus arteriosus in the transition from intrauterine to extrauterine existence. *Stippling*, deoxygenated blood; *no stippling*, oxygenated blood.

mal during the puerperium. Fibrinogen (factor I) increases to a level of 400 to 500 mg/dL. There is an increase in fibrin split products and in factors VII, VIII, IX, and X. Prothrombin (factor II) and factors V and XII remain unchanged during pregnancy. *Bleeding time* and *clotting time* do not change during a normal pregnancy.

The normal pregnant patient requires a total of 1000 mg of additional iron: 500 mg are used to increase maternal red cell mass, 300 mg are transported to the fetus, and the additional 200 mg are utilized to compensate for normal iron loss. Iron use in pregnancy is intended to prevent iron deficiency in the mother. It is not intended either to

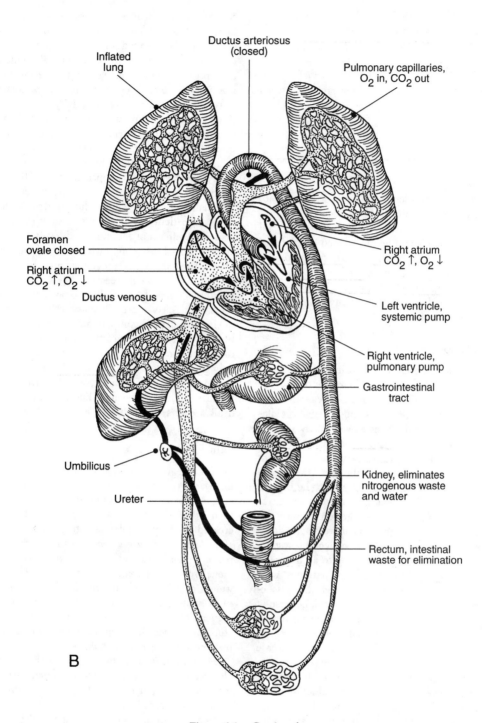

Figure 4.1. Continued.

Table 4.5.
Key Renal Changes in Pregnancy

Increases	Does Not Change
Renal plasma flow	Urinary output
Glomerular filtration rate	24-hr protein excretion
Renin	
Angiotensin I and II	
Renin substrate	

prevent iron deficiency in the fetus or to maintain maternal hemoglobin (Hb) concentration. Because iron is actively transported to the fetus, fetal hemoglobin levels will be maintained despite maternal anemia. To supply her needs, 60 mg of elemental iron is recommended daily for the nonanemic patient. This is provided in 300 mg of ferrous sulfate. Patients who are anemic should receive twice this dose.

Renal Changes

Kidneys enlarge about 1 cm during pregnancy as measured on intravenous pyelography or ultrasonography. This is the result of an increase in interstitial volume as well as distended renal vasculature. Both the renal pelves as well as the ureters are dilated during pregnancy, because of the relaxing effect of progesterone. Typically, the right ureter is more dilated than the left. Mechanical compression of the ureters — by both the ovarian venous plexus and the enlarging uterus — contributes to dilation. Because progesterone also decreases *bladder* tone, there is increased residual volume and, with the dilated collecting system, urinary stasis results, predisposing to an increased incidence of pyelonephritis in patients with asymptomatic bacteriuria. There is also loss of urinary control as pregnancy advances, because of the enlarging uterus. Bladder capacity decreases, resulting in urinary frequency (Table 4.5).

Renal plasma flow (RPF) begins to increase early in the first trimester and increases to as much as 75% over nonpregnant levels at term. Similarly, *glomerular filtration rate* (GFR) increases to 50% over the nonpregnant state. The *creatinine clearance* is markedly increased in pregnancy, with 150 to 200 mL/min being considered normal. Serum levels of creatinine, uric acid, and blood urea nitrogen decrease in normal pregnancy. *Plasma osmolality* is decreased, primarily because of reduc-

tion in the serum *sodium concentration*. The tendency to lose sodium, as a result of the increased GFR, and the elevated levels of progesterone are compensated for by an increase in renal tubule reabsorption of sodium as well as by the increased levels of aldosterone, estrogen, and desoxycorticosterone. The plasma renin activity is up to 10 times that of the nonpregnant state. Similarly, renin substrate (angiotensinogen) is increased approximately fivefold. Angiotensin levels are also increased approximately fivefold. During pregnancy, the body retains approximately 1000 mEq of sodium in the fetus, placenta, and maternal intravascular and extracellular fluid spaces. Normal pregnant patients are relatively resistant to the hypertensive effects of the increased levels of renin-angiotensin-aldosterone, whereas patients with hypertensive disease of pregnancy are not.

Because of the increase in GFR, there is a greatly increased load of glucose presented to the renal tubules. As a result, *glucose excretion* increases in virtually all pregnant patients. Therefore, quantitative urine glucose measurements are not clinically useful in managing patients with diabetes, as they do not reflect blood glucose levels.

There is no significant increase in *protein loss* in the urine during pregnancy. There are increases in urinary excretion of vitamin B_{12} and folate.

Skin Changes

During pregnancy, *vascular spiders* (spider angiomata) are most common on the upper torso, face, and arms. *Palmar erythema* occurs in more than 50% of patients. Both are caused by increased levels of circulating estrogen and regress after delivery. *Striae gravidarum* can be either purple or pink initially and appear on the lower abdomen, breasts, and thighs. They are not related to weight gain but solely the result of the stretching of normal skin. There is no effective therapy to prevent these "stretch marks," nor can they be eliminated once they appear. They do eventually become white or silvery in color.

Hyperpigmentation is believed to be the result of elevated levels of estrogen and melanocyte-stimulating hormone. It commonly affects the umbilicus and perineum, although it may affect any skin surface. The lower abdomen linea alba darkens to become the linea nigra. The "mask of pregnancy," or *chloasma* (melasma), is also common. *Skin nevi* can increase in size and pigmentation but resolve after pregnancy. Removal of rapidly changing nevi is recommended during pregnancy. *Eccrine sweating* and *sebum production* are increased during normal pregnancy, with many patients complaining of *acne*. Melasma may never disappear completely.

Hair growth during pregnancy is maintained. The anagen (growth) phase normally lasts up to 6 years. Fewer follicles are in the telogen (resting) phase. Late in pregnancy, the number of hairs in telogen is approximately one-half of the normal 20%, so that postpartum, the number of hairs entering telogen increases, thus there is significant hair loss 2 to 4 months after pregnancy. Hair growth typically returns to normal 6 to 12 months after delivery.

Breast Changes

Blood flow increases to the breast as the breasts develop to support lactation. Some patients may complain of breast tenderness and a tingling sensation. Estrogen stimulation also results in ductal growth, with alveolar hypertrophy being a result of progesterone stimulation. Montgomery's follicles, the small elevations surrounding the areolae, enlarge and become more prominent during pregnancy. During the latter portion of pregnancy, a thick yellow fluid can be expressed from the nipples. This *colostrum* is more common in parous women. Ultimately, lactation will depend on synergistic actions of estrogen, progesterone, prolactin, human placental lactogen, cortisol, and insulin.

Musculoskeletal Changes

As pregnancy progresses, a compensatory lumbar lordosis is apparent. As a result, virtually all women complain of low back pain. Beginning early in pregnancy, the effects of relaxin and progesterone result in a relative laxity of the ligaments. The pubic symphysis separates at approximately 28 to 30 weeks. Patients often complain of an unsteady gait and may fall more commonly during pregnancy than during the nonpregnant state, as a result of both these changes and an altered center of gravity.

To provide for adequate calcium supplies to the fetal skeleton, mobilization of calcium stores occurs. Maternal serum ionized calcium is unchanged from the nonpregnant state, but maternal total serum calcium decreases. There is a significant increase in maternal parathyroid hormone, which acts to maintain serum calcium levels by increasing absorption from the intestine and de-

creasing the loss of calcium through the kidney. The skeleton is well maintained, despite these elevated levels of parathyroid hormones. This may be because of the effect of calcitonin. Although the rate of bone turnover increases, there is no loss of bone density during a normal pregnancy.

Ophthalmic Changes

The most common visual complaint of pregnant women is blurred vision. This is primarily caused by swelling of the lens and resolves after pregnancy. Changes in corrective lens prescriptions should, therefore, not be encouraged during pregnancy.

Reproductive Tract and Abdominal Wall Changes

The effects of pregnancy on the *vulva* are similar to the effects on other skin. Because of an increase in vascularity, *vulvar varicosities* are very common. These usually regress after delivery. An increase in vaginal transudation as well as stimulation of the vaginal mucosa result in a thick profuse *vaginal discharge*. The epithelium of the endocervix everts onto the ectocervix, with an associated mucus plug being produced. The *uterus* undergoes an enormous increase in weight from the 70-g nonpregnant size to approximately 1100 g at term, primarily through hypertrophy of existing myometrial cells. Similarly, the uterine cavity, which in the nongravid state has a volume of less than 10 mL, increases up to as much as 5 liters. Cardiac output to the uterus is less than 2% in the nongravid state but increases to 15 to 20% at term, i.e., 500 to 700 mL/min. There is also increasing pressure caused by intraabdominal growth of the uterus, resulting in an exacerbation of *hernia defects*, most commonly seen at the umbilicus and in the abdominal wall (diastasis recti).

Endocrinologic Changes

Carbohydrate Metabolism

Several hormones secreted by the placenta are responsible for the *diabetogenic effect of pregnancy*. Human placental lactogen (HPL) increases the resistance of peripheral tissues and liver to the effects of insulin. Because HPL is secreted in proportion to placental mass, resistance to insulin increases as pregnancy progresses. Progesterone and estrogen also contribute to insulin resistance during pregnancy, and insulin is broken down by

Table 4.6.
Key Endrocine Changes in Pregnancy

Gland/Organ	Increases	Does Not Change	Decreases
Thyroid	Total T$_4$ Total T$_3$ TBG	 Free T$_3$ Free T$_4$	
Adrenal	CBG Cortisol Androstenedione DOC Aldosterone		 DHEAS
Pituitary	Prolactin Adrenocorticotropic hormone (ACTH)	TSH Oxytocin	Follicle-stimulating hormone (FSH)
Ovaries and placenta	Progesterone 17-hydroxyprogesterone Estradiol Estriol HPL hCG (peak increase at 8–10 weeks gestation)		

the placental production of insulinase. *Pregnancy is characterized by hyperglycemia, hyperinsulinemia, hypertriglyceridemia, and reduced tissue response to insulin.* The typical fasting glucose level is lower than that in the nonpregnant state, as the fetoplacental unit serves as a constant drain on maternal glucose levels. As a result, in response to maternal starvation, the patient demonstrates exaggerated hypoglycemia and hypoinsulinemia. Delivery of glucose from the mother to the fetus occurs by facilitated diffusion, and as a result, fetal glucose levels depend on maternal levels. The fetus does not, however, depend on the mother for insulin, as fetal insulin is apparent at 9 to 11 weeks of gestation (Table 4.6).

The major change in blood glucose levels in the pregnant woman is a lower fasting level with a prolonged elevation of glucose values after a glucose load is administered. The lower fasting levels result from the constant diffusion to the fetus, where glucose is used as the primary energy source. In addition, there is hypertrophy of the β cells of the maternal pancreas, which secrete two to three times the nonpregnant level of insulin late in pregnancy.

Thyroid Function

Several changes in the pregnant patient relate to thyroid function, with the net effect being that the normal pregnant woman is euthyroid. Estrogen induces an increased level of thyroxine-binding globulin (TBG), resulting in an increase in total thyroxine (T$_4$) and total 3,5,3'-triiodothyronine (T$_3$) beginning early in pregnancy. Free T$_4$ and free T$_3$, the active hormones, are unchanged from the normal range for nonpregnant patients (Table 4.6).

Adrenal Function

During pregnancy, there is an estrogen-induced increase in the plasma concentration of corticosteroid-binding globulin (CBG), resulting in elevated levels of plasma cortisol. Like thyroid hormone, only the portion of cortisol that is unbound is metabolically active. Unlike thyroid hormone, however, the concentration of free plasma cortisol is elevated, progressively increasing from the first trimester until term. There is also increased plasma concentration of deoxycorticosterone (DOC), whereas dehydroepiandrosterone sulfate (DHEAS) is decreased (Table 4.6).

FETAL PHYSIOLOGY

Circulation (Fig. 4.1)

The umbilical vein, which carries oxygenated blood (80% saturated) from the placenta, enters the portal system of the fetus and gives off branches to the left lobe of the liver. It then becomes the origin of the ductus venosus. Another branch joins blood flow from the portal vein that is flowing to the right lobe of the liver. Fifty percent of the umbilical blood supply goes through the ductus venosus. The blood flow from the left hepatic vein is mixed with the blood in the inferior vena cava and is directed toward the foramen ovale. As a result, the well-oxygenated umbilical vein blood enters the left ventricle and supplies the carotid arteries. The relatively less oxygenated blood in the right hepatic vein, having entered the inferior vena cava, flows through the tricuspid valve into the right ventricle. Blood from the superior vena cava also preferentially flows through the tricuspid valve to the right ventricle. Blood from the pulmonary artery primarily flows through the ductus arteriosus into the aorta. Less than 10% of cardiac output goes to the lung, with blood flow through the foramen ovale accounting for approximately one-third of the cardiac output.

The proximal aorta supplies highly saturated blood (65% saturated) to the brain and upper body. It is joined in its descending portion by the ductus arteriosus. The descending aorta then supplies blood to the lower portion of the fetal body, with a major portion of this blood being delivered to the umbilical arteries, which carry deoxygenated blood to the placenta.

Placenta

Glucose is the primary substrate for placental metabolism. It is estimated that as much as 70% of the glucose transferred from the mother is used by the placenta. The glucose that crosses the placenta does so by facilitated diffusion. Other solutes that are transferred from the mother to the fetus depend on the concentration gradient as well as on their degree of ionization, size, and lipid solubility. In regard to respiratory gases, fetal uptake of O_2 and excretion of CO_2 depend on the maternal and fetal blood-carrying capacities for these gases and on uterine and umbilical blood flows. There is active transport of amino acids, resulting in levels that are higher in the fetus than in the mother. Free fatty acids have very limited placental transfer, with resultant fetal levels that are lower than in the mother.

Hemoglobin and Oxygenation

Although the partial pressure of oxygen in fetal arterial blood is only 20 to 25 mm Hg, the fetus is adequately oxygenated because of its higher cardiac output in organ blood flow. In addition, the higher hemoglobin concentration in the fetus than in the adult and the higher oxygen saturation are responsible for the oxygenation of the fetus. At any given oxygen tension, the fetal blood has a higher oxygen saturation than does adult blood.

Kidney

The fetal kidney forms urine and, as a result, amniotic fluid. Fetal urine is hypotonic compared with that of a newborn.

Liver

The fetal liver is not fully functional even at term. Bilirubin is primarily eliminated through the placenta.

Thyroid Gland

The fetal thyroid gland develops without direct influence from the mother. The placenta does not transport thyroid-stimulating hormone (TSH), and only minimal amounts of T_3 and T_4 cross the placenta.

Gonads

The primordial germ cells migrate during the 8th week of gestation from the endoderm of the yolk sac to the genital ridge. At this point, the gonads are undifferentiated. Differentiation into the testes occurs 6 weeks after conception, if the embryo is 46,XY. This testicular differentiation appears to depend on the presence of the H-Y antigen. The Y chromosome is also necessary for testicular differentiation. If the Y chromosome is absent, however, an ovary develops from the undifferentiated gonad. Development of the fetal ovary begins at about 7 weeks. The development of other genital organs depends on the presence or absence of specific hormones and is independent of gonadal differentiation. If the fetal testes are present, testosterone and müllerian inhibitory factor (MIF) inhibit the development of female external genitalia. If these two hormones are not present, the female genitalia develop with regression of the wolffian ducts.

IMMUNOLOGY OF PREGNANCY

Although the maternal immune system is not altered in pregnancy, the antigenically dissimilar fetus is able to survive in the uterus without being rejected. This fetal allograft appears to be somehow protected in this privileged immunologic site.

The placenta serves as an effective interference between the maternal and fetal vascular compartments by keeping the fetus from direct contact with the maternal immune system. The placenta also produces estrogen, progesterone, hCG, and HPL, all of which may contribute to suppression of maternal immune responses on a local level. The placenta is, in addition, the site of origin for blocking antibodies and masking antibodies, which alter the immune response.

The mother's systemic immune system remains intact as evidenced by leukocyte count, B and T cell count and function, and immunoglobin levels. Because IgG is the only immunoglobin that can cross the placenta, maternal IgG comprises a major proportion of fetal immunoglobin both in utero and in the early neonatal period. It is in this fashion that passive immunity can be passed to the fetus.

Fetal lymphocyte production begins as early as 6 weeks of gestation. By 12 weeks of gestation, IgG, IgM, IgD, and IgE are present and are produced in progressively increasing amounts throughout pregnancy.

CASE STUDIES

Case 4A

A 28-year-old G3 P2002 who has lived until recently in Murfee, Arkansas, presents for prenatal care at 24 weeks of pregnancy. Her fundal height and gestational age correspond, her general physical examination is normal. Her first two pregnancies were normal except for an anemia. She and her husband have negative past medical and family histories, and they are attorneys and have recently joined a firm in your town.

Upon receipt of her prenatal laboratory information, you notice a hemogram showing a Hb of 7.2, a Hct of 27, and hypochromic microcytic erythrocytes on smear.

Questions Case 4A

What additional laboratory tests would you order:

A. Repeat complete blood count (CBC)
B. Reticulocyte count
C. Serum Fe/total iron-binding capacity (TIBC)
D. Erythrocyte sedimentation rate (ESR)
E. Rapid plasma reagent (RPR)

Answer: B, C

An iron-deficiency anemia is documented, with a low Fe and high TIBC.

Further questioning of the patient on her next visit should include specific questions about:

A. Family history of iron-deficiency anemia
B. Family history of bleeding disorders
C. Personal history of bleeding disorders
D. Dietary history
E. History of prescription medicines in the last 2 years

Answer: C

While a bleeding disorder is a possible cause of this anemia, there is no history of such. Diet may account for such an anemia, and indeed, upon further questioning, the patient admits to starch pica during each pregnancy.

Case 4B

A 32-year-old G1 P1001, whom you followed through a normal pregnancy and delivery of a healthy boy about 2 weeks earlier, presents with concern about her hair falling out. Upon questioning, you learn that relatively large amounts of hair are coming loose during her normal morning hair-brushing routine. She has made no changes in shampoo, cosmetics, or diet. She is concerned and afraid that she has cancer.

Question Case 4B

What are your next most appropriate actions?

A. Urgent referral to a dermatologist for evaluation and treatment
B. Urgent referral to a medical oncologist for evaluation and treatment
C. Cortisone ointment to be applied to the scalp daily after meals
D. Reassurance, explaining that some permanent hair loss is part of being a mother and that she will probably keep enough hair to avoid using a wig
E. All the above
F. None of the above

Answer: F

Some transitory hair loss in the 2nd to 4th postpartum week is normal, but it resolves without permanent loss.

chapter 5

ANTEPARTUM CARE

The purpose of antepartum care is to help achieve as good a maternal and infant outcome as possible. Complete obstetric care includes the correct diagnosis of pregnancy followed by an initial thorough assessment early in pregnancy; periodic examinations and screening tests as appropriate through the course of gestation; patient education addressing pregnancy care, labor and delivery, nutrition, exercise, and early infant care; and management of the patient during labor, delivery, and the postpartum period. Antepartum care ends with a final visit, generally 6 weeks following delivery.

Most pregnant women will deliver healthy infants without any prenatal care. Therefore, obstetric care is designed to promote good health throughout the course of normal pregnancy, while screening for and managing any complications that may develop. The American College of Obstetricians and Gynecologists (ACOG) has prepared a standardized antepartum care form (Figs. 5.1 and 5.2). It is suggested that the reader refer to these forms as the details of antepartum care are discussed. Specific conditions to which poor maternal and neonatal outcomes are often attributed include

1. Preterm labor;
2. Preterm or postterm delivery;
3. Perinatal infections;
4. Intrauterine growth retardation;
5. Hypertension;
6. Diabetes mellitus;
7. Birth defects.

Ideally, obstetric care should commence before pregnancy with a *preconception visit*, during which a thorough family and medical history for both parents and a physical examination of the prospective mother is done. Preexisting conditions that may affect conception and/or pregnancy are identified and appropriate management plans formulated with the goal of a "healthy" subsequent pregnancy.

Unfortunately, preconceptual counseling is not commonly employed; instead, most women seek care only after one or more periods have been missed and pregnancy has already begun. All too many pregnant women have only episodic care, which contributes to increased perinatal and maternal morbidity and mortality. Educating patients on the benefits of regular, early care and motivating them to seek it is one of the most important public health goals of our time. For these reasons, obstetric care should be designed (*a*) to provide easy access to care, (*b*) to promote patient involvement, (*c*) to provide a team approach to ongoing surveillance and education for the patient and her fetus, and (*d*) to establish protocols for screening for high-risk conditions, along with an organized plan to address any complications that may arise.

DIAGNOSIS OF PREGNANCY

The *diagnosis of pregnancy* should not be made based solely on the nonspecific symptoms and equivocal physical findings that are common in early pregnancy. A pregnancy test is used to make an accurate diagnosis. Once a positive pregnancy test is identified, the physician and patient must be aware of signs and symptoms of *spontaneous abortion, ectopic pregnancy,* and *trophoblastic disease,* which may complicate the course of what is otherwise expected to be a normal intrauterine pregnancy.

In a woman with regular menstrual cycles, a history of one or more missed periods, especially if associated with fatigue, nausea/vomiting, and breast tenderness, strongly suggests pregnancy. Urinary frequency caused by the enlarging uterus pressing on the bladder is another common finding.

On *physical examination,* softening and enlargement of the pregnant uterus become apparent 6 or more weeks after the last normal menstrual period. A *pelvic examination* in early pregnancy is one of the better ways to establish a due date (esti-

Patient Addressograph

ACOG ANTEPARTUM RECORD

DATE _____

NAME _____
      LAST   FIRST   MIDDLE

ID # _____ HOSPITAL OF DELIVERY _____

NEWBORNS PHYSICIAN _____ REFERRED BY _____

BIRTHDATE	AGE	RACE	MARITAL STATUS	ADDRESS:
MO DAY YR		W B O	S M W D SEP	
OCCUPATION			EDUCATION	ZIP: PHONE:
☐ HOMEMAKER			(LAST GRADE COMPLETED)	MEDICAID # / INSURANCE
☐ OUTSIDE WORK _____				
☐ STUDENT		Type of Work		

EMERGENCY CONTACT:		RELATIONSHIP:	PHONE:

TOTAL PREG	FULL TERM	PREMATURE	ABORTIONS INDUCED	ABORTIONS SPONTANEOUS	ECTOPICS	MULTIPLE BIRTHS	LIVING

PAST PREGNANCIES (LAST SIX)

DATE MO / YR	GA WEEKS	LENGTH OF LABOR	BIRTH WEIGHT	TYPE DELIVERY	ANES.	PLACE OF DELIVERY	PERINATAL MORTALITY YES / NO	TREATMENT PRETERM LABOR YES / NO	COMMENTS / COMPLICATIONS

PAST MEDICAL HISTORY

	O Neg + Pos.	DETAIL POSITIVE REMARKS INCLUDE DATE & TREATMENT			
DIABETES			RH SENSITIZED		
HYPERTENSION			TUBERCULOSIS		
HEART DISEASE			ASTHMA		
RHEUMATIC FEVER			ALLERGIES (DRUGS)		
MITRAL VALVE PROLAPSE			GYN SURGERY		
KIDNEY DISEASE / UTI			OPERATIONS / HOSPITALIZATIONS (YEAR & REASON)		
NERVOUS AND MENTAL			ANESTHETIC COMPLICATIONS		
EPILEPSY			HISTORY OF ABNORMAL PAP		
HEPATITIS / LIVER DISEASE			UTERINE ANOMALY		
VARICOSITIES / PHLEBITIS			INFERTILITY		
THYROID DYSFUNCTION			IN UTERO DES EXPOSURE		
MAJOR ACCIDENTS			STREET DRUGS		
HISTORY OF BLOOD TRANSFUSION			OTHER		
USE OF TOBACCO		# CIGS / DAY PRIOR TO PREG _____ # CIGS / DAY NOW _____ AGE ONSET SMOKING _____ YEARS	USE OF ALCOHOL		# DRINKS / WK PRIOR TO PREG _____ # DRINKS / WK NOW _____ AGE ONSET DRINKING _____ YEARS

INFECTION SCREENING	YES	NO	PATIENT OR PARTNER HAVE HISTORY OF GENITAL HERPES?		
HIGH RISK AIDS?			RASH OR VIRAL ILLNESS SINCE LAST MENSTRUAL PERIOD?		
HIGH RISK HEPATITIS B?			HISTORY OF STD, GC, CHLAMYDIA, HPV, SYPHILIS?		
LIVE WITH SOMEONE WITH TB OR EXPOSED TO TB?			OTHER?		

GENETICS SCREENING
INCLUDES PATIENT, BABY'S FATHER, OR ANYONE IN EITHER FAMILY WITH:

	YES	NO		YES	NO
1. PATIENT'S AGE ≥ 35 YEARS?			10. HUNTINGTON CHOREA?		
2. ITALIAN, GREEK, MEDITERRANEAN, OR ORIENTAL BACKGROUND (MCV < 80)?			11. MENTAL RETARDATION?		
3. NEURAL TUBE DEFECT (MENINGOMYELOCELE, OPEN SPINE, OR ANENCEPHALY)?			IF YES, WAS PERSON TESTED FOR FRAGILE X?		
4. DOWN SYNDROME (MONGOLISM)?			12. OTHER INHERITED GENETIC OR CHROMOSOMAL DISORDER?		
5. JEWISH (TAY SACH'S)?			13. PATIENT OR BABY'S FATHER HAD A CHILD WITH BIRTH DEFECT NOT LISTED ABOVE, ≥ 3 FIRST TRIMESTER SPONTANEOUS ABORTIONS, OR A STILLBIRTH?		
6. SICKLE CELL DISEASE OR TRAIT?					
7. HEMOPHILIA?			14. MEDICATIONS OR STREET DRUGS SINCE LAST MENSTRUAL PERIOD?		
8. MUSCULAR DYSTROPHY?			IF YES, AGENT(S)		
9. CYSTIC FIBROSIS?					

COMMENTS _____

PRESENT PREGNANCY

	O Neg + Pos.	DETAIL POSITIVE REMARKS INCLUDE DATE & TYPE RX.			
1. VAGINAL BLEEDING			5. HEADACHE		
2. VAGINAL DISCHARGE/ODOR			6. ABDOMINAL PAIN		
3. VOMITING			7. URINARY COMPLAINTS		
4. CONSTIPATION			8. FEBRILE EPISODE		
			9. OTHER		

COMMENTS _____

_____ INTERVIEWER'S SIGNATURE_____

INITIAL PHYSICAL EXAMINATION

DATE ___ / ___ / ___   PRE-PREGNANCY WEIGHT ___   HEIGHT ___   BP ___

1. HEENT	☐ NORMAL	☐ ABNORMAL	12. RECTUM	☐ NORMAL	☐ ABNORMAL	
2. FUNDI	☐ NORMAL	☐ ABNORMAL	13. VULVA	☐ NORMAL	☐ CONDYLOMA	☐ LESIONS
3. TEETH	☐ NORMAL	☐ ABNORMAL	14. VAGINA	☐ NORMAL	☐ INFLAMMATION	☐ DISCHARGE
4. THYROID	☐ NORMAL	☐ ABNORMAL	15. CERVIX	☐ NORMAL	☐ INFLAMMATION	☐ LESIONS
5. BREASTS	☐ NORMAL	☐ ABNORMAL	16. UTERUS	☐ NORMAL	☐ ABNORMAL	☐ FIBROIDS ___WEEKS
6. LUNGS	☐ NORMAL	☐ ABNORMAL	17. ADNEXA	☐ NORMAL	☐ MASS	
7. HEART	☐ NORMAL	☐ ABNORMAL	18. DIAGONAL CONJUGATE	☐ REACHED	☐ NO	___ CM
8. ABDOMEN	☐ NORMAL	☐ ABNORMAL	19. SPINES	☐ AVERAGE	☐ PROMINENT	☐ BLUNT
9. EXTREMITIES	☐ NORMAL	☐ ABNORMAL	20. SACRUM	☐ CONCAVE	☐ STRAIGHT	☐ ANTERIOR
10. SKIN	☐ NORMAL	☐ ABNORMAL	21. ARCH	☐ NORMAL	☐ WIDE	☐ NARROW
11. LYMPH NODES	☐ NORMAL	☐ ABNORMAL	22. PELVIC TYPE	GYNECOID	☐ YES	☐ NO

COMMENTS (Number and explain abnormals) _____

_____ EXAM BY: _____

Figure 5.1B. ACOG antepartum record, part 1, page 2: initial evaluation.

Patient Addressograph

ACOG ANTEPARTUM RECORD

DATE _____

NAME _____
LAST   FIRST   MIDDLE

ID # _____

PROBLEMS/PLANS (DRUG ALLERGY:)	MEDICATION LIST: Start date Stop date
1.	1.
2.	2.
3.	3.
4.	4.

EDD CONFIRMATION

INITIAL EDD:

LMP _____/_____/_____   = EDD _____/_____/_____
INITIAL EXAM _____/_____/_____ = _____ WKS. = EDD _____/_____/_____
ULTRASOUND _____/_____/_____ = _____ WKS. = EDD _____/_____/_____
INITIAL EDD _____/_____/_____   INITIALED BY _____

LMP □ DEFINITE   MENARCHE_____ (AGE ONSET)
     □ NORMAL AMOUNT/DURATION   MENSES MONTHLY □ YES □ NO
     □ APPROXIMATE (MONTH KNOWN)   FREQUENCY Q _____ DAYS
     □ UNKNOWN   PRIOR MENSES _____ DATE
         ON BCP'S AT CONCEPTION □ NO □ YES

HCG − _____/_____/_____   HCG + _____/_____/_____

18-20 WEEK EDD UPDATE:

QUICKENING _____/_____/_____ + 22 WKS. = _____/_____/_____
FUNDAL HT. AT UMBIL. _____/_____/_____ + 20 WKS. = _____/_____/_____
FHT W/FETOSCOPE _____/_____/_____ + 20 WKS. = _____/_____/_____
ULTRASOUND _____/_____/_____ = _____ WKS. = _____/_____/_____

FINAL EDD _____/_____/_____   INITIALED BY _____

32-34 WEEK EDD - UTERINE SIZE CONCORDANCE

± 4 OR MORE CMS. SUGGESTS THE NEED FOR ULTRASOUND EVALUATION

VISIT DATE (YEAR _____)											
WEEKS GEST. BEST EST.											
HT FUNDUS (CM.)											
PRESENTATION - VTX, BR, TRANSVERSE											
FHR PRESENT: F=FETOSCOPE O=ABSENT D=DOPTONE											
FETAL MOVEMENT: +=PRESENT D=DECREASED O=ABSENT											
PREMATURITY: SIGNS/SYMPTOMS: + PRESENT O ABSENT — VAGINAL BLEEDING											
MUCUS SHOW / DISCHARGE											
CRAMPS / CONTRACTIONS											
DYSURIA											
PELVIC PRESSURE											
CERVIX EXAM (DIL./EFF./STA.)											
BLOOD PRESSURE — INITIAL											
REPEAT											
EDEMA + PRESENT O ABSENT											
WEIGHT											
CUMULATIVE WEIGHT GAIN											
URINE: (GLUCOSE/ALBUMIN/KETONES)											
NEXT APPOINTMENT											
PROVIDER											
TEST REMINDERS	8-18 WEEKS CVS/AMNIO/MSAFP			24-28 WEEKS GLUCOSE SCREEN/RhIG							

Figure 5.2A. ACOG antepartum record, part 2, page 1: antepartum visits.

GUIDELINES: EDUCATION AND LABORATORY

INITIAL LABS	DATE	RESULT	REVIEWED	COMMENTS / ADDITIONAL LAB
BLOOD TYPE	/ /	A B AB O		
RH TYPE	/ /	+ / –		
ANTIBODY SCREEN	/ /	– / +		
HCT / HGB	/ /	_____ % _____ gm / dl		
PAP SMEAR	/ /	NORMAL / ABNORMAL / _____		
RUBELLA	/ /	– / +		
VDRL	/ /	– / +		
GC	/ /	– / +		
URINE CULTURE / SCREEN	/ /	– / +		
HB S AG	/ /	– / +		

8 - 18 WEEK LABS (WHEN INDICATED)	DATE	RESULT		
ULTRASOUND	/ /			
MSAFP	/ /	_____ MOM		
AMNIO / CVS	/ /	– / +		
KARYOTYPE	/ /	46, XX OR 46, XY / OTHER _____		
ALPHA-FETOPROTEIN	/ /	NORMAL _____ ABNORMAL _____		

24 - 28 WEEK LABS (WHEN INDICATED)	DATE	RESULT		
HCT / HGB	/ /	_____ % _____ gm / dl		
DIABETES SCREEN	/ /	1 HR. _____		
GTT (IF SCREEN ABNORMAL)	/ /	___ FBS ___ 1 HR. ___ 2 HR. ___ 3 HR.		
RH ANTIBODY SCREEN	/ /	– / +		
RhIG GIVEN (28 WKS)	/ /	SIGNATURE _____		

32 - 36 WEEK LABS (WHEN INDICATED)	DATE	RESULT		
ULTRASOUND	/ /	– / +		
VDRL	/ /	– / +		
GC	/ /	– / +		
HCT / HGB	/ /	_____ % _____ gm / dl		

OPTIONAL LAB (HIGH RISK GROUPS)	DATE	RESULT		
HIV	/ /			
HGB ELECTROPHORESIS	/ /	AA AS SS AC SC AF		
CHLAMYDIA	/ /	– / +		

PLANS / EDUCATION

	COUNSELED YES NO		COUNSELED YES NO
TOXOPLASMOSIS PRECAUTIONS (CATS / RAW MEAT)_____		TUBAL STERILIZATION_____	
CHILDBIRTH CLASSES_____		VBAC COUNSELING_____	
PHYSICAL ACTIVITY_____		CIRCUMCISION_____	
PREMATURE LABOR SIGNS_____		TRAVEL _____	
NUTRITION COUNSELING_____		**REQUESTS** _____	
METHOD OF ANESTHESIA_____			
BREAST OR BOTTLE FEEDING_____		**OTHER** _____	
NEWBORN CAR SEAT_____			
POSTPARTUM BIRTH CONTROL_____		**TUBAL STERILIZATION** DATE INITIALS	
ENVIRONMENTAL / WORK HAZARDS_____		CONSENT SIGNED ___ / ___ / ___ _____	

Figure 5.2B.   ACOG antepartum record, part 2, page 2: antepartum visits.

mated date of confinement [EDC] or estimated date of delivery [EDD]). Beginning at about 12 weeks of gestation (12 weeks from the onset of the last menstrual period), the uterus is enlarged sufficiently to be palpable in the lower abdomen. Other genital tract findings early in pregnancy include congestion and a bluish discoloration of the vagina (Chadwick's sign) and softening of the cervix (Hegar's sign). Increased pigmentation of the skin and the appearance of striae on the abdominal wall occur later in pregnancy. *Palpation of fetal parts and the appreciation of fetal movement and fetal heart tones* are diagnostic of pregnancy, but at a far more advanced gestational age. The patient's initial perception of fetal movement (called "quickening") is not usually reported before 16 to 18 weeks of gestation.

Detection of *fetal heart tones* is also evidence of a viable ongoing pregnancy. With a traditional, nonelectronic fetoscope, auscultation of fetal heart tones is possible at or beyond 18 to 20 weeks gestational age. The commonly used electronic Doppler devices can detect fetal heart tones at approximately 12 weeks of gestation. With this device, the patient and her family can also hear the fetal heart beat, a strong bonding experience that also can provide reassurance.

Several types of *urine pregnancy tests* are available, all of which measure *human chorionic gonadotropin* (hCG) produced in the syncytiotrophoblast of the growing placenta. Because hCG shares an α subunit with luteinizing hormone (LH), interpretation of any test that does not differentiate LH from hCG must take into account this overlap in structure. The concentration of hCG necessary to evoke a positive test result must, therefore, be high enough to avoid a false-positive diagnosis of pregnancy, i.e., a positive test result even though the patient is not pregnant. *Standard laboratory urine pregnancy tests become positive approximately 4 weeks following the 1st day of the last menstrual period,* i.e., around the time of the missed period. Home urine pregnancy tests have a low false-positive rate but a high false-negative rate (the test result is negative even though the patient is pregnant). All urine pregnancy tests are best performed on early morning urine specimens, which contain the highest concentration of hCG.

Serum pregnancy tests are more specific and sensitive because they test for the unique β subunit of hCG. This allows detection of pregnancy very early in gestation, even before the patient has missed a period. Further information about a

pregnancy may be obtained by the quantification of hCG. Figure 5.3 is a graphic presentation of the normal quantitative values of β-hCG and the expected rate of production. This can help differentiate normal from abnormal pregnancies. These more reliable and sensitive serum tests are also more expensive and difficult to perform.

Progesterone concentrations are also useful in determining pregnancy viability. Generally, serum progesterone levels less than 5 ng/mL are not consistent with a viable pregnancy, intrauterine or extrauterine, whereas levels greater than 25 ng/mL are usually consistent with a viable intrauterine pregnancy.

Ultrasound examination can detect pregnancy early in gestation. With abdominal ultrasound, a gestational sac is initially seen 5 to 6 weeks after the beginning of the last normal menstrual period (corresponding to β-hCG concentrations of 5000 to 6000 mIU/mL). Transvaginal ultrasound can detect a pregnancy at 3 to 4 weeks gestation (corresponding to β-hCG concentrations of 1500 to 2500 mIU/mL). If the β-hCG concentration is greater than 2000 mIU/mL, the embryo should be visualized by all techniques and cardiac activity usually detected.

INITIAL ANTENATAL EVALUATION

After the diagnosis of pregnancy has been established, a prenatal appointment is made, at which time a comprehensive history is taken, focusing on previous pregnancy outcome and any medical or surgical conditions that may affect pregnancy. The details of a recommended history include a history of past pregnancies, past medical history with specific attention to issues that may affect pregnancy,

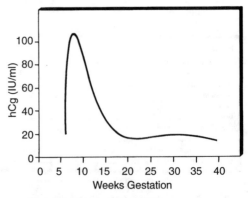

Figure 5.3.   hCG concentrations in pregnancy.

Table 5.1.
Routine Obstetric Laboratory Tests[a]

Test	Discussion
Initial Laboratory Tests — Routine	
1. Complete blood count	To determine hematologic status; to rule out anemia
2. Urinalysis and urine culture and sensitivity	To evaluate for UTI and renal function
3. Blood group, Rh	To determine blood type, Rh status, and risk of isoimmunization
4. Antibody screen	To detect maternal antibodies, which may damage fetus or make procurement of compatible blood for transfusion more difficult; the antibody screen is usually negative; anti-I and anti-Lewis are seen in about 1% of patients and are of no consequence to the fetus
5. Serologic test for syphilis (RPR, VDRL)	To detect previous/current infection; if positive, specific treponemal test required (e.g., FTA-ABS or MHA-TP)
6. Hepatitis B surface antigen	To detect carrier status or active disease; if positive, further testing indicated
7. Rubella titer	Approximately 85% of mothers have evidence of prior infection; if patient is seronegative, special precautions are needed to avoid infection, which can severely affect the fetus; vaccination is then required postpartum
8. Cervical cytology (Pap smear)	To screen for cervical dysplasia/cancer
9. Cervical culture for *N. gonorrhoeae* and *C. trachomatis*	To screen for infection; both cause neonatal conjunctivitis; association with premature labor and postpartum endometritis
10. Sickle-cell test	To detect sickle-cell trait (HbSA), associated with higher risk for UTI, and sickle-cell disease (HbSS), at risk for multiple fetal and maternal complications
11. Glucose screening (usually l-hr Glucola)	To screen for glucose intolerance
12. HIV titer by ELISA; Western blot if HIV+ by ELISA	Should be offered to all patients at risk (multiple sexual partners, drug use, or sexual contact with drug users); may be offered to all patients at physician's discretion
Subsequent Assessments	
13. MSAFP at 15 to 18 weeks	Elevated levels seen with neural tube defects, gastroschisis, and omphalocele; low levels associated with Down syndrome
14. Hematocrit at 24 to 28 weeks	To rule out anemia
15. Glucose screening (usually 1-hr Glucola) at 24 to 28 weeks	To screen for glucose intolerance

[a] *UTI*, urinary tract infection; *RPR*, rapid plasma reagin; *VDRL*, venereal disease research laboratory test; *FTA-ABS*, fluorescent treponemal antibody absorption test; *MHA-TP*, microhemagglutination assay-*Terponema pallidum*; *ELISA*, enzyme-linked immunoabsorbent assay; *MSAFP*, maternal serum α-fetoprotein.

information pertinent to genetic screening, and information about the course of the current pregnancy (see Fig. 5.1). Special attention is also given to diet; the use of tobacco, alcohol, and medications; and substance abuse. Routine laboratory studies are ordered (Table 5.1; see Fig. 5.2), and the patient is given instructions concerning routine prenatal care, warning signs of complications, whom to contact with questions or problems, and nutritional and social service information. A complete physical examination is performed, including a Pap test and a cervical culture for *Neisseria gonorrhoeae* and *Chlamydia trachomatis*.

If medical or obstetric problems are identified during the initial assessment or at any subsequent visit, the pregnancy is designated "at risk," and appropriate specific management is initiated.

INITIAL ASSESSMENT OF GESTATIONAL AGE: THE EDC

Every effort is made to assess accurately gestational age from which the EDC (due date or EDD) is calculated (see Fig. 5.2). This information is crucial to obstetric management, as it is needed to manage situations such as possible preterm labor or postdates pregnancy. Initial assessment of gestational age is made by obtaining a thorough *menstrual history*. "Normal" pregnancy lasts 40 ± 2 weeks, calculated from the 1st day of the last normal menses (*menstrual or gestational age*). Calculation of the EDC is accomplished by adding 7 days to the first day of the last normal menstrual flow and counting back 3 months. In a patient with an idealized 28-day menstrual cycle, ovulation occurs on day 14, so that the *fertilization age* or *conception age* of the normal pregnancy is actually 38 weeks. The use of the first day of the last menses as a starting point for gestational age assignment is standard, and gestational age is most commonly used.

To establish an *accurate* gestational age, the date of onset of the last normal menses is crucial. A light bleeding episode should not be mistaken for a normal menstrual period. A history of irregular periods or taking medications that alter cycle length — such as oral contraceptives, other hormonal preparations, and psychoactive medications — can confuse the menstrual history. If sexual intercourse is infrequent, or timed for conception based on basal body temperature readings, a patient may know when conception is most likely to have occurred, thus facilitating an accurate calculation of gestational age.

Pelvic examination by an experienced examiner is accurate in determining gestational age within 1 to 2 weeks until the second trimester, at which time the lower uterine segment begins to form, thereby making clinical estimation of gestational age less accurate. From 16 to 18 weeks of gestation until 36 weeks of gestation, the fundal height in centimeters is roughly equal to the number of weeks of gestational age in normal singleton pregnancies.

Obstetric ultrasound examination is the most accurate measurement available in the determination of gestational age. In the first trimester, transvaginal and transabdominal techniques allow gestational age determination with ±1 to 2 weeks accuracy by using measurements of the gestational sac and embryo/fetus. In the second trimester, accuracy is still high, in the ±2-week range. In the latter portions of the third trimester, however, accuracy decreases to ±2 to 3 weeks.

SUBSEQUENT ANTENATAL EVALUATION

For a patient with a normal pregnancy, *periodic antepartum visits* at 4-week intervals are usually scheduled until 32 weeks, at 2-week intervals between 32 and 36 weeks, and weekly thereafter. Patients with high-risk pregnancies or those with ongoing complications are usually seen more frequently, depending on the clinical circumstances. At each visit, patients are asked about how they are feeling and if they are having any problems, such as vaginal bleeding, nausea/vomiting, dysuria, or vaginal discharge. After quickening, patients are asked if they continue to feel fetal movement and if it is the same or less since the last antepartum visit. Decreased fetal movement is a warning sign requiring further evaluation of fetal well-being.

The only routine laboratory test performed at every prenatal visit is *determination of glucosuria and proteinuria*. A trace of glucosuria is a normal finding in pregnancy and requires no further evaluation. More marked glucosuria requires further evaluation, especially if there is a family history or previous obstetric history of glucose intolerance. Anything other than the presence of trace proteinuria should be considered abnormal and warrants further evaluation.

Maternal physical findings measured at each prenatal visit include blood pressure, weight, and assessment for edema. *Blood pressure* generally declines at the end of the second trimester, rising again in the third trimester. Compared with baseline levels, however, any increase in the systolic pressure of more than 30 mm Hg or any increase in the diastolic pressure of more than 15 mm Hg suggests pregnancy-associated hypertension. The *maternal weight* is compared with the pregravid weight and to the generally prescribed recommendation of a 25- to 30-pound weight gain through the course of pregnancy. There is usually a 3- to 4-pound increase between monthly visits. Significant deviation from this trend may require nutritional assessment and further evaluation. The presence of significant *edema* in the lower extremities and/or hands is very common in pregnancy and, by itself, is not abnormal. Fluid retention can be associated with hypertension, however, so that blood pressure as well as weight gain and edema must be evaluated in the clinical context before the findings are presumed to be innocuous.

Obstetric physical findings made at each visit include assessment of the uterine size by pelvic examination or fundal height measurement, documentation of the presence and rate of fetal heart tones, and determination of the presentation of the fetus. Until 18 to 20 weeks, the *uterine size* is generally stated as *weeks size*, such as "12 weeks size," "16 weeks size," etc. After 20 weeks of gestation (when the fundus is palpable at or near the umbilicus) the uterine size can be assessed with the use of a tape measure, which is the *fundal height measurement*. In this procedure, the top of the uterine fundus is identified and the zero end of the tape measure is placed at this uppermost part of the uterus. The tape is then carried anteriorly across the pregnant uterus to the level of the symphysis pubis.

Until 36 weeks in the normal singleton pregnancy, the number of weeks of gestation approximates the fundal height in centimeters. Thereafter, the fetus moves downward into the pelvis beneath the symphysis pubis ("lightening"), and fundal height measurement is less reliable. If the fundal height measurement is significantly greater than expected (i.e., "large for dates"), possible considerations include incorrect assessment of gestational age, multiple pregnancy, macrosomia (large fetus), hydatidiform mole, and excess accumulation of amniotic fluid (hydramnios). A fundal height measurement less than expected (i.e., "small for dates") suggests the possibility of incorrect assessment of gestational age, hydatidiform mole, fetal growth retardation, inadequate amniotic fluid accumulation (oligohydramnios), or even intrauterine fetal demise.

Fetal heart activity should be verified at every visit, by direct auscultation or by the use of a fetal Doppler device. The normal fetal heart rate is 120 to 160 beats per minute (bpm); the maternal pulse may also be detected with the Doppler device, so that simultaneous palpation of maternal pulse and auscultation of fetal pulse may be necessary to differentiate the two. Deviation from the normal rate or occasional arrhythmias must be evaluated carefully.

Several determinations concerning the fetus can be made by *palpation of the pregnant uterus.* The most important of these is identifying the presentation, or "presenting part" of the fetus, i.e., what part of the fetus is entering the pelvis first. This is especially important after 34 weeks. Before that time, breech, oblique, or transverse presentations are not uncommon, nor are they significant, as they may vary from day to day. At term, more than 95% of fetuses will be in the cephalic presentation (head down), with other presentations rather uncommon: breech (bottom first) about 3.5% and shoulder less than 1%. Unless the fetus is in a transverse lie (the long axis of the fetus is not parallel with the mother's long axis), the presentation will be either the head (vertex, cephalic) or the breech (buttocks).

The head is hard and well defined by ballottement, especially when the head is freely mobile in the fluid-filled uterus; the breech is softer and, therefore, more difficult to outline. If a breech presentation is noted between 34 and 37 weeks, the option of external cephalic version (ECV) must be entertained and discussed with the patient. This procedure involves turning the fetus from the breech presentation to a vertex presentation, thereby avoiding the potential adverse consequences of a vaginal breech delivery.

SPECIFIC TECHNIQUES OF FETAL ASSESSMENT

[handwritten margin note: GROWTH MATURITY WELLBEING]

Evaluation of the fetus can be conveniently categorized as assessment of fetal (*a*) growth, (*b*) well-being, and (*c*) maturity. The appropriate interpretation of these tests in light of the natural course of any antenatal problem provides a firm base on which decisions are made.

Assessment of Fetal Growth

Fetal growth can be assessed by fundal height measurement and ultrasonography. The increase in fundal height through pregnancy is predictable. Deviation of more than 2 cm in fundal height measurement from that expected at a particular gestational age between 18 and 36 weeks should prompt repeat measurement and may lead to further evaluation. A deviation of 4 cm or more requires further evaluation, including ultrasound in many cases.

Ultrasonography is the most valuable tool in assessing fetal growth. In early pregnancy, determination of the gestational sac diameter and the crown-rump length correlate very closely with gestational age. Later in pregnancy, measurement of the biparietal diameter of the skull, the abdominal circumference, the femur length, and the cerebellar diameter can be used to assess gestational age and, using various formulas, to estimate fetal weight. The range of normal values for these measurements increases significantly as pregnancy advances so that a specific assessment of gestational age in the third trimester may be ±3 weeks of the actual age. Earlier in pregnancy there is less deviation in normal values and the information derived is of greater accuracy. Measurements in the late first and early second trimesters are most reliable, generally ±1 to 2 weeks.

Assessment of Fetal Well-being

Assessment of *fetal well-being* includes maternal perception of fetal activity and several tests employing electronic fetal monitors and ultrasonography. Tests of fetal well-being have a wide range of uses, including *the assessment of fetal status at a particular time* and *prediction of fetal status for varying time intervals*, depending on the test and the clinical situation.

An active fetus is generally a healthy fetus, so that *quantification of fetal activity* is a common test of fetal well-being. A variety of methods can be used to quantify fetal activity, including the time necessary to achieve a certain number of movements each day, an average of the number of fetal movements in a given period of time repeated several times a day, or counting the number of movements in a given hour. If, for example, the mother detects more than four fetal movements while lying comfortably and focusing on fetal activity for 1 hr, the fetus is considered to be healthy. This type of testing has several advantages — it is reliable, it is inexpensive, and it involves the patient in her own care. For these reasons, fetal movement testing is frequently a part of routine obstetric care late in pregnancy, or earlier if high-risk conditions warrant.

Techniques using *electronic fetal monitoring* and *ultrasonography* are more costly but also provide more specific information. The most common tests used are the nonstress test, the contraction stress test (called the oxytocin challenge test if oxytocin is used), and the biophysical profile.

The *nonstress test* (NST) measures the response of the fetal heart rate to fetal movement. With the patient in the left lateral position and the elec-

tronic fetal monitor transducer placed on her abdomen to record the fetal heart rate, the patient is asked to note fetal movement, usually accomplished by pressing a button on the fetal monitor, which causes a notation on the monitor strip. Interpretation of the nonstress test depends on whether the fetal heart rate accelerates in response to fetal movement. A *normal, or reactive, NST* occurs when the fetal heart rate increases by at least 15 bpm over a period of 15 sec following a fetal movement (Fig. 5.4*A*). Two such accelerations in a 20-min span is considered reactive, or normal. The absence of these accelerations in response to fetal movement is a *nonreactive NST* (Fig. 5.4*B*). A reactive NST is generally reassuring in the absence of other indicators of fetal stress. Depending on the clinical situation, the test is repeated every 3 to 4 days or weekly. A nonreactive NST must be immediately followed with further assessment of fetal well-being.

Whereas the nonstress test evaluates the fetal heart rate response to fetal activity, the *contraction stress test* (CST) measures the response of the fetal heart rate to the stress of a uterine contraction. With uterine contractions, uteroplacental blood flow is temporarily reduced. *A healthy fetus is able to compensate for this intermittent decreased blood flow, whereas a fetus who is compromised is unable to do so, demonstrating abnormalities such as fetal heart rate decelerations.* To perform a CST, a tocodynamometer is placed on the maternal abdomen along with a fetal heart rate transducer. If contractions are occurring spontaneously, the test is known as a contraction stress test; if oxytocin infusion is required to elicit contractions, the test is called an *oxytocin challenge test* (OCT). The normal fetal heart rate response to contractions is for the baseline fetal heart rate to remain unchanged and for there to be no fetal heart rate decelerations. Decelerations, especially of the late variety (see Chapter 17), are nonreassuring. Repetitive decelerations following each contraction when three contractions occur in a 10-min window constitute a positive, or abnormal, CST or OCT. This is usually an indication for delivery.

Tests of fetal well-being have a significant incidence of false-positive results, i.e., the test suggests that the fetus is in jeopardy but the fetus is actually healthy. For this reason, these tests must be interpreted together with other assessments and are often repeated within 24 hr to verify the results. In addition, interpretations of the NST and OCT/CST are often combined. Because posi-

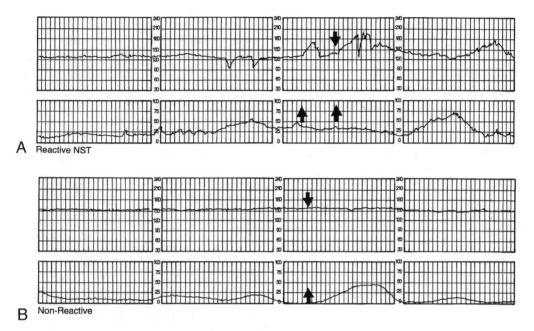

Figure 5.4. Nonstress testing. **A,** Reactive NST; note fetal heart rate acceleration in response to fetal movement. **B,** Nonreactive NST; note lack of fetal heart rate acceleration in response to fetal movement.

tive OCTs are common, fetal heart rate reactivity can have a significant impact on the final interpretation of the tests. If an OCT is positive, evidence for "reactivity" is sought (see Chapter 17). If the NST is reactive, the OCT result may be interpreted as a false-positive result. If, however, the positive OCT is accompanied by a nonreactive NST, the combination is considered especially worrisome, and a nonreassuring fetal status is likely to occur when labor begins.

The *biophysical profile* is a series of five assessments of fetal well-being, each of which is given a score of 0 or 2 (Table 5.2). The parameters include a reactive nonstress test, the presence of fetal breathing movements, the presence of fetal movement of the body or limbs, the finding of fetal tone (flexed extremities as opposed to a flaccid posture), and an adequate amount of amniotic fluid volume. Perinatal outcome can be correlated with the score derived from these five parameters. A score of 8 to 10 is considered normal, a score of 6 is equivocal requiring further evaluation, and a score of 4 or less is abnormal, usually requiring immediate intervention.

The importance of adequate amniotic fluid volume is well established. Diminished amniotic fluid is thought to represent decreased fetal uri-

nary output caused by chronic stress and shunting of blood flow away from the kidneys. The decreased amniotic fluid provides less support for the umbilical cord, which may be more frequently compressed, reducing blood flow and resulting in chronic fetal stress. Changes in fetal tone, breathing movements, and fetal movements are more likely to be signs of acute stress to the central nervous system.

Assessment of Fetal Maturity

In some high-risk obstetric situations, the maternal or fetal status is so grave that immediate delivery is required, regardless of gestational age; in others, a decision must be made as to whether the mother and fetus are at greater risk by continued antepartum management or whether delivery is best. If the pregnancy is viable but less than 36 weeks, the questions are, "How premature is the pregnancy?" and, more specifically, "Will the risk of prematurity-associated problems such as respiratory distress syndrome (RDS) be greater than those of continued intrauterine life?"

Because the respiratory system is the last fetal system to mature functionally, many of the *tests available to assess fetal maturity* focus on this organ system. Such tests, termed *direct tests* if they specif-

Table 5.2.
Biophysical Profile

Biophysical Variable	Score	Explanation
Fetal breathing movements (FBM)	Normal = 2	At least 1 FBM of at least 30-sec duration in 30 min
	Abnormal = 0	No FBM of at least 30-sec duration in 30 min
Gross body movement	Normal = 2	At least 3 discrete body/limb movements in 30 min
	Absent = 0	2 or less discrete body/limb movements in 30 min
Fetal tone	Normal = 2	At least 1 episode of active extension with return to flexion of fetal limbs/trunk or opening/closing of hand
	Absent = 0	Either slow extension with return to partial flexion or movement of limb in full extension or no fetal movement
Reactive fetal heart rate	Normal = 2	Reactive NST
	Absent = 0	Nonreactive NST
Qualitative amniotic fluid volume	Normal = 2	At least 1 pocket of amniotic fluid at least 1 cm in two perpendicular planes
	Absent = 0	No amniotic fluid or no pockets of fluid greater than 1 cm in two perpenndicular planes

ically measure substances associated with lung maturity, are routinely employed, although not all tests are used in all hospitals. Other tests measure parameters from which the likelihood of maturity can be estimated; these are termed *indirect tests,* the most common being ultrasonography.

Neonatal RDS is the inability of the newborn to ventilate successfully because of the immaturity of the lungs. RDS results from lack of a group of phospholipids, collectively known as *surfactant,* which decreases the surface tension within alveolar sacs and thereby promotes easy ventilation by maintaining patency of these sacs. In utero, production of these phospholipids remains low until 32 to 33 weeks, after which production increases. There is a great variation in this process. Gestational age alone does not reliably predict surfactant production or lung maturity. RDS is manifest by signs of respiratory failure — grunting, chest retractions, nasal flaring, and hypoxia — possibly leading to acidosis and death. Management consists of skillful support of ventilation and correction of associated metabolic disturbances until the neonate can ventilate successfully without assistance. Recently, administration of synthetic or semisynthetic surfactant

to the neonate has been under investigation and offers additional hope for an improved outcome for these infants.

The fetus breathes in utero, and phospholipids enter the amniotic fluid where they can be obtained by amniocentesis and measured. Direct tests that measure components of surfactant are listed in Table 5.3. Use of fluid obtained vaginally after spontaneous rupture of membranes is not as common, although such fluid can be used for certain tests in some instances.

Ultrasonographic determination of gestational age and estimated fetal weight are common indirect tests performed to help assess maturity. Unfortunately, ultrasonographic assessment of gestational age and fetal size do not sufficiently correlate with maturity to allow for reliable prediction, especially in the marginal maturational period between 28 and 35 weeks of gestation. Performed correctly, any test that indicates fetal maturity is associated with the subsequent development of RDS in 2% or less of cases. The predictive value of these tests is much less helpful. Overall, only 50% of infants who are delivered shortly after test results indicate immaturity will develop RDS.

Table 5.3.
Tests of Fetal Lung Maturity

Test	Endpoint for Maturity	Comment
Lecithin:sphingomyelin (L:S) ratio	≥2.0	Lecithin is the major component of surfactant; this test measures its production compared with sphingomyelin, a substance with constant production throughout pregnancy; the L:S ratio was the first reliable test of fetal lung maturity; the method is methodologically involved and labor intensive; it has been replaced by less costly tests in many laboratories
Phosphatidylglycerol	Present	A minor phospholipid that "appears" late in pregnancy; it can be measured by several methods, thus results are reported in different ways
Foam stability index	≥47	Measures the ability of amniotic fluid surfactant to maintain foam at the meniscus of a solution of amniotic fluid and alcohol

OTHER CONSIDERATIONS AND COMMON QUESTIONS IN PREGNANCY

Employment

In normal pregnancy there are few restrictions concerning work, although it is beneficial to moderate activity and to allow for additional periods of rest. Strenuous work should be avoided. A physician's note asking employers to transfer pregnant patients to less physically demanding activities is often needed.

The traditional time designated for maternity leave is approximately 1 month before the expected date of delivery and extending until 6 weeks after birth. This may be modified, depending on complications of pregnancy, the work involved, the employer attitude, the rules of the health care system under which the patient receives care, and the wishes of the patient.

Exercise

Moderate exercise programs can be continued during pregnancy. Overly strenuous exercise, especially for prolonged periods, should be avoided. Patients unaccustomed to regular exercise should not undertake vigorous new programs during pregnancy.

Nutrition and Weight Gain

Concerns about adequate nutrition and weight gain during pregnancy are common and appropriate. Poor nutrition, obesity, food faddism, and prob-

lems such as *pica* are associated with poor perinatal outcome. Concerns about the retention of weight gained during pregnancy are also common.

A complete nutritional assessment is an important part of the initial antepartum assessment, including history of dietary habits, special dietary issues or concerns, and weight trends. Regular weighing is an important part of antepartum care. Calculation of body mass index (BMI) is useful, because it relates weight to height, allowing a better indirect measurement of body fat distribution than is obtained with weight measurement alone.

Recommendations for total weight gain during pregnancy and the rate of weight gain per month appropriate to achieve it may be made based on a BMI calculated for the prepregnancy weight (Table 5.4). The "components" of an average weight gain in a normal singleton pregnancy are listed in Table 5.5. The maternal component of this weight gain starts in the first trimester and is most prominent in the first half of pregnancy. Fetal growth is most rapid in the second half of pregnancy, with the normal fetus tripling its weight in the last 12 weeks of pregnancy.

Published recommended daily allowances (RDAs) for protein, minerals, and vitamins are useful approximations (Table 5.6). It should be kept in mind, however, that the RDAs are a combination of estimates and clinical research data and are not averages or means but, rather, values adjusted near the top of the normal ranges to encompass the estimated needs of most women.

Table 5.4.
Recommended Weight Gain in Pregnancy[a]

	Weight Gain (kg)		Weight Gain (pounds)	
Maternal Classification	Total	Rate (kg/4 weeks)	Total	Rate (pounds/4 weeks)
Prepregnant BMI[b]				
Underweight (<19.8)	12.7–18.2	2.3	28–40	5.0
Normal weight (19.8–26.9)	11.4–15.9	1.8	25–35	4.0
Overweight (26.1–29.0)	6.8–11.4	1.2	15–25	2.5
Obese (>29.0)	6.8	0.9	15	2.0
Twin gestation	15.9–20.4	2.7	35–40	6.0

Adapted from Nutrition during Pregnancy. Washington, DC: National Academy Press. 1990.
[a] Rate has been adjusted to second trimester.
[b] Pregnant weight (kg) ÷ height (cm) × 100.

Thus many women have an adequate diet for their individual needs, even though it does not supply all the RDAs. RDAs are useful guidelines, but they must be considered in the light of individual nutritional assessment.

A balanced, adequate diet usually supplies all the vitamins needed in pregnancy. Vitamin supplementation is appropriate for specific therapeutic indication such as a patient's inability or unwillingness to eat a balanced, adequate diet or clinical demonstration of specific nutritional risk. Except for iron, mineral supplementation is likewise not required in otherwise healthy women. Guidelines for vitamin and mineral supplementation when required are presented in Table 5.7.

Financial problems and the inability to get to a grocery store may prevent some women from obtaining adequate foodstuffs. The federal supplemental food program for women, infants, and children (WIC), food stamp programs, and Aid for Families with Dependent Children are resources that may help in these situations.

Tobacco

Smoking should be prohibited during pregnancy because of the established risks to both mother and fetus. In addition to the adverse maternal effects, metabolites from burning tobacco and paper covering are quickly transferred from the patient to her fetus. Infants born to women who smoke weigh less than those born to nonsmokers. Even exposure to passive smoking is associated with high levels of tobacco metabolites. At times, the gastrointestinal discomforts of early pregnancy are associated with a decreased interest in cigarette smoking. The patient should take advantage of this opportunity to cease smoking.

Sexual Intercourse

Sexual activity is not restricted during a normal pregnancy. It may be restricted or prohibited under certain circumstances, when it is known to have special risks, e.g., placenta previa, premature rupture of membranes, and preterm labor.

Travel

Travel is not prohibited during pregnancy, although it is customary for patients to avoid distant travel in the last month of pregnancy. This is not because of substantial risk to either mother or fetus but rather because of the likelihood that labor may ensue away from home and customary health care providers. When traveling, patients are advised to avoid long periods of immobilization such as sitting. Walking every 1 to 2 hr, even for short periods, promotes circulation, especially in the lower legs, and decreases the risk of thromboembolic problems.

Headaches

Headaches are common in early pregnancy and may be severe. The etiology of such headaches is not known. Treatment with acetaminophen in usual doses is recommended.

Nausea and Vomiting

The majority of pregnant women experience some degree of upper gastrointestinal symptoms in the first trimester of pregnancy. Classically, these symptoms are worse in the morning (the so-called morning sickness). However, patients may experience symptoms at other times or even throughout the day. Treatment consists of frequent small meals, avoidance of an "empty stomach" by ingesting crackers or other bland carbohydrates, and patience. Medication specifically for nausea and vomiting during pregnancy (Bendectin) was removed from the market by the manufacturer several years ago because of growing litigation concerning congenital anomalies. This occurred even though the safety of the drug had actually been well established. Components of that drug — pyridoxine (vitamin B_6) and an antihistamine — have subsequently been used successfully to treat nausea and vomiting. A variety of other antinausea agents are sometimes used in patients unresponsive to conservative treatment.

Fatigue

In early pregnancy, patients often complain of extreme fatigue that is unrelieved by rest. There is no specific treatment, other than adjustment of the patient's schedule to the extent possible to accommodate this temporary lack of energy. Patients can be reassured that the symptoms disappear in the second trimester.

Leg Cramps

Leg cramps, usually affecting the calves, are common during pregnancy. A variety of treatments including oral calcium supplement have been pro-

Table 5.5.
Components of Average Weight Gain in a Normal Singleton Pregnancy

Organ, Tissue, Fluid	Weight (g)
Maternal	
Uterus	970
Breasts	405
Blood	1,250
Water	1,680
Fat	3,345
Subtotal	7,650
Fetal	
Fetus	3,400
Placenta	650
Amniotic fluid	800
Subtotal	4,650
Total	*12,500*

Table 5.6.
Recommended Daily Allowances (RDAs)

Nutrient	Nonpregnant			Pregnant	Lactating (first 6 months)
	15–18 years	19–24 years	25–50 years		
Protein (g)	44	46	50	60	65
Calcium (mg)	1200	1200	800	1200	1200
Phosphorus (mg)	1200	1200	800	1200	1200
Magnesium (mg)	300	280	280	300	355
Iron (mg)	15	15	15	30	15
Zinc (mg)	12	12	12	15	19
Vitamin A (μg RE)	800	800	800	800	1300
Vitamin D (μg)	10	10	5	10	10
Vitamin E (mg α-TE)	8	8	8	10	12
Vitamin C (mg)	60	60	60	70	95
Thiamin (mg)	1.1	1.1	1.1	1.5	1.6
Riboflavin (mg)	1.3	1.3	1.3	1.6	1.8
Niacin (mg NE)	15	15	15	17	20
Vitamin B_6 (mg)	1.5	1.6	1.6	2.2	2.1
Folic acid (μg)	180	180	180	400	280
Vitamin B_{12} (μg)	2	2	2	2.2	2.6

posed over the years, none of which is universally successful. Massage and rest are often advised.

Back Pain

Achy lower back pain is common, especially in late pregnancy. The altered center of gravity caused by the growing fetus places unusual stress on the lower spine and associated muscles and ligaments. Treatment focuses on heat, massage, and analgesia. A specially fitted girdle may also help.

Varicose Veins and Hemorrhoids

Varicose veins are *not caused* by pregnancy but often first appear during the course of gestation. Besides the disturbing appearance to many patients, varicose veins can cause an aching sensation, especially when patients stand for long periods of time. Support hose can help diminish the discomfort, although they have no effect on the appearance of the varicose veins. Popular brands of support hose do not provide the relief that prescription elastic hose can. *Hemorrhoids* are varicosities of the hemorrhoidal veins. Treatment consists of sitz baths and local preparations. Varicose veins and hemorrhoids regress postpartum, although neither condition may abate completely. Surgical correction of varicose veins or hemorrhoids should not be undertaken for about the first 6 months postpartum, to allow for the natural involution to occur.

Vaginal Discharge

The hormonal milieu of pregnancy often causes an increase in normal vaginal secretions. These normal secretions must be distinguished from vaginitis, which has symptoms of itching and malodor, and spontaneous rupture of membranes, for which thin, clear fluid appears.

Table 5.7.
Supplementation in Pregnancy

Nutrient	Recommended Supplementation	
Vitamins		
Vitamin B$_6$	2	mg
Folate	300	μg
Vitamin C	50	mg
Vitamin D	5	μg
Minerals		
Iron	30	mg
Zinc	15	mg
Copper	2	mg
Calcium	250	mg

OBSTETRIC STATISTICS

The rates of maternal and fetal mortality are of importance in evaluating the natural history of disease and in the quality of obstetric care. Four statistics are commonly used for this purpose. *Maternal death* occurs during pregnancy; it is *direct* if the cause of death is an obstetric disease and *indirect* if the cause of death is a disease coexisting with pregnancy. If death is caused by accident, it is classified as *nonmaternal.* The *maternal death rate* is the number of deaths of obstetric cause per 100,000 live births. *Fetal death* is synonymous with *stillbirth* and is the number of infants born without any signs of life. It is expressed as the *fetal death rate*, or *stillbirth rate*, which is number of stillbirths per 1,000 infants born. *Neonatal death* refers to an infant's death within the first 7 days of life and is expressed as the *neonatal mortality rate* (the number of neonatal deaths per 1,000 live births). *Perinatal death* is the number of fetal deaths plus the number neonatal deaths and is expressed as the *perinatal mortality rate* (deaths per 1,000 total births).

More pleasant statistics are the *birth rate*, which expressed as the number of births per 1,000 people in the total population, and the *fertility rate*, which is expressed as the number of live births per 1,000 females aged 15 to 45 in the population.

CASE STUDIES

Case 5A

A 14-year-old girl with an unknown interval of amenorrhea, a positive urinary pregnancy test, and morning sickness presents for prenatal care.

Questions Case 5A

What questions are useful in determining her gestational age?

A. If, and when, quickening was noted
B. Last menstrual period (LMP)
C. Past menstrual period (PMP)
D. Contraceptive use, if any
E. Menstrual cycle regularity

Answer: All

Items B–E are important in establishing her EDC by dates. Quickening would suggest a pregnancy in the late first or early second trimester.

The patient has not experienced fetal movement and thinks her last menstrual period was 2 or 3 months ago. She has never used contraception apart from condoms.

What laboratory tests are useful to further ascertain her gestational age and EDC?

A. Qualitative β-hCG
B. Quantitative β-hCG
C. Obstetric ultrasound
D. Pelvic examination
E. CT scan

Answer: B, C, D

With a positive urinary pregnancy test, a qualitative serum pregnancy test is redundant. CT scans are not used in gestational age estimation. Pelvic examination by an experienced practitioner provides useful information, especially in the first trimester. Quantitative β-hCG will allow determination of mode, transvaginal or transabdominal, of ultrasound is most useful. Intrauterine pregnancy is usually identifiable on transvaginal ultrasonography when the β-hCG is 1500 to 2500 mIU/mL and on transabdominal ultrasonography when above 5000 mIU/mL.

Case 5B

A 27-year-old G1 P0 at 37 weeks calls saying her baby is moving much less than it did a few days ago. Upon review of her antepartum record, you note no medical problems, normal fetal growth, and normal laboratory values as well as a normal obstetric ultrasound at 18 weeks.

Questions Case 5B

Your most appropriate action(s) is/are

A. Because she has an unremarkable antepartum record, reassure the patient that she is just inexperienced and that everything is okay
B. Suggest the patient come to the hospital for induction of labor
C. Suggest the patient come to the hospital for an NST
D. Suggest the patient come to the hospital for an OCT
E. None of the above, because the call is silly and should be ignored to avoid raising concerns on the mother's part

Answer: C

Answers A and E will only raise the patient's concerns and do not address the problem of proper evaluation of decreased fetal movement. An NST is the least invasive and most cost-effective test. An OCT is also a good measure of fetal well-being but is more invasive and costly than is warranted in a patient with no risk factors. Induction is not indicated.

The patient comes to the hospital and receives an NST. It is nonreactive. Your most appropriate action is to suggest which of the following?

A. A biophysical profile
B. A repeat NST in 1 week
C. An induction of labor
D. A nutrition consult to avoid hypoglycemia associated decreased fetal movement
E. Cordocentesis for fetal blood gas analysis

Answer: A

Cordocentesis is risky and not indicated, nor is induction. A biophysical profile is the least invasive and most cost-effective test of fetal well-being as follow-up to a nonreactive NST. An OCT would also serve as a test of fetal well-being, but it does not measure amniotic fluid volume and is more costly and invasive.

chapter 6

MEDICAL AND SURGICAL CONDITIONS OF PREGNANCY

Virtually any maternal medical or surgical condition can complicate the course of a pregnancy and/or be affected by pregnancy. Accordingly, physicians providing obstetric care must have a thorough understanding of the effect of pregnancy on the natural course of a disorder, the effect of the disorder on a pregnancy, and the change in management of the pregnancy and/or disorder caused by their coincidence. In this chapter, selected common medical and surgical complications that may be encountered during the course of obstetric care are discussed. Only a small portion of possible medical-surgical disorders are included here; more detailed and inclusive coverage is the province of textbooks of maternal-fetal medicine, medicine, and surgery.

The following 17 disorders or groups of disorders in pregnancy are discussed in this chapter.

1. Anemias;
2. Urinary tract infection;
3. Renal disease;
4. Respiratory disease;
5. Cardiac disease;
6. Glucose intolerance and diabetes mellitus;
7. Endocrine disease;
8. Infectious disease;
9. Thromboembolic disorders;
10. Neurologic disease;
11. Gastrointestinal disease;
12. Dental disease;
13. Hepatobiliary diseases;
14. Abdominal surgical conditions and abdominal trauma;
15. Substance abuse;
16. Coagulation disorders;
17. Cancer

1. ANEMIAS IN PREGNANCY

The plasma and cellular composition of blood changes significantly during the course of pregnancy because of an expansion of plasma volume proportionally greater than that of the red blood cell (RBC) mass (Table 6.1). On the average, there is a 1000 mL increase in plasma volume and a 300 mL increase in red cell mass (a 3:1 ratio). Since the hematocrit (Hct) reflects the proportion of blood made up primarily of red blood cells, Hct demonstrates a "physiologic" decrease during pregnancy (the so-called *physiologic anemia of pregnancy*). This decrease in hematocrit is not actually an anemia. *Anemia in pregnancy is generally defined as a hematocrit less than 30% or a hemoglobin of less than 10 g/dL*. Because of monthly blood loss with menstrual flow and contemporary dietary practices, which may lack sufficient iron and protein, women often enter pregnancy with a lowered iron store and sometimes a lowered hematocrit. When faced with the expansion of the maternal red cell mass and fetal iron needs, additional demands on the mother for iron outstrip the stores that are available; the result is *iron-deficiency anemia*. It is for these reasons that supplemental iron is appropriately prescribed for pregnant women. Iron-deficiency anemia is by far the most frequent type of anemia seen in pregnancy, accounting for 90% or more of all cases.

Because iron deficiency is the most common form of anemia in pregnancy, extensive evaluation of anemic pregnant patients should be delayed until an empiric trial of iron therapy is given and the effect observed. If the presumed iron-deficiency anemia is severe, the classic findings are small, pale erythrocytes manifest on

Table 6.1.
Hematologic Laboratory Values in Pregnancy

Test	Nonpregnant	Pregnant
Hb (g/dL)	12–16	10–13
Hct (%)	37–45	30–39
RBC (mL/mm³)	4.2–5.4	3.8–4.4
WBC (1000/mm³)	4.7–5.4	6–16
MCV (f/L)	80–100	70–90
MCH (pg/cell)	27–37	23–31
MCHC (d/dL/RBC)	32–35	32–35
Reticulocyte count (%)	0.5–1.0	1.0–2.0
Serum iron (μg/dL)	50–110	30–100
TIBC (μg/dL)	250–300	280–400
Transferrin saturation (%)	25–35	15–30
Serum folate (ng/mL)	4–16	4–10
Serum vitamin B_{12} (ng/mL)	70–85	70–500

blood smears (microcytic, hypochromic) and red cell indices that indicate a low mean corpuscular volume (MCV) — generally <80 f/liter) — and low mean corpuscular hemoglobin concentration (MCHC) — generally <30%. Further laboratory studies usually demonstrate a decreased serum iron (generally <50 μg/dL), an increased total iron binding capacity, and a decrease in serum ferritin. A recent dietary history is also highly suggestive, especially if *pica* exists (the consumption of nonedible substances such as starch, ice, or dirt). Such dietary indiscretion may contribute to iron deficiency by decreasing the amount of nutritious food and iron consumed.

Iron therapy is generally given in the form of ferrous sulfate or fumarate taken two times a day. Each 325-mg tablet provides approximately 60 mg of elemental iron. The uptake of iron is increasingly efficient as pregnancy progresses, 10% initially to 25% in the second trimester to nearly 30% in the last trimester. A response to therapy is first seen as an increase in the reticulocyte count approximately 1 week after the institution of iron therapy. Because of the plasma expansion associated with pregnancy, the hematocrit may not increase significantly but rather stabilizes or increases only slightly.

The second most common form of anemia seen in pregnancy is *folate deficiency* (or *megaloblastic anemia*). Although folate is found in green leafy vegetables, the demands of fetal and maternal growth during pregnancy (150 to 300 μg/day) outstrip the usual adult intake of 50 to 100 μg/day, requiring folate supplementation. Folate deficiency is especially likely in multiple gestation or when patients are taking medications such as phenytoin (Dilantin), nitrofurantoin, pyrimethamine, or trimethoprim or drinking ethanol in large quantities. Folate deficiency on blood smear is characterized by hypersegmented neutrophils and indices that suggest large cell volume (macrocytic anemia). Serum folate levels <4 ng/mL and erythrocyte folate activity <20 ng/mL are diagnostic. Treatment of folate deficiency anemia is 1 mg of folate orally on a daily basis, the amount generally found in most prenatal vitamin supplements. Because gastrointestinal absorption of folate is low (only 10 to 20 μg every 8 hr), divided doses may increase absorption in severe cases. With especially severe disease or in the case of malabsorption (malabsorption syndrome, surgical resection of the upper bowel), parenteral administration may be indicated.

With a *mixed iron and folate deficiency anemia*, the microcytic changes of iron deficiency negate the megaloblastic changes of folate deficiency, resulting in a normocytic and normochromic anemia. In such cases, treatment with either iron or folate alone will not be followed by a rise in red cell production.

Vitamin B_{12} deficiency also causes a macrocytic megaloblastic anemia, although it is quite rare (1/6000 to 1/8000 pregnancies). Because the normal adult female has a multiple-year store of vitamin B_{12}, this disease is usually seen in women with chronic malabsorption from disease (such as sprue, pancreatic disease, Crohn's disease, or ulcerative colitis) or surgical resection. Parenteral vitamin B_{12} is a rapid and effective treatment.

The hereditary hemolytic anemias are also rare causes of anemia in pregnancy. Some examples are hereditary spherocytosis, an autosomal dominant defect of the erythrocyte membrane; glucose 6-phosphate dehydrogenase deficiency; and pyruvate kinase deficiency.

Thalassemia trait may also present as microcytic, hypochromic anemia, but unlike iron-deficiency anemia, the serum iron and total iron binding capacity are normal. In addition, hemoglobin A_2 (HbA₂) is elevated.

The direct fetal consequences of anemia are minimal, although infants born to mothers with iron deficiency may have diminished iron stores as neonates. The maternal consequences of anemia

Table 6.2.
The Hemoglobinopathies

Characteristic	Sickle-Cell	HbSC Disease	Sickle-cell–β-Thalassemia	α-Thalassemia	β-Thalassemia
Globin abnormality	HbS (valine substituted for glutamic acid at the sixth position) in one or both chains	One globin is HbS and the other is HbC (lysine substituted for valine at the position)	One globin is HbS and one globin allele codes for β-thalassemia; decreased synthesis of HbA	Normal hemoglobins; decreased production of α globin chains	Normal hemoglobin; decreased production of β globin chains
Genetics	Autosomal recessive Sickle-cell trait: heterozygous (one chain affected); <40% HbS; 1 in 12 black Americans Sickle-cell disease: homozygous (both chains affected); 1 in 500 pregnancies in black Americans	Autosomal recessive; 1 in 700 patients at risk	Autosomal recessive; 1 in 1700 pregnancies; severity of disease depends on β allele — from no HbA production (severe disease) to moderate production (milder disease)	Autosomal recessive; severity of disease (microcytic, hypochromic anemia) depends on expression and amount of α globin produced — from none (homozygous) to 25–75% (heterozygous)	Autosomal recessive; point mutations cause decreased β chain synthesis Homozygous: β-thalassemia major (Cooley's anemia); no HbA produced; most is HbF or HbA$_2$; severe disease Heterozygous: β-thalassemia or β-thalassemia minor; one normal and one abnormal β globin allele; usually mild to moderate disease
Risk groups	African, Mediterranean, Turkish, Arabian, and East Indian heritage			Asian, African, East Indian, and Mediterranean heritage	Mediterranean, Middle Eastern, African, East Indian, and Asian heritage

are those associated with any adult anemia. If the anemia is corrected, the woman with an adequate red cell mass enters the labor and delivery process with additional protection against the need for transfusion.

The *hemoglobinopathies*, including the *sickle-cell diseases* and the *thalassemias*, are disorders of polypeptide chains that comprise the oxygen-carrying hemoglobin molecule found in the blood cells (Table 6.2). These disorders usually involve abnormalities of the β globulins; the oxygen-carrying capacity of the hemoglobin molecule, including its structural integrity under conditions of low oxygen tension, is impaired. When this results in

deformity of the normal spheroid shape of the RBC, vasoocclusive "crisis" ensues.

These disorders may be grouped into those with minimal maternal and fetal morbidity (sickle-cell trait, HbSA; sickle-cell–β-thalassemia disease, HbS–β-thal) and those with considerable maternal morbidity and occasional mortality (sickle-cell disease, HbSS; sickle-cell — hemoglobin C, HbSC). Patients with sickle-cell disease (defined as less than 40% HbS on quantitative hemoglobin electrophoresis) are inclined to maternal urinary tract infections, particularly asymptomatic bacteriuria. Otherwise the pregnancies of patients with HbSA and HbS–β-thal are generally unaffected.

Patients who are HbSS or HbSC, in contrast, may suffer vasoocclusive episodes ("crisis") with acute episodes of uteroplacental insufficiency and morbidity, such as prematurity and intrauterine growth retardation.

Although prophylactic maternal red cell transfusions have been popular, the risks of multiple blood transfusions and the general improvement in outcome in patients with hemoglobinopathies without transfusion have shifted the therapeutic emphasis to conservative management. Transfusions are, for the most part, reserved for complications of hemoglobinopathies such as congestive heart failure, sickle-cell disease crises, and severely low levels of hemoglobin. Careful antenatal assessment of fetal well-being and growth using standard techniques is an important part of managing patients with hemoglobinopathies.

2. URINARY TRACT INFECTION IN PREGNANCY

Urinary tract infections are common in pregnancy. Approximately 8% of all women (pregnant and nonpregnant) will have greater than 10^5 colonies of a single bacteria on a midstream culture. Approximately 40% of the pregnant portion of this group will develop an acute, symptomatic urinary tract infection. Compared with nonpregnant women with similar colony counts on urine culture, *asymptomatic bacteriuria* in pregnancy is more likely to be symptomatic, as are cystitis and pyelonephritis. The increased incidence of asymptomatic bacteriuria during pregnancy is thought to be due to pregnancy-associated urinary stasis and glucosuria. This relative urinary stasis in pregnancy is a result of progesterone-associated decreased ureteral tone and motility, mechanical compression of the ureters at the pelvic brim, and compression of the bladder and ureteral orifices. Also, the pH of the urine is increased because of increased bicarbonate excretion, which enhances bacterial growth, as does the mild glycosuria common in pregnancy.

It is standard to obtain a urine culture at the onset of prenatal care and to treat patients with asymptomatic bacteriuria. Ampicillin (500 mg p.o. q.i.d.), sulfisoxazole (Gantrisin; 1 g p.o. q.i.d.), or nitrofurantoin (Macrodantin; 50 mg p.o. q.i.d.) for 7 to 10 days is usually quite effective, as the most common organism is *Escherichia*

coli. In the third trimester, sulfas should be avoided as they compete with bilirubin for albumin-binding sites in the fetus and theoretically may produce hyperbilirubinemia of the newborn. Nitrofurantoin should be avoided in late pregnancy because of the risk of hemolysis as a result of deficiency of erythrocyte phosphate dehydrogenase in the newborn.

Approximately 25 to 30% of patients not treated for asymptomatic bacteriuria will proceed to symptomatic urinary tract infection (UTI), hence this treatment should prevent approximately 70% of symptomatic UTIs in pregnancy. However, 1.5% of patients with initial negative cultures will also develop symptomatic UTIs in pregnancy. Suppressive antimicrobial therapy (nitrofurantoin, 50 to 100 mg p.o. q.d.) is indicated if there are repetitive urinary tract infections during pregnancy or following pyelonephritis during pregnancy. Consideration should be given to postpartum radiology evaluation of these patients to identify renal parenchymal and urinary collecting duct abnormalities.

Acute cystitis occurs in about 1% of pregnancies. Patients complain of urinary frequency, urgency, dysuria, and bladder discomfort. Occasionally, hematuria is also seen. Fever is unlikely, and its presence should suggest upper urinary tract infection. The treatment of cystitis is the same as that of asymptomatic bacteriuria.

Patients with *pyelonephritis* are acutely ill, with fever, costovertebral tenderness, general malaise, and often dehydration. Approximately 20% of these ill patients will demonstrate increased uterine activity and preterm labor, and approximately 10% will have positive blood cultures if they are obtained in the acute febrile phase of the disease. Pyelonephritis occurs in 2% of all pregnant patients and is one of the most common medical complications of pregnancy requiring hospitalization.

After obtaining a urinalysis and urine culture, patients are treated with intravenous hydration and antibiotics, commonly a first-generation cephalosporin or ampicillin. Uterine contractions may accompany these symptoms; if uncontrolled, preterm labor may ensue. Contractions usually cease but specific tocolytic therapy may be required. It is known that *E. coli* can produce phospholipase A, which in turn can promote prostaglandin synthesis, resulting in an increase in uterine activity. Fever is also known to induce contractions so that antipyretics are required for a temperature greater than 100°F. Attention must

Table 6.3.
Chronic Renal Disease and Pregnancy

Outcome	Preserved/Mildly Impaired Renal Function (Serum Cr <1.4 mg/100 mL)	Moderate Renal Insufficiency (Serum Cr 1.4–2.5 mg/100 mL)	Severe Renal Insufficiency (Serum Cr >2.5 mg/100 mL)
Successful obstetric outcome	>95% (85%)[a]	90% (60%)	50% (10%)
Long-term renal sequelae	<3% (10%)	25% (70%)	50% (90%)

[a] Values in parentheses apply when complications occur before 28 weeks gestation.

be paid to the patient's response to therapy and her general condition; sepsis occurs in 2 to 3% of patients with pyelonephritis. If improvement does not occur within 48 to 72 hr, urinary tract obstruction or urinary calculus should be considered along with a reevaluation of antibiotic. A "single-shot" intravenous pyelogram and/or ultrasonography with attention to the ureters and kidneys is an integral part of the evaluation.

The organisms most commonly cultured from the urine of symptomatic pregnant patients are *E. coli* and other Gram-negative aerobes. Follow-up can be with either frequent urine cultures or empiric antibiotic suppression with an agent such as nitrofurantoin.

Recurrent symptoms or failure to respond to usual therapy suggests another etiology for the findings of concurrent urinary tract disease. In these patients, a complete urological evaluation 6 weeks after pregnancy may be warranted.

Urinary calculi are identified in approximately 1 in 1500 patients during pregnancy, although pregnancy per se does not promote stone development. A persistently alkaline urine also is frequently associated with patients with urinary calculi, as is urinary tract infection with *Proteus* species. Symptoms similar to those of pyelonephritis but without fever are suggestive of urinary calculi. Microhematuria is more common with this condition than in uncomplicated urinary tract infection. Although typically renal colic pain may be found, it is seen less frequently in pregnancy than in the nonpregnant state.

Usually, hydration and expectant management, along with straining of urine in search of stones, will suffice as management. Occasionally, however, the presence of a stone can lead to infection and/or complete obstruction, which may require drainage by either ureteral stent or percutaneous nephrostomy. When the diagnosis of urinary calculi is uncertain, a limited exposure intravenous pyelogram may be obtained.

3. RENAL DISEASE IN PREGNANCY

Pregnancy has profound effects on renal function, including a nearly 50% increase in glomerular filtration. The normal nonpregnant values for serum creatinine (Cr) and urea nitrogen decrease from a mean of 0.8 and 13 mg/100 mL, respectively, to mean values of 0.6 and 9 mg/100 mL.

Pregnancy in patients with preexisting renal disease is encountered frequently, because treatments such as dialysis and transplantation allow these patients health sufficient to support ovulation and pregnancy. *During preconception counseling*, these patients should be advised of the significant risks involved in a pregnancy and that pregnancy should be avoided unless their blood creatinine levels are ≤2 mg/100 mL and their diastolic blood pressure is <90 mm Hg.

Pregnancy often has no adverse effect on patients with chronic renal disease (Table 6.3). In general, patients with mild renal impairment (serum Cr <1.4 mg/dL) have relatively uneventful pregnancies provided other complications are absent. Patients with moderate renal impairment (serum Cr >1.4 to <2.5 mg/dL) have a more guarded prognosis with an increased incidence of deterioration of renal function. In about 50% of patients with renal disease, proteinuria manifests. An increase in proteinuria during pregnancy is not, by itself, a serious consequence. A brief review of the effect of pregnancy on common chronic renal disease is presented in Table 6.4. *The presence of hypertension before pregnancy or the development of hypertension*

Table 6.4.
Effect of Pregnancy on Common Chronic Renal Diseases

Renal Disease	Effects
Chronic pyelonephritis	No effect on renal lesion Increased incidence of symptomatic UTI
Urolithiasis	No direct effect on renal lesion UTI more frequent in some cases
Diabetic nephropathy	No effect on renal lesion Increased incidence UTI, preeclampsia
Chronic glomerulonephritis	No effect on renal lesion in the absence of hypertension Increased incidence UTI
Systemic lupus erythematosus	Often no effect on renal lesion, although about 33% of patients show some worsening of renal function Prognosis improves if SLE is in remission more than 6 months
Polycystic disease	No effect on renal lesion
Scleroderma	Unusual association with pregnancy, because onset of disease is more common in 4th or 5th decades No effect on preexisting renal lesion Disease may be fulminant if onset during pregnancy; postpartum exacerbation common
Periarteritis nodosa	Maternal and neonatal mortality rates high, because of frequent association with malignant hypertension; poor prognosis Therapeutic abortion should be presented as an option of management

during pregnancy is a more worrisome finding with respect to both the course of the patient's renal disease and the pregnancy.

Chronic renal disease is associated with an increased risk of first trimester spontaneous abortion. When pregnancy continues, there is an increased incidence of intrauterine growth retardation, so that serial assessment of fetal well-being and growth is recommended in most cases. Pregnancy following renal transplantation is generally associated with a good prognosis if at least 2 years have lapsed since the transplant was performed and thorough renal assessment reveals no evidence of active disease or rejection.

4. RESPIRATORY DISEASE IN PREGNANCY

The mechanical and hormonal changes associated with pregnancy alter the functional characteristics of the respiratory system (Fig. 6.1). Most women experience dyspnea of pregnancy in the latter half of pregnancy because of changes such as increased abdominal pressure associated with the expanding uterus, which cause decreased diaphragmatic excursion. Reassurance and advice to sleep in a semisitting position usually suffice for this problem.

Upper Respiratory Infections and Pneumonia in Pregnancy

Associated with the rhinovirus, adenovirus, coronavirus, parainfluenza virus, and respiratory syncytical virus, the incidence and severity of the viral common cold (upper respiratory infection; URI) is unchanged in pregnancy. After appropriate diagnosis excludes more serious problems such as influenza, mycoplasma pneumonia, and streptococcal pharyngitis, supportive care emphasizing hydration, rest, good diet, and antipyretics (e.g., acetaminophen) usually suffice. Decongestants such as pseudoephedrine should be avoided if possible in pregnancy, but they may be used sparingly if absolutely needed for symptomatic relief. Fetal involve-

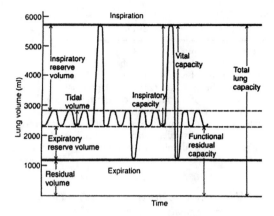

Figure 6.1. Respiratory changes in pregnancy.

ment is extremely uncommon because these mild viral respiratory illnesses do not have a viremic phase.

Pneumonia is an uncommon but serious complication in pregnancy. It is a major cause of nonobstetric maternal death, with a reported mortality of 3 to 4%. The most common causative organisms are *Streptococcus pneumoniae* and *Mycoplasma pneumoniae*, although *Haemophilus influenza*, and the fungi are seen infrequently. A rare but life-threatening pneumonia is caused by varicella. Beyond routine diagnostic steps, including chest radiographs, Gram staining of the sputum, complete blood count (CBC), electrolytes, and urinalysis, blood gas determinations are important to exclude maternal hypoxia that may adversely affect the fetus.

Management includes hydration, antipyretics (on a regular schedule when the maternal temperature is above 101°F), antibiotic therapy, respiratory toilet and oxygen supplementation if needed (as with low maternal Po_2, fetal tachycardia, and/or maternal respiratory distress), and evaluation of fetal well-being. Uncomplicated pneumococcal pneumonia is treated with penicillin G (600,000 units q. 12h. for 7 to 10 days); mycoplasma and Legionella pneumonia, with erythromycin (500 mg p.o. q.i.d. for 14 days); varicella pneumonia, with acyclovir if needed; and fungal infections with antifungal agents such as amphotericin B.

Asthma

Bronchial asthma is encountered in approximately *1% of pregnant patients*, approximately 15% of whom will have one or more severe asthma attacks during pregnancy. Edema of the bronchial walls, thick secretions, and smooth muscle contractions lead to reduced airway diameter, increased resistance, decreased expiratory flow rate, increased effort in breathing, and altered blood gases. The *effect of asthma on pregnancy is variable*, but includes increased risks of chronic hypoxia, intrauterine growth retardation, and rarely intrauterine fetal demise. Because of these associations, the management of asthma in pregnancy is directed toward minimizing the likelihood of exacerbations coupled with prompt treatment of any acute respiratory symptoms and serial assessment of fetal well-being.

Patients with *infrequent, mild asthmatic exacerbations* may be followed with minimal evaluation or treatment. These patients should be encouraged to avoid undue physical exertion and to obtain adequate rest, to avoid dehydration and exposure to allergens, and to seek immediate medical evaluation if symptoms of respiratory infection develop.

Patients with more *severe asthma* should be maintained on their prepregnancy medical regimens. Pregnant patients with an acute exacerbation require rapid fetal and maternal evaluation. Electronic fetal monitoring and/or biophysical profile will identify the fetus in stress, allowing appropriate intervention. Maternal evaluation includes physical examination, blood gas analysis, and chest x-ray. Eosinophils on sputum Gram stain suggest an allergic cause of the attack, whereas neutrophils suggest an infectious cause. Oxygen should be given if there is fetal tachycardia or the maternal Po_2 is <70 to 80 mm Hg.

A rapid response to inhalers containing β-adrenergic receptor stimulants such as epinephrine and isoproterenol (Isuprel) may be expected. Parenteral sympathomimetic therapy (epinephrine or terbutaline, 0.3 mL of a 1:1000 dilution s.c.) is also efficacious and may be repeated every 20 min. The addition of a xanthine preparation such as theophylline (which inhibits phosphodiesterase, increasing cAMP and controlling bronchospasm) or a β$_2$-receptor stimulator (such as terbutaline) is often helpful to reduce the frequency and severity of exacerbations. Theophylline may be conveniently given intravenously as a loading dose of 6 mg/kg over 20 to 30 min, followed by an maintenance dose of 0.9 mg/kg/hr, pending transition to oral therapy. Therapeutic serum theophylline levels range from 10 to 20 μg/mL. Antibiotics should be administered if there is maternal fever, purulent sputum, or an infiltrate on chest x-ray. If a patient is dehydrated, such an infiltrate may be obscure on x-ray for 12 to 24 hr until hydration is achieved.

Patients with severe asthma often require glucocorticoids: hydrocortisone, 7 mg/kg i.v. as a loading dose, followed by a maintenance infusion of 100 to 300 mg every 4 to 6 hr. Glucocorticoids cross the placental barrier and are associated with intrauterine growth retardation, a risk already exacerbated by the chronic hypoxia of severe asthma. Serial fetal evaluation for growth and acute monitoring for fetal well-being during exacerbations are essential.

Tuberculosis in Pregnancy

Tuberculosis is uncommon in pregnancy in the United States, and less than 200 cases of congenital tuberculosis have been reported. The causative agent, *Mycobacterium tuberculosis*, is acquired primarily by inhalation of droplets produced by infected individuals. Inactive infection (positive skin test and negative chest x-ray) is treated by isoniazid (300 mg p.o. q.d. for 1 year). Active infection (positive cultures, symptomatic infection) is treated by isoniazid (5 mg/kg/day p.o.) plus rifampin (10 mg/kg/day) as well as pyridoxine to combat the neuropathy often associated with isoniazid.

Sarcoidosis in Pregnancy

Maternal sarcoidosis is very uncommon in pregnancy, which is usually unaffected unless there is serious maternal cardiopulmonary dysfunction. Mild asymptomatic sarcoidosis requires no special maternal or fetal intervention, whereas severe disease (e.g., vital capacity <1 liter, pulmonary hypertension, Pa_{O_2}<55 mm Hg, dyspnea) requires vigorous maternal therapy and surveillance of fetal well-being.

Smoking in Pregnancy

It is estimated that 33% of pregnant women smoke, despite vigorous public education programs that explain the risks to the smoker (cancer, heart disease, etc.) and fetus. Pregnant smokers also place their infants at increased risk of decreased birth weight, intrauterine growth retardation, abruptio placentae, and perhaps long-term neurologic abnormalities (Table 6.5). *Patients*

Table 6.5.
Reproductive Effects of Smoking

Decreased fertility
Increased risk of spontaneous abortion
Increased risk of ectopic pregnancy
Decreased birth weight (average = 1 pound)
Increased risk of preterm delivery (preterm labor, premature rupture of membranes)
Increased risk of abruptio placentae and placenta previa
Increased risk of sudden infant death syndrome
Increased risk of developmental problems

should be counseled to stop or significantly reduce smoking during pregnancy.

5. CARDIAC DISEASE IN PREGNANCY

In the past, most pregnant patients with cardiac disease had rheumatic heart disease; patients with congenital heart disease usually died before reaching reproductive age. Presumably, modern treatment of congenital and acquired heart disease allows many patients to reach their reproductive years and become pregnant. As a result, patients with rheumatic heart disease and acquired infectious valvular heart disease (often associated with drug use) comprise only 50% of pregnant cardiac patients. Considering that pregnancy is associated with a cardiac output increase of 40%, the risks to mother and fetus are often profound for patients with preexisting cardiac disease. Ideally, cardiac patients should have preconceptional care directed at maximizing cardiac function. They should also be counseled about the risks their particular heart disease poses in pregnancy. Some patients may choose to avoid pregnancy; others may choose to terminate a pregnancy rather than assume the risks to themselves and/or their fetus; still others may choose to continue pregnancy under intense medical and obstetric management.

The *classification of heart disease* of the New York Heart Association is useful to evaluate all types of cardiac patients with respect to pregnancy (Table 6.6). It is a functional classification, which is independent of type of heart disease. Patients with septal defects, patent ductus arteriosus, and mild mitral and aortic valvular disorders often are in classes I or II and do well throughout pregnancy. Primary pulmonary hypertension, uncorrected tetralogy of Fallot, Eisenmenger syndrome, and certain other conditions are associated with a much worse prognosis (frequently death) through the course of pregnancy. For this reason, patients with such disorders are advised not to become pregnant.

General management of the pregnant cardiac patient consists of avoiding conditions that add additional stress to the workload of the heart beyond that already imposed by pregnancy, including prevention and/or correction of anemia, prompt recognition and treatment of any infections, a decrease in physical activity and strenuous work, and proper weight gain. A low sodium diet and resting in the lateral decubitus position to promote diuresis are especially helpful interventions. Adequate rest is essential. For patients with class I or II heart disease, increased rest at home is advised. In more severe classes, hospitalization and treatment for cardiac failure are often required. Coordinated management between obstetrician, cardiologist, and anesthesiologist is necessary for patients with significant cardiac dysfunction.

The fetuses of patients with functionally significant cardiac disease are at increased risk for low birth weight and prematurity.

The antepartum management of pregnant cardiac patients includes serial evaluation of maternal cardiac status as well as fetal well-being and growth. Anticoagulation, antibiotic prophylaxis for subacute bacterial endocarditis (SBE), invasive cardiac monitoring, and even surgical correction of certain cardiac lesions during pregnancy can be all accomplished if necessary (Tables 6.7–6.9). The *intrapartum and postpartum management of pregnant cardiac patients* includes consideration of the increased stress of delivery and postpartum physiological adjustment. Labor in the lateral position to facilitate cardiac function is often desirable. Every attempt is made to facilitate vaginal delivery, given the increased cardiac stress of cesarean section. Because cardiac output rises by 40 to 50% during the second stage of labor, shortening this stage by the use of forceps is often advisable. Conduction anesthesia to reduce the stress of labor is also recommended. Even with patients who are stable at the time of delivery, it must be remembered that an additional rise in cardiac output is manifest in the puerperium because of the additional 500 mL added to the maternal blood volume as the uterus contracts to a nonpregnant configuration. Indeed, the majority of obstetric patients who die with cardiac disease do so following delivery.

Table 6.6.
New York Heart Association Functional Classification of Heart Disease

Class I	No cardiac decompensation
Class II	No symptoms of cardiac decompensation at rest Minor limitations of physical activity
Class III	No symptoms of cardiac decompensation at rest Marked limitations of physical activity
Class IV	Symptoms of cardiac decompensation at rest Increased discomfort with any physical activity

Table 6.7.
American Heart Association (AHA) Recommendations for Prevention of Bacterial Endocarditis in Patients Undergoing Genitourinary Procedures

Drug	Regimen
	Standard Regimen
Ampicillin, gentamicin, and amoxicillin	Ampicillin 2 g i.v. or i.m.; gentamicin 1.5 mg/hr i.v. 30 min before procedure, not to exceed 80 mg, followed by amoxicillin, 1.5 g p.o. 6 hr later, or repeat paraenteral regimen 8 hr later
	Penicillin Allergic Regimen
Vancomycin, gentamicin	Vancomycin 1.0 g over 1 hr i.v. plus gentamicin 1.5 mg/hr 1 hr before procedure, not to exceed 80 mg; repeat 8 hr after initial regimen

Table 6.8.
Anticoagulation with Heparin

Loading dose	5000 U i.v. by rapid administration
Continuous infusion	Hourly rate to achieve 30,000–35,000 U/24 hr; adjust rate to achieve a PTT 1.5–2.5 times control
Long-term anticoagulation	17,5000 U every 12 hr; adjust dose to achieve aPTT 1.5–2.5 times control at 6 hr

Mitral valve prolapse may occur in as many as 5% of pregnancies. Occurring when the mitral valve prolapses into the left atrium during systole, this condition is usually asymptomatic except for a late stystolic murmur sometimes associated with a

Table 6.9.
Commonly Prescribed Cardioactive Drugs in Pregnancy

Drug	Indication	Adverse Fetal Effects	FDA Pregnancy Category[a]	Adverse Maternal Effects
Digitalis (digoxin)	Heart failure; arrhythmias, especially atrial fibrillation	Toxicity; neonatal death with overdosage	C	Arrhythmias; conduction disturbances; anorexia; emesis
Loop diuretics (furosemide, bumetanide)	Heart failure; hypertension; constrictive pericarditis	Growth retardation	C	Electrolyte disturbances
Thiazides (hydrochlorothiazide, direct acting)	Hypertension, heart failure, pulmonary	Neonatal jaundice; thrombocytopenia; hemolytic anemia; hypoglycemia	C	Electrolyte disturbances
Vasodilators (hydralazine, isosorbide)	Hypertension; angina	Teratogenic in animals; thrombocytopenia; leukopenia reported in newborn	C	Hypotension; nausea; diarrhea; headache
β-Adrenergic (propranolol, metropolol)	Angina; hypertrophic cardiomyopathy; hypertension; mitral valve prolapse; arrhythmia	During delivery: bradycardia; hypotension; oliguria; hypogycemia	C	Uterine contraction; bradycardia; hypotension; bronchospasm
Calcium-channel (nifedipine, verapamil)	Angina; hypertension; arrhythmia (verapamil)	Teratogenicity in small animals; no controlled human studies	C	Constipation (verapamil); bradycardia; conduction disturbances; hypotension
Antiarrhythmics Quinidine	Arrhythmia	Neonatal thrombocytopenia	C	Thrombocytopenia; life-threatening arrhythmia
Disopyramide			C	Arrhythmia
Lidocaine			C	Anticholinergic
Mexilitine			B	Epilepsy; drowsiness; confusion
Propafenone			C	GI disturbances; tremor; light-headedness; arrhythmia
Flecanide		Embryotoxic in animals	C	
Moricizine		Teratogenic in rabbits	C	GI disturbances; dizziness; AV block; arrhythmia

[a] B, negative animal studies; no human studies showing risk; should be used in pregnancy only if clearly indicated; C, animal studies show teratogenic effects; no human studies; should be used in pregnancy only if the potential benefit justifies the potential risk to the fetus.

late systolic click. Pregnancy is unaffected in this situation, with SBE prophylaxis being of questionable value. In a minority of patients, regurgitation is severe with left atrial and ventricular enlargement and dysfunction. Echocardiography will help determine the severity of disease. Blockage of β-adrenergic receptors with propranolol may aid in management of associated symptoms such as chest pain, palpitations, tachycardia, dysrhythmia, and anxiety.

Rheumatic heart disease remains a common cardiac disease in pregnancy. As the severity of the associated valvular lesion increases, these patients are at higher risk for thromboembolic disease, subacute bacterial endocarditis, cardiac failure, and pulmonary edema. A high rate of fetal loss is also seen in women with rheumatic heart disease. About 90% of these patients have mitral stenosis, whose associated mechanical obstruction worsens as cardiac output increases during pregnancy. Mitral stenosis associated with atrial fibrillation has an especially high likelihood of congestive failure.

Maternal cardiac arrhythmias are occasionally encountered during pregnancy. Paroxysmal atrial tachycardia is the most commonly encountered maternal arrhythmia and is usually associated with too strenuous exercise. Underlying cardiac disease such as mitral stenosis should be suspected when atrial fibrillation and flutter are encountered.

Peripartum cardiomyopathy is a rare but especially severe pregnancy-associated cardiac condition. It occurs in the last month of pregnancy or the first 6 months following delivery and is difficult to distinguish from other cardiomyopathies except for its association with pregnancy. A myocarditis is responsible for some of these cases, whereas in other cases no apparent etiology can be determined.

A classic patient at increased risk for peripartum cardiomyopathy is one who is black, multiparous, and over 30 years of age and who has a history of twins or preeclampsia. Management includes bed rest, digoxin, diuretics, and in some cases, anticoagulation. The mortality rate is high. The best clinical sign related to prognosis is cardiac size 6 months after diagnosis. In patients with persistent cardiomegaly, the risk of death in the near future is great. In patients in whom the heart size has returned to normal, the prognosis is better, although recurrence in a subsequent pregnancy is likely. Counseling the patient about the benefits of sterilization is warranted.

There are several uncommon cardiac conditions seen in pregnancy that warrant discussion. *Marfan's syndrome* is inherited in an autosomal dominant trait manner and is manifest by abnormality of the connective tissue. It is characterized by aortic aneurysm, ectopia lentis, and long extremities. Patients suffer dyspnea and chest pain and demonstrate an aortic disastolic murmur and midsystolic click. Rupture of the aneurysm makes pregnancy especially dangerous for these patients, as there is a 25 to 50% risk of maternal mortality

and a 50% chance that the offspring will inherit the disease. *Idiopathic hypertrophic subaortic stenosis* (IHSS) is an autosomal dominant trait with variable penetrance that results in significant aortic outflow tract obstruction. The normal fall in peripheral resistance in pregnancy is associated with an increase in this obstruction, leading to syncope congestive heart failure and sudden death. Echocardiography findings are diagnostic and include marked thickening of the ventricular septum and abnormal systolic movement of the mitral valve. Treatment is aimed at avoiding hypovolemia and maintaining venous return when a patient decides to continue a pregnancy.

6. GLUCOSE INTOLERANCE AND DIABETES MELLITUS IN PREGNANCY

Approximately 2% of pregnancies are complicated by diabetes that either develops during pregnancy or was antecedent to pregnancy. In either case, diabetes has significant implications for pregnancy, and conversely, pregnancy significantly affects diabetes.

Classification of Diabetes Mellitus

The White classification was used for many years to group cases of diabetes during pregnancy on the basis of age at onset of diabetes, duration of diabetes, and complications such as vascular disease. In recent years, the simpler *classification of the American Diabetic Association* (ADA) has become more commonly used (Table 6.10). In the ADA classification, three forms of glucose intolerance are identified. *Type I diabetes* refers to diabetes diagnosed in childhood and is often brittle and difficult to control. It is thought to result from an immunologic destruction of β cells of the pancreas. Diabetic ketoacidosis (DKA) is common in patients with this type of diabetes. *Type II diabetes* refers to the patient who has adult-onset glucose intolerance. These patients are frequently overweight and can often be controlled with a carefully followed diet. This type of diabetes is thought to result from exhaustion of the β cells rather than their destruction. *Gestational diabetes* refers to a new glucose intolerance identified during pregnancy. In most patients it is a reversible condition, although glucose intolerance in subsequent years occurs more frequently in this group of patients.

Table 6.10.
Classifications of Diabetes in Pregnancy

ADA Classification

Type I diabetes	Diagnosed in childhood, often brittle and difficult to control
Type II diabetes	Adult-onset glucose intolerance
Gestational diabetes	Glucose intolerance identified during pregnancy

The diabetic status is then described, e.g., type II diabetes with mild vascular disease

White Classification

A Gestational diabetes; onset in pregnancy

B Onset after age 20
Duration less than 10 years
No vascular disease

C Onset between ages 10 and 19
Duration 10–19 years
No vascular disease

D Onset under age 10
Duration >20 years
Some vascular disease; retina, legs

E Pelvic arteriosclerosis by x-ray

F Vascular nephritis

R Proliferative retinopathy

T Transplantation

Interrelationships between Pregnancy and Diabetes Mellitus

Effects of Pregnancy on Glucose Metabolism/Diabetes

Dietary habits are frequently changed during pregnancy, most notably with a decrease in food intake early in pregnancy because of nausea and vomiting and altered food choices. Several pregnancy-associated hormones also have a major effect on glucose metabolism. Most notable of these is *human placental lactogen* (HPL), which is produced in abundance by the enlarging placenta. HPL affects both fatty acid and glucose metabolism. It promotes lipolysis with increased levels of circulating free fatty acids and causes a decrease in glucose uptake and gluconeogenesis. In this manner, HPL can be thought of as an antiinsulin. The increasing production of this hormone as pregnancy advances generally requires ongoing changes to be made in insulin therapy to adjust for this effect.

Other hormones that have demonstrated lesser effects include *estrogen* and *progesterone*, which interfere with the insulin-glucose relationship, and *insulinase*, which is produced by the placenta and degrades insulin to a limited extent. These effects of pregnancy on glucose metabolism make the management of pregnancy-associated diabetes difficult. DKA, for example, is more common in pregnant patients.

Effects of Glucose Metabolism/Diabetes on the Gravida

With increased renal blood flow, the simple diffusion of glucose in the glomerulus increases beyond the ability of tubular reabsorption, resulting in a normal *glucosuria* of pregnancy, commonly of about 300 mg/day. With diabetics this may be much higher, but because of poor correlation with blood glucose concentrations, using urinary glucose is of little value in glucose management during pregnancy. This glucose-rich urine is also an excellent environment for bacterial growth so that pregnant diabetics have twice the incidence of *urinary tract infection* that nondiabetics have.

In addition to the added difficulties of glucose management and the increased risk of DKA during pregnancy, diabetics have a twofold increase in the incidence of *pregnancy-induced hypertension (PIH)*, or *preeclampsia*, over nondiabetics. Diabetic *retinopathy* worsens in about 15% of pregnant diabetics, some proceeding to proliferative retinopathy and loss of vision if the process remains untreated by laser coagulation (Table 6.11).

Effects of Glucose Metabolism/Diabetes on the Neonate

Infants of diabetic mothers (IDM) are at a three-fold increased risk of congenital anomalies over the 1 to 2% baseline risk of all patients. The most commonly encountered anomalies are cardiac and limb deformities. Sacral agenesis is a unique but rare anomaly for this group. *Excessive fetal growth, or macrosomia* (usually defined as a fetal weight in excess of 4500 g), is more common in diabetic pregnant patients because of the fetal metabolic effects of increased glucose transfer across the placenta. This excessive neonatal size can lead to problems with fetopelvic disproportion, requiring cesarean section or causing shoulder dystocia at the time of attempted vaginal delivery.

The *neonatal hypoglycemia* often encountered in these infants is thought to result from the sudden change in the steady-state arrangement, wherein increased glucose crossing the placenta was countered in the fetus by an increase in insulin levels. Once separated from the maternal supply of glucose, the higher level of insulin causes a significant neonatal hypoglycemia. In addition, these newborns are subject to an increased incidence of *neonatal hyperbilirubinemia, hypocalcemia,* and *polycythemia.*

Another complication of pregnancy in diabetic patients is an amniotic fluid volume increased above 2000 mL, a condition known as *hydramnios, or polyhydramnios.* Encountered in about 10% of diabetics, the increases in amniotic fluid volume and uterine size are associated with an increased risk of abruptio placentae and preterm labor. This condition is also a predisposing factor for *postpartum uterine atony.*

The risk of *spontaneous abortion* is similar in well-controlled diabetics and nondiabetics, but the risk is significantly increased if glucose control is poor. There is also an increased risk of *intrauterine fetal demise* and *stillbirth,* especially when diabetic control is inadequate (Table 6.11).

IDMs also tend to have a fivefold to sixfold increased frequency of *respiratory distress syndrome.* The usual tests of lung maturity are often poorly predictive for these infants.

Laboratory Diagnosis of Glucose Intolerance/Diabetes in Pregnancy

Approximately *1% of all pregnant patients are known to have been diabetic before pregnancy.* For these patients, obstetric diabetic management ideally begins before conception with the goal of optimal glucose control before and during pregnancy. Although there is controversy as to whether or not this causes a reduction in the risk of congenital anomalies, other maternal and neonatal benefits make it clear that a diabetic woman entering pregnancy should be at optimum glucose control if at all possible.

Gestational diabetes is usually identified by prenatal screening of all pregnancy patients, although it may be suspected in patients with known *risk factors* for gestational diabetes, including a history of giving birth to a infant weighing >4000 g, a history of repeated spontaneous abortions, a history of unexplained stillbirth, a strong family history of diabetes, obesity, and/or persistent glucosuria. *Of patients identified as having gestational diabetes, however, 50% do not have such risk factors.* This is the rationale for universal glucose screening in pregnancy.

The most commonly used screening test for glucose intolerance during pregnancy does not require the patient to be in a fasting state: 1 hr after consuming 50 g of glucose solution (Glucola), blood is drawn for plasma glucose determination. The currently recognized upper limit of normal for the *1-hr Glucola test* is 140 mg/100 mL. Patients whose glucose value exceed this limit generally require a 3-hr glucose tolerance test. After adequate carbohydrate loading for 3 days (generally, 150 g of carbohydrate/day), the first step in a *3-hr glucose tolerance test* is a fasting plasma glucose sample. Thereafter, the patient consumes 100 g of glucose in the form of Glucola and has blood drawn at 1, 2, and 3 hr thereafter for determination of plasma glucose levels. The upper limits of normal for the 3-hr Glucola test at 0, 1, 2, and 3 hr are, respectively, 105, 190, 165, and 145 mg/100 mL plasma (or for blood glucose, 90, 165, 145, and 125 mg/100 mL, respectively). Two or more abnormal values make the diagnosis of gestational diabetes. One abnormal value is considered suspicious, and testing is repeated in 4 to 6 weeks, depending on the gestational age at the time of the initial test. The standards are summarized in Table 6.12., which includes values in the more common international notation of millimoles per liter (equal to milligrams per 100 milliliters divided by 18).

In patients lacking any risk factors, the *1-hr Glucola screening is usually performed between 24 and 28 weeks gestation,* since glucose intolerance is generally manifest after that time. In patients with factors suggesting possible glucose intolerance, the testing is performed at the onset of prenatal care and, if normal at that time, repeated as the third trimester commences. Using this screening method, approximately 15% of patients will have an abnormal screening test. Of those patients who then proceed to have the standard 3-hr oral glucose tolerance test, approximately 15% will be diagnosed as having gestational diabetes.

Table 6.11.
Maternal and Fetal Complications of Pregnancy Associated with Maternal Diabetes

Maternal effects
  Hyperglycemia and glucosuria
  Diabetes ketoacidosis
  Increased incidence of urinary tract infection
  PIH/preeclampsia
  Retinopathy

Fetal/neonatal effects
  Congenital anomalies
  Macrosomia
  Hypoglycemia
  Hyperbilirubinemia
  Hypocalcemia
  Polycythemia
  Hydramnios
  Intrauterine fetal demise/spontaneous abortion

Table 6.12.
Glucose Tolerance Tests in Pregnancy

1-hr Glucola screening test
  50-g glucose challenge with no glucose preparation
  and with sampling at 1-hr postchallenge

Normal value: <140 mg/100 mL (<7.8 mM/L) plasma
glucose

3-hr glucose tolerance test
  100-g glucose challenge after 3 days glucose
  preparation with sampling as shown

Normal values:

	Less than stated mg/100 mL (mM/L) at:			
Time (hr)	Fasting	1	2	3
Plasma glucose	105	190	165	145
	(5.8)	(10.6)	(9.2)	(8.1)
Blood glucose	90	165	145	125
	(5.0)	(9.2)	(8.1)	(6.9)

Management of Diabetes during Pregnancy

Often overlooked in the overall management of a patient whose pregnancy is complicated by diabetes mellitus is the importance of *patient education.* The long-standing diabetic should realize that much tighter control of her glucose levels is advised during pregnancy, with greater attention and more frequent glucose monitoring. The impact of pregnancy on diabetes and vice versa must also be emphasized to the pregnant diabetic patient. The newly diagnosed diabetic should receive general diabetic counseling along with information about the unique features of the combination of diabetes and pregnancy. With either type of patient, intense management may be quite stressful, and all those involved with obstetric care should be mindful of the need for extra attention that many of these patients need.

The overall goal of management is to control glucose values within fairly circumscribed limits, to serially evaluate fetal well-being, and to time delivery to maximize outcome for both mother and fetus/neonate. *The mainstay of diabetes management is nutritional counseling about an appropriate diet.* Although the recommended increase in daily caloric intake has been proposed as 30 kcal/kg of ideal body weight, most pregnant diabetics end up on a daily caloric recommendation of 2300 to 2400 cal, composed of approximately 25% fat, 25% protein, and 50% complex carbohydrates. With careful attention to diet, most gestational diabetics do not require insulin.

Patients are generally followed with morning fasting and 2-hr postbreakfast plasma glucose de-

terminations, optimally obtained the morning of their office visit. For "ideal" control, the fasting plasma glucose should be maintained in the 90 to 100 mg/100 mL range and the 2-hr postbreakfast plasma glucose maintained at less than 120 mg/100 mL, although values up to 140 mg/100 mL may be acceptable in selected circumstances. Home glucose monitoring is now widely available in convenient kits that require a level of sophistication that most patients can achieve.

For patients who do not need exogenous insulin, the perinatal outcome is good. Pregnancy is allowed to continue to term with delivery planned at that time. Careful evaluation of fetal weight by ultrasonography is important, as the incidence of macrosomia remains increased in these patients.

Insulin therapy is required for the patient whose plasma glucose values exceed the limits noted for glucose tolerance testing or exceed the "ideal" levels for dietary management. Insulin does not cross the placenta and, therefore, does not directly affect the fetus. Instead, enough insulin is given to maintain normal blood glucose levels, because glucose does cross the placenta and in excessive concentration can harm the fetus. A mixture of short- and long-acting insulin is given in morning and evening injections so that there is insulin activity at all times, thus maintaining a uniform blood glucose level. A common method is to administer two-thirds of the dose in the morning and one-third in the evening. The insulin requirements of a pregnant patient are expected to increase because of increased "insulin resistance" as pregnancy progresses.

Once the patient has begun insulin therapy, plasma glucose values are obtained four times a day, typically at 7:00 AM, 11:00 AM, 4:00 PM, and 10:00 PM. Insulin doses are adjusted to maintain a fasting level under 100 mg/100 mL and other levels under 140 mg/100 mL. Understanding the duration of action of each type of insulin will provide a logical framework for adjusting insulin doses if needed. The fasting glucose reflects the dose of NPH insulin given before dinner on the previous evening. The 11:00 AM plasma glucose value reflects the morning regular insulin received 3 to 4 hr earlier. The 4:00 PM plasma glucose value reflects the morning NPH, and the 10:00 PM plasma glucose value reflects the evening doses of regular insulin. Incremental changes in glucose administration should be about 1 to 3 units at a time to avoid rapid changes in glucose values. A flow sheet is kept by the patient showing time and dosage of insulin and self-blood-sugar determinations as well as any comments about reactions, etc. (Fig. 6.2).

A fraction of hemoglobin known as hemoglobin A_{Ic} reflects glucose values over the preceding 6 to 8 weeks. This test has been used to monitor glucose control and to predict the likelihood of congenital anomalies in diabetics early in pregnancy. Overall, the value of this test has been disappointing in clinical use. Fructosamine, which reflects glucose values over the shorter interval of 2 to 3 weeks, also has limited clinical value.

Pregnant diabetics, especially type I diabetics, are prone to diabetic ketoacidosis. This serious complication can usually be avoided with frequent monitoring of blood glucose levels, attention to diet, careful insulin administration, and the avoidance of infections. Management of diabetic ketoacidosis is not different from management of DKA in nonpregnant patients and consists of adequate fluids, insulin, glucose, and electrolyte stabilization. Fetal death can accompany DKA, so electronic fetal monitoring of the fetus is essential until the maternal metabolic status is stabilized. At the other end of the spectrum, hypoglycemia is encountered at times, especially early in pregnancy, when nausea and vomiting interfere with caloric intake. Although hypoglycemia does not have untoward effects on the fetus, the symptoms and potential trauma that the patient may experience should be avoided.

Infections are more frequently encountered in pregnant diabetics. Periodic urine cultures should be obtained to detect asymptomatic bacteriuria, as the risk of urinary tract infection and pyelonephritis is twice that of the nondiabetic gravida. Patients should also be told to promptly report any other symptoms that suggest infection, so that aggressive treatment can be initiated.

Because of the risk of progressive retinopathy, pregnant diabetics should have an initial ophthalmologic evaluation and serial examinations during their pregnancies.

Fetal Assessment in Diabetic Pregnancy

Beginning at about 30 to 32 weeks of gestation, various measures to evaluate the fetal growth and well-being are undertaken. *Daily fetal kick counts* are an inexpensive and reliable screening test. Serial *nonstress testing and/or biophysical profile* measurements are also initiated, usually on a once or twice weekly schedule, but more frequently if clinical indicators warrant. Serial *ultrasonography* is performed to detect fetal anomalies and developing polyhydramnios and to follow fetal growth. Both intrauterine growth retardation and macrosomia are seen in IDM. When the estimated fetal weight by ultrasound is >4500 g, *macrosomia* is diagnosed; when >5000 g, cesarean section for delivery is recommended to avoid the risk of shoulder dystocia and similar birth trauma.

Delivery in Diabetic Pregnancy

In general, the goal is for the pregnant diabetic to deliver a healthy child vaginally. The adequacy of glucose control, the well-being of the infant, estimated fetal weight by ultrasound, the presence of hypertension or other complications of pregnancy, the gestational age, the presentation of the fetus, and the status of the cervix are all factors involved in decisions regarding delivery. In the *well-controlled diabetic with no complications, induction at term (38 to 40 weeks) is often undertaken.*

If an *earlier delivery* is deemed necessary for either fetal or maternal indications, fetal maturity studies are performed before effecting delivery. To avoid the potential delivery of an infant who might suffer respiratory distress syndrome, some clinicians require that two or more tests indicate fetal lung maturity, instead of a single test used for nondiabetics. Ideally, the presence of phosphatidylglycerol confirms the presence of fe-

DATE	INSULIN			BLOOD SUGARS				DIET/COMMENTS
				Fasting	Breakfast	Lunch	Dinner	
	NPH	AM	PM		AM	PM	PM	
	REGULAR							
	NPH	AM	PM		AM	PM	PM	
	REGULAR							
	NPH	AM	PM		AM	PM	PM	
	REGULAR							
	NPH	AM	PM		AM	PM	PM	
	REGULAR							
	NPH	AM	PM		AM	PM	PM	
	REGULAR							
	NPH	AM	PM		AM	PM	PM	
	REGULAR							
	NPH	AM	PM		AM	PM	PM	
	REGULAR							
	NPH	AM	PM		AM	PM	PM	
	REGULAR							
	NPH	AM	PM		AM	PM	PM	
	REGULAR							

Figure 6.2. Diabetic flow sheet.

tal lung maturity, but this phospholipid might not be present in detectable amounts even late in pregnancy.

The route of delivery is influenced by the estimated fetal weight. If the estimated fetal weight is >4500 g, cesarean section rather than attempted vaginal delivery may be considered, depending on maternal factors such as pelvic size. When the estimated fetal weight is >5000 g, the risk of birth trauma is significantly increased and cesarean delivery is usually recommended.

Whether the patient's labor begins spontaneously or is induced, *intrapartum glucose control* is generally managed by a constant glucose infusion of a 5% dextrose solution at 100 mL/Hr with frequent plasma glucose assessments. Short-acting insulin may be administered if needed, either by constant infusion or by intermittent injection. Somewhat surprisingly, patients whose glucose has been difficult to control through pregnancy often have very satisfactory levels of glucose in labor when so managed.

Postpartum Management in Diabetic Pregnancy

With delivery of the placenta, the source of the "antiinsulin" factors is removed. Human placental lactogen has a short half-life, and its effect on plasma glucose is evident within hours. Many patients do not require any insulin whatsoever in the first several days postpartum, and routine management generally consists of frequent glucose determinations using a sliding-scale approach with minimal insulin injections. For patients with gestational diabetes, no further insulin is required postpartum. In patients with preexisting diabetes, insulin is generally resumed at 50% of the prepregnant dose once a patient is taking a normal diet. Thereafter, insulin can be adjusted over the ensuing weeks, with requirements usually reaching the prepregnancy level.

Over 95% of gestational diabetics will return to a completely normal glucose status postpartum. Glucose tolerance screening is advocated 2 to 4 months postpartum for these patients to detect the 3 to 5% who remain diabetic and require treatment.

Diabetic women are best advised to have their pregnancies early in their reproductive lives, before the development of serious vascular complications. Contraception is best accomplished by barrier methods or intrauterine devices, as oral contraceptives may adversely affect maternal blood vessels.

7. ENDOCRINE DISEASE IN PREGNANCY

Thyroid Disease in Pregnancy

Thyroid function in pregnancy remains normal, although some clinical manifestations of pregnancy, e.g., warm skin and palpitations, may mimic thyroid dysfunction. The diagnosis of thyroid disease in pregnancy depends on the interpretation of laboratory tests. Total thyroxine (T_4) and $3,5,3'$-triiodothyronine (T_3) serum concentrations are elevated, and the $3,5,3'$-triiodothyronine resin uptake (T_3RU) is lowered during pregnancy because of estrogen-induced increases in thyroxine-binding globulin (TBG). Free T_4 (FT_4) and free T_3 (FT_3)

concentrations are unchanged, however. Calculation of the index for FT_3 and FT_4 aids in the diagnosis of hyperthyroidism and hypothyroidism, as a high value is consistent with hyperthyroidism and a low value, with hypothyroidism. Thyroid-stimulating hormone (TSH) concentration is unchanged in pregnancy (Table 6.13).

Hyperthyroidism complicates about 0.2% of pregnancies, and in 85% of cases it is associated with Graves disease, with the remainder of cases associated with acute and subacute thyroiditis, chronic lymphocytic thyroiditis (Hashimoto's disease), toxic nodular goiter, and hydatidiform mole and choriocarcinoma. Diagnosis is suspected with the classic stigmata of hyperthyroidism (nervousness, palpitations, heat intolerance, weakness, diarrhea, tachycardia, hyperreflexia, tremor, exophthalmos, and skin and hair changes), with or without goiter and confirmed by elevated thyroid function studies. Infants of hyperthyroid mothers are at increased risk for low birth weight.

Treatment with Propylthiouracil (PTU) blocks intrathyroid synthesis of T_4 as well as peripheral conversion of T_4 to T_3 and has the additional advantage of less placental transfer to the fetus than the other common medicine methimazole (Tapazole). Hyperthyroidism is usually brought under control in 3 to 4 weeks via the usual regimen of propylthiouracil: an initial dose of PTU of 300 to 400 mg/day in oral divided doses. After the patient is clinically euthyroid, the dosage may be tapered and the patient followed for evidence of relapse. PTU should be tapered to <100 mg/day at term. Skin rash, pruritis, fever, and nausea are complications in about 3% of patients, and if severe, methimazole may be substituted (30 to 40 mg/day in divided doses as initial therapy and 10 mg/day as the tapering target for the time of term pregnancy).

Fortunately, the dangerous complications of PTU therapy — granulocytopenia and agranulocytosis — are rare (0.2% of cases) and usually resolve with alternate therapy. The FT_4 is the first thyroid function parameter to fall, followed in a few weeks by FT_3I. Since the plasma half-life of T_4 is 7 days, laboratory testing at intervals of less than 1 week is not rewarding. Although *neonatal hypothyroidism* may result from suppression of the fetal thyroid with PTU, PTU has minimal transfer to breast milk and may be safely used while nursing. On the contrary, methimazole is secreted in breast milk and is not recommended during nursing.

Radioactive iodine is contraindicated during pregnancy because of its effect on the fetal thy-

Table 6.13.
Thyroid Function Studies during Pregnancy

Test	Nonpregnant Normal	Pregnant		
		Normal	Hyperthyroid	Hypothroid
Total T$_4$	Normal	Increased	Increased	Decreased
FT$_4$	Normal	Normal	Increased	Decreased
FT$_4$I	Normal	Normal	Increased	Decreased
Total T$_3$	Normal	Slightly increased	Normal to slightly increased	Normal to slightly decreased
FT$_3$I	Normal	Normal	Normal to increased	Normal to increased
T$_3$RU	Normal	Decreased	Increased	Decreased
TSH	Normal	Normal	Normal to decreased	High
TSAb[a]	Negative	Negative	Often positive	Negative

[a] TSAb, thyroid-stimulating antibody.

roid. Surgical therapy is rarely warranted during pregnancy.

Hypothyroidism is rarely encountered in pregnancy, as it is associated with anovulation and infertility. Diagnosis is suspected with the classic stigmata of hypothyroidism (tiredness, lethargy, weakness, cold intolerance, and constipation), with or without goiter, and confirmed by lowered thyroid function studies. Management with replacement thyroxine (Synthroid) is indicated (0.1 to 0.2 mg/day in a single oral dose to achieve clinical euthyroidism). TSH levels take 8 weeks to return to normal after initiation of therapy and hence have limited clinical value.

Parathyroid Disease in Pregnancy

The developing fetus requires the accumulation of up to 30 g of calcium before delivery. The placenta functions as a calcium pump that maintains fetal levels at about 1 mEq/liter higher than the maternal levels to fuel this requirement. Maternal extracellular calcium levels are in turn maintained by the balance of dietary calcium intake and excretion in urine and feces and calcium exchange from the maternal bone mass, regulated by parathyroid hormone (which shifts calcium into the blood) and calcitonin (which inhibits this shift). The diet of most Americans contains sufficient calcium in normal circumstances.

Hyperparathyroidism is rare in pregnancy but associated with significant perinatal morbidity and mortality. Neonates are often low birth weight, and more than 50% develop neonatal tetany when the maternal calcium supply is removed. Surgical

removal of the parathyroid adenoma found in 50% of cases or of the hyperplastic parathyroid glands is the treatment of choice. Oral phosphate therapy is used when surgery is contraindicated.

Hypoparathyroidism, even rarer than hyperparathyroidism in pregnancy, is usually associated with inadvertent removal of the parathyroids during thyroid surgery. Treatment includes vitamin D and calcium supplementation.

Other Endocrinopathies in Pregnancy

Adrenocortical insufficiency (Addison's disease), Cushing's syndrome, congenital adrenal hyperplasia, and hyperpituitarism and hypopituitarism are exceedingly rarely associated with pregnancy. *Diabetes insipidus* is also rarely encountered and has no direct effect on pregnancy. Patients with pituitary tumors are now being seen because of effective medical treatment of prolactinomas with bromocriptine. Bromocriptine may be discontinued in pregnancy and the patient followed closely for evidence of tumor growth (headache, changes in visual field), at which time surgical therapy may be indicated on an individual basis.

8. INFECTIOUS DISEASES IN PREGNANCY

Group B Streptococcus

The group B β-hemolytic streptococci are important causes of perinatal infections. Asymptomatic cervical colonization occurs in up to 30% of pregnant women, but cultures may be positive only intermittently even in the same patient. Approximately 50% of infants exposed to the organism in the lower genital tract will become colonized. For most of these infants, such colonization is of no consequence, but for about 2 to 3 infants per 1000 live births, significant clinical infection occurs.

There are two manifestations of clinical infection of the newborn. *Early-onset infection* is manifest as septicemia and septic shock, pneumonia, and/or meningitis. Such an infection is much more likely in premature infants than in term gestations. The mortality rate exceeds 50%. *Late-onset infection* occurs up to 4 weeks after delivery. Meningitis is the most common specific infection and the mortality in these cases is approximately 25%. Prematurity is not a factor for late-onset infection.

Routine cervical culture of patients and treatment for all cultures positive for group B streptococcus have failed to eliminate neonatal infections because of the ubiquitous nature of this organism. A common method of preventing group B streptococcus infections involves frequently obtaining cultures from patients in whom premature delivery is likely, i.e., those with premature rupture of membranes or those with preterm labor. While awaiting culture results, empiric treatment with penicillin or ampicillin is generally prescribed. Some centers recommend treatment of all patients with positive cultures, even those patients at term.

In the mother, postpartum endometritis may be caused by infection with group B streptococcus. The onset is often sudden and within 24 hr of delivery. Significant fever and tachycardia are present; sepsis may follow.

Syphilis

Syphilis is caused by the motile spirochete *Treponema pallidum*, which survives only in vivo. The spirochete is transmitted by direct contact, invading intact mucus membranes or areas of abraded skin. *T. pallidum* is generally considered to cross the placenta to the fetus after 16 weeks of gestation, although transmission has been documented at as early as 6 weeks of gestation.

Abortion, stillbirth, and neonatal death are more frequent in any untreated patient, whereas neonatal infection is more likely in primary or secondary rather than latent syphilis. Infants with congenital syphilis may be asymptomatic or have the classic stigmata of the syndrome, although

most infants do not develop evidence of disease for 10 to 14 days after delivery. Early evidence of disease includes a maculopapular rash, snuffles, mucous patches on the oropharynx, hepatosplenomegaly, jaundice, lymphadenopathy, and chorioretinitis. Later signs include Hutchinson's teeth, mulberry molars, saddle nose, and saber shins.

Serologic testing is the mainstay of diagnosis. Nontreponemal tests identify antibodies developed in response to nonspecific antigens from the immunologic inflammatory response to the spirochete. Test results are reported in quantitative titers, e.g., 1:8; the higher the titer, the greater the inflammatory response. Because false-positive venereal disease research laboratory (VDRL) and rapid plasma reagin (RPR) tests can be seen in chronic diseases such as leprosy, autoimmune diseases (e.g., lupus), and in drug addiction, treponemal-specific tests are used to confirm infection and identify antibody specific against *T. pallidum*. A positive result indicates either active disease or previous exposure. Darkfield microscopy can be used to identify the spirochete directly.

Treatment consists of a single 2.4-million-unit i.m. benzathine penicillin injection for primary and secondary infection or latent disease of <1-year duration. For latent disease of >1-year duration, three injections are given at weekly intervals. Patients with known penicillin sensitivity generally require desensitization, as penicillin is the only antibiotic that will cross the placenta in adequate amounts to treat the fetus. Posttreatment titers should be followed serially for 2 years. A fourfold rise in serologic titer indicates inadequate treatment or reinfection, and retreatment is indicated in either case. Response to therapy is again evaluated by following serologic titers.

Gonorrhea

Routine antepartum screening for *Neisseria gonorrhoeae* is universal. Recovery rates vary from 1 to 8%, depending on the population screened. Infection above the cervix, i.e., of the uterus (including the fetus) and the fallopian tubes, is rare after the first weeks of pregnancy. At delivery, however, infected mothers may transmit the organism, causing gonococcal ophthalmia in the neonate. In the past, such infection was a prominent cause of blindness, but currently used routine prophylactic treatment of the newborn's eyes with silver nitrate or tetracycline is very effective in preventing neonatal gonorrhea.

Bacterial Vaginosis

Bacterial vaginosis (BV) is the current term for vaginitis previously called *nonspecific vaginitis, Haemophilus vaginalis vaginitis, Corynebacterium vaginalis vaginitis,* and *Gardnerella vaginalis vaginitis*. The multiple names demonstrate the present understanding that bacterial vaginosis is a syndrome that involves a marked change in the vaginal flora, resulting in a loss of lactobacilli, an elevated pH, and an increase in other flora — particularly *G. vaginalis, Mycoplasma hominis,* and various anaerobic bacteria such as *Bacteroides, Peptostreptococcus,* and *Mobiluncus* species. As this is not an inflammatory vaginitis, increased numbers of white blood cells (WBCs) are not seen on wet preparation of the discharge (Table 6.14). Predisposing factors include but are not limited to multiple sexual partners, longer history of coital experience, and the presence of other sexually transmitted diseases, especially *Trichomonas vaginalis*. The evidence for the sexual transmission of bacterial vaginosis is unclear, as the treatment of male partners has not affected the incidence in their partners.

About 50% of women with bacterial vaginosis are asymptomatic. The others have variable complaints, including an increase in the amount of discharge and a "fishy" or "musty" vaginal odor and sometimes a thin gray to white discharge that stains the undergarments. Vulvar and vaginal pruritus are uncommon, because bacterial vaginosis is not an in-

flammatory condition. The diagnosis is made by finding three of four signs: (*a*) a thin homogeneous discharge that tends to adhere to the vaginal walls, (*b*) a vaginal pH elevated above 4.5, (*C*) a positive potassium hydroxide (KOH) "whiff" test, and (*d*) the presence of *clue cells* on microscopic examination. A whiff test is performed by mixing a few drops of 10% KOH with the vaginal secretions; if positive, the characteristic fishy odor is easily discovered. Clue cells, which are epithelial cells studded with large numbers of bacteria that obscure the cell border, are the single most reliable diagnostic criterion (Fig. 6.3).

Bacterial vaginosis has been associated with an increased incidence of pelvic inflammatory disease, posthysterectomy infection, postabortal pelvic inflammatory disease, preterm labor and delivery, premature rupture of membranes, amniotic fluid infection, and postpartum endometritis. Treatment with intravaginal or oral metronidazole (Flagyl; 500 mg p.o. b.i.d. for 7 days, or 1 g p.o. b.i.d. for 1 day; 1 applicatorful b.i.d. for 5 days) is effective therapy, although recurrence is common.

Genital Herpes

Herpes simplex virus (HSV) is a DNA virus that poses significant risk to the fetus/neonate. Herpes infections are categorized as either primary or recurrent; it is the primary form that poses the greatest risk to the fetus. Delivery through a lower geni-

Table 6.14.
Common Vaginal Infections

Characteristic	Normal	Infection		
		Bacterial Vaginosis	Candida Vulvovaginitis	Trichomonas Vaginitis
Common patient complaint	None	Discharge; fishy odor, possibly worse after intercourse	Itching, burning, discharge	Frothy discharge, bad odor, vulvar pruritus, dysuria
Vaginal pH	3.8–4.2	>4.5	<4.5 (usually)	>4.5
Discharge appearance	White, flocculent	Thin, homogenous, white, gray, adherent, often increased amount over normal	White, curdy ("cottage cheese"), sometimes increased amount over normal	Yellow, green, frothy, adherent, increased amount over normal
Amine odor (KOH whiff test)	Absent	Present (fishy)	Absent	Often present (fishy)
Microscopic	Lactobacilli	Clue cells, coccobacillary bacteria, no WBCs	Mycelia budding, yeast, pseudohyphae with KOH preparation	Trichomonads, WBCs >10 pf

tal tract with primary herpes virus infection is associated with neonatal infection in 50% or more of cases, a neonatal mortality of approximately 50% of those infected, and serious neurologic sequelae in nearly 75% of survivors. The risk of neonatal infection is much lower with recurrent infections, presumably because of a decreased inoculum size.

The diagnosis of HSV infection is suspected when clinical examination shows the characteristic tender vesicles with ulceration followed by crusting. Confirmation is by cell culture, with most positive results reported within 72 hr. Multinucleated giant cells can be seen on Pap smears or with the use of a Tzanck test in roughly 50% of cases.

If infection with herpes virus is suspected during the course of pregnancy, a culture from a lesion is generally obtained to confirm the diagnosis. In such patients, or any patient with a history of herpes virus infection, careful visualization of the lower genital tract is important at the onset of labor or when rupture of membranes occurs. If no lesions are identified, vaginal delivery is deemed safe. Cesarean delivery is recommended if herpes lesions are identified on the cervix, in the vagina, or on the vulva at the time of labor or spontaneous rupture of membrane (SROM). This is true whether or not the lesions are associated with primary or recurrent infection. Serial culturing for HSV near term does not predict if a patient will be shedding virus at delivery and hence should be abandoned as a routine antenatal test. Despite this, 1 of 20 infants delivered by cesarean section for this reason develop HSV infection. Acyclovir is used if symptoms are serious, although its safety in pregnancy has not been fully ensured.

Cytomegalovirus

Cytomegalovirus (CMV) infection affects 1% of births in the United States and is the most common congenital infection. CMV is a DNA virus that may be transmitted in saliva, semen, cervical secretions, breast milk, blood, or urine; CMV infection is often asymptomatic, although it can cause a short febrile illness. Like the herpes virus to which it is related, CMV may have a latency period, only to reactivate at a later time. Maternal seronegativity, and hence susceptibility, is inversely proportional to socioeconomic status.

Either primary or recurrent maternal infection is associated with a 0.5 to 1.5% risk of intrauterine infection, although severely affected infants are more often associated with primary seroconversion during pregnancy. About 10% of infected infants will demonstrate congenital defects of varying severity, including microcephaly with or without intracranial calcifications, intrauterine growth retardation, or hepatosplenomegaly. About 10% of asymptomatic CMV-infected infants will subsequently develop sensoneural hearing loss, chorioretinitis, mild neurologic effects, and dental defects.

The diagnosis is clinical and by exclusion. There is no reliable serologic testing presently available.

There is no treatment for maternal or neonatal CMV infection. Prevention of infection by habits emphasizing personal cleanliness and selectivity of personal contacts is important. Unlike herpes, active lower genital tract infection is not associated with increased risk to the neonate and is not an indication for cesarean section.

Rubella

Rubella (German or 3-day measles) is an RNA virus with important perinatal impact if infection occurs during pregnancy. Approximately 15% of reproductive-age women lack immunity to this virus and are susceptible to infection. A history of prior infection is unreliable in 50% of cases. The virus is spread by airborne droplets, with an in-

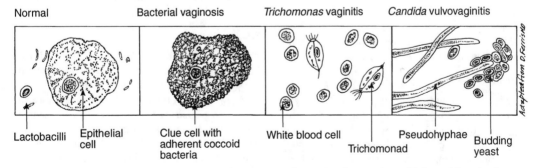

| Normal | Bacterial vaginosis | *Trichomonas* vaginitis | *Candida* vulvovaginitis |

Lactobacilli   Epithelial cell   Clue cell with adherent coccoid bacteria   White blood cell   Trichomonad   Pseudohyphae   Budding yeast

Figure 6.3. Wet mount of normal vaginal secretion and secretion from patient with bacterial vaginosis.

Toxo ZNFECTION
MORE SEVERE
MORE LIKELY

cubation period of 14 to 21 days postexposure. Clinical disease is associated with communicability from approximately 7 days before rash development through 4 days after the onset of rash. Once infection occurs, immunity is lifelong.

If a woman develops rubella infection in the first trimester, there is an increased risk of both spontaneous abortions and congenital rubella syndrome. Although 50 to 70% of babies with congenital rubella appear normal at birth, many subsequently develop signs of infection. Common defects associated with the syndrome include congenital heart disease (e.g., patent ductus arteriosus), mental retardation, deafness, and cataracts. The risk of congenital rubella is related to the gestational age at the time of infection such that up to 90% of babies acquire the syndrome if infection occurs at less than 11 weeks; 33% at 11 to 12 weeks; 25% at 13 to 14 weeks; 10% at 15 to 16 weeks; and 5% in the third trimester. Primary infection can be diagnosed using acute and convalescent sera for IgM and IgG antibodies.

Because of the fetal implications, prenatal screening for IgG rubella antibody is routine. Young women should be vaccinated remote from pregnancy if they are found to be susceptible. The vaccine uses a live attenuated rubella virus that induces antibodies in more than 95% of vaccinations. Because there is a 5% failure rate, the patient should be rechecked 6 weeks after vaccination to ensure antibody response. It is recommended that pregnancy be delayed 3 months following immunization. In women whose prenatal screen identifies a lack of rubella antibody, vaccination at the time of hospital discharge postpartum is recommended. Such management poses no risk to the newborn or other children; breast-feeding is not contraindicated.

Because there is no effective treatment for a pregnant patient infected with rubella, patients who do not have immunity are advised to avoid potential exposure. Human immune γ-globulin will not prevent or lessen the effect of infection; no antiviral therapy is available. Maternal treatment is supportive.

Toxoplasmosis

Infection with the intracellular parasite *Toxoplasma gondii* occurs primarily through ingestion of the infectious tissue cysts in raw or poorly cooked meat or through contact with feces from infected cats, which contain infectious sporulated oocytes. The latter may remain infectious in moist soil for more than 1 year. Only cats who hunt and kill their prey are reservoirs for infection, not those who exclusively eat prepared foods. Asymptomatic infection is common. Approximately 33% of reproductive-age women have antibodies to toxoplasmosis.

Infection in the first trimester causes more severe fetal disease than infection in the third trimester, but conversely, the rates of infection are less in the first than in the third trimester. About 60% of infants whose mothers are infected during pregnancy have serologic evidence of infection. Of these, 75% show no gross evidence of infection at birth. However, congenital disease can cause severe mental retardation with chorioretinitis, blindness, epilepsy, intracranial calcifications, and hydrocephalus.

Because infection is usually asymptomatic, diagnosis depends on serologic testing. Unfortunately, these tests cannot predict the time of infection with accuracy, so that the routine screening of patients is not recommended. Furthermore, such testing is of limited value in specific clinical situations. Fetal blood testing is possible when infection is likely to have occurred.

Treatment for suspected first trimester infection focuses on counseling about the risks of serious congenital infection and the potential option of therapeutic pregnancy termination. Treatment for patients for whom pregnancy termination is not an option or for those suspected of being infected later in pregnancy is a combination of sulfadiazine and pyrimethamine. However, pyrimethamine is teratogenic in laboratory animals in the first trimester so that its use is not recommended during this time.

Prevention of infection should be an important part of prenatal care, including the suggestion that all meats be thoroughly cooked and that cats be kept indoors and fed only store-bought foods. If a cat is kept outside, others should feed and care for the cat and its wastes.

AIDS

Approximately 10% of Americans infected with human immunodeficiency virus (HIV) are women, the group whose infection rate is rising most rapidly. Over 50% of these women are of childbearing age. The primary acquisition routes for women are sexual contact and intravenous drug abuse. More than 80% of pediatric HIV infection is the result of vertical transmission from mother to fetus.

Table 6.15.
Zidovudine Therapy to Reduce Vertical HIV Transmission

Regimen	Administration
Antepartum	500 mg p.o. daily from 14 to 34 weeks of gestation until labor
Intrapartum	i.v. administration during labor: 2 mg/kg loading dose followed by a continuous infusion at 1 mg/kg/hr until delivery
Postpartum	Oral administration of zidovudine syrup, 2 mg/kg, every 6 hr for 6 weeks

HIV is a single-stranded RNA-enveloped human retrovirus that has the ability to become incorporated into cellular DNA. The virus attaches to cells with high CD4 surface receptor concentrations such as lymphocytes, monocytes, and some neural cells. Via a reverse transcriptase, the virus encodes for DNA production, hence viral replication.

A few weeks after infection, most individuals have an acute seroconversion reaction. Antigen appears in a few weeks, followed quickly by antibody in most cases. Thereafter, the usual estimated latency period is almost 11 years. HIV infection becomes acquired immunodeficiency syndrome (AIDS) as the helper (CD4) lymphocyte count falls and the host becomes more susceptible. The presence of a defining opportunistic infection or a CD4 count <200 mm^3 is diagnostic of AIDS, after which the prognosis is poor, with survival more than 2 years uncommon.

The diagnosis of HIV infection is suspected with the receipt of a positive enzyme-liked immunosorbent (ELISA) test, based on an antigen-antibody reaction. The Western blot test, which identifies antibodies to specific portions of the virus, is performed to confirm the ELISA. Approximately 10% of patients will have an indeterminate Western blot, but when repeated in 4 to 6 months, the test is usually positive. The sensitivity and specificity of the combined tests are about 99%. Pretest counseling is important given the health, social, and financial ramifications of a positive test. Testing should be offered to women at high risk, especially those with multiple sexual partners and those who abuse drugs or consort with those who do. Given the reluctance of some women to reveal such behaviors, it may be prudent to offer all women testing in areas of low HIV infection prevalence but to recommend routine testing in areas with high prevalence.

Independent of other problems such as drug abuse, HIV infection appears to have no direct effect on pregnancy, including birth weight, gestational age at delivery, or abortion rates. Conversely, pregnancy does affect the immune system and may affect the course of HIV infection, although the effect is probably small.

Transplacental intrauterine transmission of HIV infection is the most significant means of fetal transmission. Between 25 and 33% of infants born to an HIV infected mother will become HIV infected. There is no advantage of cesarean section over vaginal birth, although the use of fetal scalp electrodes, fetal scalp blood sampling, and the like should be avoided in labor. The administration of zidovudine (SDV or AZT) to the mother during the antepartum and intrapartum periods and to the infant postpartum has been associated with a decrease in the rate of transmission of HIV from mother to infant, to under 10% (Table 6.15). Likewise, breast-feeding should be discouraged when the mother is infected, although the risk of breast-feeding is unclear.

9. THROMBOEMBOLIC DISORDERS IN PREGNANCY

An increase in key coagulation factors and venous stasis as a result of relaxed vasculature contribute to the development of thromboembolic disorders during pregnancy and the puerperium. This group of disorders includes phlebitis, both superficial and deep vein, and pulmonary embolism.

Superficial thrombophlebitis is the most common thromboembolic disorder in pregnancy, occurring in 1/500 to 1/750 pregnancies; three-fourths of cases occur in the initial 72 hr following delivery. With superficial phlebitis, redness and tenderness are accompanied by palpable veins in the involved area, usually the calves. Superficial phlebitis offers little maternal risk beyond discomfort and is treated with elevation of the legs, rest, heat, and mild analgesics.

Table 6.16.
Heparin Anticoagulation for Deep Vein Thrombophlebitis during Pregnancy

Route	Loading Dose	Maintenance	Subcutaneous Continuation of Therapy
Intravenous	100 U/kg	Continuous infusion: 1,000 U/hr to maintain a PPT that is prolonged 1.5–2 times the baseline for 7–10 days	Maintenance during the remainder of pregnancy (after acute therapy): 10,000–20,000 U every 12 hr s.c. and for first 6 weeks postpartum
Subcutaneous	150 U/kg	15,000–20,000 U s.c. every 12 hr to maintain a midinterval PTT of 1.5 times the baseline	Same as above

MEASURES DIAMETERS & LESS ✓Δ

The risk of *deep venous thrombosis* is probably increased in pregnancy and is also increased in the postpartum period from 0.15 to 3%. The clinical presentation may be varied, depending on the level of involvement in the lower extremities. Calf pain with tenderness to manipulation and edema can be present in differing degrees. Popliteal tenderness may be noted. Various techniques of diagnosis are available, none of which is entirely satisfactory. The gold standard is venography, but Doppler examination and impedance plethysmography can be helpful. The differential diagnosis includes rupture of a Baker cyst, muscle strain or hematoma, arterial insufficiency, arthritis, lymphangitis, myositis, bone disease, varicose veins, and superficial thrombophlebitis.

Treatment of deep venous thrombosis is with heparin anticoagulation (Table 6.16). Coumadin is reserved for the postpartum state, since it can be teratogenic in early pregnancy and may cause fetal bleeding in later pregnancy. With heparin, rest, and analgesia, symptoms of deep venous thrombosis subside in approximately 1 week, but heparin is continued well into the postpartum period.

Deep venous thrombosis is often a forerunner of *pulmonary embolism* (PE), although the initial presentation can be pulmonary in nature. Unfortunately, clinical findings of tachypnea, shortness of breath, ECG changes, and other so-called classic signs may be misleading. The differential diagnosis includes muscle strain, acute anxiety attack, and atelectasis.

When a pulmonary embolus is suspected, arterial blood gases should be obtained. Pao_2 <80 mm Hg suggests pulmonary embolism. Regardless of cause, patients with a diminished Pao_2 need oxygen therapy. The ventilation/perfusion lung scan is helpful in diagnosing pulmonary embolism. Results are often given as "low" or "high" probability

for PE; at times, pulmonary angiography is necessary to confirm the diagnosis.

Two-thirds of patients who die from a pulmonary embolism do so within 30 min of the acute event. The mortality of pulmonary embolism in pregnancy may be reduced to <1% with prompt anticoagulation. Initial anticoagulation is by intravenously administered heparin (100 to 120 U/kg loading dose, followed by a continuous infusion to maintain the PTT at twice its normal value). Coumadin may be used postpartum to maintain a therapeutic prothrombin time of 1.5 to 2.5 times the normal (e.g., 21 to 35 sec when the control is 14 sec). If the patient develops recurrent embolus despite anticoagulation therapy, vena cava ligation or insertion of a balloon/filter distal to the renal veins may be considered postpartum.

Septic pelvic thrombophlebitis occurs postpartum, the result of bacterial infection in the uterus, with spread to the ovarian veins, typically on the right. Patients under treatment for pelvic infection may have persistent fever spikes despite improvement in other aspects of infection, such as uterine tenderness. In some cases, a palpable and tender mass representing the right uterine vein can be identified. Response to heparinization is prompt, although spontaneous resolution can also occur.

10. NEUROLOGIC DISEASE IN PREGNANCY

Neurologic disease is relatively uncommon in pregnancy, occurring in <1% of cases. Most neurologic disease predates pregnancy, with some disorders being more common in pregnancy, including certain seizure disorders, cerebrovascular accidents, Guillain-Barré syndrome, Bells palsy, and herniation of an intervertebral disc. There is also a group of disorders directly associated with pregnancy: eclampsia, peripheral nerve compression syndrome, and chorea gravidarum.

Epilepsy in Pregnancy

Epilepsy occurs in approximately 0.5% of pregnant women and is characterized by paroxysmal changes in sensory, cognitive, emotional, or psychomotor function as a result of disordered brain function. Epilepsy may be caused by neurological injury, brain lesions, or idiopathic dysfunction. During pregnancy, elevated estrogen levels excite seizure foci, whereas elevated progesterone levels counteract this effect. As a result, epileptic activity is unchanged in 50% of patients, increased in 40% of patients, and decreased in 10% of patients. Prepregnancy frequency of seizures is the best predictor of seizure activity during pregnancy. Only 25% of patients who have been seizure free in the 9 months before pregnancy may expect a worsening of their condition.

Patients with epilepsy appear to have a three-fold to fourfold increased risk (6 to 10%) of bearing children with congenital anomalies. However, because many standard anticonvulsants also have teratogenic effects, the cause-and-effect relationships are uncertain. There is also an increased incidence of seizure disorders in the offspring of epileptic mothers (1/30). During a seizure, there is the additional risk of acute uteroplacental insufficiency and abruptio placentae.

Phenytoin (Dilantin) has been the standard anticonvulsant for the management of epilepsy. Its use during pregnancy is associated with the *fetal hydantoin syndrome*, which includes microcephaly, facial clefts and dysmorphism, limb malformations, and distal phalangeal and nail hypoplasia. Phenobarbital is also associated with cleft lip and palate, albeit at a reduced frequency. Because of these concerns for teratogenesis, *the most commonly used anticonvulsant in pregnancy is carbamazepine (Tegretol)*, which appears to be relatively safe with respect to congenital anomalies. Most anticonvulsants also cause bone marrow suppression and depression of vitamin K-dependent clotting factors so that there is a higher risk of fetal and neonatal hemorrhage. Supplemental folate and neonatal administration of vitamin K are indicated.

Cerebrovascular Accidents in Pregnancy

During pregnancy, the 4 in 100,000 incidence of cerebrovascular accidents (CVAs) in patients un-der age 35 and 25 in 100,000 in patients aged 35 to 45 is increased 13-fold. Resulting from several abnormalities such as aneurysms or vascular malformations, cerebral embolism, or central venous thrombosis, CVAs are usually of sudden onset with headache and visual disturbance followed by seizure or loss of consciousness and cardiovascular instability. Diagnosis is suspected from history and physical examination and is confirmed by imaging studies such as computed tomography and arterial angiography.

General treatment includes cardiorespiratory support for the mother and evaluation of fetal well-being when pregnancy is at a viable gestational age.

Specific treatment depends on the etiology of the CVA. Vascular aneurysms are often silent until rupture and more common after 30 years of age. The most common of these congenital defects of the media elastica of the vessels is the "berry aneurysm," which occurs at the circle of Willis. Aneurysms are more likely to rupture as pregnancy advances. Treatment is supportive and surgical if needed. Arteriovenous shunts are usually recognized in younger patients; treatment is surgical. Cerebral embolism is the most common cause of stroke in pregnancy. Predisposing factors include mitral stenosis with atrial fibrillation or cardiomyopathy with mural thrombi, cerebral vasculitis, thrombotic thrombocytopenic purpura, polycythemia, and sickle-cell disease. Treatment is identification and remedy of the underlying cause.

Myasthenia Gravis in Pregnancy

Myasthenia gravis is an autoimmune disease characterized by muscular weakness and easy fatigability as a result of circulating antibodies to acetylcholine receptors. The course of this uncommon complication of pregnancy (about 1 in 20,000 patients) is variable during pregnancy, with a tendency for exacerbation postpartum. Treatment consists of anticholinesterases (such as neostigmine or pyridostigmine) and avoiding neuromuscular blocking agents that might precipitate a crisis, especially magnesium sulfate. About 10% of infants will have transient myasthenic symptoms because of placental transport of maternal antibodies.

Multiple Sclerosis in Pregnancy

Multiple sclerosis is an autoimmune demyelination disease seen in about 5 in 10,000 pregnancies. It is characterized by a variable course dur-

Table 6.17.
Alterations of Gastrointestinal Function in Pregnancy and Their Clinical Manifestations

Alteration of GI Function	Characteristics	Clinical Manifestation
Esophageal	Reduced resting lower esophageal sphincter (LES) pressure Altered esophageal motility	Gastroesophageal reflux Heartburn Erosive esophagitis
Gastric	Decreased gastric emptying Increased residual volume	Increased risk of anesthesia-associated aspiration Decreased incidence of duodenal ulcer
Small bowel	Altered propulsive motility Increased transit time Increased activity/efficiency of brush borders	Stasis/bacterial overgrowth Pseudo-obstruction Sequestration of bile salts Increased absorption of some nutrients
Large bowel/colon	Reduced contractility Increased water and sodium absorption	Constipation Pseudo-obstruction

ing pregnancy and a threefold relapse rate in the postpartum period. Treatment is supportive. Infants of multiple sclerosis victims have a 3% lifetime risk of developing the disease compared with a 0.1 to 0.5% lifetime risk for the general population.

11. GASTROINTESTINAL DISEASE IN PREGNANCY

In response to incursion of the enlarging uterus into the abdominal cavity as pregnancy advances, the hormonal milieu of pregnancy, and increased nutritional needs, gastrointestinal function is markedly altered during pregnancy. Symptoms and findings may be associated with these physiological changes or may be related to disease. Alterations of gastrointestinal function and their clinical manifestations are reviewed in Table 6.17.

Nausea and Vomiting in Pregnancy and Hyperemesis Gravidarum

The majority of women experience some degree of nausea and vomiting during pregnancy. At least 66% of women experience nausea and 50% emesis in the first trimester, with the frequency of these symptoms lessening as the second and third trimesters ensue. Classically, symptoms are predominately present in the morning ("morning sickness"), but they may occur throughout the day and evening. A variety of causes have been suggested for these symptoms, although none has been clearly determined. Frequent small feedings and avoidance of foods that are unpleasant to the patient will

usually relieve symptoms to a manageable level. Prenatal vitamin supplements may aggravate these gastrointestinal symptoms and can be withheld during this time.

Symptoms of nausea and vomiting in early pregnancy should not be presumed to be morning sickness. It is necessary to rule out other more serious causes of such symptoms. Fortunately, nausea and vomiting in pregnancy is short lived and most patients can look forward to cessation of symptoms as the second trimester begins.

A variety of antiemetics can be prescribed if the above measures fail to provide adequate relief, but unfortunately, none is completely effective and all carry risks (Table 6.18). Of historical interest is the compound medication Bendectin, a combination of the antihistamine doxylamine and vitamin B$_6$ (pyridoxine), which was reasonably effective as an antiemetic in pregnancy. Although there is no evidence to support an increased teratogenic risk for the compound, medicolegal concerns led the manufacturer to withdraw the medication from the market.

Hyperemesis gravidarum (intractable emesis during pregnancy) is a more severe form of nausea and vomiting, occurring in approximately 4 out of 1000 pregnancies; it is associated with severe symptoms as well as weight loss, dehydration, ketosis, and electrolyte disturbances. Hospitalization and treatment with balanced crystalloid solutions and necessary electrolytes and "NPO status" will generally eliminate symptoms and correct metabolic disturbances in a short time. Diet can then be reinstituted slowly and progressively. Recurrences sometimes necessitate repeat hospitalizations.

Table 6.18.
Antiemetics in Pregnancy

Antiemetic	Action	Regimen	FDA Pregnancy Category[a]
Metoclopramide (Reglan)	Stimulates motility of upper GI tract and increases LES	10 mg p.o. q.i.d., p.c. and h.s.	B
Meclizine (Antivert)	Antihistamine; inhibits spasmogenic effects of histamine	12.5–25 mg p.o. q.i.d.	B
Promethazine (Phenergan)	A phenothiazine derivative with lessened psychoactive action; an H_1 receptor blocker; also has sedative and antiemetic effect	25 mg q. 4–6h. p.o. or p.r.	C

[a] B, negative animal studies; no human studies showing risk; should be used in pregnancy only if clearly indicated; C, animal studies show teratogenic effects; no human studies; should be used in pregnancy only if the potential benefit justifies the potential risk to the fetus.

Gastroesophageal Reflux in Pregnancy

At least 50% of patients experience gastroesophageal reflux in the third trimester of pregnancy. It does not alter the course of pregnancy, nor is it detrimental to the fetus; it is, however, uncomfortable for the patient. The cause is a combination of decreased intraabdominal space and increased pressure from the enlarging uterus as well as the effect of progesterone to decrease lower esophageal sphincter tone. ↑Gastric Retention Time

Treatment includes reassurance, elevating the head of the patient's bed, small more frequent meals, and liberal use of antacids at bedtime and after meals. Metoclopramide (Reglan) is especially useful as it increases lower esophageal sphincter (LES) and is an antiemetic (see Table 6.18). Antacids such as magnesium and aluminum hydroxide preparations (15 to 30 mL p.o. q.h.s. and p.c.) are also helpful.

Peptic Ulcer Disease in Pregnancy

Peptic ulcer disease is an uncommon new diagnosis in pregnancy, more often encountered as a preexisting condition. Peptic ulcers usually either improve somewhat or remain symptomatically unchanged. The diagnosis is suggested by a history of dyspepsia, which includes epigastric pain relieved by food or antacids. Empiric treatment with antacids is appropriate; upper gastrointestinal radiographs or endoscopy should be used when such therapy does not cause improvement. Small more frequent meals and avoiding irritating foods, alcohol, and cigarettes are also mainstays of management.

Gastrointestinal (GI) hemorrhage resulting from peptic ulcer is managed by nasogastric suction and ice water lavage, blood replacement as needed, monitoring of fetal well-being as appropriate by gestational age, and surgery if the bleeding is unresponsive to these medical managements.

Ptyalism in Pregnancy

Ptyalism, or excessive salivation, is especially annoying for a small number of patients, sometimes approaching 1 liter production per day. Medical treatment with tincture of belladonna or atropine alter ptyalism only slightly so that reassurance of the time-limited nature of the problem is a mainstay of management.

Pica

Pica, a craving for nonfoodstuffs such as laundry starch, ice, dirt, or clay, is common in pregnancy. It is attributed to certain ethnic groups but its true incidence is hidden in denial. Pica can be deleterious when ingestion of the materials interferes with needed food and mineral intake, resulting in anemia and/or sequelae of poor nutrition. Treatment consists of detection, counseling, encouragement to control pica, and replacement therapy, including iron, folic acid and prenatal vitamins.

Pancreatitis in Pregnancy

Pancreatitis complicates less than 0.1% of pregnancies, usually in the third trimester during the peak rise in plasma triglycerides or in patients with cholelithiasis, alcohol abuse, severe pregnancy-induced hypertension, and preexisting liver disease. There is considerable maternal morbidity (congestive heart failure, pulmonary effusion, hypotension, hyperglycemia, and acidosis) and mortality (estimated at 10%); the perinatal mortality rate is 10 to 40%.

The diagnosis is suspected in patients with nausea, emesis, and epigastric pain radiating to the back. Physical examination is usually unremarkable, although epigastric left upper quadrant or flank tenderness, flani ecchymosis (Grey-Turne's sign), and fever may be noted. The differential diagnosis includes preeclampsia, cholecystitis, hepatitis, duodenal ulcer, gastroenteritis, and intestinal obstruction. Laboratory confirmation includes a transient rise in serum amylase and lipase levels — to >200 U/100 mL within the first 12 hr after the onset of pain, with return to normal levels within 48 hr — as well as hypocalcemia. Treatment includes supportive care; nothing by mouth, to suppress pancreatic secretions; nasogastric suction; intravenous fluid therapy, to correct electrolyte imbalance, hyperglycemia (with insulin), or hypocalcemia (with calcium gluconate) and to prevent hypovolemia; and analgesia. Antibiotics are indicated if there is a fever, usually ampicillin (2 g q. 6h. i.v.). Surgical resection and drainage of pseudocysts and abscesses and/or intraperitoneal lavage to reduce intraperitoneal irritation may be required in severe cases. Vigorously treated, however, pancreatitis is usually self-limited in pregnancy.

Appendicitis in Pregnancy

Appendicitis complicates about 0.1% of pregnancies and is the most common surgical emergency in pregnancy. Maternal mortality is 2% in the first and second trimesters and approaches 10% in the third trimester compared with 0.25% in nonpregnant patients. The increased mortality is due primarily to delay in diagnosis and to a doubling in the rate of perforation during pregnancy. Premature labor is the most common perinatal complication.

The diagnosis is suspected when nausea and vomiting is preceded by anorexia and associated with periumbilical or right lower quadrant pain. The gravid uterus may mask the diagnosis by altering the position of the appendix and sequestering inflammatory exudate. The differential diagnosis in the first trimester includes ectopic pregnancy, salpingitis, ruptured corpus luteum cyst, dermoid cyst, and adnexal torsion. Late in preg-

nancy, round ligament pain, preterm labor, abruptio placentae, and degenerating leiomyoma of the uterus are more likely diagnostic possiblities.

Appendectomy with or without vigorous antibiotic therapy is necessary. Electronic fetal monitoring during and after surgery is essential with tocolysis if labor ensues in a preterm pregnancy. Whether to administer tocolytics prophylactically when operating on a preterm patient is controversial.

Inflammatory Bowel Disease in Pregnancy

Regional enteritis is seen in about 0.02% and ulcerative colitis in about 0.01% of childbearing women and is also seen on occasion in pregnancy. The morbidity of the former is related primarily to abdominal abscesses or intestinal obstruction and the latter to toxic megacolon, colonic perforation, and colonic stricture.

Regional enteritis is a chronic inflammatory condition of the bowel that causes diarrhea and pain and malabsorption of iron and vitamin B_{12} if the terminal ileum is involved. Regional enteritis appears to be unaffected by pregnancy and vice versa. Treatment consists of rest and a high-calorie, high-protein, low-fat diet. Antidiarrheals such as diphenoxylate (Lomotil; 10 mL q. 6–8h.) help with that symptom. Prednisone can be used for acute exacerbations. Cesarean birth should be considered if there are perirectal abscesses and fistulae.

Ulcerative colitis is a more acute condition than regional enteritis and is associated with bloody, watery diarrhea. Pregnancy does not exacerbate the disease, whereas severe ulcerative colitis is associated with an increased risk of spontaneous abortion and premature labor. Treatment consists of a low residue diet, antidiarrheals such as diphenoxylate, steroids, and sulfasalazine (Azulfidine; starting with 1 mg/day p.o. and increasing to 2 to 4 mg/day) for its antiinflammatory and immunosuppressive effect.

12. DENTAL DISEASE IN PREGNANCY

Pregnancy-associated gingivitis is encountered in about 50% of pregnancies. The gums are hypertrophied, red, and inflamed because of the hormonal changes of pregnancy. They are uncomfortable, bleed easily, and are more susceptible to poor dental hygiene. Pregnancy-associated gingivitis is related to poor dental hygiene combined with the hormonal changes of pregnancy. Occasionally an inflammatory growth will appear in the papilla area between the teeth. Misnamed "pregnancy tumor," this is simply a pyogenic granuloma that exacerbates the pregnancy-associated gingivitis. Good dental hygiene and astringent mouthwashes offer some relief to this problem, which regresses with the end of pregnancy.

Emergency and routine dental care can be provided as usual, although many dentists try to minimize intervention during pregnancy. *Local anesthetics without epinephrine offer little risk*. Other modalities such as nitrous oxide are best avoided during pregnancy.

13. HEPATOBILIARY DISEASES IN PREGNANCY

Hepatitis

Hepatitis is the major cause of jaundice (bilirubin >4 mg/dL) during pregnancy. Viral hepatitis takes several forms, including the more common hepatitis A (HAV), hepatitis B (HBV), and hepatitis C (HCV; parenterally transmitted non-A, non-B hepatitis) and the less common hepatitis D (HDV; also called the δ agent) and hepatitis E (HEV; formerly known as epidemic or waterborne non-A, non-B hepatitis). Hepatitis A is spread by ingestion of contaminated food or water and by fecal-oral transmission and accounts for approximately 10% of cases of hepatitis in pregnancy. It has an incubation period of 15 to 50 days, and the symptoms and signs are often vague. There is little, if any, effect on pregnancy. Pregnant women exposed to hepatitis A can be given γ-globulin, following the guidelines for nonpregnant adults.

Hepatitis C often follows transfusion with blood or blood components and has an incubation period of approximately 50 days. It can also spread through sexual contact. Many cases of hepatitis C are mild; its effects on pregnancy are similar to but much less severe than hepatitis B. Hepatitis D is uncommon but often associated with a fulminant hepatitis. Hepatitis E is clinically similar to hepatitis A but milder, except in pregnancy where maternal mortality may be quite high. Hepatitis C, D, and E combined account for approximately 10% of cases of hepatitis in pregnancy.

Hepatitis B is the most common hepatitis in pregnancy, accounting for approximately 80% of cases. It is spread by infected blood or serous body products via percutaneous or permucosal routes and has an incubation period of 15 to 50 days. Groups at special risk for HBV include intravenous drug users, homosexuals, health care workers and others who come in contact with potentially infected materials on a regular basis, and individuals with multiple sexual partners or whose partners include high-risk individuals. Hemophiliacs and others receiving blood components regularly are also at risk.

The course of hepatitis B infection is not significantly affected by pregnancy. There is a wide range of clinical presentations, from asymptomatic illness through a mild episode with low-grade fever and nausea to hepatic failure, coma, and death in unusual circumstances. Serum chemistry abnormalities include elevated serum transaminase levels, often above 1000 mU/mL, and an increased serum albumin. Most patients recover completely within 3 to 6 months, and less than 10% develop chronic infection with circulating HBV antigens.

Vertical transmission to the fetus at delivery is now recognized to pose significant danger to the neonate. Untreated, the majority of infants who are infected become chronic carriers capable of transmitting the infection to others. Hepatic carcinoma and cirrhosis are other unusual sequelae. These adverse outcomes have led to the recent institution of universal screening of all pregnant patients for the presence of the hepatitis B surface antigen (HBsAg). Women so identified should also undergo testing for antibodies and for the presence of the envelope (e) antigen, which is associated with an 80% risk of fetal transmission and of the infant becoming a chronic carrier.

If its mother is identified as a carrier or develops hepatitis B during pregnancy, the neonate should receive both active immunization for hepatitis (hepatitis B vaccine) and passive immunization with hepatitis B immunoglobulin (HBIG). Hepatitis B recombinant vaccine is recommended for pregnant women who are at high risk for contracting HBV. HBIG should be given to susceptible pregnant women within 48 hr of exposure to HBV.

During pregnancy, the diagnosis of hepatitis is made on the basis of liver function studies as well as the presence or absence of antigens and corresponding antibodies. Treatment is supportive, with hospitalization usually being recommended until patients are capable of maintaining good nourishment.

Cholestasis in Pregnancy

Cholestasis of pregnancy (pruritus gravidarum) occurs in <0.1% of pregnancies and is the second most common cause of jaundice in pregnancy. It usually occurs in the third trimester, although it is encountered throughout pregnancy. The etiology is unclear but probably involves an increased hepatic sensitivity to estrogen, resulting in cholestasis without the hepatocellular damage seen in cholecystitis or cholelithiasis.

Patients present with generalized, often intense, pruritus associated with fatigue, jaundice, and often dark urine. Laboratory evaluation reveals serum bile acid levels elevated to 10 to 100 times normal, elevated serum alkaline phosphatase to 10 times normal, and bilirubin levels elevated up to 5 mg/mL.

The main effect of cholestasis of pregnancy is the discomfort of intense pruritis. Occasional coagulation abnormalities as a result of decreased vitamin K absorption have been reported.

Treatment consists of antipruritics such as diphenhydramine hydrochloride (Benadryl) or hydroxyzine hydrochloride (Vistaril), topical skin preparations containing lanolin as a base, and reassurance. Cholestyramine may decrease the bile acid levels but is associated with gastrointestinal disturbances. Phenobarbital may be tried if cholestyramine is not effective in inducing hepatic microsomal function. Recurrence in future pregnancies and with use of oral contraceptives is likely.

Cholelithiasis in Pregnancy

Cholelithiasis occurs at the same incidence of 0.1% in pregnancy as without pregnancy. Properly treated, maternal and fetal outcomes are uncompromised, whereas failure to treat cholelithiasis effectively is associated with an increased fetal mortality rate. The pathogenesis and pathophysiology in pregnancy is also unchanged, with supersaturation of bile with cholesterol being followed by crystallization and formation of gallstones, uncomfortable distention of the gallbladder, and blockage of the cystic duct, which causes biliary colic and jaundice. An association with fatty food intake is noted. In pregnancy, increased estrogen/progesterone concentrations may increase the

concentration of cholesterol and the rate of stone formation.

The clinical history of food-associated colic and laboratory evidence of elevated liver enzymes and bilirubin is confirmed by ultrasonography of the gallbladder.

Asymptomatic cholelithiasis in pregnancy requires no treatment except admonitions about fatty food intake. Biliary colic is treated with nasogastric suction, hydration, analgesia, and antibiotics if needed. Lack of improvement or the development of pancreatitis is usually indication for cholecystectomy.

Acute Fatty Liver of Pregnancy

Acute fatty liver of pregnancy is a rare complication of pregnancy, but its severity and maternal mortality rate of 30% make its timely diagnosis and treatment of importance. Acute fatty liver usually occurs late in pregnancy in primigravidas and is characterized by vague gastrointestinal symptoms becoming worse over several days' time. Thereafter headache, mental confusion, and epigastric pain may ensue, and if untreated, there may be rapid development of coagulopathy, coma, multiple organ failure, and death. Laboratory findings include an initial modest elevation in bilirubin and an elevation of transaminase levels, but the magnitude of these elevations is not great and the disease may be misdiagnosed as being minor in nature. Treatment of this serious complication is correction of coagulopathy and electrolyte imbalances, cardiorespiratory support, and delivery as soon as feasible by the vaginal route, if possible.

14. ABDOMINAL SURGICAL CONDITIONS AND ABDOMINAL TRAUMA IN PREGNANCY

Abdominal Surgical Conditions in Pregnancy

Careful management of patients with surgical conditions should provide optimal care for the mother and consideration for optimal perinatal outcome. Any pregnant patient presenting with a potential surgical condition should be fully evaluated regardless of her pregnant status, i.e., necessary radiographic or other studies should not be avoided just because the patient is pregnant. For procedures such as x-rays of the chest, an abdominal shield may be used to avoid unnecessary exposure to the fetus. In general, exposure to low doses of radiation are considered safe for the fetus, especially when compared with the misdiagnosis of a serious surgical condition.

The fetus should be monitored as thoroughly as possible consistent with the stage of gestation and need for intervention. For a viable pregnancy this means electronic fetal monitoring for fetal heart tones and the possibility of uterine activity. The supine position should be avoided, if possible, to prevent the supine hypotensive syndrome. Oxygen administration may be helpful and is certainly not harmful. In general, those caring for these patients should be constantly aware of both maternal and fetal considerations. For example, in pregnancy the residual lung volume is diminished, providing less reserve for respiratory function. As another example, delayed gastric emptying makes aspiration more likely should surgery be necessary.

Abdominal Trauma in Pregnancy

Abdominal trauma, regularly encountered in pregnancy, is most commonly associated with automobile accidents, falls, and interpersonal violence. Prevention includes wearing of seat belts (both lap and shoulder harness) and avoiding situations and activities in which falls are likely.

A special type of trauma that must be kept in mind is physical abuse. This may occur in up to 10% of pregnant patients and may not be divulged by the patient. Frequently, a variety of somatic complaints, including abdominal symptoms, may be offered or excuses given for obvious signs of trauma.

From an obstetric viewpoint, the most important consideration about abdominal trauma is the possibility of abruptio placentae. Direct trauma to the uterus is not necessary for a shearing effect on the placenta to occur. Patients whose pregnancies have proceeded beyond the point of viability must be monitored for several hours following abdominal trauma to detect possible fetal heart rate abnormalities, resulting from diminished oxygenation because of the abruption. Because of this risk, these patients should be monitored while lying on their side so as to deflect the large uterus away from the great vessels where pressure may impede cardiac function and hence uteroplacental blood flow.

Monitoring for vaginal bleeding is important, although the bleeding may be concealed in some cases. Uterine tenderness may be a sign of abruption. Some degree of fetal-maternal hemorrhage may occur in 5 to 25% of cases; it is usually of insignificant volume. A test to detect fetal-maternal hemorrhage, such as the Kleihauer-Betke test, should be performed, and RhoGAM administered as appropriate. In some cases, coagulation studies are obtained to detect subtle changes associated with placental abruption. Tetanus toxoid should be administered to pregnant patients following the same guidelines as those for nonpregnant patients.

Uterine rupture is usually associated with only very severe direct abdominal trauma. Diagnosis and treatment is as described for uterine rupture associated with labor. Fetal injury from abdominal trauma is very rare, with fetal death usually being associated with impaired maternal status or abruptio placentae.

15. SUBSTANCE ABUSE IN PREGNANCY

The use of a variety of legal and illicit drugs and legal but potentially harmful substances during pregnancy has climbed at an alarming rate in recent years. Management of patients involved in the use and abuse of these materials is compounded by a variety of social problems, frequently inadequate prenatal care and poor nutrition. Despite these frustrations, help and encouragement to these patients must be given at every opportunity, as the consequences are so significant to the mother and her offspring.

Smoking

A decrease in the incidence of smoking has occurred more slowly in women than in men, and regrettably, young women now appear to be initiating smoking at an earlier age than in years past. It is estimated that 25 to 30% of reproductive-age women smoke, the incidence doubling if there is concurrent use of other substances of abuse. A variety of adverse pregnancy outcomes have been associated with cigarette smoking (see Table 6.5). These complications result from the effects of carbon monoxide and altered placental perfusion caused by vasoconstriction induced by nicotine. The pregnant woman who smokes endangers not only herself but also her unborn child. For some women, pregnancy provides a unique opportunity to cease or at least reduce smoking, an incentive that may be aided by the diminished appetite and nausea seen in pregnancy.

Alcohol

Ethyl alcohol is a potent central nervous depressant that has social uses which are found pleasant by many and has great potential for overuse and abuse by others. One beer, one glass of wine, or one standard mixed drink contains approximately 0.5 oz of absolute ethyl alcohol. A total of 75% of American use alcohol to some extent, including an unknown percent of pregnant women. With the ingestion of approximately 3 oz of alcohol daily during pregnancy, *fetal alcohol syndrome* is observed (Table 6.19); effects consist of prenatal and postnatal growth deficiency, mental retardation, behavioral disturbances, and congenital defects such as craniofacial anomalies.

In theory, lesser consumption in pregnancy is associated with lesser effects — described as *fetal alcohol effects* — which include minor anomalies, moderate growth deficiency, "mild" mental retardation, and subtle behavioral changes. In fact, it is unknown what the lower threshold for safe use of alcohol in pregnancy is, so that the best recommendation is abstinence during pregnancy. *Indeed, excluding genetic causes, alcohol use in pregnancy is the most common cause of mental retardation.* The performance defects associated with fetal alcohol syndrome include an average IQ of 60 to 70 for severely affected infants, fine motor dysfunction, infant irritability, and hyperactivity in later childhood. The risk of spontaneous abortion is also increased in patients consuming alcohol.

Ethanol freely crosses the placenta and fetal blood-brain barrier, presumably causing its deleterious effects by direct toxicity of ethanol and its metabolites such as acetaldehyde. Toxicity appears to be dose related and is greatest in first trimester exposure.

Cocaine

Cocaine has become the drug of choice in the United States because of easy accessibility and relatively low cost. This effective local anesthetic also has profound sympathomimetic action by dopamine potentiation (it blocks the reception of dopamine and norepinephrine), making it a very potent central nervous stimulant, which has led directly to its great potential for addiction and abuse.

This highly addictive substance causes multiple medical problems, both directly and as a result of sequelae of the lifestyle associated with drug dependence. The former include acute myocardial infarction, cardiac arrhythmias, aortic rupture, stroke, seizures, bowel ischemia, hyperthemia, and sudden death syndrome. The latter includes poor diet and hygiene; chronic lack of health care; increased risk of physical and emotional violence; and for women, sexual promiscuity/prostitution with associated risks of sexually transmitted diseases.

Cocaine use is associated with an increased incidence of spontaneous abortion and in utero fetal demise. Cocaine abusers are at increased risk for premature rupture of membranes (20%), preterm labor and delivery (25%), intrauterine growth retardation (25 to 30%), meconium-stained amniotic fluid (30%), and placental abruption (6 to 10%). In utero cerebral infarction has been reported in cocaine-abusing women. Cocaine use is associated with congenital anomalies such as segmental intestinal atresia, limb-reduction defects, disruptive brain anomalies, congenital heart defects, prune-belly syndrome, and urinary tract anomalies. Surviving infants are at higher risk for sudden infant death syndrome (SIDS), poor learning performance, and behavioral problems.

Table 6.19.
Fetal Alcohol Syndrome

Mental retardation
  Performance defects
  Lowered IQ

Growth
  Prenatal and postnatal growth retardation

Congenital anomalies
  Brain defects
  Cardiac defects (especially ventricular septal defects)
  Spinal defects

Craniofacial anomalies
  Flattened nasal bridge
  Absent to hypoplastic philtrum
  Broad upper lip
  Hypoplastic upper lip vermillion
  Micrognatia
  Microphthalmia
  Short nose
  Short palpebral fissure

Marijuana

Between 5 and 15% of pregnant women are thought to use marijuana or hashish during pregnancy. The active component — 9-tetrahydrocannabinol (THC) — is a highly active psychotropic compound that is teratogenic in animal models but equivocally so in human studies. Its use should be avoided in pregnancy.

Opiates

Heroin abuse is associated with a threefold to sevenfold increase in the rates of stillbirth, fetal growth retardation, premature labor and delivery, and neonatal mortality, probably as a result of both drug effects and the dangers of the narcotic abuser's lifestyle. Methadone treatment in pregnancy is associated with improved outcomes.

Newborn narcotic withdrawal syndrome is seen in up to 66% of infants and is potentially fatal. The syndrome is less frequently seen in the offspring of methadone-treated women, but its severity is the same for neonates of untreated women. Neonatal withdrawal syndrome is characterized by high-pitched cry, poor feeding, hypertonicity, tremor, hyperirritability, sneezing, diarrhea, and seizures. Neonatal symptoms usually appear in 1 to 2 days, although the syndrome can appear up to 10 days after birth, when the infant has been discharged from direct patient care.

Hallucinogens

There is no good evidence of direct chromosomal damage or untoward pregnancy outcome from the use of lysergic acid diethylamide (LSD) or other hallucinogenic substances. However, there are very few studies of this type of drug abuse in pregnancy. The use of hallucinogenics, in or out of pregnancy, should be actively discouraged.

16. COAGULATION DISORDERS IN PREGNANCY

Thrombocytopenia in Pregnancy

Thrombocytopenia is generally diagnosed when the platelet count is less than 100,000/mm³, although thrombocytopenia-associated bleeding usually occurs at platelet concentrations of less than 20,000/mm³. While leukemia and other neoplastic processes may be responsible for thrombocytopenia, these conditions are fortunately quite rare in obstetric patients. Drugs are common causes of thrombocytopenia. The list of drugs that cause thrombocytopenia is extensive and includes acetaminophen and a variety of antibiotics (Table 6.20). Because pregnant women consume various drugs, it may be difficult to assign the cause of thrombocytopenia to a specific drug, and an empiric withdrawal of medications may be required to make a diagnosis of drug-associated disease.

Immune thrombocytopenic purpura (ITP) is an autoimmune disorder characterized by the development of an IgG class antiplatelet antibody, occurring in 1 to 2 out of 1000 pregnancies. The diagnosis is suspected with thrombocytopenia and confirmed direct essay of platelet-associated IgG and C3 with radioactively labeled IgG antisera. Bone marrow aspiration reveals megakaryocyte hyperplasia.

Maternal treatment of ITP is initially with corticosteroids (usually Prednisone, 1.0 to 1.5 mg/kg/day). If unsuccessful, γ-globulin may be administered instead of performing a splenectomy, which formerly was the second-line treatment for this disorder. Because transfused platelets have a half-life of minutes to 2 to 3 days, compared with the normal half-life for platelets of 7 to 12 days, transfusion is not a useful therapy.

Because the maternal IgG antiplatelet antibodies cross the placenta, the fetus is also at risk, especially from trauma associated with vaginal delivery. Controversy exists over when cesarean section is appropriate. One approach is to use percutaneous umbilical blood sampling, with cesarean section being used for fetuses with a platelet count of >50,000/mm³. Fetal scalp electrodes should not be used in the labor of patients with ITP. A variation of this theme is isoimmune thrombocytopenia, in which there is maternal production of platelet antibodies directed against fetal platelet antigens that the mother's platelets do not have. Occurring in about 1/1000 pregnancies, fetal morbidity is reduced by maternal corticosteroid therapy and liberal use of cesarean delivery.

Systemic lupus erythematosus (SLE) can have thrombocytopenia as one of its manifestations. Patients with low platelet counts should be evaluated for this autoimmune disorder. Thrombocytopenia is also seen in the *hypertensive-associated HELLP syndrome* (hemolysis, elevated liver enzymes, and low platelet count).

Disseminated intravascular coagulopathy (DIC) in obstetrics is associated with placental abruption, retention of a dead fetus, sepsis, preeclampsia, and amniotic fluid embolism. Patients with these conditions must be carefully monitored for evidence of DIC. Findings include prolonged bleeding, decreased clotting factors, and elevated fibrin degradation products.

Lupus anticoagulant refers to immunoglobulins that interfere with phospholipid-related coagulation tests that were initially discovered in patients with SLE. Subsequently, it has been found that some patients with this clotting inhibitor lack other evidence of the more commonly seen SLE. The problem in these patients is that abnormal intravascular clotting occurs in the arterial system. Paradoxically, the activated partial thromboplastin time (aPTT) is prolonged, owing to the interference in this test by the immunoglobulins.

Patients with lupus anticoagulant have a rate of reproductive wastage in excess of 90%. Spontaneous abortions and intrauterine growth retardation are commonly seen. Second or third trimester fetal loss without apparent etiology may be associated with this antiphospholipid syndrome. Screening of patients with poor reproductive histories includes the aPTT and a test for anticardiolipin antibodies, which have been shown to be associated with this clinical picture. Treatment of patients with these disorders includes steroids and low-dose aspirin.

Hereditary Coagulation Defects

Hemophilia A and hemophilia B are X-linked recessive disorders caused by low factor VIII coagulant activity or deficiency of factor IX, respectively, exclusively affecting males. The importance of these disorders in obstetrics involves providing genetic counseling to women at risk for delivering an affected male fetus. *Von Willebrand's disease* is an inherited defect of coagulation in which the von Willebrand factor portion of the factor VIII complex is abnormal. Occurring in approximately 1/10,000 pregnancies, a bleeding diathasis and family history is confirmed by a prolonged bleeding time, low facor VIII level, and abnormal platelet adhesion. Factor VIII-rich cyroprecipitate is given if the factor VIII level is not >50% of normal at labor or delivery. *Antithrombin III deficiency* is an autosomal dominant deficit affecting the production of the regulatory protein that inhibits thrombin, factor Xa, and other serine proteases. More than 50% of the 1/2,000 who have this disease will also develop a deep vein thrombosis. Per-

ipartal heparin anticoagulation is required for these patients.

17. CANCER IN PREGNANCY

About 1 in 1000 pregnancies are complicated by cancer. The most common malignancies include cervical cancer, breast cancer, melanoma, ovarian cancer, leukemia/lymphoma, and colorectal cancer. Management must balance the maternal risks of the cancer and its treatment against the perinatal risks of treatment or lack thereof.

Cervical Dysplasia and Carcinoma in Pregnancy PAP → Colposcopy

Abnormal cervical cytology is encountered in 3% of pregnant women. A small number of these patients will have cervical dysplasia, and an even smaller number, cervical carcinoma. Colposcopic evaluation of all patients with high-grade squamous intraepithelial lesion (HGSIL) is essential; however, as with the nonpregnant patient, the timing of colposcopy for less severe classifications is controversial. When colposcopy is undertaken in pregnancy, it is essentially the same as in the nonpregnant patient with the exception that endocervical curettage (ECC), with its risk of iatrogenic rupture of membranes, and biopsy, with its increased bleeding, are used more sparingly. Treatment of cervical dysplasia is expectant during the pregnancy, usually

Table 6.20.
Drugs Associated with Thrombocytopenia or Abnormal Platelet Function

Antiinflammatory Agents	Destruction
Aspirin	Chlorothiazide
Ibuprofen (Motrin)	Diazepam (Valium)
Indomethacin	Diphenylhydantoin
Mefenamic acid	(Dilantin)
(Ponstel)	Quinidine
	Sulfisoxazole
Antibiotics	(Erythromycin)
Ampicillin	
Penicillin G	Others
Gentamicin	Acetaminophen
Nitrofurantoin	Chlorpromazine
	(Thorazine)
Cardiovascular drugs	Cimetidine
Dipyrimadole	Furosemide (Lasix)
(Persantine)	Heparin
Propranolol	Phenylbutazone
Theophylline	Sulfonamides
Immune-mediated	Tolbutamide
platelet	

deferred until 6 to 8 weeks after delivery, at which time reevaluation is undertaken. The healing of the cervix that occurs postpartum may lead to some resolution of cytologic abnormality.

Carcinoma in situ of the cervix is evaluated with the same method as is dysplasia, i.e., serial Pap smear and colposcopies are used to rule out progression of disease. Treatment is then based on the evaluation during the postpartum period.

Microinvasive cervical carcinoma (invasion is less than 3 mm in depth and there is no lymphatic or vascular involvement) is evaluated by conization in the second or third trimester to exclude the possibility of invasive cervical cancer. If the depth of invasion is less than 1 mm on conization, the conization is generally considered curative as well as diagnostic, whereas the treatment of invasion between 1 and 3 mm is more controversial. Postpartum hysterectomy is advocated for invasion from 1 to 3 mm.

The management of invasive cervical cancer depends on the extent of the disease, gestational age, fetal lung maturity, and ultimately the desires of the patient and her family. With a single focus of invasion 3 to 5 mm in depth and no lymphatic or vascular invasion, delay until fetal maturity followed by radical hysterectomy is often advocated. When invasion exceeds 5 mm and/or there is lymphatic or vascular involvement, pregnancy termination and treatment of the cancer are generally advocated at less than 24 weeks gestation and delay until lung maturity followed by delivery and therapy at greater than 24 weeks gestation. The prognosis, stage for stage, of cervical cancer in pregnancy compares favorably with that in nonpregnant patients. It is uncertain whether vaginal delivery through a cancerous cervix worsens the prognosis of the cancer, but abdominal delivery in this situation is usually recommended primarily on theoretical grounds.

Breast Cancer in Pregnancy

About 3 in 10,000 pregnancies are complicated by breast cancer. The relationship between breast cancer and pregnancy is uncertain. Diagnosis of breast cancer during pregnancy is made more difficult by the change of breast size and consistency. The diagnosis may, therefore, be delayed. To date, the stage-for-stage survival rates for breast cancer are unaffected by pregnancy.

Treatment of breast cancer must be individualized. Pregnancy termination has no recognized advantage in the treatment of localized breast can-

cer. Disseminated breast cancer is often responsive to hormonal ablation so that pregnancy termination in early pregnancy may be advisable, whereas in later pregnancy awaiting fetal lung maturity before delivery may pose an acceptable risk to the patient. Chemotherapeutic agents can be administered to the pregnant patient in the second and third trimesters in selected cases. There is no evidence that breast cancer adversely affects the pregnancy.

Ovarian Cancer

Ovarian carcinoma is quite rare in pregnancy, seen in about 1 in 10,000 to 20,000 pregnancies. Although ovarian carcinoma must be considered in the differential diagnosis of an adnexal mass in pregnancy, more common causes are corpus luteum cysts, pedunculated uterine fibroid, ectopic pregnancy, functional ovarian cyst, and a congenital abnormality such as a rudimentary uterine horn. Ultrasonography is useful in determining the diagnosis. Surgical intervention for an ovarian mass is best deferred until after the 16th week of pregnancy because most functional cysts will regress by this time and the risk of fetal wastage as a result of surgery and/or anesthesia is less. Surgical intervention may be required before 16 weeks if the mass undergoes torsion or rupture and is indicated if ectopic pregnancy is considered the likely diagnosis. Solid ovarian neoplasms have a higher risk of malignancy and should be evaluated more aggressively than cystic ones.

Melanoma

Melanoma is encountered in 1 in 100,000 pregnancies and is one of the few malignancies that may be adversely affected by pregnancy, because some melanomas have estrogen receptors and melanocyte-stimulating hormone is increased in pregnancy. Most originate from preexisting pigment-producing melanocytes in nevi. Treatment is determined by the stage of the lesion with survival, stage for stage, similar to that in patients who are not pregnant. While malignant metastasis to the fetus is extremely uncommon in all cancers, perhaps 33% of these rare occurrences involve malignant melanoma.

Colorectal Cancer

Colorectal carcinoma is uncommon in women under 40 years of age and is encountered in an estimated 1 in 100,000 pregnancies. The prognosis is determined by the stage and grade of tumor; the cancer is unaffected by pregnancy and vice versa.

Lymphoma and Leukemia in Pregnancy

Hodgkin's disease has a bimodal peak incidence with the first peak between 15 and 35 years of age; hence it is the most common lymphoma in pregnancy, perhaps 1 in 6,000 to 10,000 pregnancies. As this tumor is responsive to radiotherapy and chemotherapy, depending on stage, individualized treatment is appropriate. Pregnancy does not adversely affect Hodgkin's lymphoma and therapy may be individualized in many cases to provide insignificant risk to the fetus. Pregnant women with this disease are at high risk for infection and sepsis.

Non-Hodgkin's lymphoma is seen more frequently than Hodgkin's lymphoma in pregnancy because of its increased incidence in patients with AIDS, 5 to 10% of whom will develop a lymphoma.

Leukemia is extremely uncommon in pregnancy. Multiagent chemotherapy is usually given as soon as the diagnosis of leukemia is made. There is no evidence that pregnancy has a deleterious effect on leukemia, but termination may be considered in early pregnancy because of the risk of teratogenesis from the chemotherapy.

CASE STUDIES

Case 6A

A 23-year-old G1 is seen at 8 weeks gestational age for obstetric care. Her mother is an insulin-dependent diabetic.

Questions Case 6A

Which, if any, of the following laboratory studies should be performed?

A. Fasting blood sugar (FBS) at initial prenatal testing
B. Fasting blood sugar at the 28-weeks laboratory testing
C. 1-hr Glucola at initial prenatal testing
D. 1-hr Glucola at the 28-weeks laboratory testing
E. 3-hr glucose tolerance test (GTT) at initial prenatal testing
F. 3-hr GTT at the 28-weeks laboratory testing

Answer: C

Given the patient's family history of diabetes, testing before 28 weeks is indicated. The most commonly performed test would be a 1-hr Glucola. A fasting blood sugar would be less desirable, as it might miss an early

glucose intolerance. Glucose tolerance testing is inappropriate as an initial screening test.

The 1-hr Glucola is reported as 181 mg/100 mL. Appropriate management steps include

A. A 2500-cal ADA diet
B. 1-hr Glucola at the 28-weeks laboratory testing
C. 3-hr GTT
D. 3-hr GTT at the 28-weeks laboratory testing
E. Routine obstetric care

Answer: A, C

The 1-hr Glucola is above the 140 mg/100 mL screening limit, so glucose tolerance testing is required. Delay to 28 weeks is inappropriate, as the effects of glucose intolerance/diabetes are additive over time and, perhaps, more profound in early pregnancy. For this reason, the presumptive addition of an ADA diet is an also excellent precaution.

A 3-hr GTT is performed, and the results are 150, 199, 256, and 199 mg/100 mL. The ADA diet was begun immediately after the GTT was performed, 3 days ago. What will your management plan include?

A. FBS and 2-hr PP blood glucose in 1 to 2 weeks
B. FBS and 2-hr PP blood glucose at 28-weeks laboratory testing
C. 3-hr GTT in 1 to 2 weeks
D. 3-hr GTT at 28-weeks laboratory testing

Answer: A

Further GTTs are not required as the diagnosis is made. The question is whether diet alone will control the patient's blood sugars or whether insulin therapy will be required. Thus testing in 1 or 2 weeks is required, because a wait to 28 weeks may expose the fetus to abnormal blood sugars for an excessive period of time.

Case 6B

A 19-year-old G2 P1001 at 35 weeks of gestational age complains of a backache following an automobile accident. While she was driving to work, her automobile was hit from behind, buffeting her against the restraints of her lap/shoulder harness. Her abdomen hit the steering wheel lightly. Her antepartum course has heretofore been unremarkable. She notes nothing amiss except a sore back and a bruise over the lower part of her abdomen.

Question Case 6B

Physical examination is entirely normal except for the bruise she has mentioned. Her cervix is closed and there is no vaginal bleeding. Appropriate management includes

A. Obstetric ultrasound within 1 week
B. Obstetric ultrasound at this time
C. Electronic fetal monitoring within 1 week
D. Electronic fetal monitoring at this time
E. Amniocentesis

Answer: B, D

Abruptio placentae and preterm labor may manifest some hours after trauma to the gravid abdomen. Monitoring for uterine and fetal status is necessary, perhaps for 24 hr, according to some authorities. Ultrasound examination for abruptio placentae and biophysical profile are useful.

Case 6C

A 20-year-old G1 presents for prenatal care after missing her menstrual period the previous month. Her medical history and physical examination are all unremarkable except:

1. She had a short episode of drug use in her midteens, but successfully completed a drug rehabilitation program 4 years ago. She reports being drug free since.

2. She has a friable cervix and reports recurrent yeast infections.

Questions Case 6C

Which of the following problems is a special concern in this case?

A. Gonorrhea
B. Syphilis
C. Hepatitis
D. HIV infection
E. Bacterial vaginosis

Answer: D

Her history of involvement with the drug culture puts her at higher risk for any sexually transmitted disease (STD), and the friable cervix could be associated with cervicitis; however, cervical dysplasia is more frequent in patients with HIV infection.

Upon review of the prenatal laboratory evaluations, you note

1. ELISA and Western blot are both HIV+
2. Gonorrhea culture is positive
3. Urine toxicology positive for cocaine and THC
4. Pap smear reveals HGSIL

Immediate management includes which of the following:

A. Discussion of therapeutic termination of the pregnancy

B. Discussion of the risk of HIV transmission to the baby
C. Discussion of HIV infection for the patient
D. Discussion of drug rehabilitation
E. Discussion of the evaluation of the HGSIL positive PAP smear
F. Discussion of sexual practices, partners, and STDs

Answer: All

Vertical transmission of HIV to the fetus is approximately 10% with proper treatment, while the mother's ultimate prognosis is less comforting. Therapeutic abortion or plans for caring for a well or a sick infant must be discussed. The patient clearly needs further drug rehabilitation and treatment for infection.

Case 6D

An 18-year-old G2 P1001 at 30 weeks of gestation by dates and midtrimester ultrasound complains of a dull right lower quadrant and low back pain for 48 hr, associated with lack of appetite, mild nausea, no emesis, and frequent runny stools. Her pregnancy has so far been unremarkable, with the exception of hyperemesis in the first trimester (which resolved spontaneously) and a bout of the flu 1 week ago associated with nausea and diarrhea.

On physical examination, her temperature is 99.9°F, pulse 80, and blood pressure 110/75. Her fundal height is 31 cm and her uterus slightly tender. There are palpable fetal movements, the fetal heart rate (FHR) is 150 with a reactive NST, there is mild right CVA tenderness, and there are minimal bowel sounds and mild tenderness in both lower quadrants and the right upper quadrant. Her cervix is long and closed.

Question Case 6D

The more likely elements of your differential diagnosis include

A. Gastroenteritis
B. Ectopic pregnancy
C. Pyelonephritis
D. Diverticulitis
E. Appendicitis
F. Regional enteritis

Answer: A, C, E

This patient's relatively generalized discomfort is consistent with a renewed flu-gastroenteritis, early appendicitis, and early pyelonephritis. Ectopic pregnancy is extremely unlikely because of the gestational age, diverticulitis because of the patient's age and lack of previous symptoms, and regional enteritis because of the nature of the pain and its chronology.

chapter 7

PREMATURE RUPTURE OF MEMBRANES

Beginning early in pregnancy, amniotic fluid is produced continuously as the result of passage of fluid across the fetal membranes and across the skin, fetal urine production, and fetal pulmonary effluent. Amniotic fluid provides protection against infection, protects the fetus from trauma, and provides protection from umbilical cord compression. It also allows for fetal movement and fetal breathing, which, in turn, permits full fetal respiratory development. Decreased or absent amniotic fluid can lead to compression of the umbilical cord and decreased placental blood flow. Disruption (rupture) of these fetal membranes is associated with loss of protective effects of amniotic fluid.

Premature rupture of membranes (PROM) is defined as rupture of the chorioamniotic membrane before the onset of labor. PROM occurs in approximately 10 to 15% of all pregnancies. The primary risk of PROM is preterm labor and delivery, which, in turn, is associated with neonatal complications such as respiratory distress syndrome, intraventricular hemorrhage, neonatal infection, necrotizing enterocolitis, and sepsis. About 5% of patients with PROM will give birth preterm. The second most common complication is infection (chorioamnionitis), the incidence of which is increased with decreasing gestational age at PROM and positive cervical cultures for *Neisseria gonorrhoeae* and group B streptococcus. Other complications include prolapsed umbilical cord and abruptio placentae.

Because the consequences of PROM differ dramatically, depending on the gestational age at the time of rupture, the term *preterm PROM* is used to signify patients whose infants face the additional consequences of prematurity. PROM at or before 26 weeks of gestation is associated with pulmonary hypoplasia. Oligohydramnios at this very early gestational age is associated with incomplete alveolar development. Infants born with pulmonary hypoplasia cannot be adequately ventilated and soon succumb to hypoxia and barotrauma from high-pressure ventilation.

The *cause of PROM* is not clearly understood. Sexually transmitted diseases (STDs) play a role, since such *infections* are more commonly found in women with premature rupture of membranes than in those without STD. However, intact fetal membranes and normal amniotic fluid do not fully protect the fetus from infection, because it appears that subclinical intraamniotic infection may be responsible for PROM in certain cases. Metabolites produced by bacteria may either weaken the fetal membranes or initiate uterine contractions through stimulating prostaglandin synthesis.

The relationship between PROM and preterm contractions also is unclear. It is theorized that preterm contractions may cause dilation of the cervix, thereby exposing the fetal membranes to infective agents, which may then cause spontaneous rupture of the membranes. There is also uncertainty about the impact of gestational age and the length of time since membrane rupture on the likelihood of intrauterine infection. This *triad of PROM, preterm labor, and infection* remains an important clinical consideration but requires further research.

Chorioamnionitis poses a major threat to the mother and may cause fetal sepsis. Patients with intraamniotic infection can experience significant fever (generally, >100.5°F), tachycardia (maternal and fetal), and uterine tenderness. Purulent cervical discharge is usually a very late finding. The maternal white blood cell (WBC) count is generally elevated, but this finding may be misleading for two reasons: (*a*) the WBC count rises somewhat in normal pregnancy, with the upper range of normal being 12,000 to 13,000/mm^3; and (*b*) the WBC normally rises with uterine contractions and labor, at times to a level exceeding 20,000/mm^3. Patients with chorioamnionitis frequently enter spontaneous and often tumultuous labor. Once the diagnosis of chorioamnionitis is made, treatment consists of antibiotic therapy and prompt delivery by induction or augmentation of labor if needed.

DIAGNOSIS

Fluid passing through the vagina must be presumed to be amniotic fluid until proven otherwise. At times, patients will describe a "gush" of fluid, whereas at other times they note a history of steady leakage of small amounts of fluid. *Intermittent urinary leakage* is common during pregnancy, especially near term, and this can be confused with PROM. Likewise, the normally increased vaginal secretions in pregnancy as well as perineal moisture (especially in hot weather) may be mistaken for amniotic fluid.

The *Nitrazine test* uses pH to distinguish amniotic fluid from urine and vaginal secretions. Amniotic fluid is quite alkaline, having a pH above 7.0; vaginal secretions in pregnancy usually have pH values of less than 6.0. To perform the Nitrazine test, a sample of fluid obtained from the vagina during a speculum examination is placed on a strip of Nitrazine paper. The paper turns dark blue in response to amniotic fluid. Cervical mucus, blood, and semen are possible causes of false-positive results (Table 7.1).

The *"fern test"* is also used to distinguish amniotic fluid from other fluids. It is named from the pattern of arborization that occurs when amniotic fluid is placed on a slide and is allowed to dry in room air. The resultant pattern, which resembles the leaves of a fern plant, is caused by the sodium chloride content of the amniotic fluid. The ferning pattern from amniotic fluid is fine with multiple branches, as shown in Figure 7.1; cervical mucus does not fern or, if it does, the pattern is thick with much less branching. This test is considered more indicative of ruptured membranes than the Nitrazine test but, as with any test, it is not 100% reliable.

Ultrasound can be helpful in evaluating the possibility of rupture of membranes. If ample amniotic fluid around the fetus is visible on ultrasound examination, the diagnosis of PROM must be questioned; however, if the amounts of amniotic fluid leakage is small, sufficient amniotic fluid will still be visible on scan. When there is less than the expected amount of fluid seen on ultrasound, the differential diagnosis of oligohydramnios must also be considered.

The differential diagnoses for PROM include urinary incontinence, increased vaginal secretions in pregnancy (physiologic), increased cervical dis-

charge (pathologic, infection), exogenous fluids (such as semen or douche), and vesicovaginal fistula.

EVALUATION AND MANAGEMENT

Patients with PROM are *hospitalized for their initial evaluation* and further management. In the hospital environment, evaluations may proceed quickly and efficiently so that delivery may be accomplished if needed. *Factors to be considered in the management of the patient with premature rupture of membranes include* the gestational age at the time of rupture, the presence of uterine contractions, the likelihood of chorioamnionitis, the amount of amniotic fluid around the fetus, and the degree of fetal maturity.

The patient's history as well as the management factors listed above must be carefully evaluated for information relevant to the diagnosis. Abdominal examination includes palpation of the uterus for tenderness and fundal height measurement for evaluation of gestational age and fetal lie.

A sterile speculum examination is performed to assess the likelihood of vaginal infection and to obtain cervical cultures for *N. gonorrhoeae*, β-he-

Table 7.1.
Causes of False-positive and False-negative Nitrazine Tests

False-positive	False-negative
Basic urine	Remote PROM with no residual fluid
Semen	
Cervical mucus	Minimal amniotic fluid leakage
Blood contamination	
Some antiseptic solutions	
Vaginitis (esp. trichomonas)	

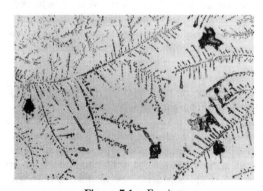

Figure 7.1. Ferning.

molytic streptococcus, and possibly *Chlamydia trachomatis.* The cervix is visualized for its degree of dilation as well as for the presence of free-flowing amniotic fluid. Fluid is obtained from the vaginal vault for Nitrazine and/or fern testing. If there is fluid pooled in the vaginal vault, it may be sent for *fetal maturity testing* if the gestational age warrants. The test for phosphatidylglycerol (PG) is considered the most reliable indicator of fetal lung maturity, since PG is not found in vaginal secretions or blood. *Because of the risk of infection, intracervical digital examination should be avoided unless, and until, the patient is in active labor.*

Ultrasound examination can be helpful in determining gestational age, verifying the fetal presentation, and assessing the amount of amniotic fluid remaining within the uterine cavity. It has been shown that labor is less likely to occur when an adequate volume of amniotic fluid remains within the uterus.

If the gestational age is thought to be in the transitional time of fetal maturity (i.e., from 34 to 36 weeks) or if there is clinical suspicion for the presence of uterine infection, amniotic fluid may be collected by amniocentesis from any pocket of fluid located on ultrasound. Fluid can be assessed for the presence of infection by Gram staining and culture, and tests of fetal maturity can be performed. The presence of bacteria on Gram stain is a better predictor of infection than the presence of white blood cells.

If the evaluation suggests *intrauterine infection,* antibiotic therapy and delivery are indicated. The antibiotic prescribed should have a broad spectrum of coverage, because of the polymicrobial nature of the infection. Delivery is usually accomplished by induction of labor or, if the infant is a preterm breech, possibly by cesarean delivery. If the patient is beginning to have uterine contractions or if the cervix is dilated beyond about 3 cm, labor is usually allowed to proceed. As in cases of labor not related to PROM, oxytocin augmentation may be necessary. Persistent contractions after PROM may be a manifestation of infection, possibly subclinical, so that most clinicians do not attempt to inhibit labor when such contractions begin spontaneously.

If the fetus is significantly preterm and in the absence of infection, expectant management is generally chosen. Patients are assessed carefully on a daily basis for uterine tenderness as well as maternal or fetal tachycardia. WBC counts are obtained frequently, usually daily for several days. Frequent

ultrasound assessment helps to determine amniotic fluid volumes, since amniotic fluid may reaccumulate around the fetus. Daily fetal movement monitoring by the mother can also be helpful to assess fetal well-being. In the absence of sufficient amniotic fluid to buffer the umbilical cord from external pressure, compression of the cord can lead to fetal heart rate decelerations. If these are frequent and severe, there should be early and expeditious delivery to avoid fetal compromise or death. Electronic fetal monitoring is used frequently during the initial evaluation period to search for any fetal heart rate decelerations.

While the evidence supporting the use of *steroids to enhance fetal pulmonary maturity* in patients with PROM is not conclusive, the majority of clinicians give an agent such as betamethasone. Despite the immunosuppressive property of steroids, they do not seem to predispose the mother or fetus to infection.

At times, the leakage of amniotic fluid will cease, DO and *the fetal membranes are said to "seal over."* NOT Should this occur, patients can be monitored at DK MOMS home, with careful attention to temperature and = PROM uterine tenderness as noted above. Unfortunately, this circumstance is unlikely. Much more common is the onset of uterine contractions and frank labor in the 1st week following rupture of membranes. For this reason, it is the exceptional patient who can expect to be discharged home with documented premature rupture of membranes.

PROM at very early gestational ages, such as before 25 to 26 weeks of gestation, presents additional problems. Along with the risks of prematurity and infection already discussed, the very premature fetus faces the further hazards of *pulmonary hypoplasia* and the *amniotic band syndrome.* The relationship of PROM with both of these entities is both interesting and important. For normal fetal lung development to occur, it is necessary that fetal breathing movements take place. During intrauterine life, the fetus normally inhales and exhales amniotic fluid. This adds substances generated in the respiratory tree to the amniotic fluid pool, including the phospholipids that form the basis for many of the fetal maturity tests. If rupture of fetal membranes occurs before 25 to 26 weeks of gestation, the lack of amniotic fluid interferes with this normal breathing process and, therefore, with pulmonary development. The result is a failure of normal growth and differentiation of the respiratory tree. If severe, the fetus is said to have *pulmonary hypoplasia.* Neonatal death then occurs because of an inability to maintain ventilation. The development of pulmonary hypoplasia is not necessarily an all-or-none phenomenon but rather represents a spectrum of disordered development.

The *amniotic band syndrome* is a constellation of findings associated with entanglement of fetal parts with the amniotic membranes that can collapse around the fetus once rupture of membranes occurs. These bands may cause virtually any type of deformity or anatomic disruption, including amputation of extremities or fingers. Patients with ruptured membranes early in pregnancy are exposed to these additional risks if expectant management is chosen. On the brighter side, PROM that occurs early in pregnancy, sometimes following genetic amniocentesis, has a greater likelihood of sealing over with reaccumulation of amniotic fluid.

CASE STUDIES

Case 7A

A 25-year-old G1 at 30 weeks of gestational age by menstrual history and early pelvic and ultrasound examinations presents with a history of "water leaking from my vagina" for the last 4 hr. Her pregnancy has been unremarkable except for a positive cervical *C. trachomatis* culture at the time of her initial obstetric visit at 8 weeks of gestational age. The infection was treated and a repeat culture was negative.

Questions Case 7A

Which of the following should be included in the initial evaluation of this patient?

A. Sterile speculum examination
B. Sterile vaginal examination
C. External electronic fetal monitoring
D. Cervical cultures for *N. gonorrhoeae* and *C. trachomatis*
E. Transabdominal ultrasonography
F. Amniocentesis

Answer: A, C, D, E

The initial evaluation should be focused to determine if PROM has occurred. Thus a sterile speculum examination to look for fluid is appropriate, but not a digital examination, which may increase the risk of infection. Fern and Nitrazine tests can be made on the fluid. Cultures from the cervix can be taken, which are especially important in this patient who has a previous history of *Chlamydia* infection. Similarly, external fetal monitoring

(EFM) and ultrasonography are valuable and offer no risk, whereas amniocentesis is unnecessarily invasive at this time.

Examination shows no fluid coming from the os or in the vaginal vault. The Nitrazine test is negative. Ultrasound shows adequate fluid. EFM shows a reassuring fetal heart rate (FHR) pattern, without evidence of uterine activity. Which of the following are likely explanations of fluid coming from this patient's vagina?

A. Involuntary urination
B. Normally increased vaginal secretions in pregnancy
C. Perineal moisture (especially in hot weather)
D. Patient anxiety

Answer: All

All of these sources of fluid leakage from the vagina are commonly encountered in pregnancy.

Case 7B

A 36-year-old infertility patient, who conceived after being administered clomiphene citrate, is now at 26 weeks of gestation based on last menstrual period (LMP) and early physical examination and ultrasonography. She presents with a history of a gush of fluid from her vagina 1 hr ago. She is now feeling "little twinges" in her uterus, a new and disturbing sensation. She is very frightened.

Speculum examination shows fluid coming from the cervical os, which is Nitrazine and fern positive. The patient's cervix appears to be about 1 cm dilated. On EFM the fetal heart rate is 170 and there are occasional uterine contractions. The patient is afebrile, and her uterus is not tender. Her WBC is found to be 16,000/mm³.

Questions Case 7B

Which of the following are likely problems in this case?

A. Premature labor
B. Intrauterine infection
C. Pulmonary hypoplasia
D. Amniotic band syndrome

Answer: All

All of these are serious clinical considerations for this patient and her fetus. At 26 weeks of gestation, survival in a neonatal ICU is likely but so is significant short- and long-term morbidity.

You and your patient decide to wait 24 hr, at which time — as you hoped — there is no evidence of intrauterine infection for premature labor. Obviously, this patient has gone to great lengths to be pregnant. Now she is faced with difficult decisions and your advice is important. Will you recommend tocolysis if uterine activity increases and steroids to help with pulmonary maturity?

A. Yes
B. No

Answer: A or B

Regarding medications, either answer could be correct in consultation with your patient. The issues of tocolysis and steroid therapy with premature rupture of membranes are controversial. The argument against is that the risk of intrauterine infection is increased, with the subsequent delivery of a premature and infected newborn outweighing the advantages of increased maturity. The argument for this therapy is that tocolysis would delay delivery and allow time to administer steroids to improve the chance of pulmonary maturity.

Will you place this patient on antibiotic therapy?

A. Yes
B. No

Answer: A

Antibiotic therapy is generally recommended, although the intrauterine space is relatively sequestered so that treatment has limitations.

chapter 8

PRETERM LABOR AND PRETERM BIRTH

Because *preterm birth* resulting from *preterm labor* (PTL) is the most common cause of perinatal morbidity and mortality, its prevention and treatment are major concerns in obstetric care. The *consequences of preterm labor and preterm birth* occur with increasing severity and frequency the earlier the gestational age of the newborn. Besides perinatal death in the very young fetus, common complications of PTL include respiratory distress syndrome (RDS; also called hyaline membrane disease), intraventricular hemorrhage, necrotizing enterocolitis, sepsis, and seizures. Long-term morbidity associated with preterm labor and delivery includes bronchopulmonary dysplasia and developmental abnormalities. The significant impact of preterm birth is best summarized by this fact: *The 10% of babies born prematurely account for more than 50% of all perinatal morbidity and mortality in the United States.*

In the consideration of the consequences of preterm delivery, it is important to *separate the concepts of low birth weight and prematurity.* Prematurity reflects gestational age, whereas low birth weight is based on the single parameter of weight, usually 2500 g or less. For example, a growth-retarded fetus of a hypertensive patient may weigh well under 2500 g at 40 weeks gestation. Such an infant is a low birth weight infant but not preterm and will suffer the consequences associated with low birth weight and maternal hypertension, but not of premature birth. Likewise, an infant of a diabetic mother may be delivered before term, weigh in excess of 2500 g and still have the significant perinatal morbidities of preterm birth.

Many preterm births are the result of deliberate intervention for a variety of pregnancy complications and hence are unavoidable perinatal complications. A major cause of preterm birth, however, is preterm labor. *Preterm labor* (PTL) is defined as the presence of *regular uterine contrac-*tions, occurring with a frequency of 10 min or less between 20 and 36 weeks gestation, with each contraction lasting at least 30 sec. This uterine activity is accompanied by cervical effacement, cervical dilation, and/or descent of the fetus into the pelvis. However, variations of this definition are commonly used, so it is often difficult to know when a patient is really in PTL. This presents a problem because treatment appears to be more effective when initiated early in the course of preterm labor; waiting for cervical changes to occur to establish a definitive diagnosis may limit successful therapy.

ETIOLOGY AND PREVENTION OF PRETERM LABOR

A number of causes and associated factors have been implicated in PTL (Table 8.1). Unfortunately, in most cases, preterm labor is idiopathic, i.e., no cause can be identified.

Patient and physician education has focused on *recognition of the signs and symptoms* that suggest PTL (Table 8.2). Patients with such symptoms should be strongly advised to seek prompt medical attention, and physicians and nurses providing obstetric care must carefully evaluate all such patients. Patient education to help recognize these signs and symptoms is an important part of care, although maternal recognition of uterine activity that leads to premature cervical changes is often inaccurate. There are indicators that often precede PTL. Patients destined to develop frank preterm labor may have increased uterine irritability and more frequent contractions in the weeks before the actual diagnosis of labor. At times they experience a sensation of pelvic pressure. Electronic fetal monitoring (periodic monitoring at home along with frequent contact with personnel trained in recognition of preterm labor) has been suggested as being beneficial for patients at high risk for preterm labor.

Table 8.1.
Factors Associated with Preterm Labor

Dehydration

Premature rupture of membranes (PROM)

Incompetent cervix
  Primary
  Secondary to surgery, e.g., cone biopsy of cervix

Infections
  Urinary
  Cervical
    β-hemolytic streptococcus, especially
    Bacterial vaginosis
  Intraamniotic

Excessive uterine enlargement
  Hydramnios
  Multiple gestation

Uterine distortion
  Leiomyomas
  Septate uterus

Placental abnormalities
  Abruptio placentae
  Placenta previa

Maternal smoking (strong implications)

Substance abuse

Iatrogenic: induction of labor

As *early asymptomatic dilation and effacement of the cervix seems to be associated with an increased likelihood of preterm labor,* a pelvic examination between 24 and 28 weeks gestation is now a common part of prenatal care. For patients at higher risk for preterm labor, evaluations are performed earlier in pregnancy and more frequently through the second half of gestation.

EVALUATION OF A PATIENT IN SUSPECTED PRETERM LABOR

Once a patient describes symptoms and signs suggestive of preterm labor, evaluation should be prompt. Application of an *external electronic fetal monitor* may help to quantify the frequency and duration of contractions; the intensity of uterine contractions is assessed very poorly on an external monitor, but abdominal palpation by experienced personnel can prove helpful. The status of the cervix should be determined, either by visualization with a speculum or by gentle digital examination. Changes in cervical effacement and dilation on subsequent examinations are important in the evaluation of both the diagnosis of PTL and the effectiveness of management. Subtle changes are often of great

Table 8.2.
Symptoms and Signs of Preterm Labor

Menstrual-like cramps

Low, dull backache

Abdominal pressure

Pelvic pressure

Abdominal cramping (with or without diarrhea)

Increase or change in vaginal discharge (mucous, watery, light bloody discharge)

Uterine contractions, often painless

clinical importance so that serial examinations by the same examiner are optimal although not always practical.

Because urinary infections can predispose to uterine contractions, a careful *urinalysis and urine culture* should be obtained. At the time of speculum examination, cervical cultures should be taken for group B β-streptococcus and, when indicated by history or physical examination findings, for *Chlamydia* and *Neisseria gonorrhoeae. Chlamydia* has been implicated in some cases of preterm labor. A normal saline wet preparation is also useful to evaluate for bacterial vaginosis, which is associated with premature labor and premature rupture of the membranes.

Ultrasound examination can be useful in assessing the gestational age of the fetus, estimation of the amniotic fluid volume (spontaneous rupture of membranes with fluid loss may precede preterm labor and may be unrecognized by the patient), fetal presentation, and placental location. The technique also can reveal the existence of fetal congenital anomalies. Because placenta previa and abruptio placentae may lead to preterm contractions, patients should also be monitored for bleeding.

Because either clinical or subclinical infection of the amniotic cavity is thought to be associated with preterm labor in some cases, *amniocentesis* may be performed. The presence of bacteria in amniotic fluid is correlated not only with preterm labor but also with the subsequent development of infection, which is less responsive to therapy. The presence of white cells in the amniotic fluid increases the likelihood of infection developing. Antibiotic therapy before delivery is instituted if infection is diagnosed or strongly suspected. At the time of amniocentesis, additional amniotic fluid may be obtained for

Table 8.3.
Agents Used in Treating Preterm Labor

Class (Example)	Action	Comments
Magnesium sulfate	Competes with calcium for entry into cells	High degree of safety; often used as first agent; may cause flushing or headaches; at high levels may cause respiratory depression (12–15 mg/dL) or cardiac depression (>15 mg/dL)
β-adrenergic agents (ritodrine, terbutaline)	Increase cAMP in cell, which decreases free calcium	β-receptors are of two types: $β_1$-receptors predominate in the heart and intestines and $β_2$-receptors predominate in the uterus, lungs, and blood vessels; side effects include hypotension, tachycardia, anxiety, chest tightening or pain, ECG changes; increased pulmonary edema occurs very infrequently but is possible, especially with fluid overload
Prostaglandin synthetase inhibitors (indomethacin)	Decrease prostaglandin (PG) production by blocking conversion of free arachidonic acid to PG	Premature constriction of ductus arteriosus possible especially after 34 weeks; bradycardia and growth retardation hypoglycemia are reported earlier, but concern has decreased with broader experience
Calcium channel blockers (nifedipine)	Prevent calcium entry into muscle cells	Newest tocolytic; possible decrease in uteroplacental blood flow, fetal hypoxia, and hypercarbia; more experience is needed.

pulmonary maturity studies, which could have bearing on subsequent management. Tocolysis, the suppression of uterine contractions by pharmacologic means, may not be appropriate if there is indication of fetal lung maturity.

MANAGEMENT OF PRETERM LABOR

The purpose in treating preterm labor is to delay delivery, if possible, until fetal maturity is attained. Management involves *two broad goals:* (*a*) the detection and treatment of disorders associated with preterm labor and (*b*) therapy for the preterm labor itself. Although it is fortunate that more than 50% of patients with preterm contractions have spontaneous resolution of abnormal uterine activity, this complicates the evaluation of treatment. First, one may not know whether there was actual preterm labor or simply normal preterm uterine activity. It may be difficult to know whether it was the treatment that stopped the preterm labor or whether it would have stopped without therapy.

Because dehydration has been known to lead to uterine irritability, *therapy often begins with intravenous hydration.* In a significant number of patients, this therapy alone will cause cessation of uterine contractions.

Various tocolytic therapies have been used in the management of preterm labor (Table 8.3); spe-

cific regimens are detailed in Tables 8.4 through 8.6. Unfortunately, tocolytics have not been clearly shown to prolong pregnancy beyond several days. Different treatment regimens address specific mechanisms involved in the maintenance of uterine contractions, and each, therefore, may be best suited for certain patients.

Typically, *patients diagnosed as having preterm labor receive one form of therapy, with the addition or substitution of other forms if the initial treatment is unsuccessful.* As noted in Table 8.3, adverse side effects, at times serious and even life-threatening to the mother, can occur. These possibilities must be taken into account in selecting a therapy. The maturity of the fetus is a consideration in deciding how aggressively to pursue therapy, and in general, the vigor with which therapy is undertaken diminishes as the gestational age of the fetus increases. One might be more willing to accept potential adverse effects for a patient in preterm labor at 26 weeks as opposed to 35 weeks. It is customary to stop therapy at 36 weeks. Treatment sequences may vary from hospital to hospital, depending on the individual hospital experience and the success rate with various therapeutic regimens.

Contraindications to tocolysis include advanced labor, a mature fetus, an anomalous fetus, intrauterine infection, significant vaginal bleeding, conditions where the adverse effects of tocolysis

Table 8.4.
Administration of Terbutaline for Preterm Labor

- 5 mg of terbutaline is mixed in 250 mL of D$_5$W, providing a terbutaline concentration of 10 μ/mL
- Infusion via a pump is started at a rate of 5 μg/min (15 mL/hr)
- The infusion rate is increased every 10–15 min by 5 μg/min (15 mL/hr) until contractions stop or occur no more than once every 20 min
- Generally, a maximum infusion rate is 30 μg/min (90 mL/hr)

Table 8.5.
Administration of Magnesium Sulfate for Preterm Labor

- 6 g MgSO$_4$ are mixed in 100–150 mL of D$_5$W and infused over 15–20 min as a loading dose
- 40 g MgSO$_4$ is mixed in 1000 mL of D$_5$W, providing a MgSO$_4$ concentration of 1 g MgSO$_4$ in 25 mL of solution
- Using a piggyback infusion via an infusion pump, the physician usually begins infusion at 2 g/hr (50 mL/hr) and increases it in 0.5-g/hr increments as needed.

Table 8.6.
Administration of Nifedipine for Preterm Labor

- Loading dose: 30 mg; disrupts one 10-mg capsule by having patient bite capsule, two 10-mg capsules are swallowed
- Immediate tocolysis: 20 mg p.o. q. 6–8h.; may increase to q. 4h. if blood pressure remains >80/50
- Maintenance: 10–20 mg q. 8h. if necessary
- Cautions: Contraindicated in patients with myasthenia gravis, renal failure, hypoglycemia or active hepatitis and/or hepatic failure; may potentiate the effect of magnesium sulfate, leading to hypotension and respiratory depression
- Pharmacology: inhibits calcium transport through L-type or slow-type channels, causing significant reductions in systemic and pulmonary vascular resistance and tocolysis; specific uterine effects include inhibition of myometrial contractility and reduction of uterine vascular resistance; potentiates magnesium sulfate but may be used concurrently with β-blockers such as terbutaline
- Side effects: flushing is common; headache in 5–10% of patients; hypotension and tachycardia are rare; no known teratogenic effects
- Other uses: treatment of hypertension in pregnancy

may be marked, and a variety of obstetric complications that contraindicate delay in delivery.

Relatively early in the third trimester, such as 28 to 32 weeks, management may include administration of certain *steroids*, such as betamethasone, *to enhance pulmonary maturity*. Both the incidence and severity of RDS appear to be reduced with this therapy. The salutatory effect for the fetus appears to wane after 7 days, so the therapy is usually repeated weekly. In addition, sequelae of RDS such as intracerebral hemorrhage and necrotizing enterocolitis occur less frequently in infants whose mother received betamethasone or a similar agent.

CASE STUDIES

Case 8A

A 26-year-old G2 P0101 presents with complaints of vaginal discharge, urinary frequency, and a sensation of pelvic pressure. She says she may be contracting sometimes, but she isn't sure. She is at 28 weeks gestation by dates and early ultrasound examination. Her first child was delivered by cesarean section at 29 weeks gestation after tocolysis with magnesium sulfate and terbutaline had failed and the fetus was found to be

breech. Her past medical history includes three episodes of *Chlamydia* infection, the last in the first trimester of this pregnancy. Her antenatal course during this pregnancy has been otherwise unremarkable.

Questions Case 8A

Based on this history, which of the following evaluations are indicated at this time? (Choose all that apply.)

A. Urinalysis (UA), culture and sensitivity (C&S)
B. Obstetric ultrasound
C. Cervical evaluation
D. Amniocentesis
E. Cervical cultures for *Chlamydia*, *N. gonorrhoeae*, and group B β-streptococcus

Answer: A, C, E

With a history of urinary frequency and previous *Chlamydia* infection, urinalysis and appropriate cultures are important initial steps. Cervical evaluation is crucial in determining if this patient with a previous preterm labor and delivery is again in preterm labor, for which she is at high risk. Obstetric ultrasound is useful, but not immediately. Evaluation for uterine activity by electronic fetal monitor (EFM) is appropriate to assess for the presence of significant uterine contractions. Finally, amniocentesis is not indicated in the initial evaluation, since at this time the patient is not known to be in preterm labor.

The patient is found to have a long, closed cervix and irregular uterine contractions that resolve with hydration. The fetal heart rate pattern is reassuring. UA shows 40 white blood cells (WBC) per high-power field (HPF). What therapy is appropriate? Is tocolysis indicated on a prophylactic basis? Is amniocentesis indicated to rule out intrauterine infection?

Answer:

Antibiotic therapy for a "UTI" or urinary tract infection is warranted at this time. Tocolysis at this time is controversial but may be employed. The risks of amniocentesis are too high in this situation where premature lungs may be assumed and there is no clinical evidence of amniotic infection.

Case 8B

A 29-year-old G4 P2103 presents complaining of painful uterine contractions for 2 hr and a sensation of pelvic fullness. She is in the 30th week of gestation age based on last menstrual period (LMP) and two ultrasound examinations. She has had three uneventful vaginal deliveries, two at term and one at 35.5 weeks.

Cervical examination shows she is 3 cm dilated and 90% effaced, her membranes are intact, and there is a cephalic part at zero station. On EFM she is having uterine contractions every 4 min, which the nurse evaluates as moderate to strong in intensity; the fetal heart pattern is reassuring.

Questions Case 8B

Which interventions are required at this time? (Choose all that apply.)

A. i.v. fluids
B. Ultrasound to evaluate for fetal anomalies
C. Tocolysis with magnesium sulfate
D. UA, C&S, and cervical cultures
E. Amniocentesis

Answer: A, B, C, D

Immediate intravenous hydration and tocolysis with magnesium sulfate are indicated. Urinalysis and cultures provide important information for future management that can be easily obtained. After tocolytic therapy has been started, ultrasound is appropriate. If tocolysis is successful, consideration for amniocentesis may then be in order.

Tocolysis with intravenous fluids and magnesium sulfate is successful, with cervical changes arrested for the time at 3 cm dilation and 90% effacement. *For further consideration:* What will you tell the patient about the risks and benefits of steroid therapy in her situation? Will you use the same or different agents if uterine contractions reoccur? Will you consider discharge if uterine contractions do not reoccur? If so, will you send the patient home on a tocolytic? Is electronic ambulatory fetal monitoring warranted in this patient?

chapter 9

OBSTETRIC HEMORRHAGE

An estimated 5% of women will describe bleeding of some extent during pregnancy. At times, the amount of bleeding is hardly more than "spotting," whereas at other times profuse hemorrhage can lead to maternal death in a very short time. In most cases, antepartum bleeding is minimal spotting, often following sexual intercourse, and is thought to be related to trauma to the friable ectocervix. Small polyps on the cervix can also cause small amounts of bleeding. Table 9.1 is a list of causes of bleeding in the second half of pregnancy. A previous Pap test and examination of the lower genital tract should eliminate the likelihood of lower genital tract neoplasms in most cases. At times, patients may mistake bleeding from hemorrhoids or even hematuria for vaginal bleeding, but the difference is easily distinguished by examination.

The two causes of hemorrhage in the second half of pregnancy that require greatest attention, because of the associated maternal and fetal morbidity and mortality, are *placenta previa* and *abruptio placentae*. Various characteristics of these entities are compared in Table 9.2.

PLACENTA PREVIA

Placenta previa refers to an *abnormal location of the placenta over or in close proximity to the internal cervical os*. Placenta previa can be categorized as *complete or total* if the entire cervical os is covered; *partial*, if the margin of the placenta extends across part but not all of the internal os; *marginal*, if the edge of the placenta lies adjacent to the internal os; and *low lying*, if the placenta is located near but not directly adjacent to the internal os (Fig. 9.1). The etiology of placenta previa is not understood, but abnormal vascularization has long been proposed as a mechanism for this abnormal placement of the placenta. In some cases, such as in twin pregnancy or if it is hydropic, the placenta

may extend to the region of the internal cervical os because of its size alone. Increasing maternal age, increasing parity, and previous cesarean delivery are factors commonly associated with placenta previa, although recent evidence suggests that age alone is not an important factor.

The incidence of placenta previa varies with gestational age, usually reported overall as about 1 in 250 pregnancies. There is great variation in incidence, however, with parity. The incidence in nulliparas is only 1 in 1000 to 1500, whereas that in grandmultiparas is as high as 1 in 20. Women with the highest risk for placenta previa are grandmultiparas, those who have had a previous placenta previa (4 to 8%), and those who have had four or more cesarean sections. With common use of ultrasonography examinations, it has been shown repeatedly that the placenta may cover the internal cervical os in about 5% of pregnancies when examined at midpregnancy, a finding seen even more frequently earlier in gestation. Because of subsequent growth of both the upper and lower uterine segments, the placenta appears to "migrate" away from the internal os in the majority of cases. The likelihood of this apparent movement diminishes as the gestational age at first detection increases.

The average gestational age at the time of the first bleeding episode is 29 to 30 weeks. Although the bleeding may be substantial, it almost always ceases spontaneously, unless digital examination or other trauma occurs. The bleeding is caused by separation of part of the placenta from the lower uterine segment and cervix, possibly in response to mild uterine contractions. The blood that is lost is usually maternal in origin. The patient often describes a sudden onset of bleeding without any apparent antecedent signs. There is no pain associated with placenta previa in most cases, unless coincident with labor or with an abruptio placenta (approximately 5 to 10% of cases).

129

Ultrasonography has been of enormous benefit in localizing the placenta, especially when the placenta is anterior or lateral. If the placenta lies in the posterior portion of the lower uterine segment, its exact relationship with the internal os may be more difficult to ascertain. In most cases, though, ultrasonography examination can accurately diagnose placenta previa (Fig. 9.2) or, by illustrating the placenta location away from the cervix and lower uterine segment, exclude it as a cause for bleeding. In some instances, transvaginal ultrasonography may be a useful adjunct to the transabdominal approach, especially in the posterior placenta.

The basic management of patients with placenta previa includes initial hospitalization with hemodynamic stabilization, followed by expectant management until fetal maturity has occurred. Ideal expectant management would be continuous

hospitalization with enforced bedrest and immediate access to emergency care, but this is increasingly prohibited by cost issues. After initial hospital management, care as an outpatient may be considered if certain criteria are met. These include a highly motivated patient who clearly understands and will comply with instructions concerning restrictions of activity, the constant attendance of a responsible adult to assist in the event of an emergency situation, and the presence of ready transportation to the hospital.

The number of bleeding episodes is unrelated to the degree of placenta previa or to the prognosis for fetal survival. Such expectant management combined with appropriate use of blood transfusion and cesarean birth have resulted in the lowering of the maternal mortality rate from 25–30% to <1% and the perinatal mortality rate from 60–70% to <10%. If the fetus is thought to be mature by gestational age criteria or by amniocentesis for fetal lung maturity testing, there is little benefit to be gained by a delay in delivery. The further from term that bleeding from placenta previa occurs, the more important it is to delay delivery to allow for further fetal growth and maturation. The degree of bleeding and the maturity of the fetus must be constantly weighed in managing these patients. Fetal maturity is usually assessed at approximately 36 weeks, with cesarean delivery performed once the fetus is deemed mature.

In some cases, when the location of the placenta cannot be accurately determined by ultrasound and delivery is required, the route of delivery is determined by a *double setup examination*. This procedure involves careful evaluation of the

Table 9.1.
Causes of Bleeding in the Second Half of Pregnancy

Vulva	Intrauterine
Varicose veins	Placenta previa
Tears or lacerations	Abruptio placentae
	Vasa previa
Vagina	
Tears or lacerations	
Cervix	
Polyp	
Glandular tissue (normal)	
Cervicitis	
Carcinoma	

Table 9.2.
Characteristics of Placenta Previa and Abruptio Placentae

Characteristic	Placenta previa	Abruptio placentae
Magnitude of blood loss	Variable	Variable
Duration	Often ceases within 1–2 hr.	Usually continues
Abdominal discomfort	None	Can be severe
Fetal heart rate pattern on electronic monitoring	Normal	Tachycardia, then bradycardia; loss of variability; decelerations frequently present; intrauterine demise not rare
Coagulation defects	Rare	Associated, but infrequent; DIC[a] often severe when present
Associated history	None	Cocaine use; abdominal trauma; maternal hypertension; multiple gestation; polyhydramnios

[a] *DIC*, disseminated intravascular coagulation.

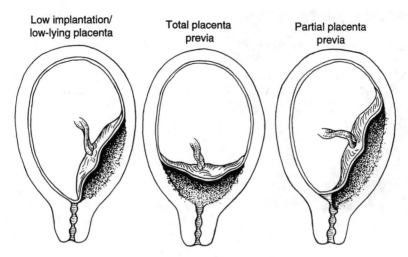

Figure 9.1. Placenta previa.

cervix in the operating room with full preparations for rapid cesarean delivery. If placental tissue is seen or palpated at the internal cervical os, prompt cesarean delivery is performed. If the placental margin is away from the internal os, artificial rupture of the membranes and oxytocin induction of labor may be performed in anticipation of vaginal delivery. Prior to the widespread utilization of ultrasound, this procedure was done more frequently than it is in modern obstetrics; nonetheless, it is still an important tool in selected cases.

An attempt at vaginal delivery of a patient with placenta previa may be indicated if the delivery can be accomplished with minimal blood loss and if the fetus is dead, has major fetal malformations, or is clearly previable. If making such an attempt is appropriate, ceasing the process and moving to cesarean delivery for maternal indication must always be considered. Placenta previa is associated with a nearly doubling of the rate of congenital malformations, the most serious including major anomalies of the central nervous system, gastrointestinal tract, cardiovascular system, and respiratory tract. At the time of diagnosis of placenta previa, a detailed fetal survey should be performed for anomalies.

Abnormal placental location can be further complicated by abnormal growth of the placental mass into the substance of the uterus, a condition termed *placenta previa accreta*. In placenta previa accreta, the poorly formed decidua of the lower uterine segment offers little resistance to trophoblastic invasion. The incidence of this severe complication is variously reported as 5 to 10% of placenta

previas, although the incidence is much higher in patients with multiple previous cesarean sections. At the time of delivery, sustained and significant bleeding may ensue, often requiring hysterectomy.

ABRUPTIO PLACENTAE

Whereas placenta previa refers to the abnormal location of the placenta, abruptio placentae, often called placental abruption, refers to the *premature separation of the normally implanted placenta* from the uterine wall. While it shares some clinical features with placenta previa, particularly vaginal bleeding, other characteristics serve to distinguish abruptio placentae from placenta previa, the most important of which are abdominal discomfort and painful uterine contractions (see Table 9.2).

Placental abruption occurs when there is hemorrhage into the decidua basalis, leading to premature placental separation and further bleeding. The cause for this bleeding is not known. Placental abruption is associated with maternal hypertension and sudden decompression of the uterus in cases of rupture of membranes in a patient with excessive amniotic fluid (hydramnios) or after delivery of the first of multiple fetuses. A more recent and serious association involves cocaine use by the mother, which leads to intense vasoconstriction and, in some cases, sudden separation of the placenta from the uterine wall. Placental abruption can also occur following trauma, even when the extent of injury is not considered serious. For example, pregnant women involved in motor vehicle accidents can sustain placental

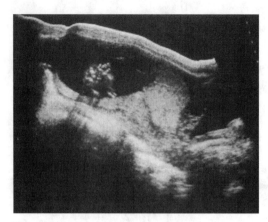

Figure 9.2.   Posterior placenta previa on transabdominal ultrasound.

abruption even though lap belts and shoulder strap restraints are used. Moreover, direct trauma to the abdomen is not required, as sudden force applied elsewhere to the body can result in coup and contrecoup injury.

The anatomic relationship between vaginal bleeding and placental abruption is shown in Figure 9.3. If the bleeding and subsequent separation of a placenta permit access to the cervical os, vaginal bleeding will be apparent. If the placental location is higher in the uterus, or if the bleeding is more central and the margins of the placenta remain attached to the underlying uterus, blood may not escape into the vagina. Thus the amount of vaginal bleeding is extremely variable, from none to heavy. The bleeding into the basalis stimulates the uterine muscle to contract, and the uterus will be painful to the patient and tender to touch. Unusually painful uterine contractions are frequent and the uterus may feel constantly tense. At times, the bleeding can penetrate the uterine musculature to such an extent that, at the time of cesarean delivery, the entire uterus has a purplish or bluish appearance, owing to such extravasation of blood (Couvelaire uterus). Despite its unusual appearance, no treatment is required, as spontaneous resolution of the condition will occur postpartum.

Because the separation of the placenta from the uterus interferes with oxygenation of the fetus, a nonreassuring fetal status is quite common in cases of significant placental abruption. Thus, in any patient in whom placental abruption is suspected, electronic fetal monitoring should be included in the initial management. Fetal death

caused by deprivation of oxygen is, unfortunately, not rare with placental abruption.

Coagulation abnormalities may also be found, thereby compounding the patient's already compromised status. Placental abruption is the most common cause of consumptive coagulopathy in pregnancy and is manifested by hypofibrinogenemia as well as by increased levels of fibrin degradation products. The platelet count can also be decreased, and prothrombin time and partial thromboplastin time can be increased as well. Such coagulopathy is a result of intravascular and retroplacental coagulation. The intravascular fibrinogen is converted to fibrin by way of the extrinsic clotting cascade. Thus not only is serum fibrinogen decreased but platelets and other clotting factors are thereby also depleted. Transfusion with crystalloid and whole blood should be implemented as soon as possible for those patients who require either volume replacement or oxygen-carrying capacity. Whole blood helps to replace not only volume but also oxygen-carrying capacity. Whole blood may also contain some clotting factors, including fibrinogen. Many experts recommend component therapy (e.g., packed red cells, platelets, fresh frozen plasma, etc.) rather than whole blood therapy (Table 9.3). The extent of placental abruption is generally categorized as the proportion of the maternal surface of the placenta on which a clot is detected at the time of delivery, e.g., 50% abruption.

Ultrasound is of little benefit in diagnosing placental abruption, except to exclude placenta previa as a cause for the hemorrhage. Relatively large retroplacental clots may be detected on ultrasound examination, but the absence of ultrasonographically identified retroplacental clots does not rule out the possibility of placental abruption, and conversely, a retroplacental echogenic area can be seen in patients without placental abruption. The diagnosis rests on the classic clinical presentation of vaginal bleeding, a tender uterus, and frequent uterine contractions with some evidence of fetal distress. The extravasation of blood into the uterine muscle causes contractions such that the resting intrauterine pressure, when measured with an intrauterine pressure catheter, is often elevated; this sign can be helpful in making the diagnosis.

Management of a patient with placental abruption when the fetus is mature is hemodynamic stabilization and delivery. Careful attention to blood component therapy is critical, and the coagulation status must be followed closely. Unless there is

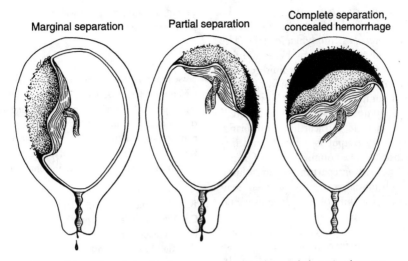

Figure 9.3. The relationship between vaginal bleeding and abruptio placentae.

Table 9.3.
Blood Replacement Products

Component (volume/unit)	Factors Present	Discussion
Packed RBC (200)	RBCs only	Replaces RBC cell mass only
Fresh-frozen plasma (200–400)	All procoagulants; no platelets	~1 g fibrinogen per unit
Cryoprecipitate (20–50)	Fibrinogen; factors VIII and XIII	Variable fibrinogen content; averages 0.25 mg/bag
Fresh whole blood (500)	RBCs and all procoagulants	Often difficult to obtain

evidence of fetal distress or hemodynamic instability, vaginal delivery by oxytocin induction of labor is preferable to a cesarean delivery, although the maternal or fetal status may require that abdominal delivery be performed. When the fetus is not mature and the placental abruption is limited and not associated with premature labor or fetal or maternal distress, observation with close monitoring of both fetal and maternal well-being may be considered while awaiting fetal maturity.

VASA PREVIA

Although rarely encountered, vasa previa presents significant risk to the fetus. In vasa previa, the umbilical cord inserts into the membranes of the placenta (rather than into the central mass of the placental tissue), and one such vessel lies below the presenting fetal part in the vicinity of the internal os. Should this vessel rupture, fetal bleeding will occur. Because of the low blood volume of the fetus, seemingly insignificant amounts of blood may place the fetus in jeopardy. A small amount of vaginal bleeding associated with fetal tachycardia may be the clinical presentation. A test to distinguish fetal blood from maternal blood, such as the Kleihauer-Betke or the APT test, can be of value when such a condition is suspected. These tests distinguish between maternal and fetal blood on the basis of the marked resistance to pH changes in fetal red cells compared with the friable nature of adult red cells in the presence of strong bases. Immediate cesarean section is the only way to save the fetus in vasa previa.

APPROACH TO A PATIENT WITH VAGINAL BLEEDING IN THE SECOND HALF OF GESTATION

In any woman with vaginal bleeding during the second half of pregnancy, fetal and maternal status should be evaluated promptly. At the same time that a search is undertaken for the cause of the bleeding, attention must be directed toward stabilization of the maternal hemodynamic state. The approach is not unlike that for any hemorrhaging patient and includes ready access for fluid replacement through one or more large-bore intravenous catheters, serial complete blood counts, type and cross-match of ample amounts of blood, and if the condition is unstable, intracardiac monitoring. Attention to urinary output is a simple and important reflection of the volume status of a patient. Because normal antepartum blood volume expansion is substantial, pregnant women may lose considerable amounts of blood before vital sign changes are apparent.

In more than half of the cases of significant vaginal bleeding in pregnancy, no specific cause can be discovered despite careful evaluation. In general, patients with significant bleeding should remain hospitalized until delivery, although in some cases minimal bleeding will cease, and the patient will appear normal in every way. Caution is advised, however, as patients with bleeding of undetermined etiology can be at greater risk for preterm delivery, intrauterine growth retardation, and fetal distress than patients with bleeding of known cause.

CASE STUDIES

Case 9A

A 26-year-old G1 at 29 weeks of gestation by last menstrual period (LMP) has phoned the hospital, saying she had an episode of bright red vaginal bleeding without other symptoms about 2 hr ago. You have not seen her previously.

Questions Case 9A

Your best instruction to her is to

A. Call back if there is another episode of bleeding
B. Come in for evaluation
C. Make an office appointment
D. Make an appointment in radiology for ultrasound evaluation

Answer: B

Immediate evaluation of fetal and maternal status is required. Placenta previa may present in this manner and, although the first bleeding episode may have been self-limited, the second may be much more profuse. Although there are no reported symptoms, abruptio placentae is still a possibility with the associated need for prompt fetal evaluation.

The patient arrives at the hospital and is found to have stable vital signs. Further history includes a fall, in which she hit her abdomen, about 6 hr before the bleeding episode. The patient's physical examination reveals a very mildly tender uterus over the area of the fall and minimal vaginal spotting, and speculum examination shows no cervical dilation or evidence of rupture of membranes. Immediate management should include

A. i.v. fluids
B. Electronic fetal monitoring
C. Ultrasound evaluation
D. Amniocentesis
E. Kleihauer-Betke test

Answer: A, B, C, E

Since the mother is hemodynamically stable, immediate evaluation of fetal status, using electronic fetal monitoring and ultrasound, is indicated because you have not established a cause of the bleeding. Ultrasound examination is often advised before any vaginal examination, although a careful speculum examination is advocated before ultrasound examination by some authorities. Venous access is indicated in the event of further bleeding. Amniocentesis may be indicated in the future, but at present it is too invasive for the information needed.

Evaluation reveals a normal 29-week fetus with normal movement and amniotic fluid volume and a partial placenta previa, which is posteriorly located. The Kleihauer-Betke test is negative. Over the next few hours, there is no more bleeding and no other symptoms. The best management at this time is

A. Cesarean birth to avoid further risk to mother and fetus
B. Amniocentesis for L:S ratio in preparation for cesarean birth
C. Resumption of normal activities, as it is only a marginal and not full placenta previa.
D. Bedrest
E. Schedule a cesarean birth for 40 weeks of gestation

Answer: D

Bedrest and pelvic rest are the basics of management. A marginal placental previa at 29 weeks may "resolve" by term, so cesarean section is not a certainty. With fetal well-being ensured for the time and no further bleeding, delivery is not indicated.

Case 9B

A 26-year-old G6 P5005 presents for her routine antepartum visit at 18 weeks' gestational age. She is distressed because at her ultrasound visit the day before she was told by the technician that her placenta was partly over the opening of her womb.

Question Case 9B

Which of the following would you tell the patient?

A. She has a placenta previa and will definitely require cesarean section
B. She has a vasa previa and will definitely require cesarean section
C. She has a placental abruption and will definitely require cesarean section
D. She has a placenta previa and may require cesarean section
E. She has a vasa previa and may require cesarean section
F. She has a placental abruption and may require cesarean section

Answer: D

The ultrasound is consistent with a partial placenta previa. Since the growth of the upper and lower uterine segments may result in the placenta "migrating away" from the cervical os, it is too early to be certain that cesarean will be required.

Case 9C

A 31-year-old G3 P1011 who believes she is about 8 months pregnant calls complaining of bright red vaginal bleeding and some cramps for the last hour. Upon questioning, you learn she has had no prenatal care, was in a drug rehabilitation program but left a few weeks ago, and is homeless.

Questions Case 9C

Your best action is which of the following?

A. Because she has had no prenatal care to this point, there is little you can do until she is in labor; thus you advise her to call again when she is in labor
B. Ask her to come in for evaluation
C. Ask her to come in for induction of labor
D. Ask her to call your office for an appointment sometime in the next 2 weeks

E. Tell her to return immediately to her drug program

Answer: B

She needs evaluation for antepartum bleeding, which may have several causes, including placenta previa, abruptio placentae, and labor. Neither induction nor any delay in evaluation is indicated.

She is evaluated, and you discover a normotensive, slightly disoriented woman with a fundal height of 30 cm and a slightly tender uterus. She has irregular uterine contractions and a baseline fetal heart rate of 150 with good beat-to-beat variability. Ultrasound shows a 30-week gestation with adequate amniotic fluid, a fundal placenta without evidence of placenta previa or abruptio placentae. Urine drug screen is positive for cocaine and alcohol. Careful pelvic examination by speculum shows her cervix to be closed with minimal bleeding and no evidence of rupture of membranes. Your most likely diagnosis is

A. Labor
B. Abruptio placentae
C. Placenta previa
D. Cervicitis
E. Cervical carcinoma

Answer: B

There is no evidence of placenta previa or labor. Although there is no evidence of abruptio placentae on ultrasound, it occurs more frequently in patients who use cocaine.

Your best management is

A. Observation at home
B. Observation in the hospital
C. Induction of labor
D. Cesarean birth
E. Discharge to the drug rehabilitation program

Answer: B

There is no evidence of maternal or fetal compromise requiring delivery. Given her drug use, noncompliance, and homeless status, observation in the hospital is especially appropriate, with serial evaluation of maternal and fetal status.

Preeclampsia

Severe

BP > 160/110

Proteinuria > 1gm/24hr
$\qquad$ 2+ on dip

Oliguria
Cerebral Disturbance / HA
Scotomata
Pulmonary Edema
Cyanosis
RUQ pain
Thrombocytopenia

Eclampsia

↑ c̄ Convulsions

chapter 10

HYPERTENSION IN PREGNANCY

Hypertensive disorders are among the most common and yet serious conditions seen in obstetrics. These disorders cause substantial morbidity and mortality for both mother and fetus, despite improved prenatal care. The etiology of hypertension unique to pregnancy remains unknown.

Hypertension in pregnancy is generally defined as a diastolic blood pressure of 90 mm Hg or greater, as a systolic blood pressure at or above 140 mm Hg, or as a rise in the diastolic blood pressure of at least 15 mm Hg or in the systolic blood pressure of 30 mm Hg or more when compared to previous blood pressures. This definition requires that the increased blood pressures be present on at least two separate occasions, 6 hr or more apart. Although this definition seems quite clear, its use in clinical practice is difficult because of various problems in obtaining a reliable assessment of blood pressure.

The position of the patient influences blood pressure. It is lowest with the patient lying in the lateral position, highest when the patient is standing, and at an intermediate level when she is sitting (Fig. 10.1). The choice of the correct size blood pressure cuff also influences blood pressure readings, with falsely high measurements noted when normal cuffs are used on large patients. Also, in the course of pregnancy, blood pressure typically declines slightly in the second trimester, rising to prepregnant levels as gestation nears term. If a patient has not been seen previously, there is no baseline blood pressure against which to compare new blood pressure determinations, thereby making the diagnosis of pregnancy-related hypertension more difficult.

Pregnancy-induced hypertension (PIH) develops in 5 to 10% of pregnancies that proceed beyond the first trimester, with a 30% incidence in multiple gestation, regardless of parity. Maternal morbidity is directly related to the severity and duration of hypertension; maternal mortality is rare, however, even when associated with such complica-

tions as abruptio placentae, hepatic rupture, or preeclampsia/eclampsia. Perinatal mortality increases progressively with each 5 mm Hg rise in mean arterial pressure, primarily associated with uteroplacental insufficiency and abruptio placentae.

HYPERTENSIVE DISEASE IN PREGNANCY

Classification

Various classifications of hypertensive disorders in pregnancy have been proposed. Table 10.1 presents the commonly used classification of the American College of Obstetricians and Gynecologists (ACOG). Since hypertensive disorders in pregnancy represent a spectrum of disease, classification systems should not be considered as rigid markers on which all management decisions are made.

Preeclampsia is defined as *the development of hypertension with proteinuria or edema (or both), induced by pregnancy, generally in the second half of gestation.* Preeclampsia is more common in women who have not carried a previous pregnancy beyond 20 weeks and is more frequent at the extremes of the reproductive years. Preeclampsia is classified as *severe* if there is a blood pressure greater than or equal to 160 mm Hg systolic or 110 mm Hg diastolic, marked proteinuria (generally >1 g/24-hr urine collection, or 2+ or more on dipstick of a random urine), oliguria, cerebral or visual disturbances such as headache and scotomata, pulmonary edema or cyanosis, epigastric or right upper quadrant pain (probably caused by subcapsular hepatic hemorrhage or stretching of Glisson's capsule), evidence of hepatic dysfunction, or thrombocytopenia. These myriad changes illustrate the multisystem alterations associated with preeclampsia.

Eclampsia is the presence of convulsions, which are not caused by neurologic disease, in a woman whose condition also meets the criteria of pre-

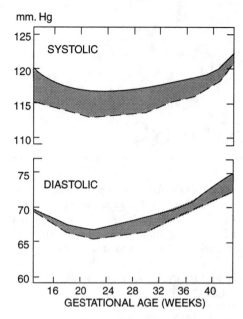

Figure 10.1. Range of blood pressures in normotensive pregnancy. Note the fall in blood pressure in the second trimester.

Table 10.1.
Hypertensive Disorders in Pregnancy[a]

Pregnancy-induced hypertension
  Preeclampsia
    Mild
    Severe
  Eclampsia

Chronic hypertension preceding pregnancy
(any etiology)

Chronic hypertension (any etiology) with superimposed
  pregnancy-induced hypertension
    Superimposed preeclampsia
    Superimposed eclampsia

[a] Classification of the ACOG.

eclampsia. This most serious aspect of hypertensive disease in pregnancy occurs in 0.5 to 4.0% of deliveries, with approximately 25% occurring in the first 72 hr postpartum.

Chronic hypertension is defined as hypertension present before the 20th week of gestation or beyond 6 weeks postpartum. Chronic hypertension can be due to a variety of causes, although the majority of cases are deemed essential hypertension. The greatest risk to a woman with chronic hypertension during pregnancy is the development of superimposed preeclampsia or eclampsia, which occurs in approximately 25% of cases. At times, it is difficult to distinguish between preeclampsia and chronic hypertension when a patient is seen late in pregnancy with an elevated blood pressure. In such cases, it is always wise to assume that the findings represent preeclampsia and treat accordingly. Finally, *preeclampsia or eclampsia superimposed upon chronic hypertension* is defined as the development of preeclampsia or eclampsia in a patient with preexisting chronic hypertension.

Not mentioned in the ACOG classification is the finding of hypertension in late pregnancy in the absence of other findings suggestive of preeclampsia. Such a condition has been termed *tran-*

sient hypertension of pregnancy or gestational hypertension. Although isolated hypertension is certainly seen in late pregnancy and in the first couple days postpartum, caution should be taken in assuming that these patients have hypertension alone.

Pathophysiology

Hypertension in pregnancy affects the mother and newborn to varying degrees, depending on the severity of disease. Given the characteristic multisystem effects, it is clear that several pathophysiologic mechanisms are involved. Unfortunately, present understanding of these mechanisms lags behind the ability to describe the clinical manifestations. One common pathophysiologic finding in hypertension in pregnancy, especially when there is progression to preeclampsia, is *vasospasm.* Although numerous theories — ranging from poor nutrition to climate changes — have been proposed to explain this vascular phenomenon, the etiology of the vasospasm remains unknown. Interestingly, it has been shown that women with uncomplicated pregnancies are extraordinarily resistant to the effects of the potent pressor angiotensin II, while those patients destined to develop preeclampsia do not demonstrate the decreased peripheral resistance normally seen in pregnancies. Hepatocellular dysfunction, coagulopathy, and renal dysfunction are also encountered, usually in severe cases of the disease.

Presumably because of vasospastic changes, placental size and function are decreased. The results are progressive fetal hypoxia and malnutrition as well as an increase in the incidence of intrauterine growth retardation, oligohydramnios, and dysmaturity. With the stress of uterine contractions during labor, the placenta is often

Table 10.2.
Laboratory Assessment of Pregnant Hypertensive Patients

Test or Procedure	Rationale
Maternal studies	
Complete blood count	Increasing hematocrit may signify worsening vasoconstriction and decreased intravascular volume
Platelet count	Thrombocytopenia and coagulopathy are associated with worsening PIH[a]
Coagulation profile (PT, PTT)[a]	
Fibrin split products	
Liver function studies	Hepatocellular dysfunction is associated with worsening PIH
Serum creatinine	Decreased renal function is associated with worsening PIH
24-hr urine for	
Creatinine clearance	
Total urinary protein	
Uric acid	
Fetal studies	
Ultrasound examination	To assess for pregnancy-associated hypertension effects on the fetus
Fetal weight and growth	IUGR[a]
Amniotic fluid volume	Oligohydramnios
Placental status	Chronic fetal stress/distress
NST/OCT	
Biophysical profile	

[a] *PT*, prothrombin time; *PTT*, partial thromboplastin time; *PIH*, pregnancy-induced hypertension; *IUGR*, intrauterine growth retardation.

incapable of supporting the fetus, resulting in intrapartum uteroplacental insufficiency with progressive fetal hypoxia and acidosis.

Evaluation

The history and physical examination are directed toward detection of pregnancy-associated hypertensive disease and its stigmata. A review of current obstetric records, if available, is especially helpful to ascertain changes or progression in findings. *Visual disturbances*, especially scotomata (spots before the eyes), or unusually severe or persistent headaches are indicative of vasospasm. *Right upper quadrant* (RUQ) *pain* may indicate liver involvement, presumably involving distention of the liver capsule. Any history of *loss of consciousness or seizures*, even in the patient with a known seizure disorder, may be significant.

The patient's weight is compared with her pregravid weight and with previous weights during this pregnancy, with special attention to excessive or too rapid weight gain. Peripheral edema is common in pregnancy, especially in the lower extremities; however, persistent edema unresponsive to resting in the supine position is not normal, especially when it also involves the upper extremities and face. Indeed, the puffy-faced, edematous hypertensive pregnant woman is the classic picture of severe preeclampsia. Careful blood pressure de-

termination in the sitting and supine positions is necessary. Fundoscopic examination may detect vasoconstriction of retinal blood vessels, presumably indicative of similar vasoconstriction of other small vessels. Tenderness over the liver attributed in part to hepatic capsule distension may be associated with complaints of RUQ pain. The patellar and Achilles deep tendon reflexes should be carefully elicited and hyperreflexia noted. The demonstration of clonus at the ankle is especially worrisome.

The maternal and fetal laboratory evaluations for pregnancy complicated by hypertension are presented in Table 10.2 and demonstrate, by the wide range of tests, the multisystem effects of hypertension in pregnancy. Maternal liver and renal dysfunction and coagulopathy are concerns and require serial evaluation. Evaluation of fetal well-being with ultrasonography, nonstress test (NST)/oxytocin challenge test (OCT), and/or biophysical profile is crucial.

Management

The goal of management of hypertension in pregnancy is to balance the management of both fetus and mother to optimize each outcome. In general, maternal blood pressure should be monitored and the mother should be observed for the sequelae of the hypertensive disease. Intervention for maternal indications should occur when the risk of permanent disability or death for the mother without intervention outweighs the risks to the fetus caused by intervention. For the fetus, there should be regular evaluation of fetal well-being and fetal growth, with intervention becoming necessary if the intrauterine environment provides more risks to the fetus than delivery with subsequent care in the newborn nursery.

MANAGEMENT OF PREECLAMPSIA

The severity of the preeclampsia and the maturity of the fetus are the primary considerations in the management of preeclampsia. Care must be individualized, but these are well-accepted general guidelines.

The mainstay of patients with *mild preeclampsia* and an immature fetus is *bed rest*, preferably with as much of the time as possible spent in a lateral decubitus position. In this position, cardiac function and uterine blood flow are maximized and maternal blood pressures in most cases are normalized. This improves uteroplacental function, allowing normal fetal growth and metabolism. For a patient with mild preeclampsia who has access to medical care and is motivated to care for herself, bed rest at home with daily weighing (if possible), fetal movement count records, and home blood pressure determinations (if available) will usually suffice. The patient is instructed to recognize the signs and symptoms that indicate worsening of the preeclampsia and to notify her physician in such an event. In the absence of significant changes in her condition, such care will allow the fetus to grow and become more functionally mature. In addition, induction of labor, if needed, is more likely to be successful as gestational age approaches term.

Hospitalization is recommended if the patient lacks either transportation for frequent prenatal visits or motivation to maintain bed rest, or for the patient in whom expectant management at home does not result in normalization of blood pressure. The same regimen is used in the hospital, but better compliance is ensured in this more controlled environment.

For the patient with *worsening preeclampsia* or the patient who has *severe preeclampsia or eclampsia*, stabilization with magnesium sulfate, antihypertensive therapy as indicated, monitoring for maternal and fetal well-being, and delivery by induction or cesarean section are required. A 24-hr delay in delivery to allow steroid administration to enhance fetal pulmonary maturity may be indicated in some cases.

For more than half a century, *magnesium sulfate* has been used to prevent convulsions. It has virtually no effect on blood pressure. Other anticonvulsants such as diazepam and phenytoin are infrequently used in obstetrics. Magnesium sulfate may be administered by intramuscular or intravenous routes, although the latter is more common. An initial 4-g loading dose is given intravenously over 20 to 30 min, followed by a constant infusion of 1 to 3 g/hr. In 98% of cases, convulsions will be prevented. Therapeutic levels are 4 to 7 mEq/liter, with toxic concentrations having predictable consequences (Table 10.3). Frequent evaluations of the patient's patellar reflex and respirations are necessary to monitor for manifestations of toxic serum magnesium concentrations. In addition, because magnesium sulfate is excreted solely from the kidney, maintenance of urine output at ≥25 mL/hr will avoid accumulation of the drug. Reversal of the effects of excessive magnesium concentrations is accomplished by the slow intravenous administration of 10% calcium gluconate along with oxygen supplementation and cardiorespiratory support if needed.

Antihypertensive therapy is indicated if the diastolic blood pressure is repeatedly above 110 mm Hg. Hydralazine (Apresoline) is the initial antihypertensive of choice, given in 5-mg increments intravenously until acceptable blood pressures are obtained. A 10- to 15-min response time is usual. The goal of such therapy is to reduce the diastolic pressure to the 90 to 100 mm Hg range. Further

Table 10.3.
Magnesium Toxicity

Serum Concentration (mg/dL)	Manifestation
1.5–3	Normal concentration
4–7	Therapeutic levels
5–10	ECG changes
8–12	Loss of patellar reflex
9–12	Feeling of warmth, flushing
10–12	Somnolence; slurred speech
15–17	Muscle paralysis; respiratory difficulty
>30	Cardiac arrest

Table 10.4.
Antihypertensive Medications Used in Pregnancy

Medication	Mechanism of Action	Effects
Thiazide	Decreased plasma volume and CO[a]	CO decreased; RBF[a] decreased; maternal electrolyte depletion; neonatal thrombocytopenia
Methyldopa	False neurotransmission, CNS[a] effect	CO unchanged; RBF unchanged; Maternal lethargy, fever, hepatitis, and hemolytic anemia
Hydralazine	Direct peripheral vasodilation	CO increased; RBF unchanged or increased; maternal flushing, headache, tachycardia, lupus-like syndrome
Propranolol	β-adrenergic blocker	CO decreased; RBF decreased; maternal increased uterine tone with possible decrease in placental perfusion; neonatal depressed respirations
Labetalol	α- and β-adrenergic blocker	CO unchanged; RBF unchanged maternal tremulousness, flushing, headache; neonatal depressed respirations
Nifedipine	Calcium channel blocker	CO unchanged; RBF unchanged; maternal orthostatic hypotension and headache (also a tocolytic); no neonatal effects known
Prazosin (Minipress)	Direct vasodilator and cardiac effects	CO increased or unchanged; RBF unchanged; maternal hypotension with first dose

[a] *CO*, cardiac output; *RBF*, renal blood flow; *CNS*, central nervous system.

Table 10.5.
Drug Therapy for Hypertensive Emergencies in Pregnancy

Drug	Regimen	Course of Action
Hydralazine (Apresoline)	10–50 mg i.m. q. 3–6h.; 5–25 mg i.v. q. 3–6h.	Onset, 10–20 min; maximum effect, 20–40 min; duration, 3–8 hr
Nifedipine	10 mg p.o. q. 4–8h.	Onset, 5–10 min; maximum effect, 10–20 min; duration, 4–8 hr
Trimethaphan camyslate (Arfonad)	i.v. infusion: 2 g/liter; 1–5 mg/min	Onset, 1–2 min; maximum effect, 2–5 min; duration, 10 min
Sodium nitroprusside	i.v. infusion: 0.01 g/liter; 0.2–0.8 mg/min	Onset, 0.5–2 min; maximum effect, 1–2 min; duration, 3–5 min
Labetalol	20–50 mg i.v. q. 3–6h.	Onset, 1–2 min; maximum effect, 10 min; duration, 6–16 hr

reduction of the blood pressure may impair uterine blood flow to rates dangerous to the fetus. Other antihypertensive agents may be used if hydralazine is not effective (Tables 10.4 and 10.5).

Once anticonvulsant and antihypertensive therapy is established, attention is directed toward *delivery*. Induction of labor is often attempted, although cesarean delivery may be needed either if induction is unsuccessful or not possible or if maternal or fetal status is worsening. At delivery, blood loss must be closely monitored, because patients with preeclampsia or eclampsia have significantly reduced blood volumes. *After delivery*, patients are kept in the labor and delivery area for 24

hr for close observation of their clinical progress and further administration of magnesium sulfate to prevent postpartum eclamptic seizures. Approximately 25% of all preeclamptic patients who have eclamptic seizures will have them before labor, about 50% during labor, and about 25% after delivery. Usually, the vasospastic process begins to reverse itself in the first 24 to 48 hr, as manifest by a brisk diuresis.

The management of patients with *chronic hypertension in pregnancy* involves closely monitoring maternal blood pressure and watching for the superimposition of preeclampsia or eclampsia and following the fetus for appropriate growth and fetal well-being. Also, the patient should be encouraged to increase the amount of time she rests. Medical treatment of milder forms of chronic hypertension has been disappointing in that no significant improvement in pregnancy outcome has been demonstrated. Antihypertensive medication is generally not given unless the diastolic blood pressure exceeds 110 mm Hg. Methyldopa is the most commonly used antihypertensive medication for this purpose. It was formerly taught that diuretics were contraindicated during pregnancy, but diuretic therapy is no longer discontinued in the patient who was already on such therapy before becoming pregnant.

MANAGEMENT OF THE ECLAMPTIC SEIZURE

The eclamptic seizure is a time of life-threatening risk for mother and fetus. Maternal risks include musculoskeletal injury (including biting the tongue), hypoxia, and aspiration. Maternal therapy consists of inserting a padded tongue blade, restraining gently as needed, providing oxygen, and gaining an i.v. access. Eclamptic seizures are usually self-limited so that medical therapy should be directed to the initiation of magnesium therapy to prevent further seizures rather than to anticonvulsant therapy with diazepam or similar drugs. Transient uterine hyperactivity for 2 to 15 min is associated with fetal heart rate (FHR) changes, including bradycardia or compensatory tachycardia, decreased beat-to-beat activity, and late decelerations. These are self-limited and not dangerous to the fetus unless they continue for 20 min or more. Delivery during this time imposes unnecessary risk for mother and fetus and should be avoided. Arterial blood gases should be obtained, any metabolic disturbance should be corrected, and a Foley catheter should be placed to monitor urinary output. If the maternal blood pressure is very high, if maternal urinary output is low, or if there is evidence of cardiac disturbance, consideration of a central monitor and continuous ECG monitoring are appropriate.

HELLP SYNDROME

HELLP is the acronym for a specific set of hypertensive patients who have *hemolysis, liver dysfunction, and low platelets*. This syndrome was recently described as a distinct clinical entity, occurring in 4 to 12% of patients with severe preeclampsia or eclampsia. Patients with HELLP syndrome are often multiparous, somewhat older than the average obstetric patient, and somewhat less hypertensive than many preeclamptic patients. The liver dysfunction may be manifest as right upper quadrant pain and is all too commonly misdiagnosed as gallbladder disease or indigestion. Maternal and fetal mortality for patients with HELLP is significant, making accurate diagnosis imperative. Unfortunately, the first symptoms are often rather vague, including nausea and emesis and a nonspecific viral-like syndrome. Treatment of these gravely ill patients is best done in a high-risk obstetric center and consists of cardiovascular stabilization, correction of coagulation abnormalities, and delivery. Parenteral analgesia in labor is appropriate, but pudendal or epidural anesthesia is contraindicated because of the risk of bleeding. Platelet transfusion before or after delivery is indicated if the platelet count is less than 20,000/mm^3, and it may be advisable to transfuse patients with a platelet count below 50,000/mm^3 before proceeding with a cesarean birth.

CASE STUDIES

Case 10A

A 38-year-old G2 P1001 presents for prenatal care at 10 weeks of gestational age by good dates and initial pelvic examination. Her obstetric history includes a normal pregnancy and delivery at age 17. She was diagnosed as having essential hypertension 4 years ago and was placed on a diuretic and methyldopa; she says her blood pressure "runs about 140/90 most of the time."

On physical examination, the patient weighs 280 pounds. A blood pressure taken with a large cuff is 135/85 supine and 140/95 sitting. She has mild arteriolar narrowing on fundoscopic examination, a normal cardiovascular examination, a 10-week-size uterus, normal deep tendon reflexes (DTRs), and 1+ lower extremity peripheral edema. Her urine sample dipstick shows 1+ protein and trace glucose.

Questions Case 10A

Your initial diagnosis is

A. Pregnancy-induced hypertension
B. Mild preeclampsia
C. Severe preeclampsia
D. Eclampsia
E. Chronic hypertension
F. Chronic hypertension with superimposed pregnancy-induced hypertension

Answer: E

This patient's hypertension precedes her pregnancy. Although her status nears the definition of mild preeclampsia, which would give her the diagnosis of chronic hypertension with superimposed mild preeclampsia, her stable history precludes this diagnosis at her initial visit.

Your initial management should include

A.   Discontinue the diuretic and methyldopa
B.   Recommend strict bed rest at home
C.   Recommend therapeutic abortion
D.   Hospitalize for the remainder of pregnancy
E.   None of these

Answer: E

Initial management should be to maximize rest, but strict bed rest at home is too much restriction at this time. Modern obstetric practice is not to change the antihypertensive medications of chronic hypertensive patients who become pregnant. Instead, the regimen is continued while maternal and fetal evaluations commence. There is no indication for hospitalization or for therapeutic abortion.

Case 10B

A 19-year-old G1 has had an unremarkable antepartum course since her first prenatal visit at 8 weeks. At the start of her 32nd week she complains of swollen hands and feet and "puffy eyes," which have been getting worse for the last 2 days. Her blood pressure is 150/95 compared with her usual blood pressure of 130/70. After resting for 30 min, her blood pressure is 145/85. Her dipstick urinary protein is 1–2+. She reports daily fetal movement that has not changed and denies headache, abdominal pain, or dizzy spells.

Questions Case 10B

Your initial diagnosis is

A.   Pregnancy-induced hypertension
B.   Mild preeclampsia
C.   Severe preeclampsia
D.   Eclampsia
E.   Chronic hypertension
F.   Chronic hypertension with superimposed pregnancy-induced hypertension

Answer: B

This patient has mild preeclampsia. Her 1–2+ proteinuria is disconcerting, but her rapid improvement in blood pressure with 30 min of rest is reassuring, as is her history of an active fetus.

Which of the following evaluations are indicated at the present time?

A.   Obstetric ultrasound
B.   NST
C.   OCT
D.   Amniocentesis for fetal lung maturity determination
E.   Pelvic examination
F.   Biophysical profile
G.   Complete blood count (CBC), coagulation profile, and liver function studies
H.   24-hr urine collection for total protein and creatinine clearance

Answer: A, B, E, F, G, H

Because there is no need to deliver the fetus at this time, fetal lung maturity is not an issue. Without evidence of fetal stress, OCT is not warranted unless the NST is not reassuring. Ultrasound can evaluate amniotic fluid volume and provide the biophysical profile. The chemical evaluations of maternal status are indicated, if for no other reason than to serve as a baseline evaluation if the mother's condition deteriorates. A pelvic examination is a wise precaution at this time to evaluate the favorability of the cervix, because the potential for induction exists if the maternal or fetal status worsens.

chapter 11

ISOIMMUNIZATION

Isoimmunization refers to the development of antibodies to red blood cell antigens following exposure to such antigens from another individual. In pregnancy, the *"other individual" is the fetus,* 50% of whose genetic makeup is derived from the father. If the mother is exposed to fetal red cells during pregnancy or at delivery, she may develop antibodies to fetal cell antigens. Later in that pregnancy, or more commonly with the subsequent pregnancy, the antibodies can cross the placenta and hemolyze fetal red cells, leading to fetal anemia. In a pregnancy complicated by isoimmunization, the manufacture of maternal antibody that destroys fetal red cells is countered by the ability of the fetus to manufacture sufficient red cells to permit survival and growth.

NATURAL HISTORY

Isoimmunization can involve many of the *several hundred blood group systems.* This disorder is frequently referred to as Rh isoimmunization, because the Rhesus (Rh) system is most frequently involved. For the sake of this discussion, the Rh system will be used as an example, although it should be remembered that isoimmunization can and does develop with many other blood systems such as Kell, Duffy, Kidd, and others.

Within the Rh system, there are several specific antigens, the one most commonly associated with hemolytic disease being the *D* antigen. If a fetus is Rh+, having received the genes for the Rh *D* antigen from its father, and the mother lacks the Rh antigen, that is, she is Rh–, the conditions exist for the development of isoimmunization. In the woman's first such pregnancy, the infant typically has no complications. At the time of delivery, however, if the mother's blood is exposed to fetal red cells, even minuscule amounts, the woman can develop antibodies to the Rh *D* antigen. Antibody development will occur in about 15% of cases of

an Rh– mother and Rh+ fetus. In a subsequent pregnancy, passage of minute amounts of fetal blood across the placenta, which occurs quite frequently, can lead to an *anamnestic response* of maternal antibody production. If the mother produces IgM-type antibodies, the molecules will not cross the placenta, because they are too large. In the case of Rh factor, however, the maternal antibody is predominantly the smaller IgG-type, which can freely crosses the placenta and enter the fetal circulation. Once in the fetal vascular system, the antibody attaches to the Rh+ red blood cells and hemolyzes them. The bilirubin produced in this hemolytic process is transferred back across the placenta to the mother and metabolized. *The condition of the fetus is determined by the amount of maternal antibody transferred across the placenta and the ability of the fetus to replace the red blood cells that have been destroyed.*

In the first affected pregnancy, the infant may be anemic at delivery and may soon develop elevated levels of bilirubin, since hemolysis continues after birth and the newborn must now rely on its own, somewhat immature, liver to metabolize the bilirubin. *In subsequent pregnancies,* with an Rh+ fetus, the process of antibody production and transfer may be accelerated, leading to the development of more significant anemia. In such cases, the fetal liver can manufacture additional red cells. However, this activity reduces the amount of proteins manufactured by the fetal liver. In turn, the reduced protein production can lead to a decreased oncotic pressure within the fetal vascular system, resulting in fetal ascites and subcutaneous edema. At the same time, the severe fetal anemia can lead to high output cardiac failure. This combination of findings is referred to as *hydrops fetalis.*

The tendency is for each subsequent baby to be more severely affected, but this is not always the case. The level of fetal disturbance may remain

Table 11.1.
Risk of Sensitization

Obstetric/Medical Event	Chance of Sensitization (percent)
Ectopic pregnancy	<1
Full-term pregnancy	1–2
Amniocentesis	1–3
Spontaneous abortion	3–4
Induced abortion	5–6
Full-term delivery, ABO compatible or incompatible	14–17
Mismatched blood transfusion	90–95

the same or, occasionally, may even be less than in the previous pregnancy. If subsequent fetuses are Rh–, which is commonly the case if the father is a heterozygote, the fetus will not be affected at all (Table 11.1).

DIAGNOSIS

Isoimmunization can often be diagnosed on the basis of *history*. A woman with a previous diagnosis of isoimmunization or with a previous birth in which the neonatal course was consistent with this disorder is at risk for recurrence. As part of routine antenatal *laboratory evaluation*, maternal blood is tested for the presence of a variety of antibodies that may cause significant disturbances in the fetus. Any significant antibodies are further evaluated for the strength of antibody response, which is reported in a titer format (1:4, 1:16, etc.). During this testing process, other antibodies may be discovered that do not cause significant fetal/neonatal problems. The two most common of these are the anti-Lewis and anti-I. When these antibodies are found, titers are not reported because of their lack of clinical importance.

MANAGEMENT

Antibody titers as described above would seem to be good markers of maternal antibody production, but in fact, such titers are of limited usefulness. In the first sensitized pregnancy, titers do seem to be helpful, but thereafter, they are of virtually no value because they do not reflect the current fetal condition. Even in the initial sensitized pregnancy, the greatest value is in distinguishing those pregnancies for which antibody production is so low as to be nonthreatening to the fetus from those

for which there are likely to be significant consequence. *A titer of 1:16 or greater is generally considered the critical point* at which there is sufficient risk of fetal jeopardy to warrant additional evaluation.

Amniotic fluid assessment is of great value in managing the isoimmunized patient. Practical use of amniotic fluid analysis became a reality in about 1960, when Liley found that *the level of bilirubin in the amniotic fluid accurately reflects the condition of the fetus.* The mechanism by which bilirubin enters the amniotic fluid from the fetal compartment is still not understood. However, in the second half of normal pregnancy, the level of bilirubin normally decreases progressively. The level of bilirubin in an affected, isoimmunized patient can be evaluated in relationship to natural decline. The level of bilirubin in the amniotic fluid is determined using a spectrophotometer. Normal amniotic fluid subjected to spectrophotometric analysis has a characteristic curve, based on optical density (OD), as shown in Figure 11.1. The presence of bilirubin causes a characteristic deviation in this curve, at 450 nm. This degree of deviation is re-

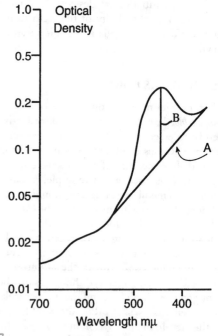

Figure 11.1 Absorption curve of amniotic fluid by spectrophotometer in a patient with isoimmunization. *A*, Anticipated curve for normal amniotic fluid; *B*, deviation of curve as a result of bilirubin in the amniotic fluid, expressed as ΔOD_{450}.

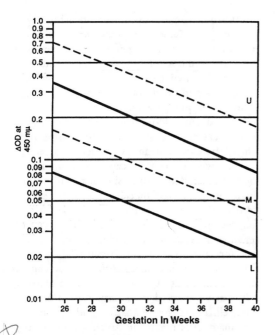

Figure 11.2. Liley curve. The ΔOD_{450} was obtained as shown in Figure 11.1 and is plotted by gestational age. The condition of fetus can be estimated by the zone in which the ΔOD_{450} falls. In the upper (U) zone, the fetus is severely affected; in the middle (M) zone, moderately affected; and in the lower (L) zone, minimally affected or not affected.

ferred to as the ΔOD_{450}. Following the pioneering work of Liley and others, normal ΔOD_{450} values have been determined (Fig. 11.2). Experience has shown how optical density relates to the severity of fetal problems, as shown in the figure.

Amniotic fluid is obtained from the patient by amniocentesis at periodic intervals between the 20th and 30th weeks of pregnancy, depending on the history of previous pregnancies. OD values are then plotted on a curve (as shown in Figure 11.2), which allows estimation of the degree of severity of the anemia in the fetus. Based on this level of severity, in conjunction with the gestational age, a decision about expected management, transfusion of the fetus, or delivery can be made. *Markedly elevated ΔOD_{450} values indicate a severely affected fetus, intermediate values indicate a moderately affected fetus, and low values represent a fetus not or only mildly affected.*

Assessment of the affected fetus by *periodic ultrasonography* can be very helpful in detecting severe signs of the hemolytic process, namely subcutaneous edema and ascites. Under ultrasound guidance, the umbilical cord can be sampled directly (percutaneous umbilical blood sampling; PUBS) and fetal blood can be taken for hematocrit determination to assess the severity of anemia. Later in pregnancy, general tests of fetal well-being are utilized in the isoimmunized patient, as the ability of an affected fetus to withstand the stresses of pregnancy and labor may be compromised.

TRANSFUSIONS

Transfusion of Rh– red blood cells to the fetus is *indicated when,* on the basis of the above assessment, it is determined that *the fetus is in significant jeopardy* for hydrops or fetal death. Traditionally, blood was transfused into the fetal abdominal cavity where absorption of the transfused cells takes place over subsequent days. More recently, direct fetal transfusions into the umbilical cord (PUBS) under ultrasonography guidance are being used more frequently, with positive results. Physicians experienced and skilled in this technique are critical to its success. The procedure carries with it a risk of fetal death of up to 3%, a risk that must be weighed against the predicted future course for the fetus in utero and the potential adverse consequences of preterm delivery. The quantity of red blood cells to be transferred can be calculated using the gestational age and size of the fetus and the fetal hematocrit. Because the transferred cells are Rh–, they are not affected by the transplacental maternal antibody. Timing of subsequent transfusions can be determined based on the severity of disease and the predicted life span of the transfused cells.

PREVENTION

Maternal exposure and subsequent sensitization to fetal blood usually occurs at delivery and much less commonly during pregnancy. In the late 1960s, it was determined that the antibody to the D antigen of the Rh system could be prepared from donors previously sensitized to the antigen. Subsequently, it was found that *administration of this antibody (Rh immune globulin) soon after delivery could, by passive immunization, prevent an active antibody response by the mother in most cases.* Rh immune globulin is effective for only the D antigen of the Rh system. No similar preparations are available for patients sensitized with the many other possible antigens. It is now standard practice for Rh– patients who deliver Rh+ infants to receive an intramuscular dose of 300 μg of Rh immune globulin (i.e., RhoGAM) within 72 hr of delivery. With this practice, the risk of subsequent sensitization decreases from approximately 15% to approximately 2%. This residual 2% was determined to be the result of sensitization occurring *during the course of pregnancy* (as opposed to at delivery), usually in the third trimester. Administration of a 300-μg dose of Rh immune globulin to Rh– patients at 28 weeks was found to reduce the risk of sensitization to about 0.2%.

Prophylaxis with Rh immune globulin in Rh– women is not necessary if the father of the pregnancy is *known with certainty* to be Rh–. Although testing of the father can be done, *if there is any question as to the paternity, prophylactic administration of Rh immune globulin should be given as described*, since the risk is negligible and the potential benefits are considerable.

In summary, Rh– pregnant patients who have no antibody on initial screening are retested at 28 weeks (to detect the rare patient sensitized earlier in pregnancy). If no sensitization has occurred, they are given Rh immune globulin to protect them from antibody formation for the remainder of pregnancy. If the father is known to be Rh–, this practice is not necessary. After delivery, the child's blood type and Rh status are determined, and if the child is Rh+, a second dose of Rh immune globulin is given to the new mother.

There are other situations where Rh immune globulin should be administered (Table 11.2). Because the amount of fetal red cells required to elicit an antibody response is minute, about 0.01 mL, *any circumstance in pregnancy in which fetomaternal hemorrhage can occur warrants Rh immune globulin administration.* Furthermore, as fetal red cell production begins with 6 weeks of conception,

Table 11.2.
Indications for Rh Immune Globulin Administration in an Unsensitized Rh-negative Patient[a]

At about 28 weeks pregnancy

Within 3 days of delivery of an Rh-positive infant

At the time of amniocentesis

After positive Kleihauer-Betke test

After an ectopic pregnancy

After a spontaneous or induced abortion

[a] Unless the father of the infant is known to be Rh–.

sensitization can occur in patients who have a spontaneous or scheduled pregnancy termination. Because the dose of antigen in such situations is low, a reduced dose of 50 μg of Rh immune globulin can be used to prevent sensitization. Amniocentesis and other trauma (e.g., from an auto accident) during pregnancy are also indications for the standard 300-μg dose of Rh immune globulin. In cases of trauma or bleeding during pregnancy, the extent, if any, to which fetomaternal hemorrhage has occurred can be evaluated using the Kleihauer-Betke test or similar test that allows the identification of fetal cells in maternal circulation. In the test, a sample of maternal blood is subjected to a strong base such as KOH. Maternal cells are very sensitive to changes in pH and, therefore, promptly lyse and become "ghost" cells. Fetal cells are much more resistant to such agents and remain intact. The ratio of fetal to maternal cells can be assessed by counting 1000 or more total cells under the microscope and determining how many cells retain the dark appearance (representing fetal cells). Then the maternal blood volume is calculated and, using the ratio just described, the total amount of fetomaternal hemorrhage is derived. Since a standard 300-μg dose of Rh immune globulin will effectively neutralize 15 mL of fetal red blood cells, the appropriate dose can then be administered.

NONRHESUS BLOOD GROUP ISOIMMUNIZATION

With a decreasing prevalence of Rhesus-isoimmunization because of Rh prevention programs, ABO hemolytic disease and non-Rh *D*/non-ABO hemolytic disease are relatively more common.

ABO hemolytic disease is associated with milder fetal kernicterus and, rarely, hydrops, probably because of the relatively smaller number of *A* and *B* antigenic sites on fetal red blood cells and because anti-*A* and *-B* are IgM and thus do not traverse the placenta well; that which does cross has a high propensity for other binding sites besides fetal red blood cells. This disease usually occurs in the first pregnancy, and amniocentesis and early delivery are rarely indicated.

Non-Rh D non-ABO hemolytic disease is frequently associated with blood transfusion, because "compatible" blood transfusion is matched only to the *ABO* and *Dd* antigens. Pregnant women who are affected by the common and uncommon antibodies that can cause hemolytic disease of the newborn are managed in the same way as those who are Rh−. Those women with antibodies that are very rarely or unassociated with hemolytic disease of the newborn need not be treated.

CASE STUDIES

Case 11A

A 22-year-old G1 P0 presents for prenatal care at 28 weeks by dates and size. Her medical and family history are negative, and her physical examination is normal and consistent with her stated gestational age. Upon review of her initial laboratory work you note that her blood type is O−. You ask her about the blood type of the father, but he has left town and she does not know what it is.

Questions Case 11A

What should your management be?

A. Offer RhoGAM on the possibility that the father is Rh+
B. Do not offer RhoGAM because the father's Rh status is unknown
C. Don't bring up the issue unless the patient asks

Answer: A

Because of the risk of isoimmunization and the low risk of administration of RhoGAM, it should be offered and given.

The patient declines as she does not want a medication unless she knows it is necessary. When she is 38 weeks, the patient learns that the father of the child is blood type O+. She asks if her baby will be damaged as a result. You respond

A. Certainly, because you failed to be treated appropriately
B. Probably, because you failed to be treated appropriately
C. Probably not, because it is the second or subsequent pregnancies that are usually affected
D. Certainly not, because it is always the second or subsequent pregnancies that are affected

Answer: C

You may reasonably reassure her and test for antibody to ascertain if any sensitization has occurred.

chapter 12

MULTIPLE GESTATION

At first glance, twin pregnancy is often considered a novelty, with pleasant images of identical children dressed alike. In fact, pregnancies with multiple fetuses pose significant medical risks for both the mother and her offspring. Special care is necessary to achieve an optimal outcome. Caring for two or more infants likewise challenges even the most devoted parents. This chapter provides an overview of twin pregnancy — its diagnosis, antepartum, intrapartum, and postpartum care — with reference to pregnancies with three or more fetuses when relevant. In general, all potential complications with twin pregnancies are somewhat more frequent and more serious as the number of fetuses increases.

INCIDENCES OF MULTIPLE GESTATION

The overall incidence of recognized twins in the United States is approximately 1 in 90, slightly higher in blacks and slightly lower in whites. Twin gestations can be characterized as dizygotic (fraternal) or monozygotic (identical). *Dizygotic twins* occur when two separate ova are fertilized by two separate sperm, and in fact, represent two siblings who happen to be born at approximately the same time. *Monozygotic twins* represent division of the fertilized ovum at various times after conception. There is a marked difference in the incidence of twinning in various populations, almost exclusively due to the incidence of dizygotic twinning. The *incidence of monozygotic twinning* is fairly constant around the world at *approximately 1 in 250 pregnancies*, whereas *dizygotic twinning* occurs as frequently as *1 in 20 pregnancies* in certain African countries. Increasing age and increasing parity are independent factors for dizygotic twinning. A familial factor is present in twinning that follows the maternal lineage. Ultrasonography, which allows early detection and serial evaluations, has provided valuable information concerning the outcome of twin pregnancies. Only about 50% of twin pregnancies detected in the first trimester result in the delivery of viable twins, with the remaining associated with death and resorption of one embryo/fetus with eventual delivery of a single fetus. Both spontaneous abortions and congenital anomalies occur more frequently in multiple pregnancies than in singleton pregnancies.

The likelihood of twinning is increased significantly if *fertility agents or other assisted reproductive technologies* are utilized. With clomiphene citrate induction of ovulation, the twinning rate is about 6 to 8%. With the use of exogenous gonadotropin therapy, the rate increases to about 25 to 35%. As in vitro fertilization programs typically insert several fertilized ova into the uterine cavity, multiple fetuses would be expected to occur in some instances; in fact, the rate of two or more fetuses is about 35 to 40%.

The incidence of three or more pregnancies may be approximated by 90 raised to the power of the number of fetuses minus one. Thus triplets are 1 in 90^2, or 1 in 8,100; quadruplets, 1 in 90^3, or 1 in 729,000; and so forth.

NATURAL HISTORY

As the number of fetuses increases, the expected *duration of pregnancy* diminishes. Compared with singleton pregnancies, which deliver at 40 weeks, twins deliver at an average of 37 weeks, triplets at 33 weeks, and quadruplets at an average of 29 weeks. Thus with each additional fetus, the length of gestation is decreased by about 4 weeks. Although all twins face certain risks, *monozygotic twins face additional risks related to the time when twinning occurs*. The developmental sequence associated with the separation of the conceptus into twins explains the basis for these problems as well as the configuration of the fetal membranes at

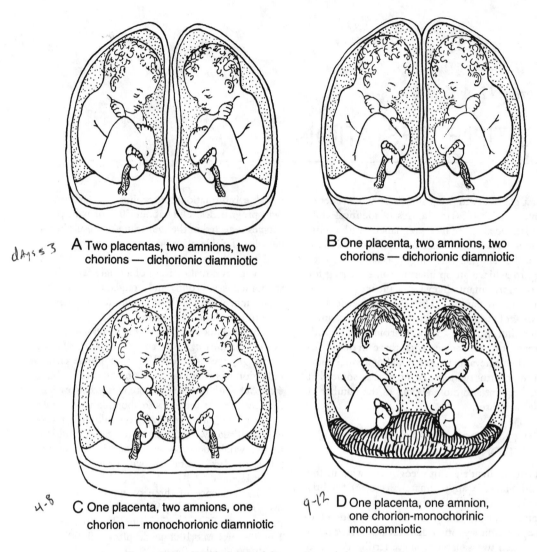

days ≤ 3   **A** Two placentas, two amnions, two chorions — dichorionic diamniotic

B One placenta, two amnions, two chorions — dichorionic diamniotic

4-8   **C** One placenta, two amnions, one chorion — monochorionic diamniotic

9-12   **D** One placenta, one amnion, one chorion-monochorinic monoamniotic

Figure 12.1.   Development of the amnion and chorion in twin pregnancies.

delivery. If division of the conceptus occurs within 3 days of fertilization, each fetus will be surrounded by an amnion and chorion, and the membranes are termed diamniotic/dichorionic. If division occurs between the 4th and 8th day following fertilization, the chorion has already begun to develop, whereas the amnion has not. Therefore, each fetus will be surrounded by an amnion, but a single chorion will surround both twins, a condition termed diamniotic/monochorionic. Division from day 9 to day 12 takes place after development of both the amnion and the chorion, and the twins will share a common sac, a condition

termed monoamniotic/monochorionic (Fig. 12.1). Division thereafter is incomplete, resulting in the development of conjoined twins, which may be fused in any of a multitude of ways, but usually at the chest and/or abdomen. This rare condition is seen in about 1 in 70,000 deliveries.

Further development can result in various vascular anastomoses between the fetuses that, in turn, can lead to a condition known as _twin-twin transfusion syndrome_. In this circumstance, blood flow of the fetuses mixes such that there is net flow from one twin to another, at times with disastrous consequences. The so-called donor twin can

Table 12.1.
Antenatal Management of Twin Pregnancies

Concern	Action
Adequate nutrition	Balanced diet; additional increase in daily caloric intake; multivitamin and mineral supplements (e.g., folate)
Increased blood loss at delivery	Prevent anemia (iron)
Fetal growth	Bedrest beginning at 24–26 weeks — the value of this is unclear, but also decreases preterm labor
Preterm labor	Educate patient on signs of labor; increase bedrest; cervical examinations every 1–2 weeks; home monitoring in select cases
Pregnancy-induced hypertension	Frequent blood pressure determinations; frequent urinary protein assessment
Fetal growth, discordant growth	Periodic ultrasonography examinations

have impaired growth, anemia, hypovolemia, and other problems. On the other hand, the recipient twin can develop hypervolemia, hypertension, polycythemia, and congestive heart failure as a result of this abnormal transfusion. A secondary manifestation involves the amniotic fluid dynamics. Because of transudate across the skin or, probably more important, increased urinary output owing to its hypervolemia, the recipient produces abundant amniotic fluid, whereas the donor twin may in fact have oligohydramnios. The hydramnios in one twin further compounds the risk of preterm labor in multifetal pregnancies. Recently, intrauterine laser ablation of the vascular anastomoses has met with some success in treating this difficult problem. Other vascular abnormalities include absence of an umbilical artery, which may be associated in 30 percent of cases with other congenital problems, especially renal agenesis. A single umbilical artery is seen in about 3 to 4% of twins, compared with 0.5 to 1% of singletons.

Multifetal pregnancy is associated with increased perinatal morbidity, three to four times that for a comparable singleton pregnancy in the case of twin gestation. The most significant cause of morbidity is preterm labor and delivery, followed by intrauterine growth retardation, polyhydraminos (in about 10% of multiple gestations, predominantly mono-

chorionic gestations), maternal disease (especially preeclampsia), congenital anomalies, and placental and umbilical cord accidents. The spontaneous abortion rate is higher in multiple gestation.

DIAGNOSIS OF MULTIPLE GESTATION

Twin pregnancy is usually *suspected when the uterine size is excessively large for the calculated gestational age.* Although there is a variation in fundal height measurements in singleton pregnancies, an increase of 4 cm between the week gestation and the carefully measured fundal height should prompt evaluation to detect twins, reassign gestational age, diagnose hydramnios, or provide other explanation for the discrepancy. In modern obstetrics, the diagnosis of twins or multiple gestation is *usually made by obstetric ultrasonography.* The differential diagnosis includes incorrect dates, leiomyoma uteri or other tumors, polyhydraminos of other etiology, and in early pregnancy, hydatidiform mole.

Once the diagnosis of twin pregnancy has been made, subsequent antenatal care addresses each of the *potential concerns* for mother and fetus listed in Table 12.1. Although the maternal blood volume is greater with a twin gestation than with singleton pregnancy, the anticipated blood loss at delivery is also greater. Anemia is more common in these patients, and a balanced diet with iron, folate, and possibly other micronutrients is important. Although the value of bedrest in prolonging gestation is controversial, it is generally advised that a woman limit her activity after 24 to 26 weeks to avoid *premature labor,* which is more common in twin gestations. Careful attention to detection of uterine contractions is important, and the patient should be cautioned about signs of preterm labor, such as low back pain, a thin vaginal discharge, and diarrhea. Cervical examinations to detect early effacement and dilation are usually done every 1 to 2 weeks. At these visits, evidence suggesting pregnancy-induced hypertension is also gathered, which includes careful measurement of blood pressure and testing for protein in the urine. Beginning at 30 to 32 weeks, daily fetal kick counts are usually begun to help assess *fetal well-being.* Although somewhat surprising, patients can almost always distinguish movements of different fetuses. Nonstress tests or other fetal monitor testing is begun as the pregnancy approaches term. Fortunately, fetal lung maturity is achieved somewhat earlier in twin pregnancies than in singleton pregnancies.

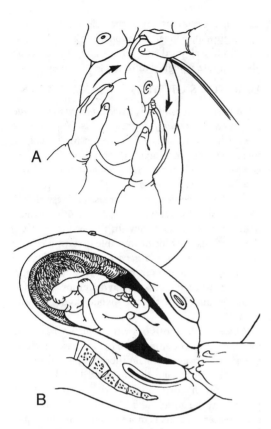

Figure 12.2. **A,** External cephalic version. **B,** Internal podalic version.

The chief antenatal assessment in twin pregnancy remains the periodic ultrasonography examination, which is done about every 4 weeks after 20 weeks gestation. At each examination, growth of each fetus is assessed and an estimate of amniotic fluid volume made. If growth is discordant, usually defined as a 20% difference in weight (the difference in weight divided by the weight of the larger fetus is 20% or more), ultrasonography may be performed more often and tests of fetal well-being (such as a nonstress test and kick counts) are begun at 30 to 32 weeks. Fetal breathing and body movements as well as body tone (elements of the biophysical profile) can also be determined with ultrasonography.

INTRAPARTUM MANAGEMENT

Intrapartum management is largely *determined by the presentation of the twins.* In general, if the first (presenting) twin is in the cephalic (vertex) presentation, labor is allowed to progress to vaginal delivery, whereas if the presenting twin is in a position other than cephalic, cesarean delivery is often performed. During labor, the heart rate of both fetuses is monitored separately. Approaches to the delivery of twins vary, depending on gestational age, presentation of the twins, and the experience of the attending physicians. Regardless of the delivery plan, access to full obstetric anesthetic and pediatric services is mandatory, in that cesarean delivery may be required on short notice.

If vaginal delivery of the first twin is accomplished and the second twin is also cephalic, delivery of the second twin generally proceeds smoothly. With proper monitoring of the second twin, there is no urgency in accomplishing the second delivery. If the second twin is presenting in any way other than cephalic, there are two primary manipulations that may effect vaginal delivery. The first is *external cephalic version* whereby, using ultrasonographic visualization, the fetus is gently guided into the cephalic presentation by abdominal massage and pressure. The second maneuver is *internal podalic version,* in which the physician reaches a hand into the uterine cavity, identifies the lower extremities of the fetus, and gently delivers the infant via breech delivery. The possibility of a prolapsed umbilical cord must always be borne in mind when delivery of twins is to be accomplished (Fig. 12.2). Postpartum, the overdistended uterus may not contract normally, leading to uterine atony and postpartum hemorrhage.

CASE STUDIES

Case 12A

At 32 weeks of gestation, a 35-year-old G1 P0 with known twins is noted to have a fundal height not commensurate with gestational age. Her weight gain and blood pressure are normal as are her antenatal laboratory studies. She says the babies are moving normally and that she feels well, although "rather large."

Questions Case 12A

Which of the following interventions, if any, are indicated?

A. Oxytocin challenge test (OCT)
B. Ultrasound
C. Nonstress test (NST)
D. Induction of labor if cephalic/cephalic presentation
E. Cesarean birth

Answer: B, C

Intrauterine growth retardation and discordant growth are both common in twin pregnancies. Measurements of each fetus for comparison may reveal abnormal development. If found, further testing with possible delivery is indicated. Evaluation of fetal well-being at the time of obstetric ultrasound and NST are noninvasive tests that yield valuable information. Given the risk of premature labor, OCT is less commonly used and would best be reserved if the NST is not reassuring. Delivery should be contemplated only if one or both fetuses is compromised.

At ultrasound her twins are noted to be monochorionic/diamniotic, with both twins moving actively in adequate amounts of amniotic fluid. Comparison of twin A to twin B shows a 25% difference in weights, with Twin A being the larger. An NST is reactive for both twins so that the biophysical profile is 10/10 for each twin. Your best explanation and recommendations are

A. Cesarean birth now, because the discordant growth is a harbinger for intrauterine fetal death in the near future for Twin B
B. Induction of labor, because the discordant growth is a harbinger for intrauterine fetal death in the near future for Twin B
C. Biweekly NSTs and weekly BPPs and evaluation for fetal growth
D. Spend as much time as possible at rest on left side
E. B, C, and D

Answer: C, D

Without evidence of intrauterine compromise, delivery is not indicated. Evaluation of fetal well-being and growth is needed, however, on a biweekly basis, with delivery being considered if the disparity in growth widens or information consistent with a nonreassuring fetal status develops.

chapter 13

FETAL GROWTH ABNORMALITIES: INTRAUTERINE GROWTH RETARDATION AND FETAL MACROSOMIA

INTRAUTERINE GROWTH RETARDATION (RESTRICTION)

The term *intrauterine growth retardation* (IUGR) is used to describe infants whose weights are much lower than expected for their gestational age. *A fetus/infant whose weight lies in the lowest 10% of the normal population is designated as having IUGR*, a determination based on standard weight/gestational age tables. By definition then, the prevalence of IUGR will be 10%. Unlike "low birth weight," IUGR is based on weight for a *specific gestational age*. Thus careful assessment of gestational age is crucial to diagnosing and, therefore managing, patients with IUGR.

The fetus with IUGR is best viewed as fragile, that is, potentially lacking adequate reserves for continued intrauterine stress or neonatal adaptation. Such infants are at greater risk for intrauterine fetal death or neonatal death, asphyxia, and fetal distress before or during labor; and once delivered, they are at risk for meconium aspiration, hypoglycemia, hypothermia, respiratory distress, and many other problems. Indeed, the perinatal mortality rate is increased 7- to 10-fold with intrauterine growth retardation, and their perinatal morbidity is exceedingly high. Because of these risks, it is important to identify such babies in utero, maximize the quality of their intrauterine environment, plan and implement their delivery using the safest means possible, and provide superb care in the neonatal period.

Etiology

For a fetus to thrive in utero, an adequate number of fetal cells must be present and differentiated properly. In addition, adequate foodstuffs, other nutrients, and oxygen must be available via an adequately functioning uteroplacental unit to allow growth in number of cells and then in size. Early in pregnancy growth is primarily by cellular hyperplasia, or cell division, so that *early-onset intrauterine growth retardation* leads to an irreversible diminution of organ size and perhaps function. This type of IUGR is associated with heritable factors, immunologic abnormalities, chronic maternal disease, fetal infection, and multiple pregnancy. Later in pregnancy, growth is more and more dependent on cellular hypertrophy rather than hyperplasia so that *delayed-onset intrauterine growth retardation* results in decreased cell size and is amenable to restoration of size with adequate nutrition. Uteroplacental insufficiency is the primary cause of this kind of IUGR.

Although a number of *causes of intrauterine growth retardation* have been recognized (Table 13.1), a definite cause of IUGR cannot be identified in approximately 50% of all cases. Therefore, IUGR must be suspected at every visit in every patient. Causes of IUGR can be conveniently grouped into maternal and fetal origins. Maternal smoking has been known for many years to be associated with decreased birth weight, to a magnitude of roughly 0.5 pound at term. Since maternal habits are important causes of growth retardation, modification of such behavior can improve outcome.

The recommended maternal *weight gain* during pregnancy is about 30 pounds. If there are marked nutritional deficiencies, however, a decrease in fetal weight has been demonstrated. In studies performed during World War II, severe famine and marked caloric restriction resulted in

157

decreased birth weights of 0.5 to 1.0 pound, depending on the nutritional status of the women before the onset of nutritional deprivation. It is difficult to define the role of less severe forms of nutritional deficiencies on fetal growth. In pregnancies with multiple fetuses, even normal nutrition may not be enough to provide adequate nutrition for all fetuses, resulting in intrauterine growth retardation.

The most common known maternal factor associated with intrauterine growth retardation is _hypertensive disease_. Vasospasm diminishes uteroplacental blood flow and hence the ability of the mother to provide adequate nutrition to the fetus through the placenta. From 25 to 30% of all cases of IUGR are associated with maternal hypertensive disease. Other maternal disorders may likewise interfere with fetal growth, notably _cyanotic heart disease_ and _hemoglobinopathies._

Fetal causes of intrauterine growth retardation include congenital infections and anomalies. The most clearly understood _fetal infections_ that interfere with growth are rubella and cytomegalovirus infections, especially at early gestational ages. These infections may be manifest only as mild "flu-like" illnesses, but their occurrence should be noted. Damage to the fetus during organogenesis can result in a decreased cell number, which is manifest by diminished growth later in gestation. Probably 5% or less of all cases of IUGR are related to early infection with these or other viral agents. Bacterial infections have not been implicated in IUGR. _Congenital anomalies_ account for up to 15% of all cases of IUGR. Chromosomal anomalies such as trisomy 21, 18, and 13 are typically associated with diminished fetal growth. Other genetic abnormalities, such as certain congenital heart defects and a variety of dysmorphic syndromes likewise result in smaller than expected infants.

Evaluation and Management

The diagnosis of IUGR is suspected from the history. A patient with a history of having a child with intrauterine growth retardation is at increased risk for a recurrence of this problem. Personal habits such as smoking and use of alcohol or other drugs of abuse such as cocaine should be part of the routine obstetric history obtained at the onset of prenatal care. Recognition of such elements in the history is important so every effort can be made to discourage such behavior. A medical history of disorders potentially interfering with fetal growth, primarily hypertension, should be obtained at the onset of prenatal care.

Physical examination is limited in usefulness in diagnosing IUGR, but it serves as an important _screening test_ for abnormal fetal growth. Maternal size and weight gain throughout pregnancy have a limited utility, but access to such information is readily available and a low maternal weight or little or no weight gain through pregnancy can suggest IUGR. Between approximately 15 and 36 weeks gestation, _fundal height measurement_ should advance in centimeter increments in close parallel with gestational age in weeks. Thus a patient at 28 weeks gestation would be expected to have a fundal height of close to 28 cm. Serial measurements, especially by the same examiner, can serve as an effective screening test for IUGR, since an increase in fundal height less than expected may suggest the diagnosis of IUGR and raise the need for additional testing. Clinical estimations of fetal weight are not very helpful in diagnosing IUGR, except when fetal size is grossly diminished.

Ultrasonography has provided an important obstetric tool to diagnose and assess intrauterine growth retardation. Measurements of various fetal structures can be compared with standardized tables that reflect normal growth. The measurement of the biparietal diameter, head circumference, abdominal circumference, and femur length are among the measurements usually obtained. Ratios of these measurements and equations can provide useful information with respect to fetal size. The diameter of the cerebellum appears to be unaltered by a number of the factors that lead to growth retardation. Accordingly, in patients with uncertain

Table 13.1.
Causes of Intrauterine Growth Retardation

Maternal	Fetal
Behavior	Infection
Smoking	Rubella
Drugs	Cytomegalovirus (CMV)
Alcohol	
	Anomalies
Nutritional deficiencies	Chromosomal
	Other genetic
Maternal disease	
Hypertension	
Cyanotic heart disease	
Others	

gestational age, measurement of the diameter of this structure may prove helpful.

By the use of ultrasonography, IUGR can be distinguished as asymmetric or symmetric. *Asymmetric IUGR* refers to an unequal decrease in the size of structures. For example, the abdominal circumference may be low, but the biparietal diameter may be at or near normal. Such asymmetry can be seen with severe nutritional deficiencies and with hypertension, when fetal access to nutrients is compromised. In *symmetrical IUGR,* all structures are approximately equally diminished in size with a relative sparing of fetal brain and heart compared with asymmetric IUGR. Congenital anomalies or early intrauterine infection can alter cell number and lead to this type of IUGR. This distinction is not always clear, but it does serve as a guide in seeking the etiology of IUGR.

In patients at increased risk for intrauterine growth retardation, a *baseline ultrasonography* examination should be obtained early in prenatal care and usually repeated periodically. As growth retardation is related to gestational age, all patients whose length of pregnancy is uncertain should be assessed with physical examination and ultrasonography to establish an accurate gestational age as early in pregnancy as possible. Ultrasonography also can identify the amount of amniotic fluid present. The combination of oligohydramnios (diminished amniotic fluid volume) and intrauterine growth retardation is especially worrisome because it is associated with severe disease and/or worsening outcome. The mechanism is thought to be decreased fetal blood volume, which diminishes renal blood flow, which in turn leads to a reduction of urine output, a primary source of amniotic fluid in the second half of pregnancy.

Direct studies of the fetus are useful in selected patients with IUGR. Fetal tissue can be obtained via amniocentesis (fetal fibroblasts floating in the amniotic fluid), chorionic villus sampling (CVS; or biopsy of placenta), direct blood sampling (percutaneous umbilical blood sampling; PUBS), or removal of fetal plasma and cells. PUBS also permits immunoglobin studies and viral cultures to be obtained in patients with suspected viral infections as a cause of IUGR. Moreover, the level of oxygenation and the acid-base status can be assessed with this technique. PUBS and to some extent CVS are less widely available than ultrasound-directed amniocentesis.

Once intrauterine growth retardation has been diagnosed, *the goal is to deliver the healthiest possible infant at the optimal time.* This involves a balance between the degree of prematurity estimated at the time of diagnosis with the degree of suspected fetal compromise. Initial management consists of a comprehensive attempt to determine a cause for the IUGR. If a correctable etiology is found, corrective action should be taken. Management of the patient with IUGR can be categorized as antepartum, intrapartum, and postpartum (or neonatal) (Table 13.2). Antepartum management consists of efforts to determine the cause of the IUGR, promote growth, and monitor carefully for fetal compromise. Ultrasonography by experienced personnel can usually identify congenital anomalies that may be associated with IUGR. Measurements of amniotic fluid volume and fetal structures can be made on a serial basis. The degree of IUGR can then be followed in the ensuing weeks. Bedrest, or at least limited activity, is often prescribed for patients with IUGR, because limitation of activity, especially with the patient lying in the left-lateral

Table 13.2.
Assessment and Management of Patient with Intrauterine Growth Retardation

Antepartum	Intrapartum	Postpartum (Neonatal)
Eliminate cause, if possible	Electronic fetal monitoring	Pharyngeal suction
Bedrest, frequent fetal movement counts	Preparation for cesarean delivery; amnioinfusion	Effective neonatal resuscitation as needed
Serial sonography	Oxygen therapy	Avoid hypoglycemia
NST; contraction stress test; BBP	Neonatal/anesthesia consultation	Avoid hypothermia; oxygen therapy, if needed
Doppler ultrasound		
Amniocentesis for maturity studies		
PUBS		

position, maximizes uterine blood flow. This has a salutary effect on fetal growth.

Determination of fetal activity by the so-called kick counts is a useful way of assessing *fetal well-being*. Various electronic fetal monitoring tests, such as the nonstress test (NST) or contraction stress test (CST), or electronic fetal monitoring combined with ultrasound (the biophysical profile; BBP) can be used once or twice a week (or even more frequently) to assess the condition of the fetus. Although these tests can be helpful if the results are normal, the high false-positive rate must be considered when management decisions regarding delivery are made. Use of these tests in combination may reduce this false-positive rate. Examination of the blood flow through the umbilical cord with Doppler ultrasound may be useful in patients with IUGR, although reports about the value of this test are inconclusive. In selected patients with IUGR of uncertain cause, fetal blood aspirated directly through PUBS can be analyzed for viral antibody titer, chromosomes, and other parameters that reflect fetal oxygenation and acid-base status. Amniocentesis for tests of fetal lung maturity may provide information helpful in selecting the timing of delivery.

The decision regarding proper *time for delivery* is based on a combination of factors. The fetus who is thought to be in marked jeopardy may be delivered by scheduled cesarean section without a trial of labor if its ability to withstand labor is questionable and an induced labor is likely to be lengthy. If induction of labor is undertaken, however, constant electronic fetal monitoring to detect signs suggestive of fetal jeopardy is important. Preparations for cesarean delivery should be made, because rapid deterioration of the fetus may occur. Consultation with anesthesia and neonatology personnel is important for optimal care of the patient and her newborn. Amnioinfusion (instillation of warmed normal saline via transcervical catheter) may be helpful if fetal heart rate decelerations thought to be due to diminished amniotic fluid volume are present. Maternal oxygen therapy may be beneficial throughout the course of labor.

Expert *neonatal care* is critical because of the reduced capacity of the fetus/infant to adapt and adjust to extrauterine life. Because of the frequent passage of meconium before delivery, the mouth and nasopharynx must be suctioned, usually with direct visualization of the vocal cords. These infants are prone to other complications such as respiratory distress, hypoglycemia, and hypothermia. Fortunately, infants who survive the neonatal period have a generally good prognosis.

FETAL MACROSCOMIA

Fetal macrosomia is defined, depending on the definition used, as >4000 or 4500 g or a fetal weight greater than the 90th percentile for a given gestational age. Identification of these fetuses is important, and when possible, the underlying cause must be treated. The physician must anticipate the potential problems of vaginal delivery of a large infant, including a prolonged second stage of labor, shoulder dystocia, and immediate neonatal injury.

Macrosomia is associated with maternal obesity, maternal diabetes, and excessive maternal weight gain during pregnancy. Diagnosis is suspected when the fundal height is >4 cm above the expected height for a given gestational age. The diagnosis is confirmed by ultrasonography. The differential diagnosis includes a large but normal fetus, multiple gestation, polyhydramnios, uterine leiomyoma or other gynecologic tumor, and in early pregnancy, molar pregnancy.

Antepartum care focuses on management of any treatable cause of macrosomia. Intrapartum management consists of choice of delivery route. Some advocate cesarean birth for macrosomic fetuses, while others argue that the perinatal outcome is the same so that the risk to the mother is not justified. When vaginal delivery is chosen, the physician must be prepared to deal with shoulder dystocia.

CASE STUDIES

Case 13A

A 36-year-old G2 P0010 is seen for her first prenatal visit at 8 weeks. Her medical history includes essential hypertension, smoking, and poor dietary habits. She had three hospitalizations for pelvic inflammatory disease and one for a cone biopsy of the cervix. Her family history includes a sister with Down syndrome, a mother and grandmother with insulin-dependent diabetes, and a sister with carcinoma of the breast.

On physical examination, the patient's blood pressure is 160/95, and she has 1+ proteinuria. She weighs 200 lb and is 5 feet 1 inch tall. Her general physical examination is normal with the following specific findings: (a) normal breast examination, (b) 2/6 holosystolic murmur without radiation or extra sounds, (c) obese abdomen without masses, (d) cervix consistent in appearance with her history, (e) retroverted 14-week-size uterus that is slightly irregular in shape, and (f) 2+ dependent edema and normal deep tendon reflexes (DTRs).

Questions Case 13A

This patient is at increased risk for a growth-retarded infant. Of the several risk factors mentioned, which pose the most likely threats?

A. Obesity
B. Poor nutrition
C. Hypertension
D. Smoking
E. Status post cone biopsy
F. History of sexually transmitted disease (STD) or infectious disease
G. Family history of Down syndrome
H. Family history of diabetes
I. Family history of breast carcinoma
J. Cardiac murmur
K. Uterus with irregular shape
L. Uterus whose size is greater than expected by last menstrual period (LMP) date

Answer: B, C, D, F, G, H

Obesity per se is not a direct risk factor for IUGR, although it may contribute to general health concerns such as hypertension and the risk of glucose intolerance. Poor nutrition is a risk, although the maternal-fetal unit is able to compensate for considerable dietary inadequacy. This patient's hypertension and smoking are major risk factors, both having great potential for diminution of placental function. A family history of Down syndrome in a 36-year-old woman is of concern, as a genetically abnormal baby may also be growth retarded. Diabetes may be associated with abnormal fetal growth, both growth retardation and macrosomia. Although a family history of breast cancer places the patient at higher risk for breast cancer, it has no direct relationship to IUGR risks. A systolic murmur is common in pregnancy and with hypertension in pregnancy, but any underlying cardiac dysfunction may be an increased risk factor for IUGR. A size/dates disparity must be resolved, and accurate dating should be established so that fetal growth may be evaluated; but this disparity is itself not a risk factor of IUGR. The irregular uterine shape suggests a fibroid uterus, but does not pose an independent risk for IUGR.

Which of the following prenatal evaluations/initial managements do you recommend to this patient, given her risk factors for IUGR?

A.   Nutrition consultation

B.   Social service consultation
C.   ECG
D.   Echocardiogram
E.   24-hr urine for creatinine clearance (CrCl) and total protein
F.   Glucose screening
G.   Genetics counseling with genetic amniocentesis
H.   STD screening (cultures, infective titers)
I.   Mammography
J.   Obstetric ultrasound
K.   Pap smear
L.   Colposcopy
M.   Counseling about smoking

Answer: A, B, E, F, G, J, M

The antenatal evaluations and initial interventions address risk factors for IUGR seen in this patient. Mammography is not indicated in this pregnant patient with a negative physical examination, but should be scheduled for the postpartum period. Colposcopy will not be necessary as long as the Pap smear is normal. ECG and echocardiogram would only be warranted if the heart murmur is felt to be clinically significant. Routine STD screening is appropriate, but extensive evaluation is not warranted.

Case 13B

A 28-year-old G2 P1001 at 32 weeks of gestational age has a fundal height of 26 cm. A late first trimester ultrasound had been consistent with her gestational age by dates. Her first baby was delivered by cesarean section for fetal distress. The baby was reportedly "too small" and had not "grown right." The baby is well at home but is suffering some difficulty in school.

Questions Case 13B

An ultrasound performed at this time should provide what information?

A.   Biophysical profile
B.   Evaluation of fetal growth
C.   Evaluation for fetal anomalies
D.   Evaluation of amniotic fluid volume
E.   PUBS for genetic evaluation

Answer: A, B, C, D

The first four choices address the issues of fetal growth and fetal well-being, both of which require assessment at this time. PUBS has a place in the evaluation of the growth-retarded fetus, but only after the diagnosis of IUGR has been made and then under specific conditions when the risk of the procedure outweighs the risk of not obtaining the information from the test. It is not yet apparent that PUBS is indicated.

Ultrasonographic evaluation shows concordant growth of fetal head and trunk, but an overall growth in the 20th percentile for the estimated gestational age. The biophysical profile is reassuring (10 of 10). How should this patient be managed? What tests will be used and how often are they to be done?

A. NST, BBP, and assessment of interval fetal growth weekly.
B. NST, BBP, and assessment of interval fetal growth biweekly
C. NST, BPP, and assessment of interval fetal growth at 36 weeks.
D. NST, BBP, and assessment of interval fetal growth when the patient goes into labor.

Answer: A

Continued growth and evidence of fetal well-being are the main issues. If data suggest a nonreassuring fetal status, delivery by appropriate means is indicated.

At her 37-week evaluation, the NST is reactive, and the BBP is 10/10. The infant has grown but is still at the 20th percentile. Your plan of management is

A. The same
B. Induction of labor
C. Cesarean birth

Answer: A

Maintain the same management because the fetus has grown, although still in the 20th percentile, and the tests show evidence of fetal well-being.

At her 38-week evaluation, the NST is reactive, and BBP is 8/10 with markedly decreased amniotic fluid. The infant has grown but is in the 18th percentile Your plan of management is

A. The same
B. Induction of labor
C. Cesarean birth

Answer: B

Oligohydraminos is an ominous sign in a growth-retarded fetus, and at 38 weeks delivery is indicated. A trial of labor is appropriate, but preparation for cesarean birth should be made because it is unknown what fetal reserves remain to deal with the stress of labor.

chapter 14

POSTTERM PREGNANCY

Macrosomic →↓Glucose ↑Bili

Normal pregnancy lasts from 38 to 42 weeks, which is considered "term." Stated another way, term is the due date or estimated date of confinement (EDC) ±2 weeks. *A patient who has not delivered by the completion of the 42nd week* (294 days from the 1st day of the last normal menstrual period) *is said to be postterm* (a common synonym is *postdates*). This condition occurs in about 8 to 10% of pregnancies and carries with it an increased risk of adverse outcome. The increased morbidity and mortality in a small percent of cases, however, warrants careful evaluation of all postterm pregnancies. In addition, postterm pregnancies can create significant stress for the patient, her family, and those caring for her. Therefore, the physician should reassure the patient and discuss with her the options for management.

ETIOLOGY

The actual *cause of postterm pregnancy* is not known, although several causes are associated with it (Table 14.1). Uterine contractility has also been shown to be diminished in some cases of postterm pregnancy, suggesting a cause intrinsic to the myometrium. Whatever the etiology, there is a tendency for recurrence of postterm pregnancy. *About 50% of patients having one postterm pregnancy will experience prolonged pregnancy with the next gestation.*

EFFECTS

The morbidity and mortality for the postterm fetus increases several-fold compared with term pregnancies because of several reasons. Approximately 20% of truly postterm newborns demonstrate some elements of *dysmaturity, or postmaturity syndrome*. Dysmature infants often are growth retarded and have loss of subcutaneous fat, giving the child a classic wizened, elderly appearance. Integumentary changes are also seen, including long nails, scaling epidermis, and meconium staining of the nails, skin, and umbilical cord. About 25% of prolonged pregnancies result in a *macrosomic infant* (i.e., birth weight >4000 g). These infants may demonstrate altered glucose and bilirubin metabolism and are at risk for hypoglycemia and hyperbilirubinemia. They also have an increased incidence of birth trauma, especially shoulder dystocia, fracture of the clavicle, and associated brachial plexus injury (Erb, or Erb-Duchenne, palsy) during vaginal delivery as well as of the need for cesarean section as a result of fetopelvic disproportion. In fetal macrosomia, there can also be maternal trauma, with lacerations of the maternal perineum or, in the case of cesarean delivery, of the uterus and other pelvic organs.

Brachial plexus injury is reported in about 1 in 500 term deliveries and is especially likely in the delivery of macrosomic infants, breech deliveries, or in difficult deliveries, although it may occur in the seemingly uneventful, easy delivery. In the *Erb (or Duchenne) palsy*, or paralysis, stretch or tear injury to the upper roots of the brachial plexus results in paralysis of the deltoid and infraspinatus muscles and flexor muscles of the forearm, causing the limb to hang limply close to the side, forearm extended and internally rotated; finger function is usually retained. Less frequently, damage is limited to the lower nerves of the brachial plexus, causing *Klumpke's paralysis*, or paralysis of the hand. As most injuries are mild, treatment is expectant, with splints and physical therapy and the anticipation of complete or nearly complete recovery in three to six months.

The *diminished amniotic fluid volume, or oligohydramnios*, associated with postterm pregnancy is largely responsible for the *increased fetal stress and distress* seen late in pregnancy and in the intrapartum period. Amniotic fluid volume reaches its maximal amount of about 1 liter at 36 to 37 weeks gestation and thereafter diminishes to an average

Table 14.1.
Factors associated with "postterm" pregnancy

Factor	Discussion
Inaccurate or unknown dates	Most common cause; high association with and major risk factor of late or no prenatal care
Irregular ovulation; variation in length of follicular phase	Results in overestimation of gestational age
Altered estrogen:progesterone ratio	
Anencephaly	Decreased production 16α-hydroxydehydro-epiandrosterone sulfate, a precursor of estriol
Fetal adrenal hypoplasia	Decreased fetal production precursors of estriol
Placental sulfatase deficiency	X-linked disease prevents placenta conversion of sulfated estrogen precursors
Extrauterine pregnancy	Pregnancy not in uterus, no labor (see Chapter 30)

of less than half that at 42 weeks. The umbilical cord normally floats freely in the amniotic fluid. The loss of significant fluid volume means a loss in protection for the umbilical cord so that impingement on the cord can occur.

Increasingly severe *placental dysfunction* with decreased transfer of water, electrolytes, glucose, amino acids, and oxygen can occur in postterm pregnancy. Approximately 40% of placentas from postterm pregnancies demonstrate placental infarcts, calcification, and fibrosis consistent with decreased functional capability. This intrauterine nutritional and respiratory deprivation may contribute to fetal stress and to the development of postmaturity syndrome.

Another special concern in postterm pregnancies is meconium passage and the possibility of aspiration of meconium (*meconium aspiration syndrome*), which can lead to severe respiratory distress from mechanical obstruction of both small and large airways as well as meconium chemical pneumonitis. Meconium passage is not limited to postterm pregnancies; it is seen in 13 to 15% of all term pregnancies. The incidence of meconium passage rises as pregnancy becomes prolonged. Since diminished amniotic fluid volume is also present in postterm pregnancy, the neonate is more likely to aspirate more concentrated solutions of this potentially toxic, particulate meconium.

DIAGNOSIS

The diagnosis of postterm pregnancy rests on establishment of the correct gestational age. Every effort should be made to accurately assess gestational age as early

as possible in pregnancy, when the parameters used for this purpose are most discriminating and reliable. With improved access to prenatal care and the greater importance placed on accurate gestational age assessment, the percentage of patients in whom postterm pregnancy is suspected but whose dates are uncertain has diminished. Nonetheless, an alarmingly high number of patients do not seek prenatal care early in pregnancy or do not have an accurate gestational age determination. Physicians should be suspicious of the presumed due date of any patient who first appears for prenatal care late in pregnancy who might be "1 or 2 months overdue." Care should be taken to properly evaluate and monitor her fetus for these problems associated with postterm pregnancy.

MANAGEMENT

The first step in management of postterm pregnancy is a careful review of the information used to establish the gestational age to be as certain as possible that the estimate is correct. *Once a patient approaches 41 weeks gestation (1 week past her due date), the management options are either to induce labor or to continue surveillance of fetal well-being until spontaneous labor occurs.*

If gestational age is felt to be firmly established, factors that influence the decision of whether to deliver or not rest with the patient's concerns and desires, the assessment of fetal well-being, and the status of the cervix. Induction of labor is appropriate if the cervix is favorable — i.e., softened, effaced, and somewhat dilated — and if the patient prefers labor induction. If the cervix is not favorable or the patient does not wish induction of labor, fetal well-being is monitored while awaiting spontaneous labor or a change in the cervix so that induction is appropriate. A variety of management schemes have been devised for this "waiting period," none of which is clearly superior. Daily fetal movement counting is included in most management plans, along with nonstress testing or oxytocin challenge testing once or twice a week and frequent assessments of amniotic fluid volume by ultrasound. A biophysical profile done twice a week is also widely used.

If the gestational age is not well established, the clinician uses whatever information is available to determine the best date. Amniocentesis is not especially helpful, as fetal lung maturity is rarely a question in the postterm evaluation. When the best date is selected, a management plan similar to that for a postterm pregnancy with well-established dates is used.

Although there is no absolute time within which labor must be induced, many physicians believe that delivery should be effected by either 42 or 43 weeks. Induction of labor can be attempted using intravenous Pitocin (oxytocin) or prostaglandin vaginal suppositories (Prostin; carboprost tromethamine). In some patients, if the cervix is quite unfavorable, cervical "ripening" can be accelerated using an intracervical or intravaginal preparation of prostaglandin, or laminaria, a hydrophilic device that dilates the cervix (see Chapter 16). Rarely, cesarean section without attempted induction may be performed. Proponents of such cutoff dates are said to favor *"aggressive management,"* citing increased morbidity and mortality after 42 or 43 completed weeks gestation. Modern methods for surveillance of fetal well-being make it less logical to be dogmatic about mandatory induction at a given gestational age. Proponents of *"expectant management"* allow pregnancy to continue for some time as long as there is evidence of fetal well-being.

Because of the risk of macrosomia-associated birth trauma, ultrasonographic estimation of fetal weight should be obtained before any induction of labor in a postterm pregnancy. If the estimated fetal weight is >4500 to 5000 g, cesarean section is often the appropriate mode of delivery.

Patients with postterm pregnancies should be advised to come promptly to the hospital when labor pains commence. Once the onset of regular contractions occurs, careful electronic fetal monitoring should be employed throughout labor because of the risk of fetal stress/distress. Intrapartum management includes the artificial rupture of membranes, when possible, to allow detection of meconium and to allow the placement of a fetal scalp electrode and intrauterine pressure catheter (IUPC). If the decreased amniotic fluid is sufficient to permit undue pressure on the umbilical cord, deceleration of the fetal heart rate may occur. Infusion of normal saline through the IUPC (amnioinfusion) may provide a buffer for the cord and eliminate these decelerations. Because of the increased risk of cesarean delivery for fetal stress and because of the potential problems associated with meconium, both anesthesia and pediatric personnel should be alerted that a postterm patient is in labor.

At the time of delivery, special precautions are taken. If meconium passage has been noted, the infant's nasopharynx and oropharynx should be suctioned before delivery of the shoulders, since compression of the chest has forced fluid within the chest upward to the pharynx. Pediatric support should be in the delivery room to provide prompt visual examination of the infant's airway to a level beneath the larynx and to suction any meconium material. This infant management significantly decreases, but does not eliminate, the likelihood of meconium aspiration syndrome. Because of the risk of macrosomia, the physician performing the delivery should be familiar with the techniques used to treat shoulder dystocia such as exaggerated flexion of the thighs (Figure 14.1) and suprapubic pressure (Figure 14.2).

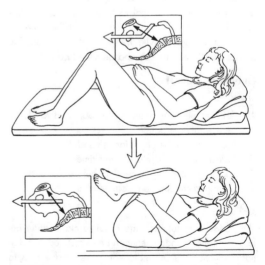

Figure 14.1. McRoberts maneuver: hyperflexion of thighs to aid in management of shoulder dystocia.

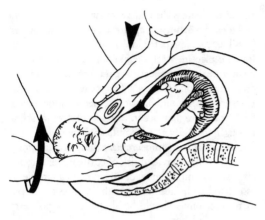

Figure 14.2. Rotation plus suprapubic pressure to aid in management of shoulder dystocia.

CASE STUDIES

Case 14A

A 35-year-old G1 P0 patient presents on June 6 for prenatal care, saying that her previous doctor said she was due "about now." The prenatal records she brings include the notation of a "light last menstrual period (LMP)" on September 20; a "period" on August 25; fetal movement "sometime just before Christmas"; a first pelvic examination on November 1, which showed an anteverted 10- 11-week-size uterus; and an ultrasound on January 4 consistent with a 15-week gestation and another on May 15 consistent with a "term" pregnancy. The patient says the baby is moving as much this week as during the previous 2 weeks. The patient has no obstetric risk factors. Physical examination is completely normal. The fundal height is 38 cm and the cervix is closed and uneffaced with the vertex at –1 station. The patient asks to be induced and delivered now.

Questions Case 14A

She should be told that

A. Another ultrasound should be obtained to clarify her gestational age
B. No action by the physician is needed
C. Induction is appropriate at this time
D. Further evaluation is needed before a course of management can be recommended

Answer: D

The patient's gestational age requires clarification before a rational management can be formulated. In addition, induction without indication poses undue risks to mother and fetus, especially with an unfavorable cervix as depicted in this case. Ultrasound is most useful in

determination of gestational age in late first and second trimesters but only relatively precise (±2 to 3 weeks) in the third trimester.

Based on the information given, the best estimate of this patient's gestational age is

A. 38 weeks
B. 39 weeks
C. 40 weeks
D. 41 weeks
E. 42 weeks
F. 43 weeks

Answer: D

The LMP of September 20 was "light," whereas that of August 25 was "normal." Although this is insufficient to establish dates, the "normal" LMP of August 25 is consistent with the first pelvic examination and midtrimester ultrasound and not inconsistent with the late trimester ultrasound. Thus setting a gestational age of 41 weeks is appropriate.

Which of the following studies are appropriate at this time?

A. Ultrasound to establish gestational age
B. Ultrasound to evaluate amniotic fluid volume
C. Biophysical profile
D. Electronic fetal monitoring of the fetus (nonstress or stress test)
E. Amniocentesis to determine fetal lung maturity

Answer: B, C, D

Ultrasound is relatively imprecise in the last trimester for gestational age measurement, although it is useful for evaluation of amniotic fluid volume and for biophysical profile measurement. Likewise, electronic fetal monitoring (e.g., nonstress test) to assess the fetal status is appropriate. Amniocentesis is not needed, as fetal lung maturity is not an issue.

All the studies performed on this patient were reassuring as to maternal and fetal status. One week later, on June 13 the patient reports that the baby is still moving well, although she feels more pelvic pressure and has been having cramps. On physical examination, the fundal height is unchanged and the cervix is 90% effaced and 3 cm dilated, with the vertex at zero station with intact membranes. The patient again requests induction of labor. She should now be told that

A. Another ultrasound to determine gestational age is necessary

B. She should not worry; she will deliver when she is ready
C. Induction of labor is appropriate
D. Further studies are necessary before a course of management can be recommended

Answer: C

The patient's cervical examination has now changed to one favorable for induction, which is now the least risky management for mother and fetus. If the cervical examination had been unchanged, continued evaluation of fetal well-being would have been appropriate. Delivery would be indicated if there were evidence of fetal distress or at 42 or 43 weeks, depending on the physician's attitude toward the maximum allowable duration of gestation.

Case 14B

A patient G1 P0 at 41 weeks confirmed by first trimester ultrasound has had an unremarkable pregnancy. Fetal well-being studies are normal. The fundal height is 45 cm. On pelvic examination, the cervix is uneffaced and closed and the cephalic part is at –3 station. After 1 week of expectant management, the patient reports good fetal movement and some mild, somewhat regular contractions. On examination, fundal height is 44 cm. fetal heart rate is 140 bpm, and pelvic examination shows the vertex at –3 station, intact membranes, and a cervix dilated to 4 cm and 100% effaced. The patient requests induction of labor.

Questions Case 14B

The patient should be told that

A. Another ultrasound will be ordered for clarification of gestational age
B. She should not worry; she will deliver when she is ready

C. Labor will be induced now
D. She is in labor

Answer: D

The duration of pregnancy is clear and no further studies are needed. A patient in early labor at 42 weeks gestation should be allowed to labor there being no contraindication to the contrary.

Which of the following studies are appropriate at this time for this patient?

A. Ultrasound to estimate fetal weight
B. Electronic fetal monitoring of the fetus
C. Amniocentesis to determine fetal lung maturity
D. Artificial rupture of the membranes

Answer: A, B

The fundal height and pelvic examination suggest the possibility of macrosomia. If macrosomia is discovered by ultrasonographic estimation of fetal weight, a clinical decision whether to try for a vaginal delivery or to proceed with cesarean section must be made based on the estimated fetal weight, the clinical pelvimetry, the status of the fetus, and the informed wishes of the parents. Electronic monitoring of the postterm fetus during labor is important because of the higher risk of uteroplacental insufficiency. Artificial rupture of the membranes will allow direct fetal heart monitoring via fetal scalp electrode and allow assessment for the presence of meconium, but this should be done when the presenting part is sufficiently into the pelvis. At –3 station, the risk of cord prolapse is higher than if the presenting part were applied to the cervix, although it is not entirely inappropriate under the circumstances.

chapter 15

NORMAL LABOR AND DELIVERY

Labor is the process by which products of conception (fetus, placenta, cord, and membranes) are expelled from the uterus. It is defined as the progressive effacement and dilation of the uterine cervix, resulting from rhythmic contractions of the uterine musculature. Cervical dilation that occurs without uterine contractions is not considered true labor. Uterine contractions without effacement and dilation of the cervix occur normally in the third trimester of pregnancy and are termed Braxton Hicks contractions, or false labor. Approximately 85% of patients will undergo spontaneous labor and delivery between 37 and 42 weeks gestation.

CHANGES BEFORE THE ONSET OF LABOR

As the patient approaches term, there is an increasing number of uterine contractions of greater intensity. Although spontaneous uterine contractions, which are not felt by the patient, occur throughout pregnancy, late in pregnancy they become stronger and more frequent, resulting in the patient's preception of discomfort. These Braxton-Hicks contractions are not associated with progressive dilation of the cervix, however, and therefore do not fit the definition of labor. It is frequently difficult for the patient to distinguish these often uncomfortable contractions from those of true labor, and as a result, it is difficult for the physician to determine the true onset of labor by history alone. Braxton Hicks contractions are typically shorter in duration and less intense than true labor contractions, with the discomfort being characterized as over the lower abdomen and groin areas. It is not uncommon for these contractions to resolve with ambulation.

True labor, on the other hand, is associated with contractions that the patient feels over the uterine fundus, with radiation of discomfort to the low back and low abdomen. These contractions become increasingly intense and frequent. The ultimate test of whether the contractions are those of true labor is if they are associated with cervical effacement and dilation.

Another event of late pregnancy is termed *lightening*. In this, the patient reports a change in the shape of her abdomen and the sensation that the baby has gotten less heavy, the result of the fetal head descending into the pelvis. The patient may also report that the baby is "dropping." The patient often notices that the lower abdomen is more prominent and the upper abdomen is flatter, and there may be more frequent urination as the bladder is compressed by the fetal head. The patient may also notice an easier time breathing, as there is less pressure on the diaphragm.

Patients often report the passage of blood-tinged mucus late in pregnancy. This *bloody show* results as the cervix begins thinning out (*effacement*) with the concomitant extrusion of mucus from the endocervical glands. Cervical effacement is common before the onset of true labor, as the internal os is slowly drawn into the lower uterine segment. The cervix is often significantly effaced before the onset of labor, particularly in the nulliparous patient. The mechanism of effacement and dilation is shown in Figure 15.1.

EVALUATION FOR LABOR

Instruction as to when to report to the hospital when labor is suspected is a routine part of antepartum care. *Patients are told to come to the hospital for any of the following reasons:* if their contractions occur approximately every 5 min for at least 1 hr, if there is a sudden gush of fluid or a constant leakage of fluid (suggesting rupture of membranes), if there is any significant bleeding, or if there is significant decrease in fetal movement. At the time of initial evaluation at the

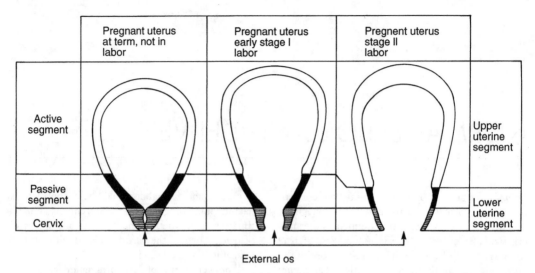

	Pregnant uterus at term, not in labor	Pregnant uterus early stage I labor	Pregnent uterus stage II labor	
Active segment				Upper uterine segment
Passive segment				Lower uterine segment
Cervix				

External os

Figure 15.1. Mechanism of effacement, dilation, and labor. With continuing uterine contractions, the upper uterus (active segment) thickens, the lower uterine segment (passive segment) thins, and the cervix dilates. In this way, the fetus is moved downward, into and through the vaginal canal.

hospital, the *prenatal records* are reviewed by the physician to (*a*) identify complications of pregnancy up to that point, (*b*) confirm gestational age to differentiate preterm labor from labor in a term pregnancy, and (*c*) review pertinent laboratory information. A *focused history* by the physician helps in determining the nature and frequency of the patient's contractions, the possibility of spontaneous rupture of membranes or significant bleeding or changes in maternal or fetal status. A *limited general physical examination* is performed (with special attention to vital signs) along with the abdominal and pelvic examinations. If contractions occur during this physical examination, they may be palpated for intensity and duration by the examining physician. Auscultation of the fetal heart tones is also of critical importance, particularly immediately following a contraction, to determine the possibility of any fetal heart rate deceleration.

The initial examination of the gravid abdomen may be accomplished using *Leopold maneuvers* (Fig. 15.2), a series of four palpations of the fetus through the abdominal wall that helps accurately determine fetal lie, presentation, and position. *Lie* is the relationship of the long axis of the fetus with the maternal long axis. It is longitudinal in 99% of cases, occasionally transverse, and rarely oblique (when the axes cross at a 45° angle, usually converting to a transverse or longitudinal lie during labor). *Presentation* is determined by the "present-

ing part," i.e., that portion of the fetus lowest in the birth canal, palpated during the abdominal examination and when a vaginal examination is performed. For example, in a longitudinal lie, the presenting part is either breech or cephalic. The most common cephalic presentation is the one in which the head is sharply flexed onto the fetal chest such that the occiput or vertex presents. *Position* is the relationship of the fetal presenting part to the right or left side of the maternal pelvis (Fig. 15.3). The fetal head may also be turned more or less toward the sacrum or symphysis, termed anterior and posterior *asynclitism*, respectively (Fig. 15.4).

The *four Leopold maneuvers* (see Fig. 15.2) include the following:

1. *Determining what occupies the fundus.* In a longitudinal lie, the fetal head is differentiated from the fetal breech, the latter being larger and less clearly defined.
2. *Determining location of small parts.* Using one hand to steady the fetus, the fingers on the other hand are used to palpate either the firm, long fetal spine or the various shapes and movements indicating fetal hands and feet.
3. *Identifying descent of the presenting part.* Suprapubic palpation identifies the presenting part as the fetal head, which is relatively mobile, or a breech, which moves the entire body. The extent to which the presenting part is felt to extend below the symphysis suggests the station of the presenting part.

4. *Identifying the cephalic prominence.* As long as the cephalic prominence is easily palpable, the vertex is not likely to have descended to 0 station.

As part of the abdominal examination, palpation of the uterus during a contraction is helpful in determining the intensity of that particular contraction. The uterine wall is not easily indented with firm palpation during a true contraction, but may be indented during a Braxton Hicks contraction.

The *vaginal examination* should be performed using an aseptic technique. In the presence of significant bleeding, the vaginal examination should be done with extreme care, if at all, because of the risk of disrupting a placenta previa (see Chapter 9). If it is unclear whether or not membranes have been ruptured, a sterile speculum examination should be performed before any digital examination of the cervix to ascertain if spontaneous rupture of the membranes has occurred (see Chapter 7). Visualization of the cervix through the speculum also allows for better identification of the source of any bleeding.

The digital portion of the vaginal examination allows the examiner to determine the degree of *cervical effacement* (expressed as percent effacement, i.e., a cervix that is thinned to one-half of its original 2-cm length is termed 50%, whereas a cervix that is virtually totally thinned is described as 100% effaced) as well as the consistency (firm or soft) of the cervix (Fig. 15.5). A cervix that is not effaced, but is softened, is more likely to

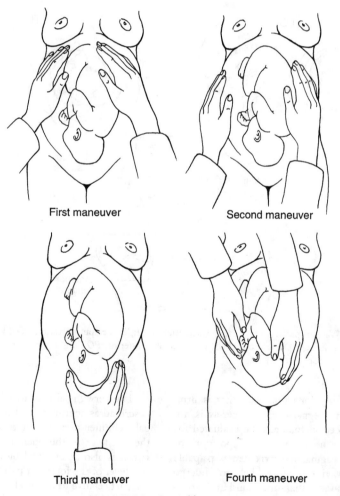

First maneuver

Second maneuver

Third maneuver

Fourth maneuver

Figure 15.2. Leopold maneuvers.

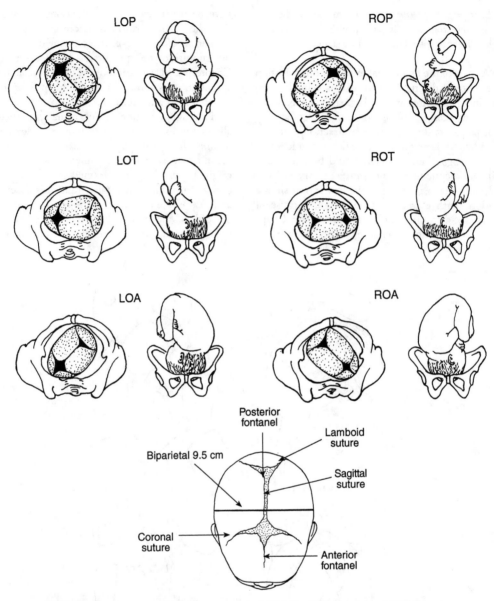

Figure 15.3. Various positions in vertex presentation. *LOP,* left occiput posterior; *LOT,* left occiput transverse; *LOA,* left occiput anterior; *ROP,* right occiput posterior; *ROT,* right occiput transverse; *ROA,* right occiput anterior.

change with contractions than one that is firm, as it is earlier in pregnancy. If the cervix is not significantly effaced, it may also be evaluated for its *relative position*, i.e., anterior, midposition, or posterior in the vagina. A cervix that is palpable anterior in the vagina is more likely to undergo change in labor sooner than one found in the posterior portion of the vagina.

The cervix is also palpated for *cervical dilation*, described as centimeters of dilation. The individual examiner uses one or two fingers to identify the diameter of the opening of the cervix. Fetal *station* is also determined by identifying the relative level of the foremost part of the fetal presenting part relative to the level of the ischial spines. If the presenting part has reached the level of the

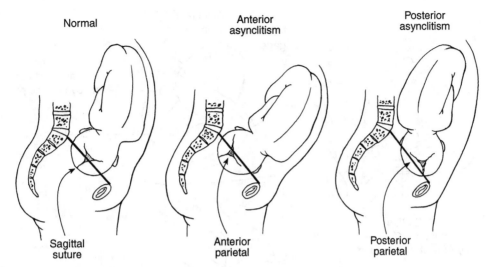

Figure 15.4. Asynclitism.

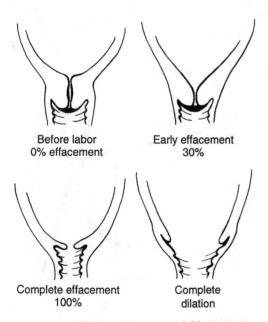

Figure 15.5. Effacement and dilation.

ischial spines, it is termed *0 station*. The distance between the ischial spines to the pelvic inlet above and the distance from the spines to the pelvic outlet below are divided into thirds, and these measurements are used to further define station. If the presenting part is palpable at the pelvic inlet, it is called −3 station, if it has descended one-third of the way to the ischial spines, it is called −2 station, etc. Descent of the fetal presenting part below the

spines is similarly defined as +1 station, +2 station, etc. (Fig. 15.6). *The clinical significance of the fetal head presenting at 0 station is that the biparietal diameter of the fetal head, the greatest transverse diameter of the fetal skull, has negotiated the pelvic inlet.*

If the patient is found not to be in active labor (i.e., <3 to 4 cm dilated) and there is no confounding medical or obstetric problems, she may be sent home to await the onset of true labor. If there is a question as to whether or not true labor has commenced, the patient may be reevaluated after approximately 1 hr. In some cases, patients are encouraged to ambulate to differentiate Braxton Hicks contractions (which may resolve) from true labor (which will continue). If the patient is in labor, she is admitted to the labor area of the hospital and active management of labor is undertaken.

STAGES OF LABOR

Although labor is a continuous process, it is divided into three functional stages. The *first stage* is the interval between the onset of labor and full cervical dilation (10 cm). The first stage is further divided into two phases. The *latent phase* encompasses cervical effacement and early dilation. The second is the *active phase*, during which more rapid cervical dilation occurs, usually beginning at approximately 3 to 4 cm. The *second stage* encompasses complete cervical dilation through the delivery of the infant. The *third stage* begins immediately after delivery of the infant and ends with the delivery of the placenta. The *fourth stage*

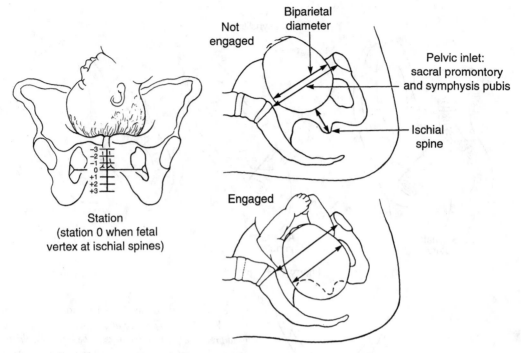

Figure 15.6. Station and engagement of the fetal head.

Table 15.1.
Mean Duration of the Various Phases and Stages of
Labor with Their Distribution Characteristics

Parity	Latent Phase (hr)	Active Phase (hr)	Maximum Dilation (cm/hr)	Second Stage (hr)
Nulliparas				
Mean	6.4	4.6	3.0	1.1
Limit[a]	20.1	11.7	1.2	2.9
Multiparas				
Mean	4.8	2.4	5.7	0.39
Limit[a]	13.6	5.2	1.5	1.1

[a] 5th or 95th percentile

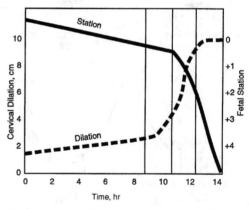

Figure 15.7. Graphic presentation of cervical dilation and station during the first and second stages of labor.

of labor is defined as the immediate postpartum period of approximately 2 hr after delivery of the placenta during which time the patient undergoes significant physiologic adjustment. Table 15.1 outlines the duration of various stages of labor, as defined by Friedman, and Figure 15.7 represents this graphically.

MECHANISM OF LABOR

The mechanism of labor (also known as the cardinal movements of labor) refers to the changes of the position of the fetus as it passes through the birth canal. The fetus usually descends in a fashion whereby the occipital portion of the fetal head is the lower-most part in the pelvis and rotates toward the largest pelvic segment. This vertex presentation occurs in 95% of term labors. As a result, the cardinal movements of labor are defined relative to this presentation. How a fetus in the breech presentation moves through the birth canal is significantly different. To accommodate to the maternal bony pelvis, the fetal head must undergo several movements as it passes through the birth canal. These movements are accomplished by means of the forceful contractions of the uterus. *These cardinal movements of labor* do not occur as a distinct series of movements but do describe in total how the fetal head adapts to the bony pelvis. These are (*a*) engagement, (*b*) descent, (*c*) flexion, (*d*) internal rotation, (*e*) extension, (*f*) external rotation, and (*g*) expulsion (Fig. 15.8).

Engagement is defined as descent of the biparietal diameter of the head below the pelvic inlet, diagnosed clinically by palpation of the presenting part below the level of ischial spines (0 station). The importance of this event is that it suggests that the bony pelvis is adequate to allow significant descent of the fetal head. It is not uncommon for the fetal head to become engaged before the onset of true labor, particularly in nulliparous patients. *Descent of the presenting part* is a necessity for the successful completion of passage through the birth canal. The greatest rate of descent occurs during the latter portions of the first stage of labor and during the second stage of labor. Figure 15.7 is a graphic demonstration of fetal descent and dilation of the cervix. *Flexion of the fetal head* allows for the smaller diameters of the fetal head to present to the maternal pelvis. *Internal rotation*, like flexion, facilitates presentation of the optimal diameters of the fetal head to the bony pelvis. *Extension of the fetal head* occurs as it reaches the introitus. To accommodate to the upward curve of the birth canal, the flexed head now extends. *External rotation* occurs after delivery of the head as the head rotates to "face forward" relative to its shoulders. *Expulsion* is the final delivery of the fetus from the birth canal.

MANAGEMENT OF LABOR

Although the patient may have undergone some education regarding the labor and delivery process, it is important to realize that the patient has significant fears that remain. The patient should not be left unattended for any significant length of time, and a support person may be allowed to remain with the patient throughout the labor and delivery process in most cases. Maternal vital signs should be taken at least every 30 min during the first stage of labor. The patient should be given nothing by mouth except for small sips of water,

ice chips, or hard candies. Laboratory information, including hematocrit, type and screen, platelet count, and urinalysis for glucose and protein, are obtained when the patient is admitted to the hospital. An intravenous line (16- to 18-gauge) is frequently inserted during the active phase of labor to provide hydration and immediate access to the intravascular space should medications be necessary. As the gastrointestinal tract significantly slows in its function during labor, hydration by means of the intravenous line rather than by mouth is optimal.

During the course of labor, descent of the fetus causes the bladder to be elevated relative to the lower uterine segment and cervix. This often results in the patient having difficulty voiding. The patient should, therefore, be encouraged to void frequently. Catheterization may become necessary if the bladder becomes distended. The use of a cleansing enema to empty the lower colon may be employed subject to the needs of the patient and local custom.

Depending on individual institutional limitations, the patient may be allowed to labor in any of several *positions.* Typically, the patients are kept at bedrest in a sitting or reclining position. The lateral recumbent position is more comfortable for some patients whereas other patients choose to ambulate or sit in a rocking chair during the first stage of labor if medical and pregnancy conditions permit. At all times, close monitoring of the fetal heart rate must be available. *Electronic fetal monitoring* is very common and often routine, but it is probably not necessary for the low-risk term pregnancy. If routine electronic fetal monitoring is not undertaken, auscultation of the fetal heart rate should be performed at least every 15 min, immediately after a uterine contractions.

During the second stage of labor, fetal heart rate auscultation should be performed after each uterine contraction. If electronic fetal monitoring is undertaken, either as routine or for patients who are considered at risk, an external tocodynamometer is initially used to assess uterine activity, providing information regarding the frequency and duration of contractions but not intensity. Internal pressure monitoring, using an intrauterine catheter, can be performed to measure intensity more accurately by directly measuring intrauterine pressure. This internal form of fetal monitoring requires rupture of the membranes and, therefore, cannot usually be accomplished until the cervix is at least 1 to 2 cm dilated.

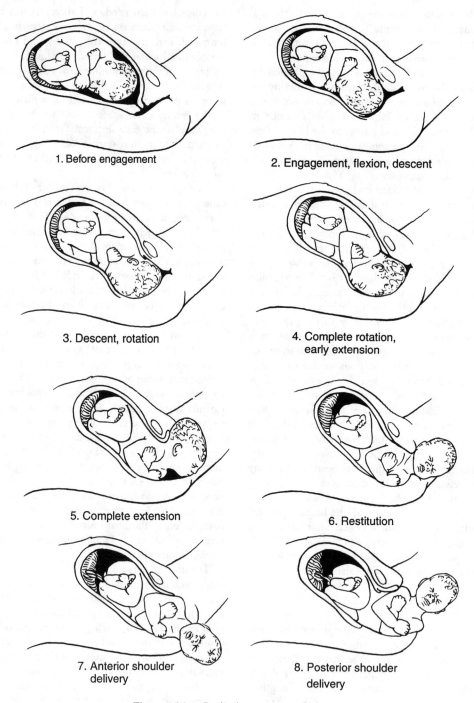

1. Before engagement

2. Engagement, flexion, descent

3. Descent, rotation

4. Complete rotation, early extension

5. Complete extension

6. Restitution

7. Anterior shoulder delivery

8. Posterior shoulder delivery

Figure 15.8. Cardinal movements of labor.

Fetal heart rate can be monitored externally by Doppler ultrasound or internally using a direct fetal electrocardiogram, which is obtained by apply-ing a scalp electrode. The latter technique allows for more detailed evaluation of subtle changes in fetal heart rate pattern (see Chapter 17). When-

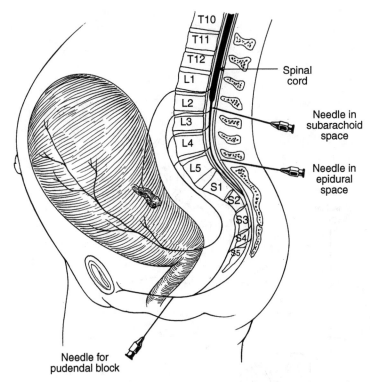

Figure 15.9. Sensory pathways for pain in labor; anatomic sites for spinal, epidural, and pudendal block.

ever artificial rupture of the membranes is to be performed, the presenting part must be well-applied to the cervix. This minimizes the risk of an iatrogenic umbilical cord prolapse.

Monitoring of maternal conditions, including pulse, blood pressure, respiratory rate, temperature, urine output, and fluid intake, should be carried out periodically throughout the course of labor.

Because the latent phase of labor may be affected by *analgesic and anesthetic agents*, these should generally not be employed until the active phase of labor. There is no evidence that either analgesics or anesthetics significantly affect the active phase of labor. Many patients have prepared for labor using childbirth education classes, during which time they are taught techniques of relaxation to deal with the pain of labor contractions. Some patients find the use of narcotic analgesics to be helpful adjuncts to these measures. In the doses typically given during labor, neonatal depression is not a major concern. Commonly used medications include the narcotic meperidine (Demerol; 5 to 20 mg slow i.v. p. q. 2–3h. or 25 to 75 mg i.m. q. 3–4h.) and the synthetic opioid agonist-antago-

nist butorphanol tartrate (Stadol; 1 to 2 mg slow i.v. p. q. 3–4h.).

Any analgesic or anesthetic technique used during the labor and delivery process should take into account those sensory pathways involved and the points at which they may be affected (Fig. 15.9). During the first stage of labor, pain results from contraction of the uterus and dilation of the cervix. This pain travels along the visceral afferents, which accompany sympathetic nerves entering the spinal cord at T10, T11, T12, and L1. As the head descends, there is also distention of the lower birth canal and perineum. This pain is transmitted along somatic afferents that comprise portions of the pudendal nerves that enter the spinal cord at S2, S3, and S4.

The anesthetic technique that provides pain relief during labor is the *epidural block*. The advantage of this technique is its ability to provide analgesia during labor as well as excellent anesthesia for delivery yet maintain the patient's sense of touch facilitating participation in the birth process. It can also be used in either vaginal or abdominal deliveries and in postpartum procedures such as tubal li-

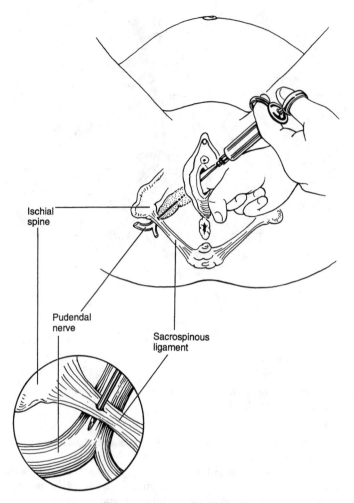

Ischial
spine

Pudendal
nerve

Sacrospinous
ligament

Figure 15.10. Pudendal block.

gation. *Spinal anesthetic* can be used for vaginal or abdominal delivery also, but it is typically given just before delivery. A *pudendal block* can be administered easily at the time of delivery to provide perineal anesthesia for a vaginal delivery (Fig. 15.10). A *local bock, i.e., local injection of anesthetic* may be used at the area of an episiotomy or tear.

Epidural anesthesia is superior to spinal anesthesia in that it can be left as a continuous source of analgesia and anesthesia during both the labor and delivery process. It avoids the risk of spinal headache in the mother and reduces the risk of sympathetic blockade, which could lead to hypotension. There is also less motor blockade than with spinal anesthesia. Although the pudendal block is easy to perform and also has the least potential risk to the mother and fetus, its utility is

also the most limited. *General anesthesia* is reserved only for cesarean sections in selected cases. The potential risk of complications such as maternal aspiration reduces its more widespread utility.

Evaluation of the patient's progress of labor is accomplished by means of a series of pelvic examinations. The number of examinations should be minimized to avoid the risk of chorioamnionitis. At the time of each vaginal examination, the perineum is cleansed and a sterile lubricant is used. Each examination should identify cervical dilation, effacement, station, position of the presenting part, and the status of the membranes. These findings should be noted graphically on the hospital record so that abnormalities of labor may be identified. During the latter portions of the first stage of labor, patients may report the urge to push. This may signify significant descent of the fetal head with pressure on the perineum. More frequent vaginal examinations during this time may be necessary. Similarly, in case of significant fetal heart rate decelerations, more frequent examinations may be necessary to determine whether or not the umbilical cord is prolapsed or if delivery is imminent.

In addition to rupturing the membranes to insert an intrauterine pressure catheter or a fetal scalp monitor, *artificial rupture of membranes* may be beneficial in other ways. The presence or absence of meconium can be identified. Blood in the amniotic fluid may also have significance (see Chapter 9). Rupture of the membranes does, however, carry some risk, as the incidence of infection may be increased if labor is prolonged or umbilical cord prolapse may occur if rupture of the membranes is undertaken before engagement of the presenting fetal part. *Spontaneous rupture of membranes* has similar risks. The fluid should be observed for meconium and blood. Fetal heart tones should be assessed after membranes spontaneously rupture.

Once the *second stage of labor* has been reached (i.e., complete, or 10 cm of, cervical dilation), voluntary maternal effort (pushing) can be added to the involuntary contractile forces of the uterus to facilitate delivery of the fetus. With the onset of each contraction, the mother is encouraged to inhale, hold her breath, and perform an extended Valsalva maneuver. This increase in intraabdominal pressure aids in fetal descent through the birth canal.

It is during the second stage of labor that the fetal head may undergo further alterations. *Molding* is an alteration in the relationship of the fetal cranial bones, even resulting in partial bone overlap. Some minor degree is common as the fetal head adjusts to the bony pelvis. The greater the disparity between the fetal head and the bony pelvis, the greater the amount of molding (Fig. 15.11). *Caput succedaneum* is the edema of the fetal scalp caused by pressure on the fetal head by the cervix. An extended second stage may last as long as 2 to 3 hr, and the prolonged resistance encountered by the fetal vertex may prevent appropriate identification of fontanels and sutures. Both caput and molding resolve in the first few days of life. If identified before the second stage of labor, these changes should be noted on the pelvic examination and may indicate a significant problem in negotiation of the birth canal.

DELIVERY

The patient should be prepared for a well-controlled delivery of the fetal head. In general, nulliparous patients take a greater amount of time to deliver than multiparous patients, once the second stage of labor has started. The position of the patient for delivery most preferred by physicians is the dorsal lithotomy position. This allows the physician to have better control of the delivery with optimal exposure for both the delivery and subsequent surgical repair, if needed. Other positions are preferred by some patients. With each successive contraction, the maternal force as well as uterine contractions cause more of the fetal scalp to be visible at the introitus. If necessary, an *episiotomy* should be performed only after the perineum has been thinned considerably by the descending fetal head (Fig. 15.12). By enlarging the vaginal outlet, an episiotomy facilitates delivery and may be indicated in cases of instrumental delivery and/or protracted or arrested descent. The role of routine prophylactic episiotomy is unclear and is, therefore, best left to the individual doctor and patient. If used, episiotomies are usually cut midline or occasionally laterally, as a mediolateral episiotomy. Advantages of the former include less pain, ease of repair, and less blood loss. The primary disadvantage is greater risk of extension into a third- or fourth-degree laceration, involving the rectal sphincter and rectal mucosa, respectively.

As the fetal head crowns, i.e., distends the vaginal opening, it is delivered by extension to allow the smallest diameter of the fetal head to pass over the perineum. This decreases the likelihood of laceration or extension of episiotomy. To facilitate this, the physician performs a modified *Ritgen maneuver* (Fig. 15.13). In this, one hand is placed over the vertex while the other exerts pressure through the perineum onto the fetal chin. A sterile towel is used to avoid contamination of this hand by contact with the anus. The chin can then be delivered slowly, with control applied by both hands.

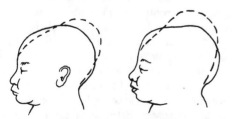

Figure 15.11. Molding of head.

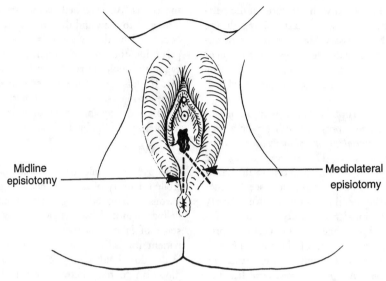

Figure 15.12. Episiotomy.

After the head is delivered, nasal and oral suction is performed with a bulb syringe. If meconium has been present, suctioning of the pharynx must also be accomplished. The neck should then be evaluated for the possible presence of a nuchal cord, which should be reduced over the fetal head if possible. If the cord is tight, it may be doubly clamped and cut. After delivery of the head, the shoulders descend and rotate to a position in the anteroposterior diameter of the pelvis. The attendant's hands are placed on the chin and vertex, applying gentle downward pressure, thus delivering the anterior shoulder. To avoid injury to the brachial plexus, care is taken not to put excessive force on the neck. The posterior shoulder is then delivered by upward traction on the fetal head (Fig. 15.14). Delivery of the body now occurs easily.

The fetus is then cradled in the attendant's arms, with the head down to maximize drainage of secretions to the oropharynx. Further suctioning is accomplished before clamping the umbilical cord. To avoid significant heat loss, the newborn should not be exposed to significant periods of ambient temperature without being completely dry. The infant should be moved to the warmer, where further care can be undertaken.

THIRD STAGE OF LABOR

Immediately after delivery of the infant, the uterus significantly decreases in size. Blood from the um-

bilical cord should be obtained and sent for type and Rh testing. Cord blood may also be used for arterial blood gases determination. *Delivery of the placenta* is imminent when the uterus rises in the abdomen, becoming globular in configuration, indicating that the placenta has separated and has entered the lower uterine segment; a gush of blood and/or "lengthening" of the umbilical cord also occur. These are the three classic *signs of placental separation.* Pulling the placenta from the uterus by excess traction on the cord should be avoided. This inappropriate application of force may result in *inversion of the uterus*, an obstetric emergency associated with profound blood loss and shock. Instead, it is appropriate to wait for spontaneous extrusion of the placenta, sometimes up to 30 min. As the placenta passes into the lower uterine segment, gentle downward pressure is applied to the fundus of the uterus, and the placenta is guided by very gentle traction on the umbilical cord (Fig. 15.15).

If spontaneous placental separation does not occur, or as a routine for some physicians, the placenta may be removed manually. This is accomplished by passing a hand into the uterine cavity and using the side of the had to develop a cleavage plane between the placenta and the uterine wall. The placenta can then be manually removed. The umbilical cord should be evaluated for the presence of the expected two umbilical arteries and one umbilical vein.

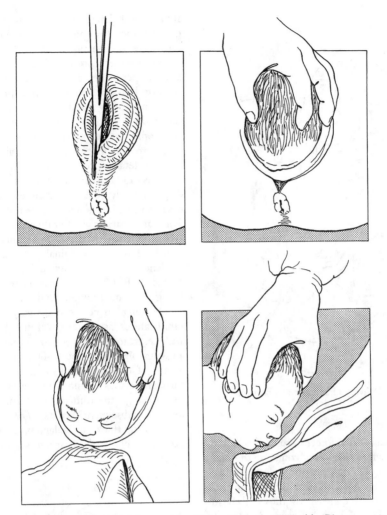

Figure 15.13. Vaginal delivery with midline episiotomy assisted by Ritgen maneuver.

After the placenta has been removed, the uterus should be palpated to ensure that it has reduced in size and become firmly contracted. Excessive blood loss at this or any subsequent time should suggest the possibility of uterine atony. The use of uterine massage as well as oxytocic agents such as oxytocin, Methergine (methylergonovine maleate), or prostaglandins may be routinely used.

Inspection of the birth canal should be accomplished in a systematic fashion. The introitus and vulvar areas, including the periurethral area, should be evaluated for lacerations. Ring forceps are commonly used to hold and evaluate the cervix. Lacerations, if present, are most commonly found at the 3 o'clock and 9 o'clock positions on the cervix. Lacerations of the vagina and/or perineum and extensions of the episiotomy are also evaluated. Repair is accomplished with an absorbable suture. Obstetric lacerations are classified in Table 15.2.

INDICATIONS FOR OPERATIVE DELIVERY

Techniques of operative delivery include obstetric forceps, vacuum extraction, and cesarean section. Forceps are primarily used to supply traction to the fetal head to augment the forces expelling the fetus when the mother's voluntary efforts in conjunction with uterine contractions are insufficient to deliver

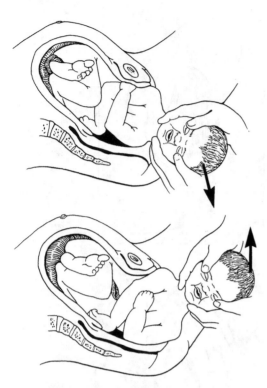

Figure 15.14. Delivery of anterior and posterior shoulders.

the infant. Occasionally, forceps are used to rotate the fetal head before traction to complete the vaginal delivery. Forceps may also be used to control delivery of the fetal head, thereby avoiding any potentially precipitous delivery of the fetal head. Proper application of obstetric forceps by an experienced clinician is necessary to avoid the potential risk of trauma to both maternal and fetal parts. Table 15.3 is a list of conditions necessary to apply forceps, and Table 15.4 is a classification of forceps.

Vacuum extraction is sometimes used in lieu of obstetric forceps. Because traction is applied only to the instrument, some believe that the delivery is more physiologic and has less potential for trauma than forceps although bruising or trauma to the fetal scalp may occur.

Cesarean section now accounts for up to 40% of births in some obstetrical units, with 20% cesarean section rates not uncommon. The rate of cesarean section was stable at less than 5% until 1965. Cesarean section rates have increased since that time for various reasons. One of the major reasons often cited is the ready availability of neonatal intensive care units, in which infants have a significantly greater survival rate than what was once the case. Another factor in the increase in the rate of cesarean sections is its use in the delivery of fetuses in breech presentations. Cesarean sections are also performed if there are signs of fetal distress or dystocias and as a repeat procedure.

An increasing number of cesarean sections are being done for dystocia and uterine inertia. In addition, increased sophistication for fetal surveillance provides more information about the possibility of fetal distress. As a result, more cesarean sections can be attributed to cases of fetal distress. Approximately 20% of the increase in the rate of cesarean sections is due to repeat cesarean births. For many years, it was felt that a previous cesarean section mandated that all future deliveries would also have to be abdominal. With the increasing tendency to attempt vaginal birth after cesarean section (VBAC), fewer cesarean sections are now being performed for this indication.

Deciding on cesarean delivery has important ramifications, as the maternal mortality associated with cesarean delivery is two to four times that of a vaginal birth, i.e., 1 per 2500 to 1 per 5000 operations. Cesarean section can be performed through various incisions in the uterus. An incision through the thin lower uterine segment allows for subsequent trials at VBAC. An incision through the thick, muscular upper portion of the uterus, a classical cesarean section, carries a

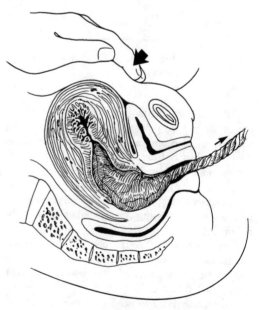

Figure 15.15. Delivery of the placenta.

greater risk for subsequent uterine rupture if labor occurs so that repeat cesarean sections for these patients is still recommended.

FOURTH STAGE OF LABOR

For the first hour or so after delivery, the likelihood of serious postpartum complications is the greatest. Postpartum uterine hemorrhage occurs in approximately 1% of patients. It is more likely to occur in cases of rapid labor, protracted labor, or uterine enlargement (large fetus, polyhydramnios). Immediately after the delivery of the placenta, the uterus is palpated to determine that it is firm. Uterine palpation through the abdominal wall is repeated at frequent intervals during the immediate postpartum period to ascertain uterine tone. Perineal pads are applied and the amount of blood on these pads as well as pulse and blood pressure are monitored closely for the first several hours after delivery to identify excessive blood loss.

CARE OF THE NEWBORN

Once the newborn has been delivered, it is transported to the warming unit, which is equipped with a radiant heat source. The neonate is dried well to minimize evaporative loss of core temperature. The nose and oropharynx are suctioned once

again as the infant is placed in the supine position with the head lowered and turned to one side. The newborn is expected to both breathe and cry within the first 30 sec of life. Suctioning as well as mild stimulation of the infant by rubbing the back or slapping the feet help to stimulate this.

The initial evaluation of the infant is carried out at 1 and 5 min, using the Apgar scoring system (Table 15.5). The Apgar score was designed as a quick assessment of the newborn and should not be used to define birth asphyxia. These scores should not be used to identify the cause of the newborn's depression, nor can they be used to predict long-term neurologic outcome. In general, a low 1-min Apgar identifies the newborn who requires particular attention, whereas the 5-min Apgar can be used to evaluate the effectiveness of any resuscitative efforts that have been undertaken.

Apgar scores of 7 to 10 are indicative of an infant who requires no active resuscitative intervention; scores of 4 to 7 are considered indicators of mildly to moderately depressed infants. The severely depressed infants with Apgar scores of less than 4 rarely require a full evaluation using the Apgar score. Instead, immediate resuscitative efforts are started, which may include endotracheal intubation and suctioning with the possible use of positive pressure oxygen.

Table 15.2.
Classification of Obstetric Lacerations

First degree	Involves the vaginal mucosa or perineal skin, but not the underlying muscle
Second degree	Involves the underlying fascia or muscle, but not the rectal sphincter or rectal mucosa
Third degree	Extends through the rectal sphincter but not into the rectum
Fourth degree	Extends into the rectal mucosa

Table 15.3.
Conditions for Forceps Application

Cervix	Fully dilated
Membranes	Ruptured
Position and station of fetal head	Known and engaged
Anesthesia	Adequate for maternal comfort
Maternal pelvis	Evaluated and found appropriate

Table 15.4.
Forceps Classification[a]

Outlet forceps	The fetal skull has reached the perineal floor, the scalp is visible between contractions, the sagittal suture is in the anteroposterior diameter or in the right or left occiput anterior or posterior position, but not more than 45° from the midline
Low forceps	The leading edge of the skull is station +2 or more
Midforceps	The head is engaged but the leading edge of the skull is above +2 station

[a] The main controversy that has surrounded forceps delivery classification has been the definition of station used. Recently the ACOG redefined *station* for the purpose of forceps delivery classification, describing the leading bony point of the fetal head in centimeters at or below the level of the maternal ischial spines (0–+5) rather than the previously used systems of third (0–+3).

Table 15.5.
Apgar Scoring System

Sign	Score		
	0	1	2
Heart rate	Absent	<100	>100
Muscle tone	Limp	Some flexion of extremities	Active motion
Respiratory effort	Absent	Slow, irregular	Good cry
Reflex activity response to stimulation	No response	Grimace	Cough, sneeze, or crying
Color	Blue or pale	Body pink and extremities blue	Completely pink

CASE STUDIES

Case 15A

A 22-year-old G1 at term comes to the labor unit complaining of increasingly severe and frequent uterine contractions for 10 hr and a gush of fluid 1 hr ago. Her prenatal records reveal an unremarkable antepartum course, with dating by last menstrual period (LMP) and second trimester ultrasound, normal fetal growth, and normal prenatal laboratory findings. Maternal examination including blood pressure are normal.

Questions Case 15A

The initial fetal management should consist of

A. Auscultation or Doppler evaluation of fetal heart rate (FHR)
B. Placement of fetal scalp electrode for evaluation of fetal heart rate
C. Palpation or tocodynamometer evaluation of uterine contractions
D. Placement of intrauterine pressure catheter for evaluation of uterine contractions
E. Leopold maneuvers to ascertain presentation and lie
F. Complete obstetric ultrasound to ascertain lie, presentation, and position (fetal status)
G. Speculum examination and evaluation of fluid, if present, by Nitrazine and slide evaluation
H. Pelvic examination

Answer: A, C, E, G, H

Auscultation, palpation, and Leopolds maneuvers will suffice as initial methods of evaluation of lie, fetal heart rate, and uterine contractions. Internal monitoring and ultrasound require more indication. Fluid should be examined to check for pH and ferning — signs of rupture of membranes — as the gush of fluid may well have been urine. Pelvic examination at term is acceptable to determine if the patient is in labor.

Leopold maneuvers reveal a normal-size fetus in cephalic presentation, palpation reveals strong uterine contractions every 3 min, fluid examination is consistent with urine, and pelvic examination reveals 3 cm and 100%, intact membranes, and a cephalic part at −1 station. FHR is 145. What stage of labor is she in?

A. First stage
B. Second stage
C. Third stage
D. Fourth stage

Answer: A

Continued management includes

A. External EFM
B. Internal EFM
C. Obstetric ultrasound
D. Induction of labor
E. Augmentation of labor

Answer: A

The patient is evidently in normal early labor with a normal pregnancy. External electronic monitoring is sufficient, and indeed, intermittent auscultation would be as satisfactory.

Labor continues for 5 hr, and cervical examination reveals dilation to 4 cm. FHR remains normal. Then spontaneous rupture of membranes occurs with meconium fluid noted. Continued management includes

A. Fetal scalp electrode (FSE)
B. Amnioinfusion
C. Intrauterine pressure catheter (IUPC)
D. Obstetric ultrasound
E. Augmentation of labor

Answer: A, B, maybe C

With the unexpected presence of meconium-stained amniotic fluid, an FSE to evaluate fetal heart rate variability and an amnioinfusion to decrease the risk of meconium aspiration are appropriate. An IUPC can be placed but is not required if external monitoring is sufficient and cervical change is progressing near the expected 1.5 cm/hr.

Case 15B

A 35-year-old G2 P0010 at term has been pushing in second stage for 3 hr; fetal heart tones are reassuring, but the patient is exhausted and demonstrating diminishing ability to push. Spontaneous uterine contractions continue every 3 min, lasting 45 sec, measuring 65 mm Hg on the average. Pelvic examination reveals a cephalic presentation in left occiput posterior presentation (LOP) at –3 station with moderate molding of the head and a marked caput succedaneum.

Question Case 15B

Your best management is

A. Continued labor
B. Augmented labor
C. Forceps delivery
D. Cesarean delivery
E. External version

Answer: D

Assuming reassuring fetal status, the old rule of limiting the second stage of labor to 2 hr is now outdated.

The information here, however, suggests molding of the head at a high station and a very tired mother. The forceps would be above the midforceps definition and, therefore, unsafe. Cesarean birth is the safest routine for mother and fetus.

Case 15C

A term infant is born by spontaneous vaginal delivery almost immediately upon arrival in the labor unit. The infant is covered with meconium fluid, is limp, has a heart rate of 100, and has some body tone and a grimace.

Question Case 15C

Your management of the newborn will include

A. Oxygen by face mask
B. Intubation
C. Warming
D. External cardiac massage
E. Blood gas sampling
F. Stimulation

Answer: B, C, F

Intubation and removal of any meconium in the nasopharynx and below the cords is important to avoid meconium aspiration syndrome. Stimulation, warming, and oxygen in the interval immediately after birth as needed after aspiration of meconium are the first appropriate steps.

chapter 16

ABNORMAL LABOR

Abnormal labor, or *dystocia* (literally, "difficult labor or childbirth"), results when anatomic or functional abnormalities of the fetus, the maternal bony pelvis, the uterus and cervix, and/or a combination of the above interferes with the normal course of labor and delivery. The diagnosis and management of dystocia is a major health care issue, because more than one-fourth of all cesarean sections are performed for this indication. Since the goal of modern obstetrics is a safe, healthy delivery for both mother and fetus, minimizing the morbidity and mortality of the labor process continues to be a primary focus of clinical attention.

Abnormal labor describes complications of the normal labor process: *slower-than-normal progress (protraction disorder)* or a *cessation of progress (arrest disorder).* The patterns of abnormal labor are summarized in Table 16.1. Less specific terms have also been applied to abnormal labor patterns and remain in common usage. *"Failure to progress"* describes lack of progressive cervical dilation and/or descent of the fetus and is similar to the arrest disorders. *"Cephalopelvic disproportion"* is a disparity between the size or shape of the maternal pelvis and the fetal head, preventing vaginal delivery, and is similar to an arrest disorder. This may be caused by the size or shape of the pelvis and/or the fetal head, or a relative disparity as a result of malpresentation of the fetal head.

CAUSES OF ABNORMAL LABOR

Correct diagnosis and management of abnormal labor requires evaluation of the mechanisms of labor: in classic terms, the "power" the "passenger," and the "passage," otherwise referred to as the uterine contractions, fetal factors (presentation, size, etc.), and the maternal pelvis, respectively.

Evaluation of the Power

The power, or *strength, duration, and frequency of uterine contractions,* may be evaluated both qualita-

tively and quantitatively. Frequency and duration of contractions can be subjectively evaluated by *manual palpation of the maternal abdomen during a contraction.* Strength of uterine contractions is often judged by how much the uterine wall can be "indented" by an examiner's finger during a contraction: strong contraction, no indentation; moderate contraction, some indentation; mild contraction, considerable indentation. Although subjective, such determinations by an experienced examiner are of value. The frequency and duration of uterine contractions may be measured more accurately by using a *tocodynamometer* while performing external electronic fetal monitoring. A tocodynamometer is an external strain gauge, which is placed on the maternal abdomen; it records when the uterus tightens and relaxes but does not directly measure how much force the uterus is generating for a given contraction.

The actual pressure generated within the uterus cannot be directly measured without the

Table 16.1.
Abnormal Labor Patterns

Prolonged latent phase
  No progress from latent to active phase of labor
    >20 hr for nulligravidas
    >14 hr for multiparas

Protraction disorders
  Prolonged active phase of labor such that
    Cervical dilation proceeds at
      <1.2 cm/hr for nulligravidas
      <1.5 cm/hr for multiparas
    Descent of the presenting part proceeds at
      <1 cm/hr for nulligravidas
      <1.5 cm/hr for multiparas

Arrest disorders   *2 4cm*
  Secondary arrest of dilation: no cervical dilation for
    >2 hr for nulligravida or multipara in the active
    phase of labor
  Arrest of descent: no descent of the presenting part
    in >1 hr in second stage of labor

use of an *internal* or *intrauterine pressure catheter* (IUPC). To use an intrauterine pressure catheter, the physician introduces a fluid-filled tube into the uterine cavity and attaches it to an external strain gauge. The actual intrauterine pressure is transmitted through the tubing to the strain gauge, which then records duration and frequency as well as the strength of the contractions in millimeters of mercury (Fig. 16.1).

For cervical dilation to occur, each contraction must generate at least 25 mm Hg of pressure, with 50 to 60 mm Hg being considered the optimal intrauterine pressure. The frequency of contractions is also important in generating a normal labor pattern; a minimum of three contractions in a 10-min window is usually considered adequate. During the first stage of labor, arrest of labor should not be diagnosed until the cervix is at least 4 cm dilated (i.e., the latent phase of labor

has been completed) and a pattern of uterine contractions that is adequate both in frequency and intensity has been established.

During the *second stage of labor*, the "powers" include both the uterine contractile forces and the voluntary maternal expulsive efforts (pushing). Maternal exhaustion, excessive anesthesia, or other conditions such as cardiac disease or neuromuscular disease may already affect these combined forces so that they are insufficient to result in vaginal delivery. Forceps or vacuum-assisted vaginal delivery or cesarean section may then be required.

Evaluation of the Passenger

Evaluation of the passenger includes *estimation of fetal weight and clinical evaluation of fetal lie, presentation, position, and attitude*. If a fetus has an estimated weight >4000 to 4500 g, the incidence of dystocias, including shoulder dystocia or

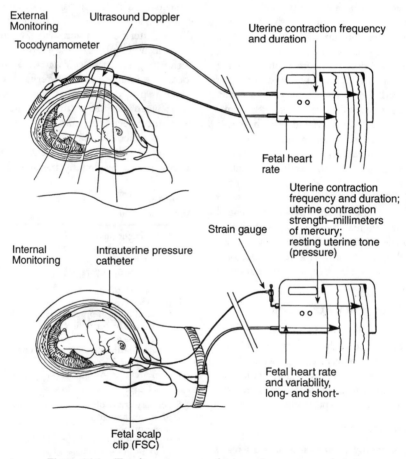

Figure 16.1. Tocodynamometers and intrauterine pressure catheters.

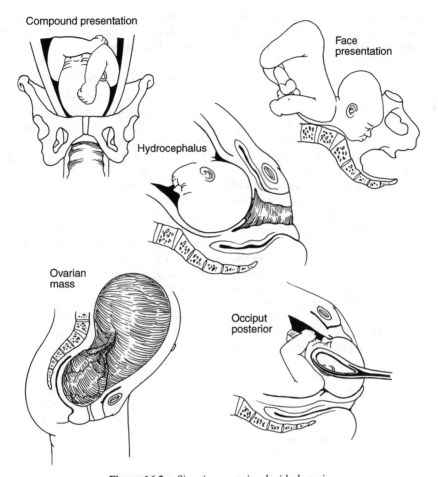

Figure 16.2.   Situations associated with dystocia.

fetopelvic disproportion, is greater. Because ultrasound estimations of fetal weight are often inaccurate by as much as 500 to 1000 g, care must be taken to use the information in conjunction with the entire clinical assessment.

If the fetal head is asynclitic (turned to one side) or if the fetal head is extended, a larger cephalic diameter is presented to the pelvis, thereby increasing the possibility of dystocia. A *brow presentation* (occurring about 1 in 3000 deliveries) will typically convert to either a vertex or face presentation, but if persistent, causes dystocia requiring cesarean section. Likewise, a *face presentation* (about 1 in 600 to 1000 deliveries) requires cesarean section in most cases, although a mentum anterior presentation (chin toward mother's abdomen) may be delivered vaginally in some instances. In cases of mentum anterior that do deliver vaginally, the chin is beneath the pubis, the head may undergo flexion,

rather than the normal extension, with subsequent delivery of the occiput over the perineum.

Persistent occiput posterior positions are also associated with longer labors (approximately 1 hr in multiparous patients and 2 hr in nulliparous patients). Occasionally, delivery from the occiput posterior position is not possible, and the vertex must be rotated to the occiput anterior position. The fetal head can be rotated manually or, if necessary, with forceps or vacuum.

In compound presentations, when one or more limbs prolapse alongside the presenting part (about 1 in 700 deliveries), the extremity usually retracts as labor continues. When it does not, or in the 15 to 20% of compound presentations associated with umbilical cord prolapse, Cesarean birth is required. When dystocia caused by the fetal position cannot be corrected either manually or with instruments, cesarean section is appropriate (Fig. 16.2).

Fetal anomalies, including hydrocephaly and soft tissue tumors, may also cause dystocia. The use of prenatal ultrasound significantly reduces the incidence of unexpected dystocia for these reasons.

Evaluation of the Passage

Unfortunately, measurements of the bony pelvis are relatively poor predictors of successful vaginal delivery. This is because of the inaccuracy of measurements as well as case-by-case differences in fetal accommodation and mechanisms of labor. *Clinical pelvimetry,* i.e., manual evaluation of the diameters of the pelvis, cannot predict whether a fetus can successfully negotiate the birth canal, except in rare circumstances when the pelvic diameters are so small as to render the pelvis "completely contracted." X-ray pelvimetry or other imaging techniques are also of minimal clinical utility when determining whether a patient will require cesarean section for dystocia. Before assuming that the bony pelvis is preventing vaginal delivery, adequate contractions must be ensured (see Table 3.1 and Fig. 3.5). In addition to the bony pelvis, there are soft tissue etiologies of dystocia, e.g., a distended bladder or colon, an adnexal mass, or a uterine fibroid. In

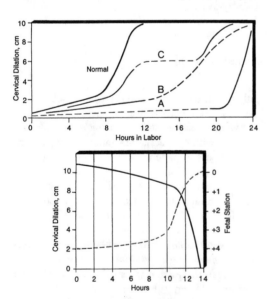

Figure 16.3. Abnormal labor. **Top,** Examples of labor patterns: *A,* prolonged latent phase; *B,* prolonged active phase; *C,* arrest of active phase. **Bottom,** Relationship of descent of presenting part of fetus (*solid line*) and progressive dilation of cervix (*broken line*).

some instances, epidural anesthesia may contribute to dystocia by decreasing the tone of the pelvic floor musculature.

EVALUATION OF ABNORMAL LABOR

Graphic documentation of progressive cervical dilation and effacement facilitates assessing a patient's progress in labor and identifying any type of abnormal labor pattern that may develop. Throughout labor, maternal and fetal well-being are continuously assessed along with the progress in labor. The mother, in particular, should be provided emotional support and encouragement as the possibility of prolonged labor is faced and the various interventions are considered. Keeping the patient and support person fully apprised of the situation is an important aspect of the management of potentially abnormal labor.

Each *vaginal examination* should provide the following information: dilation of the cervix in centimeters, percentage effacement of cervix, station of the presenting part, presence of caput or molding of the fetal head, and position of the presenting part. The results of each examination are compared with previous examinations and any changes noted. In cases of failure of descent of the fetus, clinical reevaluation of the bony pelvis and its relationships to the fetus helps to identify the potential need for operative vaginal delivery or cesarean section.

Uterine contractions can be assessed by manual palpation or by electronic fetal monitor as previously discussed. The uterine contraction pattern and/or the force of the contractions may be inadequate, either causing the abnormal labor pattern or resulting from a mechanical disorder.

In the past, *x-ray pelvimetry* was utilized to aid in the evaluation of the maternal pelvis during labor. It was thought that the size and shape of the pelvis could be visualized, as could fetal position and station. Unfortunately, this radiologic approach to managing dystocia has been shown not to be of benefit.

PATTERNS OF ABNORMAL LABOR

Abnormal labor, or dystocia, is divided into prolongation disorders and arrest disorders. These abnormal labor patterns are demonstrated graphically in Figure 16.3.

A latent phase of labor exceeding 20 hr in a primigravid patient or 14 hr in a multigravid patient is abnormal. The causes of such a *prolonged latent phase* of labor include abnormal fetal position, "unripe" cervix when labor commences, administration of excess anesthesia, fetopelvic disproportion, and dysfunctional/ineffective uterine contractions. The presence of a prolonged latent phase does not necessarily herald an abnormal active phase of labor. In addition, some patients who are initially thought to have a prolonged latent phase turn out only to have false labor. Although certainly of concern, particularly to the patient, a prolonged latent phase does not in and of itself pose a danger to the mother or fetus.

A *prolonged active phase* in the primigravid patient lasts longer than 12 hr or has a rate of cervical dilation of less than 1.2 cm/hr; for a multipara, 1.5 cm/hr. Causes of a prolonged active phase include fetal malposition, fetopelvic disproportion, excess use of sedation, inadequate contractions, and rupture of the fetal membranes before the onset of active labor. Risks associated with a prolonged active phase include increased rates of operative vaginal deliveries or cesarean section, an increased risk of intrauterine infection, and an associated increased risk of fetal compromise. In the absence of fetal distress, slow cervical dilation poses no threat to mother or fetus and can be allowed to progress, albeit slowly. On the other hand, secondary arrest of dilation should be assessed promptly and acted on.

Secondary arrest of dilation occurs when cervical dilation during the active phase of labor stops for 2 hr or more and is demonstrated by a flattening of the labor curve. Either dilation ceases because uterine contractions are no longer sufficient to maintain the progress of labor or labor arrests in spite of adequate uterine contractions, usually associated with too large an infant, a fetal lie/position/attitude that prevents progress in labor, or a too small or abnormally shaped pelvis. Since ineffective contractions can be associated with mechanical factors such as disproportion and malpresentation, careful evaluation of all factors is necessary.

In the multiparous patient, a prolonged active phase is defined as lasting more than 6 hr. Cervical dilation should occur at a rate of at least 1.5 cm/hr. Although a prolonged active phase is much less common in multiparous patients, the physician cannot be lulled into a false sense of security by the history of previous successful vaginal birth(s). Careful evaluation of all the factors is no less important in the multiparous patient than in the primiparous patient.

Active descent of the presenting part should occur progressively, beginning late in the first stage and throughout the second stage of labor. An "arrest of descent" over a 2-hr period is suggestive of either cephalopelvic disproportion or ineffective uterine contractions.

MANAGEMENT OF ABNORMAL LABOR

Induction of labor is the stimulation of uterine contractions before the spontaneous onset of labor, with the goal of achieving delivery. *Augmentation of labor* is the stimulation of uterine contractions that began spontaneously but are either too infrequent or too weak or both. Stimulation of labor is usually carried out with intravenous oxytocin (Pitocin) administered as an intravenous piggyback solution by means of a metered pump. In this way exact amounts of oxytocin may be given per minute. There are several regimens for oxytocin administration; two examples are presented in Table 16.2: a regular-dose oxytocin program and a low-dose oxytocin program. The use of an intrauterine pressure catheter to document actual strength as well as frequency and duration of uter-

Table 16.2.
Oxytocin Administration for Induction and Augmentation of Labor

Infusion	Low Dose	Regular Dose
Initial i.v. infusion	1000 mL D$_5$LR	1000 mL D$_5$LR
Piggyback infusion	20 U oxytocin in 1000 mL 0.9 N/S	20 U oxytocin in 1000 mL 0.9 N/S
Initial infusion rate	1 mU/min	1 mU/min
Interval and decrement for increasing infusion rate	1 mU q. 30min	1–2 mU q. 15–30min
Maximum infusion rate	15–20 mU/min	Three contractions/10 min; no upper limit on infusion rate

Table 16.3.
The Bishop Score for Cervical Ripening[a]

Factor	Points			
	0	1	2	3
Dilation	Closed	1–2 cm	3–4 cm	5+ cm
Effacement	0–30%	40–50%	60–70%	80+%
Station	–3	–2, –1	0	+1, +2
Consistency	Firm	Medium	Soft	
Position	Posterior	Mid	Anterior	

[a] A score of 0 to 4 points is associated with the highest likelihood of failed induction; a score of 9 to 13 points is associated with the highest likelihood of successful induction.

ine contractions stimulated by oxytocin is generally recommended.

The incidence of prolongation of the first stage of labor can be minimized by avoiding unnecessary intervention, i.e., labor should not be induced when the cervix is not well prepared, or "ripe" (softened, anteriorly rotated, partially effaced). The degree of cervical ripening, or readiness, for labor is estimated by digital examination of the cervix. The Bishop score has been used to try to quantify this determination (Table 16.3), and although not especially precise, it provides an excellent schema for cervical evaluation and a rough approximation of the likelihood of successful induction of labor and transvaginal delivery.

When a cervix is not favorable, intravaginal *prostaglandin E₂ gel (dinoprostone) gel* (Prepidil gel) has been used to ripen the cervix, and indeed, labor often ensues without the need of oxytocin stimulation. A dose of 0.5 mg of prostaglandin gel is inserted next to the cervix every 4 to 6 hr. The main concern in the use of prostaglandin is uterine hyperstimulation, which in turn may cause uteroplacental insufficiency and, rarely, uterine rupture. Prostaglandin gel is relatively contraindicated in patients with concurrent asthma. Another method to ripen the cervix is insertion of *laminaria*. Laminaria can be made from the stems of the seaweed *Laminaria japonica* or be of artificial origin. They are hygroscopic rods that are inserted into the internal os. As the rods absorb moisture and expand, the cervix is slowly dilated (Fig. 16.4). The risks associated with laminaria use include failure to dilate the cervix, cervical laceration, inadvertent rupture of the membranes, and infection.

Prolonged first stage of labor can be correctly diagnosed by accurately differentiating true labor

from *false labor*, the latter being best treated with rest and sedation (Table 16.4).

A *prolonged latent phase* can be managed by either *rest* or *augmentation of labor* with intravenous oxytocin once mechanical factors have been ruled out. If the patient is allowed to rest, one of the following will occur: She will cease having contractions, in which case she is not in labor; she will go into active labor; or she will continue as before, in which case oxytocin may be administered to augment the uterine contractions. The use of *amniotomy*, or *artificial rupture of membranes*, is also advocated for patients with prolonged latent phase. It is believed that after amniotomy the fetal head will provide a better dilating force than would the intact bag of waters. In addition, there may be a release of prostaglandins, which could aid in augmenting the force of contractions. Before amniotomy is performed, the presenting part should be firmly applied to the cervix so as to minimize the risk of causing an umbilical cord prolapse. Amniotomy is usually performed with an amniotome or "amnihook," a thin plastic rod with a sharp hook on the end. The end is guided to the open cervical os with the examiner's fingers, and the hook is used to snag and tear the amniotic sac. The fetal heart rate should be evaluated both before and immediately after rupture of the membranes.

During the *active phase of labor*, mechanical factors such as fetal malposition and malpresentation as well as fetopelvic disproportion must be considered before augmentation of uterine contractions with oxytocin. In cases in which the fetus fails to descend in the face of adequate contractions, disproportion is likely and cesarean section warranted. If no disproportion is present, oxytocin can be used if uterine contractions are judged to

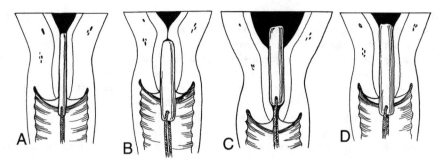

Figure 16.4. Use of laminaria. **A,** Laminaria inserted properly just beyond the internal os. **B and C,** Laminaria improperly inserted not far enough and too far, increasing the risk, respectively, of failure to dilate the cervix and inadvertent rupture of the membranes. **D,** Properly placed laminaria that has expanded, causing cervical dilation.

Table 16.4.
Differentiating Contractions of True and False Labor (Braxton Hicks Contractions)

True Labor	False Labor
Regular intervals, gradually increasing	Irregular intervals and duration
Intensity increasing	Intensity unchanged
Cervical dilation occurs	No cervical dilation
Back and abdominal discomfort	Lower abdominal discomfort
No relief from sedation	Relief from sedation

be inadequate. In cases of maternal exhaustion resulting in secondary arrest of dilation, rest followed by augmentation with oxytocin is often effective. If not already ruptured, artificial rupture of the membranes is also recommended.

Should fetal or maternal distress occur, prompt intervention is warranted. If this happens during the second stage of labor with the vertex low in the pelvis, forceps or vacuum can be used to effect a vaginal delivery. In all other cases, cesarean section may have to be carried out. Distress of either mother or baby in the first stage of labor generally mandates cesarean delivery.

MANAGEMENT OF PROLONGED SECOND STAGE

In the past, a 2-hr second stage was considered indication for cesarean section or operative vaginal delivery. Data now show that if the fetal heart rate is reassuring, it is safe to allow the mother to continue pushing in an attempt to accomplish vaginal delivery. As long as both mother and baby are doing well, the second stage of labor does not have to be concluded in any specific time frame.

Should disproportion exist, cesarean section is necessary. If not, oxytocin may be used to improve the frequency and/or strength of contractions.

Bearing down efforts by the patient in conjunction with the uterine contractions help bring about delivery. Because this is the one phase of labor over which the patient has some control, emotional support and encouragement are of great importance. In some cases, the use of an episiotomy may provide relief from the perineum that has resisted delivery. Similarly, forceps or vacuum extraction may be used to assist the necessary descent and rotation of the fetus, resulting in vaginal delivery.

RISKS OF PROLONGED LABOR

Prolonged labor can have deleterious effects on both fetus and mother. Maternal risks include infection, maternal exhaustion, lacerations, and uterine atony with possible hemorrhage. In addition, there are the attendant risks of any operative delivery. Fetal risks include asphyxia, trauma from difficult deliveries, infection, and possibly cerebral damage because of prolonged pressure to the head.

Prolonged labor (along with postdatism, growth retardation, and other situations associated with decreased amniotic fluid volume) is associated with the passage of meconium into the amniotic fluid and, subsequently, the risk of *meconium aspiration syndrome.* Fetuses who inhale meconium-stained fluid during labor or from the nasopharynx just after birth may suffer this syndrome, which includes both mechanical obstruction and chemical pneumonitis from the meconium material. Pathologic factors include atelectasis, consolidation, and barotrauma as well as some degree of

direct removal of pulmonary surfactant by free fatty acids in meconium.

Intrapartum treatment of meconium-stained amniotic fluid may include *amnioinfusion,* by which a normal saline solution is slowly infused through a tube inserted in the uterus, washing meconium-stained fluid out and replacing it with the saline solution. As the head is delivered, but before delivery of the fetal chest, careful suctioning of the nasopharynx should be performed. Postpartum examination of the area below the vocal cords with a laryngoscope and suctioning out of meconium below the cords, using an endotracheal tube, are also recommended procedures.

BREECH PRESENTATION

Breech presentation occurs in about 2 to 4% of singleton deliveries at term and more frequently in the early third and second trimesters. In addition to prematurity, other conditions associated with breech presentation include multiple pregnancy, polyhydramnios, hydrocephaly, anencephaly, uterine anomalies, and uterine tumors. The three kinds of breech presentation — *frank, complete, and*

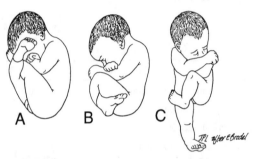

Figure 16.5. Breech presentations. **A,** Frank breech. **B,** Complete breech. **C,** Incomplete breech, single footling.

Table 16.5.
Types of Vaginal Breech Deliveries

Total breech extraction
  Entire body extracted

Partial breech extraction
  Spontaneous delivery to umbilicus, remainder of body extracted

Spontaneous breech delivery
  No traction or manipulation of the fetus, which delivers spontaneously

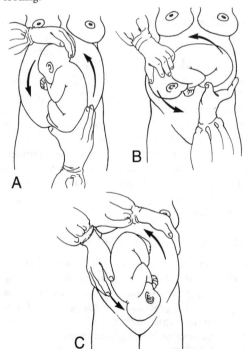

Figure 16.6. External cephalic version.

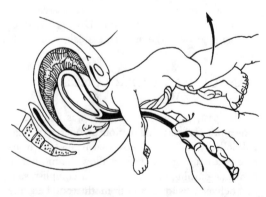

Figure 16.7. Application of Piper forceps to the aftercoming head.

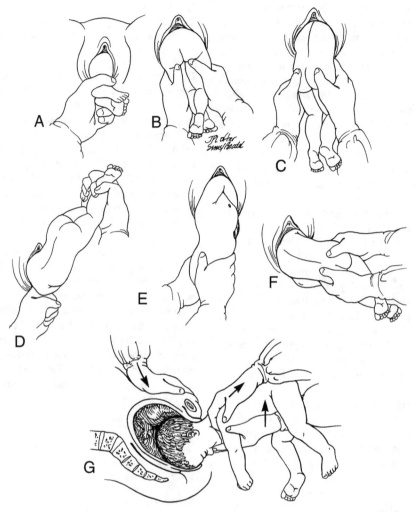

Figure 16.8. Breech extraction. **A–C,** Gentle traction on the feet and ankles, thighs, and pelvis. Note that traction is not applied above the pelvis. **D,** Gentle traction and rotation as the scapulae become visible, sweeping the posterior and then anterior arm free in the process. **E–G,** Mauriceau maneuver to deliver the head.

incomplete breech (Fig. 16.5) — are diagnosed by a combination of Leopold maneuvers, pelvic examination, radiography, and ultrasonography.

The morbidity and mortality for mother and fetus, regardless of gestational age or mode of delivery, is higher in the breech than in the cephalic presentation. This increased risk to the fetus comes from associated factors such as fetal anomaly, prematurity, and umbilical cord prolapse as well as birth trauma.

Vaginal delivery of the preterm fetus weighing <2000 g is avoided by many obstetricians because of concern about an increased risk of birth injury. Al-

though the data to support this concern are contradictory, the practice of cesarean birth for these smaller infants is common. At the other end of the spectrum, vaginal delivery of the term breech weighing >4000 to 4500 g is usually avoided, primarily because of concern about entrapment of the head after the vaginal delivery of the smaller body.

The risks of vaginal delivery of the breech at term or cesarean delivery for the breech are avoided in approximately half of appropriately selected cases by use of external cephalic version (Fig. 16.6). Selection criteria include a normal fetus with reassuring fetal heart tracing, adequate amniotic fluid, presenting part not in pelvis, no uterine operative scars, and no labor. The risks include placental abruption, cord accident, and uterine rupture. External version is more often successful in parous women. Whether or not to use tocolytics at the time of attempted version is controversial, but the use of anti-D immune globulin in D– women is recommended.

There are three types of vaginal delivery of the breech (Table 16.5). The keys to successful vaginal delivery of the term breech are appropriate selection of cases and patience during the delivery, allowing as much of the delivery as possible to be spontaneous.

The suggested criteria for a vaginal breech delivery include (*a*) a normal labor curve, (*b*) estimated fetal weight between 2000 and 4000 g in the frank breech presentation, (*c*) a reassuring fetal heart tracing, (*d*) an adequate maternal pelvis by clinical pelvimetry, and (*e*) a normally flexed fetal head. Hyperextension of the fetal head occurs in about 5% of term breeches, requiring cesarean birth to avoid head entrapment. Because of the risk of umbilical cord prolapse, vaginal delivery of the footling breech is usually avoided.

The delivery of the aftercoming fetal head assisted with Piper forceps is shown in Figure 16.7, and the technique of breech extraction is presented in Figure 16.8. The key to the vaginal delivery of the breech is not to rush the process, allowing spontaneous delivery insofar as possible before intervention.

CASE STUDIES

Case 16A

A 5-foot 8-inch, 145-pound, 19-year-old G1 at 41 weeks gestational age presents complaining of uterine contractions. Her antepartum course has been unremarkable; her baby is active. Her fundal height is 45 cm, and her uterine contractions are occurring every 6 min and judged to be mild in intensity. Fetal heart tones are normal without deceleration. Pelvic examination shows the cervix to be 30% effaced and 1 cm dilated, with a cephalic part at –2 station, and membranes intact. Clinical pelvimetry is judged adequate.

Questions 16A

Which of the following are appropriate managements at this time?

A. Monitored labor
B. Ultrasound for fetal weight determination

C. Amniotomy
D. Cesarean section for fetopelvic disproportion
E. Patient discharged home with reassurance

Answer: A, B

The patient may or may not be in labor. Monitoring will help evaluate the pattern of uterine activity and the fetal heart rate (FHR). As she is 41 weeks, there is more risk of uteroplacental insufficiency than there would have been 1 or 2 weeks earlier. Ultrasound for fetal weight may be helpful, as there is information to suggest macrosomia. Amniotomy is not advisable with a high presenting part. There is no indication for operative delivery, nor is it appropriate to send the patient home until it is known whether she is in labor and whether her fetus demonstrates heart rate evidence suggestive of fetal compromise.

The initial ultrasound shows a normal fetus in cephalic presentation with normal amniotic fluid volume and an estimated fetal weight of 7.5 lb. The patient develops regular, more intense uterine contractions and progresses to 6 cm dilation and 100% effacement with the vertex descending to –1 station. The head is felt to be right occiput transverse (ROT). Thereafter, uterine contractions become somewhat less intense and there is no further dilation for 2.5 hr. Fetal hart rate monitoring continues to demonstrate a reassuring pattern. Your diagnosis at this time is

A. Prolonged latent phase
B. Prolonged active phase
C. Secondary arrest of labor
D. Cephalopelvic disproportion
E. Failure to progress

Answer: C

Components of your management should now include

A. Artificial rupture of membranes
B. Fetal scalp electrode (FSE) application
C. Intrauterine pressure catheter application
D. X-ray pelvimetry
E. Pelvic ultrasonography

Answer: A, C

The passage and passenger are felt to be large enough and not too large, respectively. You must now assess the power (i.e., the strength as well as frequency and duration of uterine contractions). A fetal scalp electrode is commonly applied concurrent with rupture of the membranes and placement of IUPC.

Artificial rupture of membranes is performed with appreciation of clear amniotic fluid. The cervix remains

6 cm dilated and the ROT vertex is at −1/−2. An IUPC and FSE are applied. Uterine contractions are found to be occurring every 4 to 5 min, lasting 30 sec and generating 25 to 35 mm Hg pressure. The FHR remains reassuring. Your best management now is

A. Fetal scalp blood sampling
B. Forceps delivery
C. Cesarean birth
D. Induction of labor
E. Augmentation of labor

Answer: E

Without a nonreassuring FHR pattern fetal scalp sampling is unnecessary. Likewise, without evidence of fetal distress, operative delivery — transabdominal or transvaginal — is not indicated. You cannot induce labor, as it is spontaneously begun. Augmentation is appropriate.

Pitocin augmentation is begun and continued for 5 hr; for the last three the IUPC show 60 to 80 mm Hg uterine contractions that are occurring every 3 to 4 min and lasting 60 to 75 sec. The resting uterine pressure is 15 mm Hg. The FHR remains reassuring.

Over this 5-hr period pelvic examination reveals the following:

	dilation	eff.	sta.	pos.
1st hr	6 cm	90%	−1/−2	ROT
2nd hr	6–7 cm	90%	−1/−2	ROT
3rd hr	6–7 cm	100%	−1/−2	ROT
4th hr	6–7 cm	100%	−1/−2	ROT
5th hr	6–7 cm	100%	−1/−2	ROT

A large caput develops in the 4th to 5th hr. Your best management now is

A. Fetal scalp blood sampling
B. Forceps delivery
C. Cesarean birth
D. Induction of labor
E. Augmentation of labor

Answer: C

Operative vaginal delivery is contraindicated by dilation and station. Augmentation has been successful in that an adequate mechanism of labor has been demonstrated for 4+ hr without progress.

Case 16B

A 31-year-old G2 P1001, who delivered an 8.5-lb son vaginally 8 years ago, presents at term in active labor and progresses rapidly to complete dilation. She then begins to push. After 2 hr of monitored labor, the vertex has progressed from −1 station to +1 station but with a prominent caput succedaneum noted. The fetal heart rate pattern is reassuring.

Question Case 16B

Which of the following are appropriate next steps in this patient's management?

A. Forceps delivery
B. Cesarean section
C. Continued monitored labor
D. Augmentation with oxytocin

Answer: C

After this patient has had a second stage of labor prolonged beyond the traditional 2-hr limit, there has been some descent from −1 to +1 station. Continued monitored labor is appropriate if clinical evaluation indicates that the baby is not macrosomic or malformed or there is not obvious fetopelvic disproportion. If either is the case, cesarean section would be appropriate. Augmentation of the contractions would be appropriate if they were inadequate in frequency or intensity. Forceps delivery would be appropriate if either maternal or fetal condition warranted delivery and the fetus were in a position to be so delivered. In this case, at +1 station with caput succedaneum present, it is unlikely to be deliverable via forceps.

Case 16C

A 38-year-old G5 P4004 at term arrives in active labor, 5 to 6 cm dilated and 90% effaced with a presenting part at −1 station, and intact membranes. She has had no prenatal care and four previous vaginal deliveries of four boys all weighing 8.5 to 9 lb.

As there are variable decelerations and a questionable loss of long-term variability, artificial rupture of membranes is performed, at which time the patient is found to have a frank breech presentation, now 7 cm dilated with the breech at −1 station. The FHR is now reassuring. Contractions are strong, occurring every 3 min.

Questions Case 16C

Your best management would be

A. External version
B. Internal version
C. Piper forceps delivery
D. Cesarean birth
E. Monitored labor

Answer: E

There is debate of the propriety of vaginal breech delivery. Some physicians believe that the morbidity is too great for this procedure and opt for cesarean birth for all breech deliveries. Others will allow vaginal delivery of the breech in selected cases.

Which of the following should occur to select properly between vaginal and cesarean birth?

A.   Ultrasound for estimated fetal weight
B.   Clinical estimation of fetal weight
C.   Clinical pelvimetry
D.   X-ray pelvimetry
E.   Flat plate of abdomen

Answer: A, B, C, E

Estimation of fetal weight by one or both methods and clinical evaluation of the bony pelvis are required. A flat plate of the abdomen will identify an extended head, which is a contraindication to vaginal delivery. Her history of previous deliveries of infants up to 9 pounds suggest a clinically adequate pelvis.

chapter 17

INTRAPARTUM FETAL ASSESSMENT

Evidence suggesting a *nonreassuring fetal status* occurs in 5 to 10% of pregnancies, when there is concern that the function of the maternal-fetal physiologic unit is so altered that fetal death or serious injury may occur. The term *fetal distress* is also often used for this situation, but the term is imprecise and nonspecific, having a low positive predictive value even in high-risk situations and often being associated with a neonate that shows no evidence of intrauterine compromise as measured by Apgar scores and blood gas studies. Furthermore, when delivery is facilitated because of a nonreassuring fetal status, the delivery of a vigorous infant is not inconsistent. When, however, an infant is born with clinical evidence of intrauterine fetal compromise, the term *fetal asphyxia* should be used to describe the infant's status only when the situation fits the criteria suggested in the *Guidelines for Prenatal Care* of the American College of Obstetricians and Gynecologists (Table 17.1). Thus, when this concern arises, the term *nonreassuring fetal status* associated with whatever findings elicit the comment should be used rather than *fetal distress*.

It is the task of the obstetric team to recognize this situation and to intervene as needed to avoid or minimize injury to the fetus. The decision to intervene is often difficult, because fetal heart rate monitoring and fetal acid-base measurement are sometimes difficult to interpret. To help interpret these indirect measures of nonreassuring fetal status, the obstetric team correlates the intrapartum status with the patient's antepartum information, including historical risk factors (e.g., hypertension, maternal smoking), physical examination information (e.g., hypertension, fetal size), laboratory information (e.g., glucose tolerance data, ultrasound examinations), and dynamic testing information (e.g., biophysical profile determinations, NST/OCT testing). When interpreting this information, the obstetric team is especially alert for items that are known to predispose to the *three categories of causes*

of *nonreassuring fetal status:* uteroplacental insufficiency, umbilical cord compression, and fetal conditions/anomalies (Table 17.2).

The *uteroplacental unit* provides oxygen and nutrients to the fetus while receiving carbon dioxide and wastes, the products of the normal aerobic fetal and placental metabolisms. *Uteroplacental insufficiency* occurs when the uteroplacental unit starts to fail at this task. Initial fetal responses include fetal hypoxia; shunting of blood flow to the fetal brain, heart, and adrenal glands; and transient repetitive late decelerations of the fetal heart rate. *If the cause of the fetal hypoxia is progressive and is not recognized and corrected, fetal respiratory and then metabolic acidosis can ensue. These patterns of nonreassuring fetal status are usually reversible either by altering the conditions of uteroplacental function or by rapid delivery of the baby.*

If delivery occurs promptly, the 1-min Apgar score may be low, but the 5-min score is usually high. Apgar scores are a measure of fetal reactions after delivery and are scored on a 0 to 10 scale. If, however, the fetus continues to experience hypoxia, the time will come when the fetus will progressively switch over to anaerobic glycolysis, shunt more blood flow to vital organs, and progressively develop a metabolic acidosis superimposed on the respiratory one. Lactic acid accumulates as this process continues and progressive damage to vital organs occurs, especially the fetal brain and myocardium. At delivery, both the 1- and the 5-min Apgar scores are usually depressed, and if the intervention was not timely, serious and possibly permanent damage (and sometimes even death) result.

Fortunately, deleterious fetal acid-base changes are usually preceded by hypoxia manifest in fetal heart rate changes, which can be recognized by electronic monitoring or intermittent auscultation. Timely intervention is then usually possible once nonreassuring fetal status has been identified. The techniques of intrapartum monitoring are designed to discover this process as early as possible.

Table 17.1.
Criteria for Diagnosis of Fetal Asphyxia

Any neonate who had hypoxia proximate to delivery severe enough to result in hypoxic encephalopathy will show other evidence of hypoxic damage, specifically including *all* of the following:

1. Metabolic or mixed acidemia (pH less than 7.00) on an umbilical cord arterial sample, if obtained

2. Persistent Apgar scores of 0–3 for longer than 5 min

3. Evidence of neonatal neurologic sequelae such as seizures, coma, hypotonia, and one or more of the following: cardiovascular, gastrointestinal, hematologic, pulmonary, or renal system dysfunction

Table 17.2.
Causes of Nonreassuring Fetal Status

Uteroplacental insufficiency	Placental edema
	  Maternal diabetes
	  Hydrops fetalis
	  Rh isoimmunization
	Placental "accidents"
	  Abruptio placentae
	  Placenta previa ± accreta
	Postdatism
	Intrauterine growth retardation
	Uterine hyperstimulation

Umbilical cord compression	Umbilical cord accidents
	  Umbilical cord prolapse or
	    entanglement (gross, occult)
	  Umbilical cord knot
	  Abnormal umbilical cord insertion
	  Anomalous umbilical cord
	  Oligohydramnios (from any cause)

Fetal conditions/ anomalies	Sepsis (maternal/fetal; chrioamnionitis) Fetal congenital anomalies Intrauterine growth retardation Prematurity Postdatism

INTRAPARTUM MONITORING

Fetal Heart Rate Monitoring

Methods of Fetal Heart Rate Evaluation

Before the popular use of electronic fetal monitoring (EFM), intermittent auscultation of the fetal heart rate after contractions was the technique used to assess intrapartum fetal well-being. With the use of EFM, fetal heart rate patterns have been identified and associated with various fetal conditions and prognoses. In the last few years, the now generalized use of these monitors has come into question. Continuous EFM of "high-risk patients" who have a predictable increased risk of intrapartum nonreassuring fetal status is usually not questioned. The value of EFM is questioned in "low-risk patients" whose risk of intra-partum nonreassuring fetal status is known to be small, yet it is interesting that it is in this group of patients that the risk of unexpected nonreassuring fetal status is highest. Given the present widespread use of EFM, the debate will be long and vigorous, with the ultimate pattern of use of both EFM and intermittent fetal heart rate auscultation being uncertain.

Fetal Heart Rate

EFM fetal heart rates are described by rate and by pattern of variability. The techniques are described in Chapter 15. *The baseline fetal heart rate* ("normal fetal heart rate") at term is defined as 120 to 160 beats per minute (bpm), with slightly higher rates in preterm fetuses. *Baseline fetal tachycardia* is defined as >160 bpm for 10 or more minutes, being classified as mild if the baseline is between 161 and 180 bpm and severe, if more than 181 bpm. Fetal tachycardia may be transient (generally less than 10 min) and without significance, although it is sometimes associated with situations that may require various interventions to avoid permanent fetal damage.

The most common cause of fetal tachycardia is elevated maternal temperature, which is often the first evidence of developing chorioamnionitis. Because the fetal oxygen-hemoglobin dissociation curve is adversely affected by increased temperature, a fetal tachycardia coupled with increased maternal temperature should prompt adminstration of antipyretics to the mother. If there is evidence of chorioamnionitis, antibiotic therapy is indicated.

Baseline fetal bradycardia is defined as less than 120 bpm for 10 or more minutes and is classified as moderate between 80 and 100 bpm and severe as <80 bpm. Heart rates between 100 and 119 bpm, while classified as a bradycardia, are rarely associated with fetal compromise unless accompanied by other evidence of nonreassuring fetal

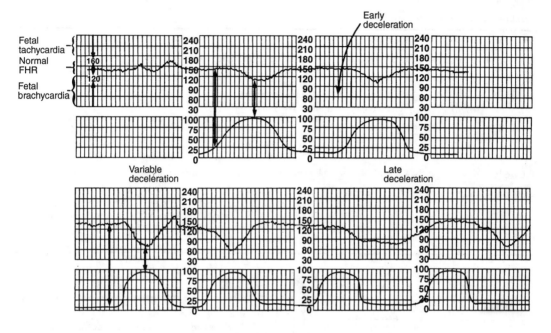

Figure 17.1.   Fetal heart rate patterns.

status. Fetal bradycardias may be associated with congenital heart block and with situations associated with severe fetal compromise such as placental abruption (Fig. 17.1 and Table 17.3).

A *sinusoidal heart rate pattern* is when the rate is 120 to 160 bpm, but there is a smooth undulating pattern of 5 to 10 bpm in amplitude (very reminiscent of a sine wave) and shortened short-term variability (Fig. 17.2). The cause of this pattern is unknown, although it has been associated with fetal anemia and Rh isoimmunization and newborns with significant compromise. Sinusoidal-like patterns are sometimes seen after analgesic administration, so that the evaluation and treatment of this pattern is difficult. *Fetal arrhythmias* are seen in <1% of monitored labors, are usually transient, and are diagnosed by fetal ECG. If they persist, evaluation of the fetus for inherent pathology (especially hydrops and congenital anomalies) is indicated, as some treatment may be needed upon delivery or, rarely, intrapartum.

Fetal Heart Rate Variability

Fetal heart rate (FHR) variability is the most reliable single EFM indicator of fetal status (fetal well-being). FHR variability results from a complex interplay of cardioinhibitory and cardioaccelerator centers in the fetal brain, which, in turn, are extremely sensitive to the fetal biochemical status (oxygenation and acid-base status). *The presence of good variability is highly suggestive of adequate fetal central nervous system (CNS) oxygenation.* Two types of variability are described (Fig. 17.3). *Short-term variability* is the variation in amplitude seen on a beat-to-beat basis, normally 3 to 8 bpm, measured from R wave to R wave by direct fetal scalp electrode. *Long-term variability* is an irregular, crude wave-like pattern with a cycle of 3 to 5 cycles per minute and an amplitude of 5 to 15 bpm. These patterns are normally encountered after approximately 28 weeks gestation, but they are difficult to interpret (especially their absence) before this gestational age.

Short-term variability is measurable only with the use of an internal fetal scalp electrode (FSE), whereas long-term variability may be measured, albeit not as well as with FSE, by Doppler measurement. Decreased variability is associated with fetal hypoxia and/or acidemia, drugs that may depress the fetal CNS (e.g., maternal narcotic analgesia), fetal tachycardia, fetal CNS and cardiac anomalies, prolonged uterine contractions (uterine hypertonus), prematurity, and fetal sleep. Care must be taken in the interpretation of decreased variability when a

Table 17.3.
Baseline Fetal Heart Rates

Fetal Heart Rate (bpm)	Description	Associated Causes
>160 for >10 min	Fetal tachycardia	Maternal fever and infection Fetal infection Fetal anemia Maternal thyrotoxicosis Fetal tachyarrhythmias Maternal treatment with sympathomimetic or parasympatholytic (e.g., atropine) drugs Fetal immaturity Fetal hypoxia
120–160	Normal FHR	Normal function of maternal-fetal unit
<120 for >10 min	Fetal bradycardia	Maternal treatment with β-blockers (e.g., propranolol) Fetal congenital heart block (as in systemic lupus erythematosus, where an antibody may be produced that crosses the placenta and damages the conduction system of the fetus) Fetal anoxia

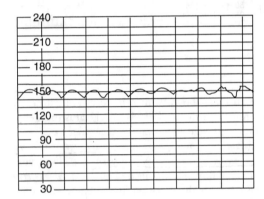

Figure 17.2. Sinusoidal fetal heart rate pattern associated with a fetal-maternal hemorrhage and severe fetal anemia.

transient cause such as fetal sleep may be involved, lest an unnecessary intervention be considered.

Periodic Fetal Heart Rate Changes

The FHR may vary with uterine contractions by slowing or accelerating in periodic patterns. These changes in FHR are in response to two mechanisms: (*a*) intrinsic reflex fetal heart rate control, especially responses to hypoxia and acidemia as well as normal reflex responses, and (*b*) fetal myocardial hypoxia. Periodic FHR changes are classified into patterns based on their shape, magnitude (in beats per minute), and relationship to the same parameters of the uterine contractions with which they are associated. These patterns have prognos-

tic value for the intrapartum evaluation of the fetus (see Fig. 17.1).

Accelerations of the FHR are defined as an increase in the fetal heart rate above the baseline of at least 15 bpm, usually of 15 to 20 sec duration, and are associated with an intact fetal mechanism unstressed by hypoxia and acidemia. *Fetal heart rate accelerations are, therefore, reassuring and generally indicative of fetal well-being.* Stimulation of the fetal scalp by digital examination will usually engender a heart rate acceleration in the uncompromised, nonacidotic fetus and is used by some obstetricians as a test of fetal well-being. External sound/vibration stimulation, also termed *acoustic stimulation*, elicits the same response and is also used for this purpose.

Early FHR decelerations are slowings of the FHR (never below 100 bpm), which begin as the uterine contraction begins, reach their nadir at the peak of the uterine contraction, and return to the baseline FHR with the end of the uterine contraction, i.e., mirror images of the uterine contraction. These early decelerations are the result of *pressure on the fetal head* (from the birth canal, digital examination, forceps application), causing a reflex response via the vagus nerve with acetylcholine release at the fetal sinoatrial node. This response may be blocked with vagolytics such as atropine. *Early FHR decelerations are considered physiologic and are not a cause of concern.*

Variable FHR decelerations are slowings of the FHR, which may start before, during, or after uterine contraction starts (hence, variable), but

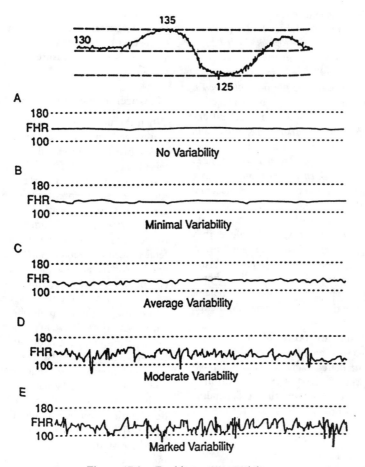

Figure 17.3. Fetal heart rate variability.

are characterized by a rapid fall in the FHR, often to below 100 bpm, and then a rapid return to baseline. These variable decelerations are also reflex mediated, usually associated with *umbilical cord compression* and mediated via the vagus nerve with sudden and often erratic release of acetylcholine at the fetal sinoatrial node, resulting in the characteristic sharp deceleration slope of these decelerations. Umbilical cord compression may result from wrapping of the cord around parts of the fetus, anomalies, or even knots in the umbilical cord and is especially associated with oligohydramnios, in which the buffering space for the umbilical cord created by the amniotic fluid is lost. These variable decelerations are the most common periodic FHR pattern. They are often correctable by changes in the maternal position to relieve pressure on the umbilical cord. Infusion of fluid unto the amniotic cavity

(amnioinfusion) has also been used effectively to relieve pressure on the umbilical cord in cases of oligohydramnios or when rupture of membranes has occurred.

If the FHR falls below 100 bpm, a sterile vaginal examination is indicated to check for a prolapsed umbilical cord, a rare but emergent cause of the sudden development of this usually benign periodic FHR pattern. If the FHR falls below 60 to 70 bpm for more than 30 sec, repetitive variable decelerations will often have a summative effect on fetal well-being, with the development of hypoxia, acidemia, and distress. If the FHR falls below 60 bpm, transient loss of fetal SA node function has been noted with transient "fetal cardiac arrest." These decelerations below 60 to 70 bpm require careful evaluation of cause. Both variable and late decelerations have been classified as mild, moderate, and severe, with the assertion that the risk of fetal hypoxia and acidosis increases with the degree of deceleration (Tables 17.3 and 17.4).

Late FHR decelerations are slowings of the FHR that begin after the uterine contraction starts, reach their nadir after the peak of the uterine contraction, and resolve to baseline after the uterine contraction is over, i.e., also a mirror image of the contraction but "late" relative to it. These late decelerations are viewed as ominous, especially if repetitive and most especially if associated with decreased variability. *Late decelerations are sometimes associated with uteroplacental insufficiency,* as a result of either decreased uterine perfusion or decreased placental function, and thus with decreased intervillous exchange of oxygen and carbon dioxide and *progressive fetal hypoxia and acidemia.* Therefore, they are associated with causes of uteroplacental insufficiency, including postdatism, placental abruption, maternal hypertension, maternal diabetes, maternal anemia, maternal sepsis, and problems with uterine contractions such as hyperstimulation or hypertonia.

Two mechanisms are postulated to associate late decelerations with fetal hypoxia and acidemia: chemoreceptor-mediated vagal reflex and hypoxic myocardial depression or both. Intervention is usually required, the nature and timing depending on full evaluation of the maternal and fetal status.

Table 17.4.
Grading of Periodic FHR Patterns

Pattern/Grade	Fall (bpm)	Duration (sec)
Variable		
Mild	Any value	<30
Moderate	<70	>30, <60
Severe	<70	>60
Late		
Mild	<15	Any duration
Moderate	15–45	Any duration
Severe	>45	Any duration

Certainly, the need to intervene increases with the progression of nonreassuring fetal status. One evaluation that is often used to help guide interventions is direct measurement of fetal acid-base status.

Measurement of Fetal Acid-Base Status

When the uteroplacental unit is functioning normally, even with the stress of uterine contractions, which cause a transient decrease in placental intervillous perfusion, fetal acid-base status is easily maintained in normal ranges. *Normal fetal acid-base status* is mirrored in the normal umbilical cord blood gas values at term (Table 17.5). When there is *uteroplacental insufficiency,* inadequate fetal oxygenation causes a switch from fetal aerobic to fetal anaerobic metabolism, resulting in the production of lactate and progressive fetal acidosis, compounding the deleterious effects of fetal hypoxia. Initially, the fetus responds by shunting blood flow to the brain and heart from other organs. With progressive hypoxia, late decelerations develop and, with the addition of acidosis, loss of beat-to-beat variability. Brain and myocardial damage follow, with subsequent high risk of other end organ damage. When there are indicators of such an ominous situation (e.g., persistent late decelerations on EFM and decreased beat-to-beat variability) direct measurement of the fetal acid-base status is an option. The most common method is fetal scalp capillary blood gas or blood pH measurement.

FETAL SCALP pH/BLOOD GAS EVALUATION

The chorioamnion must be ruptured and the presenting part descended to allow access to the presenting fetal part through the cervical os, which must be dilated at least 2 to 3 cm. Given access to the fetal part, either head or breech, a plastic or

Table 17.5.
Normal Umbilical Cord and Fetal Scalp Blood Gas Values

Umbilical Cord		Values	Fetal Scalp
Venous	Arterial		
7.34 ± 0.15	7.34 ± 0.15	pH	7.25–7.40
30 ± 15	15 ± 10	P_{O_2}	15 ± 10
35 ± 8	45 ± 15	P_{CO_2}	45 ± 15
5 ± 4	7 ± 4	Base deficit	7 ± 4

metallic cone is inserted through the os and pressed against the fetal scalp. The scalp surface is thoroughly cleaned and the cone held with enough pressure to avoid dilution of the blood with amniotic fluid. A thin layer of silicone gel is often applied to the surface, serving to provide a smooth uniform surface on which the blood droplet may form. A small incision is then made in the fetal scalp with a specialized lancet, and the drops of blood that form are collected in a heparinized capillary tube and analyzed. Pressure is applied to the incision site through one or two uterine contractions, until bleeding stops. Care must be taken not to make the incision over a fontanel or suture line. A caput succedaneum will not alter the pH information obtained (Fig. 17.4).

Scalp blood samples are often difficult to interpret because absolute parameters that mandate specific interventions do not exist. Instead, as with other measures of fetal well-being, the information obtained must be correlated with the aggregate understanding of the status of the maternal-fetal unit at the time of the measure. Some general guidelines for the use of scalp pH include (*a*) a scalp pH greater than 7.25 is generally considered reassuring, requiring no further scalp sampling unless other measures of fetal well-being worsen; (*b*) a scalp pH between 7.20 and 7.24, raises concern about the possible development of fetal hypoxia/acidemia, and generally, repeat scalp measurements are made within 15 to 30 min; (*c*) a scalp pH less than 7.20 means that fetal compromise is strongly expected, and generally, interventions are required on an immediate basis to ameliorate the cause of the nonreassuring fetal status or to effect delivery. Determining whether the acidosis is respiratory, metabolic, or mixed in origin is often useful for management decisions (Table 17.6). Although a rare situation, maternal acidosis may complicate the evaluation of scalp pH results. For comparison, a free-flowing maternal venous sample may be evaluated for pH,

with the fetal sample usually being approximately 0.1 pH unit below the maternal value.

MANAGEMENT

Interpretation of intrapartum fetal well-being measurements are made within the context of the entire obstetric situation, including maternal and fetal factors and the course and anticipated duration and outcome of labor. The number of variables to consider and the often imprecise nature of the information make these among the most difficult of medical decisions. In-depth training and experience in obstetrics are required to perform these complex tasks adequately.

Sometimes the fetal heart rate pattern will demonstrate a single pattern. If it is reassuring, no intervention is needed; if it is not reassuring, the appropriate intervention is often clear. More often, however, the observed FHR pattern is a mixture of two more patterns and variations of baseline values. In these cases, it is generally prudent to manage the obstetric situation based on the most ominous of the patterns present.

In general, if there is evidence of progressive fetal hypoxia and acidosis in a situation where the

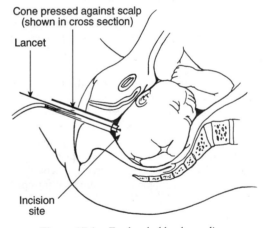

Cone pressed against scalp (shown in cross section)

Lancet

Incision site

Figure 17.4. Fetal scalp blood sampling.

Table 17.6.
Classification of Neonatal Acidemia When Umbilical Cord pH Is <7.20

Type of Acidemia	P_{CO_2} (mm Hg)	HCO_3 (mEq/liter)	Base Deficit (mEq/liter)
Respiratory	≥65 (high)	>17 (normal)	<9 (normal)
Metabolic	<65 (normal)	≤17 (low)	>9 (high)
Mixed	≥65 (high)	≤17 (low)	>9 (high)

time of vaginal delivery is remote, operative de-livery by cesarean section is indicated for fetal reasons. Awaiting vaginal delivery is appropriate if, in the judgment of the obstetric team, vaginal delivery will occur soon enough that the progres-sion of nonreassuring fetal status will not result in serious fetal injury and/or death or when ef-fective interventions to ameliorate the nonreas-suring fetal status may be taken. In general, a scalp pH greater than 7.24 is reassuring; cer-tainly, good variability on EFM is a reassuring factor. If meconium is present in the amniotic fluid, perinatal morbidity is increased by 5 to 10%, a condition that tends to dissuade contin-ued labor when other evidence of nonreassuring fetal status is also present.

While awaiting vaginal delivery or while pre-paring for cesarean delivery, one or more of the following steps are appropriate: (*a*) discontinue oxytocin infusion that may have been started for induction or augmentation; (*b*) administer oxygen to the mother, usually 5 to 6 liters/min by face mask; (*c*) check the maternal blood pressure, treat-ing any hypotension with intravenous fluids and, if needed, pressors such as ephedrine; (*d*) change the maternal position to left lateral position to decrease uterine pressure on the great vessels and thereby increase blood return to the heart, car-diac output, and uteroplacental blood flow; and (*e*) consider "intrauterine resuscitation," using an intravenous tocolytic (such as the β_2-sympathomi-metic terbutaline, 0.25 mg i.v.p. or s.c.) to relax the uterine tone and slow the contraction rate, thereby increasing uteroplacental blood flow. Um-bilical arterial and venous blood gases should be drawn immediately after the delivery from the cord attached to the placenta before placental sep-aration. The data will help the management of the newborn and shed light on the results of intrapar-tum interventions.

CASE STUDIES

Case 17A

Your patient is a 24-year-old G3 P2002 with an unre-markable antepartum course who presents at 41 weeks gestational age having uterine contractions of increas-ing severity for 8 hr before being seen. On examina-tion, the cervix is 3 to 4 cm, 80% effaced, −2 station; the fetus is in cephalic presentation with intact mem-branes. She is admitted, an intravenous line and appro-priate laboratory studies are initiated, and external elec-tronic fetal monitoring is begun. After 30 min, the sample of EFM tracing seen in Figure 17A.1 is represen-tative of her tracing.

Questions Case 17A

Which statement best describes the patient's intrapar-tum clinical situation?

A. FHR bradycardia and poor variability
B. FHR tachycardia and good variability
C. Normal FHR and good variability
D. Normal FHR and intermittent late decelerations

Answer: C

The baseline FHR is 120 to 125 bpm, within the normal range, and there is short- and long-term variability. There are no decelerations. This is a completely reassur-ing FHR tracing.

Labor continues for 4 hr and the patient's pelvic ex-amination then shows 6 to 7 cm, 100%, 0 station. Mem-branes are artificially ruptured, a FSE and an intrauter-ine pressure catheter (IUPC) are placed, and after 15 min the patient is given 25 mg of meperidine intrave-nously for pain; 30 min later, the sample of EFM tracing seen in Figure 17A.2 is representative of her tracing. Which statement best describes the patient's intrapar-tum clinical situation?

A. FHR bradycardia and poor variability
B. Normal FHR and poor variability

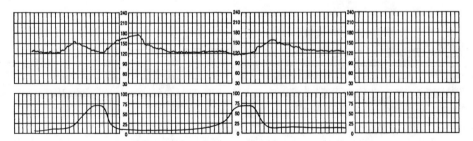

Figure 17A.1

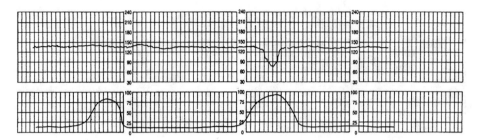

Figure 17A.2

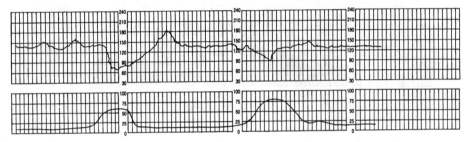

Figure 17A.3

C. Normal FHR, poor variability, and occasional variable decelerations

D. Normal FHR, poor variability, and occasional late decelerations

Answer: B

Apart from being 41 weeks gestational age, there is no further historical information suggesting reasons for fetal distress. The patient's FHR tracing before the intravenous narcotic administration was normal, and the loss of variability after narcotic administration is consistent with narcotic effect. The single variable deceleration may be explained by pressure on the fetal head, which is at 0 station.

Labor continues for 3 hr, and the patient's pelvic examination then shows 9 to 10 cm, 100%, +1 station. A representative sample of her EFM tracing at this time is seen in Figure 17A.3. Which statement best describes the patient's intrapartum clinical situation?

A. FHR tachycardia and poor variability
B. Normal FHR and poor variability
C. Normal FHR, poor variability, and occasional variable decelerations

D. Normal FHR, poor variability, and occasional late decelerations

Answer: D

This is a mixed pattern, with reassuring return of variability now that the narcotic effect is gone, but occasional late decelerations are noted. There is no indication for operative delivery, as vaginal delivery may be expected in the near future in this multipara. Conservative interventions such as oxygen administration are indicated. Because she has had a previous cesarean section, and because of the intermittent late decelerations, close observation is indicated.

Case 17B

Your patient is a 17-year-old G1 at 39 weeks who presents with premature spontaneous rupture of membranes (clear fluid) following an antepartum course remarkable only for an iron deficiency anemia, which responded to hematemic therapy. After waiting 6 hr, you begin a Pitocin (oxytocin) induction of labor. The tracing seen in Figure 17B.1 is representative of her EFM trace 3 hr later when the pelvic examination reveals a cervix dilated to shows 5 cm, 100%, vertex at 0/+1 station with a caput succedaneum, left occiput anterior (LOA), and

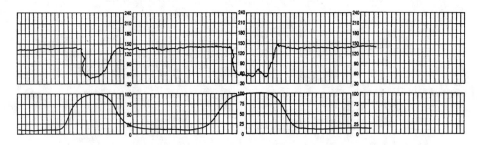

Figure 17A.4

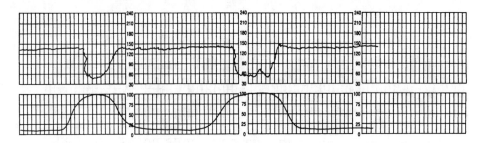

Figure 17B.1

the presence of the FSE and IUPC, which you placed before starting the induction.

Questions Case 17B

Which statement best describes the patient's intrapartum clinical situation?

A. Normal FHR baseline and variability without decelerations
B. Normal FHR baseline and variability with variable decelerations
C. Normal FHR baseline and decreased variability without decelerations
D. Normal FHR baseline and decreased variability with variable decelerations
E. Normal FHR baseline and decreased variability with late decelerations

Answer: D

Although there is a normal FHR, there is poor variability and severe variable decelerations. In a primigravida delivery, this loss of variability is not reassuring and intervention is indicated.

What is your best management now?

A. Continued monitoring, induced labor
B. Continued monitoring labor of labor, but discontinue induction
C. Fetal scalp blood sample

D. Forceps delivery
E. Cesarean birth

Answer: C

Continued labor without further evaluation of fetal wellbeing is inappropriate, as the tracing is not reassuring. Repetitive late decelerations, and especially decreased variability, are associated with fetal compromise. Forceps delivery is impossible as the patient is not fully dilated. A case could be made for cesarean delivery in this patient remote from delivery, but the evidence of fetal compromise would not be sufficient for most obstetricians to proceed with cesarean birth. Fetal scalp sampling would provide more information on which to base a discussion.

A fetal scalp blood sample is performed. The pH is 7.13. The patient is still 5 cm dilated. What is your best management now?

A. Continued monitoring, induced labor
B. Continued monitoring labor, but discontinue induction
C. Fetal scalp blood sample
D. Forceps delivery
E. Cesarean birth

Answer: E

There is now sufficient evidence of fetal compromise to warrant cesarean birth.

chapter 18

POSTPARTUM CARE

The *puerperium* is the 6-week period following birth during which the reproductive tract returns to its normal, nonpregnant state. Many of the physiologic changes of pregnancy have returned to normal within 1 to 2 weeks after delivery, whereas others may take much longer. The initial postpartum examination, traditionally scheduled at the end of this 6-week interval, is now often scheduled sooner. This is because many patients return to full nonpregnant activity in less than 6 weeks.

PHYSIOLOGY OF THE PUERPERIUM

Involution of the Uterus

The *uterus* weighs approximately 1000 g and has a volume of 5000 mL immediately after delivery compared with its nonpregnant weight of approximately 70 g and capacity of 5 mL. Immediately after delivery, the fundus of the uterus is easily palpable halfway between the pubic symphysis and the umbilicus. The immediate reduction in uterine size is a result of delivery of the fetus, placenta, and amniotic fluid as well as the loss of hormonal stimulation. Further uterine involution is caused by autolysis of intracellular myometrial protein, resulting in a decrease in cell size but not cell number. Through these changes, the uterus returns to the pelvis by 2 weeks postpartum and is at its normal size by 6 weeks postpartum. Immediately after birth, uterine hemostasis is maintained by contraction of the smooth muscle of the arterial walls and compression of the vasculature by the uterine musculature.

Lochia

As the myometrial fibers contract, the blood clots from the uterus are expelled and the thrombi in the large vessels of the placental bed undergo organization. Within the first 3 days, the remaining decidua differentiates into a superficial layer, which becomes necrotic and sloughs, and a basal layer adjacent to the myometrium, which contained the fundi of the endometrial glands and is the source of the new endometrium. The uterine discharge (*lochia*), therefore, contains blood as well as the superficial decidual layer, debris, and necrotic remnants of membranes. For the first 2 to 3 days, the lochia is red (*lochia rubra*). As hemostasis is established, the amount of blood in the lochia is reduced with a relative increase in serous secretion, resulting in a brownish color, ultimately becoming serous in appearance (*lochia serosa*) at the end of the 1st week postpartum. At this time, the lochia contains more degenerated decidual material as well as bacteria, resulting in a yellow appearance.

This discharge is fairly heavy at first and rapidly decreases in amount over the first 2 to 3 days postpartum, although it may last for several weeks. In women who breast-feed, the lochia seems to resolve more rapidly, possibly because of a more rapid involution of the uterus caused by uterine contractions associated with breast-feeding. In some patients, there is an increased amount of lochia 1 to 2 weeks after delivery because the eschar that developed over the site of placental attachment has been sloughed. By the end of the 3rd week postpartum, the endometrium is reestablished in most patients.

Cervix and Vagina

Within several hours of delivery, the *cervix* has reformed, and by 1 week, it usually admits only one finger (i.e., it is approximately 1 cm in diameter). The round shape of the nulliparous cervix is usually permanently replaced by a transverse, fish-mouth-shaped external os, the result of laceration during delivery. *Vulvar* and *vaginal tissues* return to normal over the first several days, although the

209

vaginal mucosa will reflect a hypoestrogenic state should the woman breast-feed, as ovarian function is suppressed during breast-feeding. The hymen is now represented by several tags of tissue, the *myrtiform caruncles.*

Return of Ovarian Function

Ovulation can occur as early as 4 to 5 weeks postpartum if the woman chooses not to breast-feed. The mean time to ovulation in nonlactating women is approximately 10 weeks, with 50% of women ovulating by 90 days postpartum (Fig. 18.1). Among breast-feeding women, the time to first ovulation depends on how long the woman breast-feeds. Ovulation is suppressed in the lactating woman in association with elevated prolactin levels. In these patients, prolactin remains elevated for 6 weeks, whereas in nonlactating women, prolactin levels return to normal by 3 weeks postpartum. Estrogen levels fall immediately after delivery in all patients, but begin to rise approximately 2 weeks after delivery if breast-feeding is not undertaken.

Abdominal wall

Return of the elastic fibers of the skin and the stretched rectus muscles to normal configuration occurs slowly and is aided by exercise. The silvery *striae* seen on the skin usually slowly resolve. *Diastasis recti*, separation of the rectus muscles and fascia, usually also resolves over time.

Cardiovascular System

Pregnancy-related cardiovascular changes return to normal 2 to 3 weeks after delivery. Immediately postpartum, plasma volume is reduced by approximately 1000 mL, caused primarily by blood loss at the time of delivery. During the immediate postpartum period, there is also a significant shift of extracellular fluid into the intravascular space. The increased cardiac output seen during pregnancy also persists into the first several hours of the postpartum period. The elevated pulse rate seen during pregnancy persists for approximately 1 hr after delivery but then decreases. These conditions may contribute to decompensation seen in the early postpartum period in patients with heart disease. Immediately after delivery, approximately 5 kg of weight are lost as a result of diuresis and the loss of extravascular fluid. Further weight loss varies in rate and amount from patient to patient.

Hematopoietic System

The leukocytosis seen during labor persists into the early puerperium, thus minimizing the usefulness of identifying early postpartum infection by laboratory evidence of an elevated white cell count. There is some degree of autotransfusion of red cells to the intravascular space after delivery as the uterus contracts.

Renal System

Renal function as evidenced by glomerular filtration rate (GFR) returns to normal within a few weeks postpartum although the GFR remains elevated in the first few days postpartum. Therefore, drugs with renal excretion should be given in decreased doses during this time. There may be considerable edema around the urethra after vaginal delivery resulting in transitory urinary retention.

MANAGEMENT OF THE IMMEDIATE POSTPARTUM PERIOD

Hospital Stay

The amount of time a patient remains in the hospital after delivery continues to decrease. In the past, patients were kept in the hospital for 3 days after the birth of their first child, and 2 days after subsequent deliveries. Postpartum hospital stays for cesarean section patients were routinely 4 to 5 days. The period of hospitalization for all patients has been significantly reduced. Many patients are now routinely discharged 24 hr after vaginal delivery and 72 hr after cesarean section. Figures 18.2 and 18.3 are examples of routine postpartum and postcesarean delivery orders.

Maternal-Infant Bonding

It is recognized that shortly after delivery, the parents become totally engrossed in the events surrounding the newborn infant. Any significant separation of the mother from her infant that reduces activity such as cuddling, fondling, kissing, or gazing at the infant may have a negative impact on the involvement of maternal behaviors on a long-term basis. Contemporary obstetric units have enhanced these interactions by minimizing unnecessary medical interventions while increasing participation by the father and other family members. Rooming-in (mother and newborn are cared for in the same room rather than the newborn taken to a nursery) and an environ-

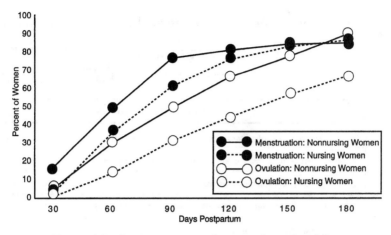

Figure 18.1. Postpartum return of menstruation and ovulation.

ment that facilitates breast-feeding also contribute to this atmosphere. Interaction between the infant and the new parents is also observed by the nursing staff with the resultant ability to identify any problems such as negative or even abusive actions toward the newborn.

Uterine Complications

The likelihood of serious *postpartum complications* is greatest immediately after delivery. Significant hemorrhage occurs in approximately 1% of patients (see Chapter 19); infection is seen in approximately 5% of patients. Immediately after the delivery of the placenta, the uterus is palpated bimanually to ascertain that it is firm. Uterine palpation through the abdominal wall is repeated at frequent intervals during the immediate postpartum period to prevent and/or identify uterine atony. Perineal pads are applied, and the amount of blood on these pads as well as pulse and pressure are monitored closely for the first several hours after delivery to identify excessive blood loss.

Analgesia

Postpartum analgesia is primarily indicated for perineal discomfort resulting from lacerations, episiotomy, and hemorrhoids or for postoperative pain from cesarean delivery or postpartum tubal ligation. Patients may also require pain medication for "afterbirth pains," the painful uterine contractions following delivery. This degree of discomfort from postpartum uterine contractions is seen more prominently in breast-feeding women because of the increased release of oxytocin during

suckling. Common medications for this include acetaminophen, aspirin, and nonsteroidal anti-inflammatory drugs.

Breast Care

Breast engorgement in women who are not breast-feeding typically occurs 3 days postpartum and may be treated with techniques such as breast binders, ice packs, and avoidance of nipple stimulation. *Bromocriptine* (Parlodel), a dopamine receptor agonist that acts to suppress prolactin release by the anterior pituitary, was previously used for lactation suppression, but is no longer recommended. Oral analgesics, such as codeine, are also useful adjuncts.

Occasionally, the breast-feeding mother may develop a *postpartum mastitis* manifest by high fever and usually chills, pain, and localized erythema and firmness of the breast. This is usually caused by *Staphylococcus aureus* arising from the nursing infant's throat and nose and transmitted during nursing. Treatment includes penicillin G or a penicillinase-resistant drug such as dicloxacillin for penicillinase-reducing strains. For patients who are allergic to penicillin, erythromycin would be an appropriate alternative. Nursing from the affected side may be continued without danger to the infant. If an abscess develops, surgical drainage of the abscess in addition to antibiotic therapy is necessary.

Immunizations

Women who do not have antirubella antibody should be immunized for *rubella* during the im-

NAME AND UNIT NUMBER	ADMISSION NUMBER	NURSING STATION	WOMEN'S HOSPITAL/PERINATAL CENTER
	ROOM OR BED NUMBER		OBSTETRIC SERVICE
	DATE		**THE MED** REGIONAL MEDICAL CENTER AT MEMPHIS

DATE	HOUR	ROUTINE POSTPARTUM ORDERS
		These orders do NOT apply to postoperative, diabetic, hypertensive or preeclamptic-eclamptic patients.
		1. Patients with caudal, spinal or epidural must be able to move legs before leaving recovery room.
		2. BP, P fundal check and blood loss assessment q 15 min x 4, 1 h x 2; oral temperature qid for 48 hours,
		then 6 A.M. only (unless febrile > 100.4); notify physician if pulse > 110; systolic BP > 150 or
		< 90 distolic BP > 100; temp. > 100.4.
		3. Continue IV at 125-150 ml q h until discontinued.
		4. NPO until stable and normal observations for 1 h, then discontinue IV and place on regular diet.
		5. UP ad lib, unless spinal, epidural or saddle block must be able to move extremities and regain sensation
		in legs before getting out of bed.
		6. Encourage daily shower.
		7. If unable to void within 4-6 hours and bladder distended, catherize with #18 Foley; if volume > 500
		ml or necessary to catherize second time, leave Foley in place 24 hours; specimen to lab for C & S
		when catheter removed.
		8. Routine perineal and breast care daily; encourage use of supportive bra.
		9. Acetaminophen #3 p.o. q 3-4 h PRN pain; notify physician if pain relief inadequate.
		10 Promethazine 25 mg IM q 4 PRN nausea; notify physician if second dose is required.
		11. Dalmane 30 mg p.o. HS PRN
		12. Dioctyl sodium sulfosuccinate 100 mg p.o. tid.
		13. Bisacodyl USP suppository PRN the p.m. of the second postpartum day if no bowel movement since
		delivery.
		14. Hct in A.M. day after delivery. Notify physician if < 30%, UA.
		15. If mother D neg., Du neg.; check ABO, Rh and Coombs of baby and record on maternal chart.
		16. Type and crossmatch for anti-D immune globulin if appropriate after laboratory evaluation.
		17. Rooming in if desired.

PHYSICIAN'S ORDERS

Figure 18.2. Routine postpartum orders.

**POST CESAREAN SECTION
PHYSICIAN'S ORDERS**

DATE	HOUR	These orders do not apply to other postoperative, diabetic, hypertensive or preeclamptic-eclamptic patients.
		1. Patients with caudal, spinal or epidural must be able to move legs before leaving recovery room.
		2. BP, P, fundal check and blood loss assessment q 15 min x 4, q 1 h x 4, then per shift; notify physician if pulse >110; systolic BP >150 or <90, diastolic BP >100.
		3. Clear liquid diet, bedrest.
		4. Turn, cough and deep breath q 2 h x 6.
		5. Temp qid; notify if <100.4.
		6. #18 Foley catheter to dependent drainage.
		7. I&O q 4 h until Foley catheter removed; notify physician if output <100 ml in any 4 h interval.
		8. Each IV to run at 125-150 ml/h; do not exceed 250 ml in any hour.
		#1 1000 cc D5LR with 10 IU oxytocin added.
		#2 1000 cc D5 1/4NS with 10 IU oxytocin added.
		#3 1000 cc D5 1/4NS with 10 IU oxytocin added.
		#4 1000 cc D5 1/4NS at 50 cc/h to keep vein open until physician discontinues.
		9. Morphine sulfate 10 mg IM q 3-4 h, PRN pain, notify physician if pain relief inadequate; acetaminophen #3 p.o. 3-4 h PRN for mild discomfort after oral intake resumed or acetaminophen 600 mgm p.o. q 3-4 h PRN for pain.
		10. Promethazine 25 mg. IM q 4-6 h PRN nausea, notify physician if second dose is required.
		11. Encourage use of supportive bra.
		12. Bisacodyl USP suppository PRN; PRN Fleet's enema if no results from suppository.
		13. Dioctyl Sodium Sulfocuccinate 100 mgm p.o. tid when oral intake resumes.
		14. Antacid 30 cc p.o. PRN.
		15. Witchazel wipes PRN for Pericare.
		16. Dalmane 30 mg. p.o. HS PRN.
		17. Hct in a.m.
		18. If mother D Neg., check ABO, RH and Coombs' on baby and record on maternal chart.
		19. Type and crossmatch for anti-D immune globulin if appropriate after laboratory evaluation.
		20. Rooming-in if desired.

Signature _____   Form No. 6091.001 (Rev. 7/84)

Figure 18.3. Routine postcesarean delivery orders.

mediate postpartum period. Breast-feeding is not a contraindication to this immunization. In some locations, a *tetanus toxoid booster* injection is also given at this time if needed. If the woman is D–, is not isoimmunized, and has given birth to a D+ infant, 300 μg of anti-D immune globulin (Rho GAM) should be administered before discharge. If the mother is *hepatitis* HbsAg+, the newborn must be immunized before discharge.

Bowel Movement and Urination

It is common for a patient not to have a *bowel movement* for the first 1 to 2 days after delivery, as patients have often not eaten for a long period of time. Stool softener (e.g., Colace, 100 mg p.o. b.i.d., or Peri-Colace, 100 mg p.o. b.i.d.) is routinely prescribed in many institutions, especially if the patient has had a fourth-degree episiotomy repair or a laceration involving the rectal mucosa. Periurethral edema after vaginal delivery may cause *transitory urinary retention*. Patients should be monitored for urination after delivery, and if catheterization is required more than twice in the first 24 hr, placement of an indwelling catheter for 1 to 2 days is advisable as well as prophylactic administration of an antibiotic such as ampicillin.

Care of the Perineum

Perineal pain is minimized using oral analgesics, the application of an ice bag to minimize swelling, and/or a local anesthetic spray. Severe perineal pain unresponsive to the usual analgesics may signify the development of a hematoma, which will require evacuation if it continues to grow in size or becomes infected. *Infection of the episiotomy* is rare (<0.1%) and usually is limited to the skin and responsive to broad-spectrum antibiotics. *Necrotizing fascitis* is a rare but extremely serious infection requiring extensive resection and debridement of the perineum, cardiovascular support, and broad-spectrum antibiotic therapy. *Dehiscence*, like infection, is uncommon with repair individualized on the basis of the nature and extent of the wound.

Contraception

Postpartum care in the hospital should always include discussion of *contraception*. As Figure 18.1 demonstrates, approximately 15% of nonnursing women are fertile at 6 weeks postpartum. All forms of contraception should be considered. Oral contraceptives are not contraindicated by breast-feeding. Once lactation is established, neither the volume nor the composition of breast milk is adversely affected by the administration of oral contraceptives (see Chapter 22).

Postpartum sterilization by tubal ligation is a popular method of permanent contraception, but generally the decision for this procedure should be made during the antepartum period and well documented in the chart. Then, if after delivery the patient still wishes sterilization, it may be performed without concern about the decision process (see Chapter 23).

Sexual Activity

Coitus may be resumed when the patient is comfortable. She should be counseled, especially if breast-feeding, that coitus may initially be uncomfortable because of a lack of lubrication and that the use of exogenous, water-soluble lubrication is helpful. The female superior position may be recommended, as the woman is thereby able to control the depth of penile penetration. The lactating patient may also be counseled to use topical estrogen to the vaginal mucosa to minimize the dyspareunia caused by coital trauma to the hypoestrogenic tissue.

Patient Education

Patient education at the time of discharge should not be solely focused on postpartum and contraceptive issues. This is a good opportunity to reinforce the value and need for preventive health care and health care maintenance for both mother and infant. This should include a review of follow-up that has been arranged for the newborn infant and frequency and scope of health care for the new mother. Previously identified high-risk behaviors such as alcohol, tobacco, and drug abuse should once again be addressed. Infant safety concerns, e.g., automobile child restraints, are also appropriate topics of discussion. Postpartum follow-up of any preexisting medical conditions should also be reviewed.

Lactation and Breast-Feeding

An increasing belief in the advantages of breast-feeding has led many physicians to recommend this form of infant nutrition. As a result, more patients breast-feed and do so for a longer period of time. Benefits of breast-feeding include increased convenience for some mothers, decreased cost, improved infant nutrition for a variable period of time, and some protection against infection and allergic reaction. Successful breast-feeding depends on several factors, particularly the motivation of the mother and her ability to include breast-feeding in her daily activities. For some women, breast-feeding may be impossible, even if desired, because of restrictions on time caused by work. *Support by family and health care providers for the decision that best fits the total needs of the mother and baby is very important.* If breast-feeding is chosen, rooming-in during the hospital stay allows the mother to begin the process in a less pressured setting while allowing the hospital staff to provide helpful recommendations and support. *The decision to breast-feed or bottle feed is best made before delivery and is facilitated by balanced discussion during the antepartum visits.*

At the time of delivery, the drop of estrogen and other placental hormones is a major factor in removing the inhibition of the action of prolactin. Also, suckling by the infant stimulates release of oxytocin from the neurohypophysis. The increased levels of oxytocin in the blood result in contraction of the myoepithelial cells and emptying of the alveolar lumen of the breast. Prolactin release is also stimulated by suckling with resultant secretion of fatty acids, lactose, and casein. Postpartum, *colostrum* is produced in the first 5 days postpartum, slowly being replaced by maternal milk. Colostrum contains more minerals and protein but less fat and sugar than maternal milk, although it does contain large fat globules, the so-called colostrum corpuscles, which are probably epithelial cells that have undergone fatty degeneration. Colostrum also contains immunoglobulin A, which may offer the newborn some protection from enteric pathogens. Subsequently, on approximately the 3rd to 6th day postpartum, milk is produced.

For milk to be produced on an ongoing basis, there must be adequate insulin, cortisol, thyroid hormone, and adequate nutrients and fluids in the diet. Nutrients and fluids are especially important, as maternal fat stores deposited during pregnancy provide only one-third of the fat and calories needed to produce 850 mL of milk each day. The remainder must be supplied by an appropriate diet and fluid intake. All vitamins except K are found in human milk, but as they are present in varying amounts, maternal vitamin supplementation is recommended. Vitamin K may be administered to the infant to prevent hemorrhagic disease of the newborn. To maintain breast-feeding, the alveolar lumen must be emptied on a regular basis (Fig. 18.4).

Nipple care is also important during breast-feeding. The nipples should be washed with water and exposed to the air for 15 to 20 min after each feeding. A water-based cream such as lanolin or vitamin A and D ointment may be applied if the nipples are tender.

Engorgement, mastitis, and plugged duct (galactocele) are the three causes of enlarged tender breast postpartum. They may be differentiated according to their signs and symptoms, presented in Table 18.1. Engorgement is treated by continued nursing or expression of milk by breast pump as well as application of heat and oral analgesics. Mastitis is associated with infection by *S. aureus*, β-*hemolytic streptocci, and Haemophilus influenza* and is treated with antibiotics (dicloxacillin, 500 mg p.o. q.i.d.) for at least 1 week. Nursing may be continued during treatment. A plugged duct is treated with warm packs and a breast pump. Rarely, incision and drainage may be required.

Drugs in the breast milk is a common concern for the breast-feeding mother. Less than 1% of the total dosage of any medication is seen in breast milk. This should be considered when any medication is prescribed by a physician or when any over-the-counter medications are contemplated by the patient (Table 18.2). Specific medications that would contraindicate breast-feeding include lithium carbonate, tetracycline, bromocriptine, methotrexate, and any radioactive substance as well as all substances of abuse such as amphetamine, cocaine, heroin, marijuana, nicotine, and phencyclidine (PCP).

ANXIETY, DEPRESSION, AND THE POSTPARTUM PERIOD

Although pregnancy and childbirth are usually joyous times, for some patients the experience is followed by significant emotional distress. Identification of specific risk factors for postpartum and antepartum anxiety and depression is an important first step in identifying and dealing with these problems. Of patients with previous postpartum mental disease, approximately 25% will have a recurrence after their next pregnancy. One-third of patients with psychiatric illness during the postpartum period have a history of psychiatric disease. The exact cause of most of the postpartum emotional changes is unknown, although suggested etiologies include changing hormone levels

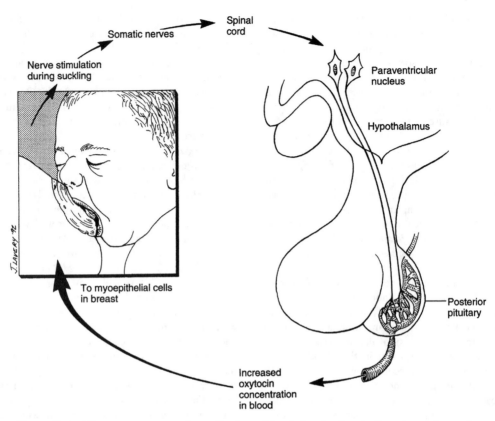

Figure 18.4. The somatosensory pathways for the suckling-induced reduced reflex release of oxytocin.

Table 18.1.
Differential Diagnosis of Enlarged Tender Breast Postpartum

Finding	Engorgement	Mastitis	Plugged Duct
Start	Gradual	Sudden	Gradual
Location	Bilateral	Unilateral	Unilateral
Swelling	Generalized	Localized	Localized
Pain	Generalized	Intense, localized	Localized
Systemic symptoms	Feels well	Feels ill	Feels well
Fever	No	Yes	No

(as is seen with premenstrual changes), difficulty adjusting to a new lifestyle, and the stresses of parenthood.

There is a wide spectrum of response to pregnancy and delivery, ranging from mild depression ("postpartum blues," which occurs in more than 50% of the deliveries, typically occurring on postpartum day 2 or 3 and subsiding within 1 to 2 weeks) to postpartum depression (approximately 10% of women) to the extreme response of intense depression with suicidal ideation (occurring in approximately 1 in 2000 deliveries). The overall incidence of depression during the postpartum period appears not to be significantly greater than at other times. Early symptoms of depression include sleeplessness, loss of self-esteem, irritability, and mood swings. More serious symptoms include anorexia, obsessive behavior, panic, and delusions. A

Table 18.2.
Medications and Breast-feeding

Medication or Substance	Reason for Concern/Effect on Lactation
Contraindicated during Breast-feeding	
Bromocriptine (Parlodel)	Supresses lactaton
Cyclophosphamide (Cytoxan)	Possible immune suppression; neutropenia; unknown effect on growth
Cyclosporine	Possible immune suppression; unknown effect on growth
Doxorubicin (Adriamycin)	Concentrated in milk; possible immune suppression; unknown effect on growth
Ergotamine (Ergotrate)	In dosages for migraine, emesis, diarrhea, convulsions
Lithium	50% therapeutic level in infant
Methotrexate	Possible immune suppression; unknown effect on growth
Substances of abuse (amphetamines, cocaine, heroin, marijuana, nicotine, and phencyclidine)	Growth retardation; neurologic damage; obstetric accidents
Uncertain Effects but of Concern when Breast-feeding	
Antianxiety medications, antidepressants, and antipsychotics	No reported effects, but may be of special concern because of primary drug effect when given to nursing mothers for long periods of time
Chloraphenicol	Idiosyncratic bone marrow suppressions
Metoclopramide (Reglan)	Concentrated in milk; dopaminergic blockade
Metronidazole (Flagyl)	In vitro mutagen; consideration to discontinuing breast-feeding for 12–14 hr to allow secretion of single-dose regimens

most disturbing symptom is the patient's estrangement from the newborn.

Both internal and external forces may result in postpartum psychiatric illness. A patient who does not cope well with stress is particularly susceptible to such potentially traumatic stimuli as previous infertility, complications of the antepartum, intrapartum, or postpartum course or conflicts in the roles of mother and wife. A supportive spouse and family can minimize the severity of any symptom complex.

Anxiety is very common during the antepartum and intrapartum periods, but can be minimized by having the patient as an active participant in the planning of and carrying out of the birthing process plan. Prepared childbirth and the rational use of minimal anesthesia at the patient's discretion may help the patient feel a sense of control. Active involvement of nursing personnel in the identification of significant anxiety and depression is also critical, because they observe the patient on a more ongoing basis than do physicians.

Treatment must be tailored to the patient's individual situation, with the vast majority of mild postpartum depression being managed by the attending physician in conjunction with the support

of hospital staff such as nursing personnel and social workers. The mother who is fearful of, or is adverse to, contact with the newborn should not be forced into contact. Both psychotherapy and medication such as antidepressants or lithium carbonate may be provided, usually in consultation with a clinical psychologist or psychiatrist. If conditions worsen despite outpatient efforts, inpatient therapy is warranted.

Whether during the antepartum, intrapartum, or postpartum period, depression and anxiety should be viewed as significant problems. It should be noted, however, that they are not necessarily solely related to pregnancy or its complications. Specifically, women are clinically depressed twice as frequently as men. Anxiety accompanies depression in three-fourths of cases. The earliest clinical clue to the diagnosis of depression may be in inability to experience pleasure or happiness (anhedonia). Women particularly susceptible to depression are those with young children, those who are living in poverty, those who are abused, and those who have professional careers.

There appears to be some evidence that there is a hereditary factor that predisposes some pa-

anxiety

tients to developing anxiety disorders. This may occur in as many as 10 to 15% of the population. Because every patient is subjected to some degree of stress, anxiety is generally seen in all patients, resulting in some shifts in mood as part of the normal life experience. As with depression, however, anxiety can become dysfunctional, with the patient seeing the world as a hostile or unsafe environment. Nonspecific nervousness, panic, irritability, and fear of losing control suggest significant anxiety disorder requiring treatment.

THE POSTPARTUM VISIT

At the time of the first postpartum visit, inquiries should be made into the following: status of breast-feeding, return of menstruation, resumption of coital activity, use of contraception, interaction of the newborn with the family, and resumption of other physical activities such as return to work. Involutional changes will have occurred in most instances. Inflammatory changes because of the healing of the cervix may result in minor atypia on a Pap smear performed at this time. Unless there is a past history of significant cervical dysplasia, repeating the Pap smear in 3 months is appropriate.

CASE STUDIES

Case 18A

A 24-year-old married woman has just delivered her first child, a healthy boy weighing 7 lb. Her antepartum and intrapartum courses were unremarkable. On the 1st day postpartum, she is noted to cry easily and to have slept poorly.

Question Case 18A

Which of the following are appropriate management steps at this time?

A. Reassure the patient that everything is okay and that feeling sad after a delivery is normal.
B. Ask the patient why she is crying.
C. Ask the nursing staff to ask the patient why she is crying.
D. Ask a psychiatrist to evaluate the patient's apparent sadness.
E. Ask a social worker to evaluate the patient's apparent sadness.

Answer: A, B, C

Discussion: Reassuring the patient is not inappropriate as a general measure, but it must be combined with some assessment of the apparent sadness. In general, this is best done at this level of distress by the physician or nursing staff; consultation to psychiatry or social services is generally not indicated.

Case 18B

A 23-year-old G1 delivers a healthy term boy by normal vaginal delivery after an unremarkable antepartum course and spontaneous labor. She decides to breast-feed, which is begun satisfactorily during her stay in the hospital. She and her new son are well at the time of discharge. Three days later she calls complaining of the worst pain she has ever had in her breasts.

Questions Case 18B

When you return her call, which of the following questions are most important?

A. Where does it hurt? One breast or both? Where on the breasts?
B. How do you feel in general?
C. Do you have a fever?
D. How is the breast feeding going? Is the baby eating well? Regularly?

Answer: All

Upon questioning, you learn that the pain is in the left side of her left breast, which is tender and swollen but does not feel especially warm to touch. Her temperature is 99°F and she feels generally well except for the pain. The most likely diagnosis is

A. Breast engorgement
B. Mastitis
C. Blocked duct

Answer: C

Appropriate initial management includes

A. Incision and drainage
B. Antibiotic therapy
C. Warm packs
D. Analgesics

Answer: C, D

chapter 19

POSTPARTUM HEMORRHAGE

Excessive bleeding in the minutes and hours following delivery is a serious and potentially fatal complication. Hemorrhage can be sudden and profuse, or blood loss can occur more slowly but be prolonged and persistent. Traditionally, postpartum hemorrhage is defined as a blood loss in excess of 500 mL of blood associated with delivery. Many patients lose considerably more blood than this and the figure of 500 mL may actually represent the average amount of blood loss after vaginal delivery, with twice this amount lost at cesarean delivery. This chapter discusses the causes of postpartum hemorrhage followed by a general approach to the patient who bleeds excessively after giving birth.

MAJOR CAUSES OF POSTPARTUM HEMORRHAGE

Uterine Atony

Uterine atony is by far the most common cause of postpartum hemorrhage. Ordinarily, the uterine corpus (or body) contracts promptly after delivery of the placenta, constricting the spiral arteries in the newly created placental bed and preventing excessive bleeding from them. This muscular contraction, rather than coagulation, prevents excessive bleeding from the placental implantation site. When contraction does not occur as expected, the resulting uterine atony gives rise to postpartum hemorrhage.

A number of *factors predispose to uterine atony* (Table 19.1). These include conditions in which there is extraordinary enlargement of the uterus, such as hydramnios or twins; abnormal labor (both precipitous, prolonged or augmented by oxytocin); and conditions that interfere with contraction of the uterus, such as uterine leiomyomas or use of magnesium sulfate. The clinical diagnosis of atony is based largely on the tone of the uterine muscle on palpation. Instead of the normally firm, contracted uterine corpus, a softer, more pliable — often called "boggy" — uterus is found. The cervix is usually open. Frequently, the uterus will contract briefly when massaged, only to become more relaxed when the manipulation ceases.

Management of uterine atony is both preventive and therapeutic. In the management of a normal delivery, it is customary to infuse oxytocin diluted in intravenous fluids (usually 20 units in 1 liter of fluid run at 125 to 165 mL/hr) starting soon after the placenta has been delivered. Oxytocin promotes contraction of the uterine corpus and decreases the likelihood of uterine atony. It is given in dilute solution because the intravenous administration of undiluted oxytocin can cause significant hypotension.

Once uterine atony occurs and is diagnosed, management can be categorized as manipulative, medical, and surgical. *Uterine massage* alone is often successful in causing uterine contraction and this should be done while preparations for other treatments are under way (Fig. 19.1). Another manipulation, which is rarely used nowadays, is packing of the uterine cavity with gauze, which serves as a temporizing measure while awaiting definitive therapy. Medical treatments include oxytocin, *Methergine* (methylergonovine maleate), and several prostaglandin preparations, administered separately or in combination. Methergine is a potent constrictor that can cause uterine contractions within several minutes. It is always given intramuscularly, since rapid intravenous administration can lead to dangerous hypertension. Prostaglandin $F_2\alpha$ may be given intramuscularly or directly into the myometrium, and prostaglandin E_2 may be given by vaginal suppository. Both result in very strong uterine contractions. Typically, oxytocin is given prophylactically as noted above; if uterine atony occurs, the infusion rate is increased, and in addition, Methergine, prostaglandin, or both are given sequentially.

Occasionally, uterine massage and oxytocics are unsuccessful in bringing about appropriate uterine

Table 19.1.
Factors Predisposing to Uterine Atony

Precipitous labor	Multiparity
General anesthesia	Oxytocin use in labor
Prolonged labor	History of postpartum
Uterine leiomyomas	hemorrhage
Macrosomia	Amniotic fluid embolus
Hydramnios	Magnesium sulfate in laboring
Twins	patient
Amnioitis (sepsis)	

contraction, and surgical measures must be utilized. Surgical management of uterine atony may include ligation of the uterine arteries or hypogastric arteries, selective arterial embolization, and hysterectomy (Fig. 19.2). At times, these procedures may be lifesaving. Management must be individualized in cases of severe uterine atony, taking into account the degree of hemorrhage, the overall status of the patient, and her future childbearing desires (Table 19.2). When hemorrhage occurs, large-bore intravenous access should be obtained, and blood should be typed and cross-matched for possible transfusion.

Lacerations of the Lower Genital Tract

Lacerations of the lower genital tract are far less common than uterine atony as a cause of postpartum hemorrhage, but they can be serious and require prompt surgical repair. *Predisposing factors* include an instrumented delivery with forceps, a manipulative delivery such as a breech extraction, a precipitous labor, and a macrosomic infant.

Although minor lacerations to the cervix in the process of cervical dilation and delivery are routinely found, lacerations of greater than 2 cm in length and those that are actively bleeding generally require repair. To minimize blood loss caused by significant cervical and vaginal lacerations, all patients with any predisposing factors or any patient in whom blood loss soon after delivery appears to be excessive despite a firm and contracted uterus, should have a careful repeat inspection of the lower genital tract. This examination may require assistance to allow adequate visualization. As a rule, repair of these lacerations is usually not difficult if adequate exposure is provided. Occasionally, however, extensive repair is required, necessitating general anesthesia (Fig. 19.3).

Retained Placenta

Separation of the placenta from the uterus occurs because of cleavage between the *zona basalis* and the *zona spongiosa*. Once separation occurs, expulsion is caused by strong uterine contractions. Retained placenta can occur when either the process of separation or the process of expulsion is incomplete. Predisposing factors to retained placenta include a previous cesarean delivery, uterine leiomyomas, prior uterine curettage, and succenturiate placental lobe.

Placental tissue remaining within the uterus can prevent adequate contractions and predispose to excessive bleeding. After expulsion, every placenta should be inspected to detect missing cotyledons, which may remain in the uterus. If retained placenta is suspected, either because of apparent absent cotyledons or because of excessive bleeding, it can often be removed by inserting two fingers through the cervix into the uterus and manipulating the retained tissue downward into the vagina. If this is unsuccessful or if there is uncertainty regarding the cause of hemorrhage, an ultrasound examination of the uterus is very helpful. A firmly contracted uterus exhibits a characteristic "stripe" on ultrasound imaging, representing the newly contracted endometrial cavity. Absence of such a stripe implies placental tissue and/or blood clots remaining within the uterine cavity. Curettage with a suction apparatus and/or a large sharp curet may remove the retained tissue. Care must be exercised to avoid perforation through the uterine fundus.

Placental tissue may also remain in the uterus because separation of the placenta from the uterus may not occur normally. At times, placental villi penetrate the uterine wall to form what is generally called *placenta accreta*. More specifically, abnormal adherence of the placenta to the superficial lining of the uterus is termed placenta accreta, penetration into the uterine muscle itself is called *placenta increta*, and complete invasion through the thickness of the uterine muscle is termed *placenta percreta*. If this abnormal attachment involves the entire placenta, no part of the placenta separates. Much more commonly, however, attachment is not complete and a portion of the placenta separates while the remainder remains attached. Major life-threatening hemorrhage can ensue. Hysterectomy is often required, although in a woman who desires more children, an attempt to separate the placenta by curettage, or other means of controlling the bleeding, is usually appropriate in trying to avoid a hysterectomy.

Table 19.2.
Management of the Patient with Postpartum Hemorrhage

Evaluate promptly once excessive bleeding is detected.	Visualize cervix and vagina in search of lacerations. Repair if present.
Review clinical course for probable cause. Any difficulty removing placenta? Were forceps used? Other predisposing factors?	Remember that postpartum hemorrhage may be from multiple causes, e.g., atony plus lacerations.
Perform bimanual examination in recovery area/ delivery room. Uterus boggy? Massage. Initiate or increase oxytocin; give Methergine, 0.2 mg i.m. Placental fragments within uterus on exploration or on ultrasound examination? If so, return to delivery room for curettage. Laceration or hematoma? Repair in delivery room.	Observe patient constantly. Repeated bimanual examination. If bleeding persists, is the blood clotting? If not, consider DIC.
	Inform patient of the problem and what measures are being taken to correct it. Get an appreciation of her desires regarding further childbearing and hysterectomy.
Monitor and maintain circulation. Large-bore intravenous catheters: 1 or 2 well-functioning lines. Type and cross-match blood. Check hematocrit and coagulation profile with platelet count for baseline.	Preoperative management options Uterine packing Prostaglandin administration
	Operative measures Ligation of vessels Hypogastric artery ligation Uterine artery ligation Selective arterial embolization Hysterectomy is treatment of last resort in patient who wants to retain her uterus
Notify obstetric physicians, nurses, and anesthesia and operating room personnel of potential need for surgical intervention.	Intensive care measures Hemodynamic, renal, and coagulation surveillance measures

OTHER CAUSES OF POSTPARTUM HEMORRHAGE

Hematomas

Hematomas can occur anywhere from the vulva to the upper vagina as a result of delivery trauma. The frequency of hematoma formation is higher for the vulva and lower vagina than the upper vagina, while, conversely, the morbidity is higher with hematomas in the less accessible upper vagina. Hematomas may also develop at the site of episiotomy or perineal laceration. Hematomas may occur without disruption of the vaginal mucosa, when the fetus or forceps cause shearing of the submucosal tissues without mucosal tearing.

Vulvar or vaginal hematomas are characterized by exquisite pain with or without signs of shock. Hematomas that are less than 5 cm in diameter and are not enlarging can usually be managed expectantly by frequent evaluation of the size of the hematoma and close monitoring of vital signs and urinary output. Application of ice packs can also be helpful. Larger and enlarging hematomas must be managed surgically. If the hematoma is at the site of episiotomy, the sutures should be removed and a search made for the actual bleeding site, which is then ligated. If not at the episiotomy site, the hematoma should be opened at its most dependent portion, the hematoma drained, the bleeding site identified, if possible, and the site closed with interlocking-hemostatic sutures. Drains and vaginal packs are often used to prevent reaccumulation of blood.

Coagulation Defects

Virtually any congenital or acquired abnormality in blood clotting can lead to postpartum hemorrhage. Abruptio placentae, amniotic fluid embolism, and severe preeclampsia are obstetric conditions commonly associated with disseminated intravascular coagulopathy (DIC). The treatment of coagulation defects is aimed at correcting the coagulation defect. When assessing a patient with postpartum hemorrhage, it should always be noted whether or not the blood that is passing from the genital tract is clotting. It also should be recalled that profuse hemorrhage itself can lead to coagulopathy.

Amniotic Fluid Embolism

Amniotic fluid embolism is a rare, sudden, and often fatal obstetric complication caused by entry of

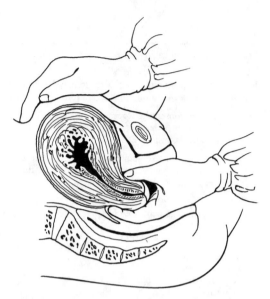

Figure 19.1. Management of uterine atony with manual massage. One hand gently massages the uterus from the abdomen while the other is inserted so that the cervix is cradled in the fingers and thumb to allow maximal compression and massage.

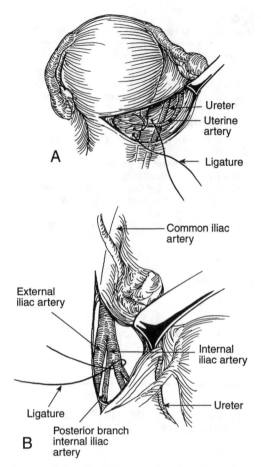

Figure 19.2. Surgical treatment of atonic uterine hemorrhage. **A,** Ligation of the uterine artery. The artery crosses over the ureter and is ligated beyond this point at the uterine corpus. **B,** Hypogastric artery ligation. Ligation of the anterior division of the internal iliac artery is performed after careful identification and retraction of the ureter, which usually overlies the bifurcation of the iliac artery into the external and internal iliac branches.

amniotic fluid into the maternal circulation. The condition results in severe cardiorespiratory collapse and usually a coagulopathy. Treatment is directed toward total support of the cardiovascular and coagulation systems.

Uterine Inversion

Uterine inversion is a rare condition; the uterus literally turns inside out, with the top of the uterine fundus extending through the cervix into the vagina and sometimes even past the introitus. Hemorrhage with uterine inversion is characteristically severe and sudden. Treatment includes administration of an anesthetic that causes uterine relaxation (such as halothane) or other agent with uterus-relaxing properties (such as terbutaline), followed by replacement of the uterine corpus. If this fails, surgical treatment, possibly including hysterectomy, may be needed (Fig. 19.4).

GENERAL MANAGEMENT OF PATIENTS WITH POSTPARTUM HEMORRHAGE

Once excessive blood loss is identified, prompt assessment is mandatory. A general approach to management is outlined in Table 19.2. Because the

vast majority of cases of postpartum hemorrhage are caused by uterine atony, the uterus should be palpated abdominally, seeking the soft, boggy consistency of the relaxed uterus. If found, oxytocin infusion should be increased and either Methergine or prostaglandins given if the excessive bleeding continues.

Other questions will help direct assessment:

Was expulsion of the placenta spontaneous and apparently complete?

Were forceps or other instrumentation used in delivery?

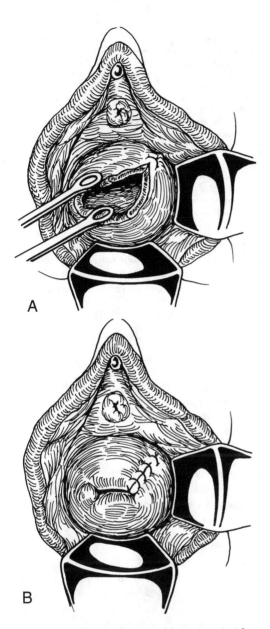

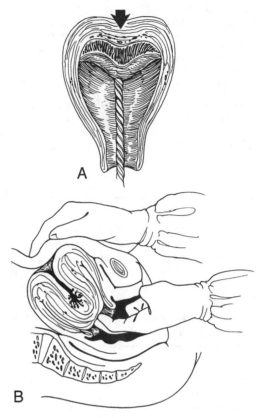

Figure 19.4. Uterine inversion. **A,** Uterine inversion occurring with fundally implanted placenta. **B,** Manual replacement of a partially inverted uterus.

Figure 19.3. Repair of a cervical laceration. **A,** After careful demonstration of the entire extent of the laceration, the first suture is placed above the apex of the laceration to prevent extension after the repair. **B,** The laceration is then repaired, whether with interrupted sutures, as shown, or with figure-of-eight or running sutures.

Was the baby large or the delivery difficult or precipitous?

Were the cervix and vagina inspected for lacerations?

Is the blood clotting?

As the cause of the hemorrhage is being identified, general supportive measures for patients with hemorrhage of any cause are initiated. Large-bore intravenous access; crystalloid infusions; type, cross-match, and administration of blood or blood components as needed; periodic assessment of hematocrit and coagulation profile; and monitoring of urinary output are all important.

The management of postpartum hemorrhage is greatly facilitated if patients at high risk are identified and preliminary preparations made before the bleeding episode. Table 19.3 reviews such precautionary measures.

CASE STUDIES

Case 19A

A 25-year-old G1 P0 has labor induced at 42 weeks gestational age. Her induction is prolonged but finally

Table 19.3.
Precautionary Measures to Prevent or Minimize Postpartum Hemorrhage

Before delivery	In delivery room
Identify any predisposing factors	Avoid excessive traction on umbilical cord
Determine baseline hematocrit	Inspect placenta for complete removal
Send blood specimen to blood bank for group and	Perform digital exploration of uterus
screen	Massage uterus
Establish well-functioning intravenous line with	Visualize cervix and vagina
large-bore catheter	Remove all clots in uterus and vagina before
Obtain baseline coagulation studies and platelet	transfer to recovery area
count if indicated	
	In recovery area
	Closely observe patient for excessive bleeding
	Frequently palpate uterus with massage
	Determine vital signs frequently

results in a forceps-assisted delivery of a healthy 9.5-lb boy. The placenta is expelled 9 min after delivery and appears to be intact. Inspection of the vagina and cervix reveals no lesions except the midline episiotomy. Intravenous oxytocin is begun in dilute solution at the time of placental delivery. During the repair of the midline episiotomy, excessive vaginal bleeding is noted. The patient is becoming tachycardic but her blood pressure is consistent with her intrapartum blood pressures.

Questions Case 19A

Which of the following causes of postpartum hemorrhage may be excluded from consideration at this time based on the information provided?

A. Coagulation defect
B. Uterine atony
C. Retained placental tissue
D. Vaginal laceration
E. None of the above

Answer: E

None can be excluded. Lacerations are sometimes missed on inspection, and placental tissue may be left behind with a placenta that appears to be intact.

Based on the information provided, which of the following is the most likely cause of this patient's postpartum hemorrhage?

A. Coagulation defect
B. Uterine atony
C. Retained placental tissue
D. Vaginal laceration
E. None of the above

Answer: B

Uterine atony is likely in this clinical situation, which includes prolonged pregnancy, Pitocin induction, pro-

longed labor, difficult delivery, and large infant. However, forceps delivery of a large baby is associated with lacerations of cervix and vagina, which are sometimes difficult to recognize without careful, complete inspection.

Your initial management should include

A. Careful but rapid reexamination for lacerations
B. Administration of oxytocin
C. Administration of prostaglandin
D. Uterine artery ligation
E. Hysterectomy
F. Uterine massage
G. Hypogastric artery ligation

Answer: A, B, C, F

Initial measures are intended to facilitate uterine contraction and hemostasis. Operative interventions are indicated if these maneuvers fail.

Case 19B

A 32-year-old G2 P0001 undergoes a spontaneous vaginal delivery of a healthy 8-lb girl after an unremarkable spontaneous labor. After 10 min without spontaneous placental delivery, traction is applied to the umbilical cord. Placental tissue is expelled with the umbilical cord but vaginal hemorrhage ensues immediately thereafter. The placenta is clearly not intact.

Questions Case 19B

What are appropriate immediate interventions?

A. Fluid resuscitation and cardiovascular support
B. Oxytocin administration
C. Manual exploration of the uterine cavity
D. Uterine massage
E. Notification of the operating room and anesthesia of a possible surgical emergency

Answer: A, B, C, D

All of these maneuvers are important for diagnostic and/or therapeutic reasons. Retained placental tissue can be assumed and treatment of an associated uterine atony should be undertaken immediately while attempts to remove the placental tissue proceed. The careful clinician should remember that lacerations are still a possible additional cause of bleeding, albeit unlikely. The need for possible surgical intervention is still remote, so that notification of the operating room is not presently necessary.

Oxytocin administration, prostaglandin administration, and uterine massage reduce but do not stop the bleeding. Vaginal examination reveals placental tissue in the uterus, but repeated attempts to dislodge it are not successful. Indeed, careful examination between the retained placental tissue and the uterine wall does not reveal a "cleavage plane." What is the most likely diagnosis?

A. Placenta previa
B. Placental abruption
C. Placenta accreta
D. Uterine inversion
E. Endometrial carcinoma

Answer: C

The description is of placenta accreta, causing vaginal hemorrhage unresponsive to oxytocic and uterine atony. Uterine inversion is unlikely given the examination results. Endometrial carcinoma is exceedingly unlikely in this situation.

chapter 20

INFECTIONS IN THE POSTPARTUM PERIOD

Infections occurring during the puerperium are a relatively frequent cause of morbidity and, rarely, even mortality in obstetric practice. This chapter addresses common causes of infections in the days and weeks following delivery.

The mode of delivery is itself a determinant of infection. Following vaginal delivery, infection occurs much less frequently than after cesarean birth. The incidence of infection varies from 10% to as high as 50% in some populations, depending on the mode of delivery and presence of factors that predispose to postpartum infection (Table 20.1). Certainly, cesarean birth is a significant factor in and of itself.

PUERPERAL FEBRILE MORBIDITY

The definition of puerperal *febrile morbidity*, as determined many years ago by the Joint Committee on Maternal Welfare, is a *"temperature of 38.0°C (100.4°F) or higher, the temperature to occur on any 2 of the first 10 days postpartum, exclusive of the first 24 hours, and to be taken by mouth by a standard technique at least four times daily."* This guideline was proposed to help distinguish true infection from minor temperature elevations commonly seen in the early puerperium and presumed to be the result of breast engorgement. *Practically speaking, significant elevations in maternal temperature even within the first 24 hr postpartum, especially when accompanied by other evidence of infection, are generally thought to represent frank infection, and treatment is often instituted.* However, this "official" definition of puerperal morbidity does serve as a reminder that not every temperature elevation reflects infection and that, in borderline cases, expectant management is warranted. A number of factors predispose to infection following delivery (see Table 20.1). After an overview of the evaluation of a patient with fever in the early puerperium, discussions of severe common types of puerperium infection are provided. After a discussion of several common types of infections, an overview of the evaluation of the patient with fever in the early puerperium is provided.

EVALUATION OF THE FEBRILE PATIENT

The "sequence" of infection sites is somewhat predictable after vaginal or surgical delivery. On the 1st day postoperatively, the lungs are the common cause of fever (atelectasis, pneumonia); on the 2nd day, the urinary tract (cystitis, pyelonephritis); on the 3rd day, the wound (superficial infection, necrotizing fasciitis); and on the 4th day, the extremities (thrombophlebitis). The common mnemonic phrase is *Wind, Water, Wound, and Walking.* The most common infection is metritis (infection of the uterine cavity and adjacent tissue), which is usually associated with the development of fever on the 1st or 2nd days postpartum. Finally, infection of the breast (mastitis) is seen in the first few weeks postpartum, usually in patients who are breast-feeding.

When evaluating a febrile patient, a *history* of the labor and delivery can be helpful. If, for example, the patient had amnionitis and was febrile through labor, one would suspect metritis as the cause of fever. A careful history regarding pulmonary symptoms, urinary tract disturbance, and abdominopelvic pain and tenderness is of paramount importance. *Examination* should include the lungs, the back (for costovertebral tenderness), palpation of the abdomen, careful inspection of the incision site, a check for the presence of bowel sounds, examination of the perineum (if an episiotomy was performed or if a laceration occurred), a pelvic examination, assessment for calf tenderness, and inspection of any intravenous site. Although a pelvic examination may not elicit any findings other than uterine tenderness, one can confirm that lochia drainage is, in fact, occurring and baseline information can be obtained concerning adnexal masses that may be important if the fever persists and an abscess develops. Blood cultures are not usually obtained unless the infection appears severe, sepsis is suspected, fever is especially high, or the response to limited therapy is delayed.

METRITIS

The most common infection following cesarean delivery is infection of the uterus. Often such infection is improperly termed *endometritis* but, in fact, these infections usually extend well beyond the thin endometrial lining into the adjacent myometrium, the loose fibroareolar tissues within the parametrium, and sometimes beyond, with pelvic abscess formation. Hence the *preferred term is metritis* for the initial "limited infection." A special case is the *postcesarean phlegmon*, when infection proceeds from the lateral aspect of the uterus laterally to the pelvic sidewall, forming a pseudomass (Fig. 20.1). The duration of labor, duration of rupture of membranes, and the presence of amnionitis during labor are the major factors leading to the development of metritis.

Fever is the characteristic feature in the diagnosis of metritis, and it may be accompanied by *uterine tenderness*. If the infection has spread to the parametrium and adnexa, tenderness may be present there as well. Signs of peritoneal irritation and diminished or absent bowel sounds, especially associated with ileus, indicate more serious infection, including the possibility of abscess formation. A leukocytosis in the range of 15,000 to 30,000 cells per mL3 is common but difficult to interpret in the presence of the normal early puerperium leukocytosis.

As with virtually all pelvic infections, metritis is polymicrobial in origin. Both aerobic and anaerobic organisms are commonly isolated, with anaerobic organisms predominating. The most common of these organisms are listed in Table 20.2. Because

Table 20.1.
Factors That Predispose to Postpartum Infections

Maternal
  Obesity
  Low socioeconomic status
  Anemia
  Immunosuppression
  Chronic disease, e.g., diabetes mellitus
  Vaginal infection, especially bacterial vaginosis

Associated with labor and delivery
  Rupture of fetal membranes
  Intraamniotic infection
  Prolonged labor
  Multiple pelvic examinations during labor
  Internal electronic fetal monitoring, fetal scalp
    electrode (FSE), and/or intrauterine pressure
    catheter (IUPC)
  Cesarean birth, especially if prolonged operating time

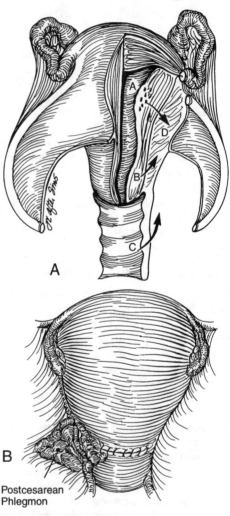

A

B

Postcesarean
Phlegmon

Figure 20.1. **A,** Metritis. Infection may extend from a placental site (*A*) or cervical/vaginal lacerations (*B, C*) into the loose parametrial tissues (*D*). **B,** Postcesarean phlegmon. Infection extends from the incision site laterally to the pelvic sidewall, seeming on pelvic examination as a firm, three-dimensional mass next to the uterus.

Table 20.2.
Common Organisms Associated with Pelvic Infections

Aerobes		Anaerobes	
Gram-positive	Gram-negative	Gram-positive	Gram-negative
Staphylococcus	*Escherichia coli*	*Peptococcus*	*Bacteroides*
Streptococcus (A, B)	*Proteus*	*Peptostreptococcus*	
Enterococcus (group D *Streptococcus*)	*Klebsiella*	Clostridium	

Table 20.3.
Antibiotic Therapy for Metritis

Single-drug regimens	
Cefazolin (Ancef)	1 g i.v. q. 8h.
Cefotetan (Cefotan)	2 g i.v. q. 12h.
Cefoxitin (Mefoxin)	1–2 g q. 8h.
Multiple-drug regimens	
Clindamycin — gentamicin	
Clindamycin (Cleocin)	900 mg i.v. q. 8h.
Gentamicin (Garamycin)	70–100 mg i.v. q. 8h.[a]
Clindamycin — azetreonam	
Clindamycin (Cleocin)	900 mg i.v. q. 8h.
Aztreonam (Azactam)	2 g i.v. q. 8h.
Cefoxitin — doxycycline	
Cefoxitin (Mefoxin)	1–2 g q. 8h.
Doxycycline	100 mg i.v. q. 8h.

[a] Adjust for impaired renal function; check serum levels for therapeutic range on 1st day.

bacteria are normally found in the vagina and endocervix, it is difficult to culture the endometrial cavity properly because sampling devices are contaminated upon transcervical sampling. On a practical basis, treatment using broad antibiotic coverage against a variety of common microorganisms is generally prescribed without cultures.

Various choices of *initial antibiotic therapy* are utilized, most of which are successful. Single-agent therapy has the benefit of ease of administration and is often cost saving; cephalosporins such as cefotetan and cefoxitin are commonly used. A combination of ampicillin and an aminoglycoside is also popular, as is the combination of clindamycin with gentamicin. Many such initial therapies have "gaps" in their total coverage, that is, one or more major pathogens are not sensitive to the antibiotic treatment. Therefore, *it is customary to provide additional antibiotic coverage if there has been no response within 48 to 72 hr.* Intravenous antibiotic administration while the patient is hospitalized is preferred for initial treatment. *Intravenous*

antibiotic therapy is continued until the patient is asymptomatic, has normal bowel function, and has been afebrile for at least 24 hr. Subsequent outpatient oral antibiotic treatment is usually unnecessary (Table 20.3).

Occasionally a *pelvic abscess* will further complicate the patient's recovery. Evidence that suggests abscess formation includes persistent fever despite antibiotic therapy, protracted malaise, delayed return of gastrointestinal function, localization of pain and/or tenderness in the abdominal cavity, and detection of a mass on pelvic/abdominal examination. Ultrasonography or other imaging scans (CT, MRI) may be helpful in diagnosing a pelvic abscess. Management of a persistent pelvic abscess includes drainage either by percutaneous techniques, culdotomy (Fig. 20.2), or laparotomy. Intraabdominal rupture of a pelvic abscess is a surgical emergency. Sepsis may occur in association with pelvic infection, with or without frank abscess formation.

Prophylactic antibiotic therapy at the time of cesarean delivery has been shown to significantly reduce the likelihood of postpartum infection. A single dose of a broad-spectrum antibiotic (for example, cefazolin sodium [Ancef], 1 g) is generally given at the time of clamping of the umbilical cord, a practice designed to avoid confounding of subsequent bacterial cultures of the infant should they be necessary. Additional doses of antibiotics given after surgery do not seem to provide added protection against infection.

RESPIRATORY COMPLICATIONS/ INFECTION

Respiratory complications are especially common in the first 24 hr after delivery, particularly if general anesthesia was used. *Atelectasis* is also common if general anesthesia was used. Training in the use of an inspiratory inhaler preoperatively and its use under supervision postoperatively will significantly reduce the incidence and severity of this complication. Atelectasis is arguably a cause of postoperative fever, but it is certainly associated with it, and its resolution often coincides with clinical defervescence. *Postoperative pneumonia* is uncommon and is usually seen in those with predelivery respiratory disease. *Aspiration pneumonia* is a feared complication of any surgery, but it is especially likely when general anesthesia is used in pregnancy, when there is relative gastric stasis and a greater likelihood of emesis.

URINARY TRACT INFECTIONS

Urinary tract infections are also commonly seen following cesarean delivery but may occur after vaginal delivery. Bladder catheterization, a practice common with both cesarean deliveries and epidural anesthesia, introduces bacteria into the lower urinary tract, which can lead to infection.

Dysuria (painful urination) is not as common in the puerperium as at other times because of a relative insensitivity of the bladder following delivery. *Frequency* of urination is also a normal occurrence postpartum, minimizing the value of this symptom during the postpartum period. *Costovertebral tenderness* may suggest an upper urinary tract infection. When a urinary tract infection is suspected, a "clean-catch" or catheterized urine sample should be obtained for urinalysis and for culture. Antibiotic treatment is begun with one of a variety of broad-spectrum agents, and if the patient is especially uncomfortable, urinary analgesia may be provided (phenazopyridine, 200 mg t.i.d). The antibiotic can be changed if the culture results obtained 24 to 48 hr later indicate resistance of the bacteria to the initial antibiotic, especially if symptoms persist (see also Chapter 31).

WOUND INFECTIONS, SEPARATIONS, AND DEHISCENCE

Infection of the *incision site* following cesarean delivery can occur but is uncommon (3 to 8% of cases in most series, reduced by 50% with prophylactic antibiotic use). Risk factors include obesity, diabetes, corticosteroid therapy, immunosuppression, anemia, and poor hemostasis from any cause with hematoma formation. Fever accompanied by pain, tenderness, and erythema around the incision are seen most frequently on the 3rd and 4th days after delivery. Induration and drainage from the incision site may also be noted. As with any wound infection, the incision must be probed to determine the

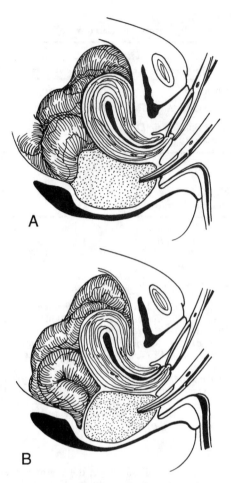

Figure 20.2. Drainage of pelvic abscess by colpotomy. **A,** Drainage of abscess in posterior cul-de-sac of Douglas by colpotomy. **B,** Drainage of rectovaginal septal abscess by colpotomy.

extent of infection, to ensure that the fascia is intact, and to permit adequate drainage of purulent or serosanguineous material. A culture of the site should be obtained, after which broad-spectrum antibiotic treatment is often initiated, although drainage alone may be adequate. Meticulous care of the open wound is also vital. If the infection disrupts the closure of the fascia, return to the operating room for debridement and reapproximation of the wound is necessary, with delayed closure of the skin being the usual management.

Infections of the episiotomy site are very uncommon (probably less than one-quarter of 1% of cases), which is somewhat surprising given the bacteriologic milieu in that area. Infected episiotomy sites are tender and swollen. Poor tissue turgor often leads to breakdown of the sutures used in the initial repair. The sutures should be removed and drainage permitted, both to limit further spread of infection and to promote healing. Sitz baths also help in healing. Subsequent repair of the episiotomy site, if necessary, can be accomplished soon after the infection has cleared.

Necrotizing fasciitis is a rare infection that may be seen on the perineum or with abdominal incisions. This especially virulent and frequently fatal infectious process involves the subcutaneous tissue, muscle, and fascia. It may spread downward along the thighs or upward onto the abdomen and chest. This necrotic tissue must be immediately debrided until healthy tissue is reached. Antibiotics, cardiovascular system support, and subsequent skin grafting comprise the overall treatment. Without such vigorous care, fatality is virtually ensured; even with treatment, approximately 50% of the patients with necrotizing fasciitis do not survive. The important key is early recognition of the possibility that a wound infection, whether perineal or abdominal, may represent this overwhelming infection.

SEPTIC PELVIC THROMBOPHLEBITIS

Septic pelvic thrombophlebitis is an uncommon infection and is a sequela of pelvic infection. The venous drainage of the pelvic organs tends to flow in a left-to-right fashion through the right ovarian vein. Venous stasis in these widely dilated veins, along with the presence of multiple bacteria if infection is present, can lead to septic thrombosis in these vessels; subsequent *microembolization* of the lungs or other organs via the inferior vena cava is possible.

Clinically, this infection is manifest as *residual fever and tachycardia* following several days of antibiotic treatment for presumed metritis. Usually the patient is asymptomatic with respect to uterine tenderness and bowel function. Although it is possible to diagnose this condition with CT scanning or other such imaging, it is customary to begin empiric treatment with *heparin*. Prompt resolution of the fever and tachycardia, usually within 24 hr, corroborates the diagnosis. Anticoagulation therapy is recommended for at least 7 and up to 30 days.

MASTITIS

In the lactating woman, breast infection occurs most commonly several days postpartum, but it can occur months later. Initially, symptoms can be misleading. Patients often complain of significant *fever* (often 103°F or more), *malaise*, and *general body aching*. Breast symptoms may be somewhat vague, although breast tenderness is described if patients are asked specifically about this. Commonly, patients think they have a generalized viral infection and call their physician seeking information regarding medications to take for the flu while lactating.

After the onset of these signs and symptoms, evidence of infection becomes more localized to the breasts over the following days. Erythema and tenderness are present, often with a brawny and indurated area to palpation, which may be segmented in orientation. The infection is virtually always unilateral. *Staphylococcus aureus* is cultured from the breast milk in about 50% of cases; no single predominant organism is identified in other cases. The origin of the infection is, in fact, the infant's pharynx; accordingly, there should be no concern on the part of the mother with respect to transmitting the infection to the infant.

It is no longer common practice to culture the breast milk. However, because of the prevalence of the *S. aureus* as the offender, an antibiotic that is penicillinase-resistant, such as *dicloxacillin* (500 mg p.o. q. 6h.) is recommended. Resolution of symptoms is generally prompt, with marked improvement within 24 to 36 hr. Patients should be cautioned to complete the full antibiotic course to prevent recurrence. It is *not necessary to withhold nursing* on the infected breast, although some patients benefit greatly from uninterrupted rest for the first day or two of therapy.

Mastitis is generally distinguished from a blocked (inspissated) duct (see Chapter 18) on the basis of fever. At times, however, it may be difficult to distinguish these two entities, and antibiotic treatment is generally begun empirically.

CASE STUDIES

Case 20A

At 9 days postpartum, a new mother complains that she feels awful, is running a fever of 99 to 100°F, and "just aches all over." She is breast-feeding, but the baby has been fretful the last 48 hr. She has no complaints of sore throat, dysuria, or pelvic pain (except the uterine cramps she has come to expect with breast-feeding), and her breasts are not especially tender. On examination, the left breast is slightly warmer to touch and slightly more tender than the right.

Questions Case 20A

The most likely diagnosis is

A. Mastitis
B. Breast abscess
C. Fibrocystic disorder
D. Squamous cell carcinoma
E. Trauma and fat necrosis

Answer: A

Appropriate management includes

A. Surgical drainage of the infected breast
B. Cannulation of the breast ducts over the affected lobules
C. Administration of an oral penicillinase-resistant antibiotic
D. Instructions to cease breast-feeding until the infection clears
E. Mammography to rule out carcinoma

Answer: C

The presumptive diagnosis is early mastitis. Mastitis usually responds readily to oral antibiotic therapy. Surgical intervention for mastitis is not indicated, although drainage of an abscess may be. There is no risk to the baby or mother from continuing breast-feeding. The risk of carcinoma is exceedingly low.

Case 20B

A 27-year-old G1 P0 is induced at 42 weeks for postdates pregnancy, undergoes induction with FSE and IUPC for 36 hr, and is delivered by cesarean section for fetal distress when she has dilated to 8 cm. The patient was afebrile before the surgery and was given one dose of prophylactic antibiotics at the time of umbilical cord clamping.

Her immediate postpartum course is unremarkable. She is bottle feeding and lactation has not begun. On the 3rd postpartum day, she develops a fever to 102.2°F with chills and lower quadrant abdominal pain. Examination reveals a tender uterine fundus and somewhat diminished but not absent bowel sounds. There is a slightly foul lochia, and the cervix is tender to manipulation. The breasts are nontender. A complete blood count reveals a hematocrit of 29 and a white blood cell (WBC) count of 14,500 with a left shift.

Questions Case 20B

The most likely diagnosis is

A. Mastitis
B. Metritis
C. Pelvic abscess
D. Septic pelvic thrombophlebitis
E. Atelectasis

Answer: B

Mastitis is unlikely in a bottle-feeding mother with normal breast findings. Metritis is highly likely given the prolonged labor with intrauterine catheter and scalp electrode and subsequent cesarean birth. Pelvic abscess is possible but it is somewhat early for this to develop. Septic pelvic thrombophlebitis is possible but likewise unlikely at this time. Atelectasis is unlikely to present 3 days after surgery with this temperature.

Your management at this time should include

A. Single-agent antibiotic therapy
B. Multiple-agent antibiotic therapy
C. Anticoagulation with heparin
D. Diagnostic laparoscopy or laparotomy
E. Observation

Answer: A

A single-agent antibiotic regimen will suffice in most cases of simple metritis. Multiple-agent regimens are best left for situations in which the response to a single agent is unsatisfactory. Anticoagulation is not indicated at this time, as the diagnosis of septic thrombophlebitis has not been made. Surgical evaluation is contraindicated with a diagnosis that is expected to respond to a simple antibiotic regimen. Observation to see if the fever continues is an option, but most clinicians will proceed with therapy given a history that includes so many factors predisposing to metritis and these physical findings.

After 72 hr the patient remains febrile and uncomfortable. Her WBC is now 19,000. Your management at this time should include

A. Single-agent antibiotic therapy
B. Multiple-agent antibiotic therapy
C. Anticoagulation with heparin
D. Diagnostic laparoscopy or laparotomy as required
E. Observation

Answer: B

Multiple-agent antibiotic therapy is now indicated to cover the full range of aerobic and anaerobic organisms that may be expected in metritis.

Multiple-agent therapy is continued for 48 hr but the patient remains febrile. Examination of the abdomen reveals a less tender uterus and pelvic examination reveals a slightly tender uterus but no masses. Ultrasound examination does not reveal an abscess. The most likely diagnosis is

A. Mastitis
B. Metritis
C. Pelvic abscess
D. Septic pelvic thrombophlebitis
E. Atelectasis

Answer: D

Without evidence of abscess, the most likely diagnosis is metritis plus septic pelvic thrombophlebitis.

Your management at this time should include

A. Single-agent antibiotic therapy
B. Multiple-agent antibiotic therapy
C. Anticoagulation with heparin
D. Diagnostic laparoscopy or laparotomy as required
E. Observation

Answer: C

chapter 21

DISORDERS OF THE BREAST

Disorders of the female breast pose unique problems for patient and physician. Our society places special significance on the female breast, especially in matters of femininity and sexuality. In addition, there are appropriate fears of breast cancer, which are confounded by normal monthly changes that may be both uncomfortable and disconcerting. Consideration of both the medical disorder and its emotional sequelae is a challenge in the management of breast disorders.

The adult female breast is actually a large, modified sebaceous gland, located within the superficial fascia of the chest wall (Fig. 21.1). It weighs between 200 and 300 g and is made up primarily of fatty tissue, fibrous septa, and glandular structures. Breast tissue is organized into 12 to 20 triangular lobes with a central duct, collecting ducts, and secretory cells arranged in alveoli. Each of these lobes drains at the nipple. The breast has a rich blood supply and lymphatic system, which facilitate metastases of malignancies (Fig. 21.2) Breast tissue may be located anywhere along "milk lines" that run from the axilla to the groin. Extra nipples (*polythelia*) are more common than true accessory breasts (*polymastia*).

Breast tissue is very sensitive to hormonal changes. The development of adult breast shape during puberty is a result of hormonal changes. The sensitivity to hormones is also responsible for cyclic changes that occur during the menstrual cycle and for the symptoms often reported by patients during therapeutic hormonal manipulations.

Each of the tissues of the breast may be the source of pathologic change. Fibrocystic changes and fibroadenomas may arise in the connective tissues of the breast. Fatty tissues may undergo necrosis in response to trauma or may harbor lipomas. The duct system of the breast may become dilated (duct ectasia or galactocele), contain papil-

lary neoplasms, or undergo malignant change. Although more common in nursing mothers, infection of the breast (mastitis) may also occur.

Breast cancer is the most common malignancy of women, accounting for roughly one-fourth of all women's malignancies. It is the leading cause of death from cancer for women between the ages of 35 and 54. With approximately 175,000 new cases and 44,500 breast cancer deaths per year in the United States, breast cancer is the most common cause of death in women in their 40s. *Roughly one woman in nine will develop breast cancer in her lifetime.* Both the incidence of and deaths from breast cancer have increased by approximately 1% per year since 1973, but newer diagnostic technologies and increased awareness promise earlier diagnosis and more successful treatment.

BENIGN BREAST DISEASE

Fibrocystic Change

The term *fibrocystic change* encompasses more than 35 different processes, including the misnomer "fibrocystic disease." Fibrocystic changes are the *most common of all benign breast conditions.* They may be present in one-third to one-half of premenopausal women and are a source of symptoms for roughly half of these women. The alterations associated with fibrocystic change may arise from an exaggerated response to hormones. Consequently, fibrocystic changes are most common during the reproductive years or occasionally during hormone replacement after menopause. Disturbed ratios of estrogen and progesterone and an increased rate of prolactin secretion have both been suggested as causes for these changes. Neither of these theories has been conclusively proven, nor is there any evidence that fibrocystic changes are caused by oral contraceptives.

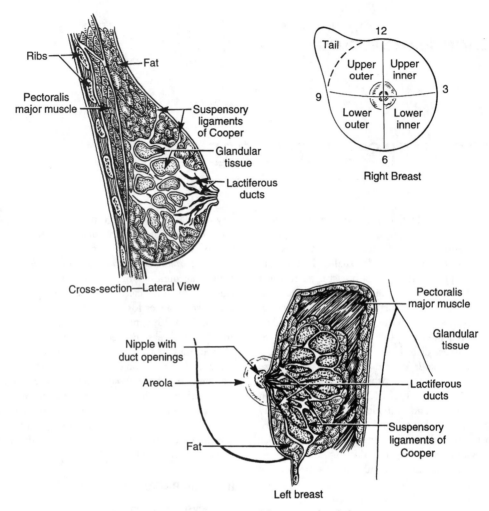

Figure 21.1. The structure of the mature female breast.

Histologically, fibrocystic changes occur in three states. Initially, there is a *proliferation of stroma,* especially in the upper outer quadrants of the breast, that leads to the induration and tenderness experienced by the patient. In the second phase, *adenosis* occurs, leading to cyst formation. During this phase, cysts range from microscopic to 1 cm in diameter. Marked proliferation of the ducts and alveolar cells occur in this stage. In the late stages of fibrocystic change, *larger cysts* are present and *less pain* occurs (unless there is rapid change in a cyst). Proliferative changes may be marked in any of the involved tissues. When atypia is found in hyperplastic ducts or apocrine cells, there is a fivefold increase in the risk of future carcinoma.

Fibrocystic changes most commonly present as cyclic, bilateral pain (mastalgia) and engorgement. The pain associated with fibrocystic changes is diffuse, often with radiation to the shoulders or upper arms. Occasionally well-localized pain will occur when a cyst expands rapidly. On examination, diffuse bilateral nodularity is typical, with larger cysts taking on the character of a balloon filled with fluid. These changes are most prominent just before menstruation.

The management of fibrocystic changes may include fine-needle aspiration of cysts, which is diagnostic and often therapeutic. Open biopsy is indicated if there are mammographic findings suggesting neoplasia, or if on fine-needle aspiration (*a*) the fluid obtained is bloody, (*b*) there is a

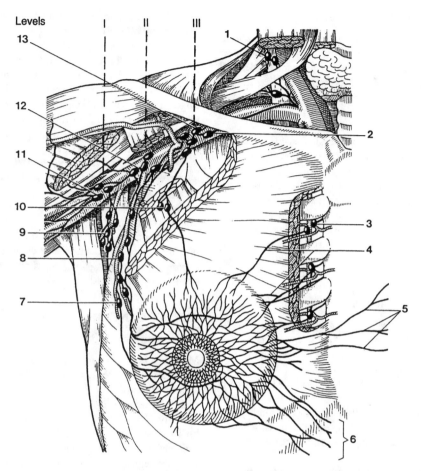

Figure 21.2. Lymphatic drainage of the breast. *I*, Low axillary nodes; *II*, central axillary nodes; *III*, subclavian nodes; *1*, deep cervical nodes; *2*, infraclavicular nodes; *3*, sternal nodes; *4*, pathway to the mediastinal nodes; *5*, pathway to the contralateral breast; *6*, pathway to the subdiaphragmatic nodes and liver; *7*, anterior pectoral lymph nodes; *8*, central axillary nodes; *9*, subpectoral axillary nodes; *10*, interpectoral nodes (Rotter's); *11*, brachial vein nodes; *12*, axillary vein nodes; *13*, subclavian vein nodes.

residual mass after aspiration is performed, or (*c*) the cyst recurs. Dietary restriction of caffeine and foods containing methylxanthines benefit some patients, while others respond to a low-salt diet, vitamin E, and/or a mild diuretic such as hydrochlorothiazide (25 to 50 mg per day for 7 to 10 days before menses). Danazol is effective in severe cases, but symptoms often resume following discontinuation of the medication. In the most severe cases, bilateral mastectomy may be required to relieve intractable, incapacitating pain.

Fibroadenoma

Fibroadenomas are the second most common form of benign breast disease. They occur most often in young women. These firm, painless, freely movable breast masses average 2 to 3 cm in diameter and are comprised of a mixture of proliferating epithelial and supporting fibrous tissues. Although generally solitary, multiple fibroadenomas develop in 15 to 20% of patients. These tumors do not change during the menstrual cycle and are generally slow growing. They are usually found during physical examination or during breast self-examination. The management of these usually benign lesions, like most similar lesions, is evaluation by examination and imaging techniques and then biopsy or excision, because the reliability of nonhistologic methods of evaluation to rule out malignancy is insufficient.

Lipomas and Fat Necrosis

The fatty tissue of the breast may be the source of benign tumors that are difficult to distinguish from malignancy. Both lipomas and fat necrosis may present as ill-defined tumors of the breast. Lipomas are generally nontender, but their diffuse character may raise suspicions of malignancy. Secondary signs suggestive of cancer (e.g., skin and nipple changes) are generally absent.

Fat necrosis is uncommon and most often the result of trauma, although the causative event frequently cannot be identified. The patient usually presents with a solitary, tender, ill-defined mass. Skin retraction is present in some patients. Direct evidence of trauma is most often lacking. Even with a history of trauma, the similarity of findings between fat necrosis and cancer (on physical examination and mammography) generally requires further evaluation and biopsy or excision to establish the diagnosis.

Intraductal Papilloma

Intraductal papillomas are polypoid epithelial tumors arising in the ducts of the breast. These fibrovascular tumors are covered by benign ductal epithelium. Although these tumors may range from 2 to 5 mm in diameter, they are typically not palpable. The patient presents with a *spontaneous bloody, serous, or cloudy nipple discharge.* Although these polyps are most often benign, the similarity of symptoms to carcinoma mandates excisional biopsy for most patients.

Mammary Duct Ectasia and Galactocele

Mammary duct ectasia may arise from chronic intraductal and periductal inflammation, which causes *dilation of the ducts and inspissation of breast secretions.* Most common in the fifth decade of life, this condition presents with a thick gray to black nipple discharge, pain, and nipple tenderness. Palpation around the nipple will elicit discharge and may reveal thickening that may be difficult to distinguish from cancer. Nipple retraction is common. Biopsy will confirm the diagnosis, and once established, no further therapy is needed unless warranted by the patient's symptoms.

Ductal obstruction and inflammation during or soon after lactation may lead to the development of a galactocele. Galactoceles are cystic dilations of a duct or ducts. These ducts contain inspissated milky secretions that may become infected and lead to acute mastitis or abscess formation. When uncomplicated by infection, needle aspiration and decompression of the ducts is curative and excision is rarely required.

BREAST CANCER

Demographics

Much has been written about factors that increase a woman's risk of breast cancer (Table 21.1), but little is known about the actual cause. *Risk factors themselves are of limited clinical value.*

Only 21% of patients aged 30 to 54 years with breast cancer are identified by risk factors. However, risk factors may be useful in planning detection strategies. For example, the incidence of breast cancer rises with age. A total of 85% of all breast cancer occurs after the age of 40 (66% over the age of 50). For this reason, current *recommen-*

Table 21.1.
Risk Factors for Breast Cancer

Factor	Relative Risk	Factor	Relative Risk
Family history of breast cancer		Other neoplasms	
First-degree relative (sister or mother)	1.2–3.0	Contralateral breast cancer	5.0
		Carcinoma of uterus or ovary	2.0
Menstrual history		Carcinoma of major salivary gland	4.0
Menarche <12 years old	1.3		
<40 menstrual years	1.5–2.0	Other conditions	
		Atypical hyperplasia	4.0–6.0
Oral contraceptive use	No effect	Previous biopsy	1.9–2.1
		North American (white or black)	5.0
Estrogen replacement <10 years	No effect	Age 60 vs. age 40	2.0
		Moderate alcohol use	1.5–2.0
Pregnancy		Radiation exposure (>90 rads)	4.0
First delivery >35 years old	2.0–3.0	Obesity	Suggested but unknown
Nulliparous	3.0	Large bowel cancer	Suggested but unknown
		Increased dietary fat	Suggested but unknown

Table 21.2.
Guidelines for Mammographic Screening

Mammography every 1–2 years from age 40 to 49

Annual mammography from age 50 on

Screening mammography before age 35 may be
  appropriate in selected high-risk patients

Table 21.3.
Simplified Classification of Breast Cancer

Mammary duct cancers
  Infiltrating (80%)
    Papillary carcinoma
    Intraductal carcinoma
    Colloid carcinoma
    Medullary carcinoma
  Noninfiltrating (5%)
    Papillary carcinoma
    Intraductal carcinoma (comedocarcinoma)
    Intracystic carcinoma

Size More Important Than Cell Type For Survival

Mammary lobule cancers
  In situ and infiltrating (12%)

Sarcomas
  Cystosarcoma phylloides
  Stromal sarcoma
  Liposarcoma
  Angiosarcoma

Lymphoma

Rare cancers
  Sweat gland carcinoma
  Tubular carcinoma
  Adenoid cystic carcinoma
  Metaplastic lesions
  Inflammatory carcinoma (2%)
  Paget's disease (1%)
  Metastatic cancers

dations for mammographic screening for breast cancer depend on the patient's age (Table 21.2).

Types of Breast Cancer

Although 80% of breast cancers are of the nonspecific infiltrating intraductal type, many different cancer types can occur (Table 21.3). Breast cancer survival depends less on cell type than it does on the size of the tumor. Most breast tumors have a long latency from onset to clinically detectable size (Fig. 21.3). For this reason, efforts to improve early detection are directed toward mammographic screening of those at high risk and increased public awareness through programs such as breast self-examination.

Symptoms

In the early stages of cancer growth, the tumor is usually painless and may feel mobile. As the tumor grows, the borders become less distinct and fixation to the supporting ligaments or underlying fascia occurs. Nipple discharge and skin changes (*peau d'orange*, or "orange peel skin") are late occurrences and are associated with a poor prognosis. Approximately 80% of breast cancers present as a mass.

Clinical Aspects

History and Physical Examination

With as many as one-fourth of all breast cancers found during routine examination, the role of the careful history and physical examination cannot be overemphasized. *A careful breast examination should be a part of every gynecological examination* (see Chapter 1). All patients should be questioned on whether they practice breast self-examination. *Breast self-examination* should be done on a monthly basis. Since *90% of breast cancers are found by the patient*, this is an opportunity both to highlight an important screening test and to obtain information that may be of help clinically. A general family, medical, menstrual, and obstetric history should be obtained for all patients. Significant risk factors are also evaluated. Even though these risk factors will identify only 25% of cancer patients, they are helpful in planning screening and surveillance.

When obtaining the *history* of a patient with breast problems, information about the presenting complaint such as pain, tenderness, mass, or discharge should be sought. The duration of symptoms and any changes in symptoms are also important. Any changes related to the menstrual cycle should especially be noted.

Physical examination of the breast should be performed by the physician annually and as a part of the evaluation of any breast complaint. The examination should begin with inspection of both breasts, looking for contour, symmetry, skin, or nipple changes. This should take place with the patient in both the upright and supine position, with the patient's arms above the head and also with her hands on her hips and contracting her pectoral muscles. Palpation of the breast tissue proceeds in a systematic way using the flat of the fingers, rolling the breast between the fingers and the underlying tissues. This may

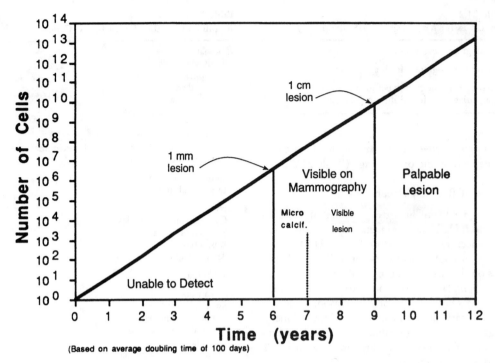

Figure 21.3. Mammographic and clinical detection of breast mass. With a presumed doubling time of 100 days, breast cancer may be detected by mammography significantly earlier than it can be identified clinically. *Micro calcif.*, microcalcification.

be carried out by quadrants or in a spiral fashion designed to ensure that the entire breast is examined. Palpation of the axilla and supraclavicular area must be included.

Evaluation

The *evaluation of any breast complaint* is based on the history and physical examination, augmented by four additional modalities: *imaging, fine needle aspiration, fine needle biopsy, and open biopsy.*

Imaging

The only nonexperimental method of breast imaging and evaluation is *mammography*. Mammography provides the best mode currently available of screening for early lesions and *has been credited with reducing the mortality rate from breast cancer by up to 30%. Breast cancer mortality could be reduced by as much as 50% if all women over the age of 40 were screened annually.*

Screening mammography (see Figure 21.4) involves compression of the breast tissue against an imaging plate in two projections — craniocaudad

and mediolateral — and the use of a small amount of radiation to form the four images comprising the standard screening mammogram (Fig. 21.4). Compression of the breast tissue is necessary to encompass the tissue and provide clear visualization of the tissue. The axillary tail of Spence is sometimes not fully visualized and this must be kept in mind in the interpretation of screening mammograms. To avoid this problem, some clinicians use a mediolateral oblique view, which tends to include more of this axillary tissue (Fig. 21.5).

Mammography, with a radiation exposure of approximately 0.5 rad, provides the opportunity to identify small, nonpalpable lesions (1 to 2 mm), microcalcifications, and other changes suspicious for malignancy (Figs. 21.6 and 21.7). It is approximately 85% accurate in diagnosing malignancy, and therefore, provides a clinically useful adjunct to clinical impressions and the definitive procedure of biopsy.

Ultrasonography has been proposed as a useful tool in the evaluation of breast pathology. Although ultrasound is very good at differentiating between cystic and solid masses, it provides little

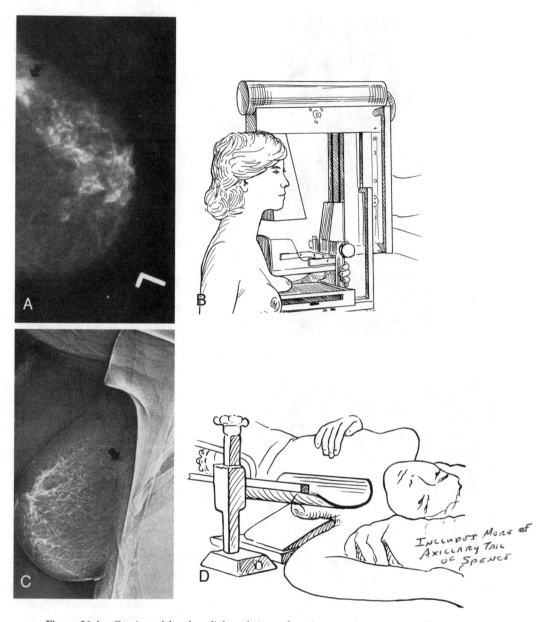

Figure 21.4. Craniocaudal and mediolateral views of routine screening mammography.

additional information in the clinical management of the patient. Thermography and breast transillumination are not useful as either screening or diagnostic tools. The role of magnetic resonance imaging is still under evaluation.

Breast Cyst Aspiration

A simple and very valuable diagnostic tool is *needle aspiration* (Fig. 21.8). If the patient has a breast mass that feels cystic, aspiration with a 22- to 25-gauge needle may be both diagnostic and therapeutic. In women over the age of 35, mammography before aspiration should be considered because of the increased incidence of malignancy. Preaspiration mammography also provides an accurate baseline appearance in the off chance that bleeding into the cyst occurs as a result of the needle aspiration.

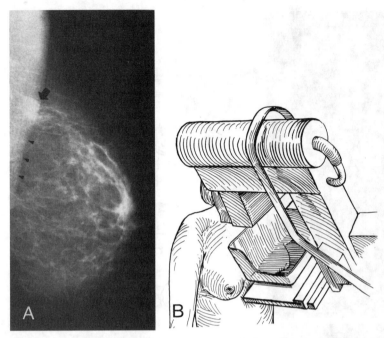

Figure 21.5. Mediolateral oblique mammogram to facilitate inclusion of axillary tail.

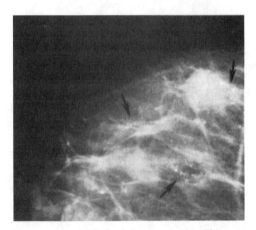

Figure 21.6. Multifocal duct carcinoma. Close-up shows multiple clusters of calcifications (*arrows*) and two masses. Only the larger mass was palpable.

Fluid aspirated from patients with fibrocystic changes will customarily be straw colored. Fluid that is dark brown or green occurs in cysts that have been present for a long time. Cytologic evaluation of the fluid obtained is generally of little value.

Fine Needle Aspiration

Fine needle aspiration of cells from a breast mass is gaining acceptance in the United States. In this procedure, a 16- to 22-gauge needle is inserted into the mass, multiple passes are made with negative pressure applied by a syringe, and cells or tissue is obtained (Fig. 21.9). The material collected is examined histologically or cytologically for signs of malignancy. This technique is 70 to 90% accurate, with a 20% false-negative rate. Therefore, if the aspiration is negative, open biopsy should still be performed. This technique depends heavily on the availability of expert cytopathology services.

Open Biopsy

The ultimate method of evaluation of any breast mass is open biopsy. This is often performed under local anesthesia through either radial or circumareolar incisions. For small lesions or those difficult to localize, preoperative identification and radiographically guided J-wire placement may be of value (so-called needle-localized biopsy). Postoperative x-ray of the pathology specimen should confirm excision of the desired tissue (see Fig. 21.10).

Differential Diagnosis by Complaint or Finding

The most common presenting complaints are pain and the presence of a mass. Both of these complaints represent sources of great distress and per-

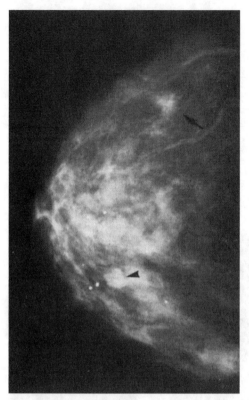

Figure 21.7. Cephalocaudal film-screen mammogram. Small scirrhous carcinoma (*arrow*) is contrasted with well-marginated fibroadenoma (*arrowhead*).

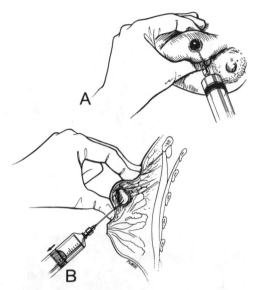

Figure 21.8. Needle aspiration of cystic breast mass. The needle is passed into cyst, which is stabilized as shown. The cyst's contents are removed by gentle suction.

ceived emergency to the patient. Therefore, they deserve prompt and considerate attention.

Diffuse, bilateral breast pain occurring before menstruation is most often caused by *fibrocystic changes*. *Dorsal radiculitis or inflammatory changes in the costochondral junction* (Tietze's syndrome) may also present in this way. Well-localized breast pain may result from rapid expansion of a *cyst, obstruction of a duct*, or inflammation (such as *mastitis*). Breast pain is a presenting complaint in <10% of patients with breast cancer.

Masses in the breast, with the attendant fear of cancer, represent one of the most emotionally charged and difficult differential diagnoses the clinician must make. Masses that are firm, round, and well demarcated are most likely to be *fibroadenomas*. Areas with a flattened, rubbery consistency are suspicious for malignancy, although other conditions such as fat necrosis may cause similar changes. In either case, *further evaluation (such as*

tissue confirmation by open or needle biopsy) is mandatory. One approach to this process is shown in Figure 21.10.

Although *bloody discharge* from the nipple is the hallmark of *intraductal papillomas*, any unilateral spontaneous nipple discharge requires a thorough evaluation. The color or clarity of the fluid does not rule out carcinoma. Cytologic evaluation of the nipple discharge is associated with a false-negative rate of almost 20%, significantly reducing its value. Mammography and biopsy are required to establish the diagnosis.

Nipple discharge associated with burning, itching, or nipple discomfort in older patients is suggestive of *ductal ectasia*. In these patients, the discharge is thick or sticky and gray to black in color. As with other sources of nipple discharge, excisional biopsy is often required.

GENERAL MANAGEMENT

Selection of Therapy

The treatment of patients with breast cancer is directed toward three goals: (*a*) control of local disease, (*b*) treatment of distant disease, and (*c*) improved quality of life. To this end, *most breast cancer is treated by surgical excision and adjunctive therapy*. Breast cancer spreads by both vascular and

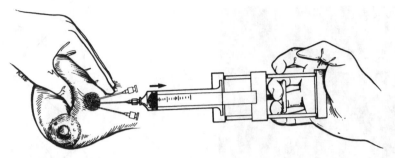

Figure 21.9. Fine needle aspiration of solid breast mass. The needle is passed into the solid mass and withdrawn at several different angles and in several different places while suction is maintained.

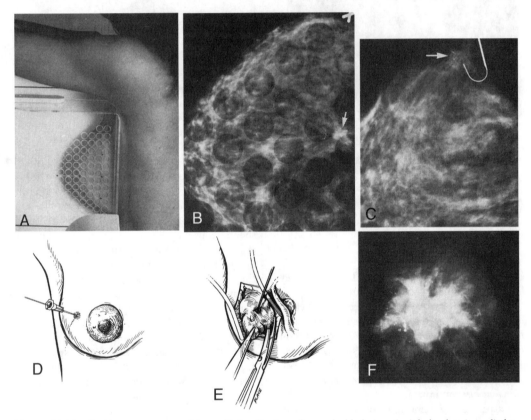

Figure 21.10. Prebiopsy mammographic needle localization of nonpalpable lesion, **A,** A hole plate is applied to the breast surface closest to the lesion. **B,** A mammogram identifies the hole over the nonpalpable stellate lesion suggestive of malignancy. **C,** A guide wire is inserted under mammographic direction. **D,** Excision of the specimen along the needle. **E,** Demonstration by mammogram of the specimen that the stellate lesion has been removed for evaluation.

lymphatic routes with some direct infiltration. Recognition of this has led away from traditional radical surgical treatment, to therapy directed at both local and distant disease simultaneously. With lo- cal disease only, 5-year survival approaches 90%. This drops to 50 to 70% when there is regional involvement. Unfortunately, roughly 50% of patients have axillary lymph node involvement at the

Table 21.4.
Staging of Breast Cancer[a]

TNM[b] classification of breast cancer	
T	Primary tumors
TIS	Paget's disease of the nipple with no demonstrable tumor
T1 T1a, T2a, T3a	Tumor >2 cm With no fixation
T2 T1b, T2b, T3b	Tumor >2–5 cm With fixation to underlying pectoral fascia or muscle
T3	Tumor >5 cm

T4
    T4a
 	
    T4b
 	
    T4c
    T4d
	Tumor of any size with direct extension to chest wall or skin
	With fixation to chest wall (including ribs, intercostal muscles, and serratus anterior muscle but not pectoral muscle)
	With edema (including peau d'orange), ulceration of skin of breast, or satellite skin nodules on same breast
	Both T4a and T4b
	Inflammatory cancer
	Dimpling of the skin, nipple retraction, or any other skin changes except those in T4b may occur in T1, T2, or T3 without changing the classification

N	Regional lymph nodes
N0	No palpable ipsilateral axillary nodes

N1
    N1a
    N1b
	Movable ipsilateral axillary nodes
	Nodes not considered to contain growth
	Nodes considered to contain growth

N2	Ipsilateral nodes considered to contain growth and fixed to one another or to other structures
N3	Ipsilateral supraclavicular or infraclavicular nodes considered to contain growth, or edema of the arm
M	Distant metastasis
M0	No known distant metastases
M1	Distant metastases present

Definition of clinical stages using TNM classification			
Stage I	T1a	N0 or N1a	M0
	T1b	N0 or N1a	M0
Stage II	T0	N1b	M0
	T1a	N1b	M0
	T1b	N1b	M0
	T2a	N0, N1a, or N1b	M0
	T2b	N0, N1a, or N1b	M0
Stage III	T3	Any N	M0
	Any T	N2	M0
Stage IV	T4	Any N	Any M
	Any T	N3	Any M
	Any T	Any N	M1

[a] Staging system of the International Union Against Cancer and American Joint Commission of Cancer Staging and End Results reporting.
[b] Tumor-node-metastasis.

time of diagnosis. Based on the stage of the disease (Table 21.4) and presence of hormone receptors, this adjunctive therapy may consist of radiation therapy, chemotherapy, hormonal manipulations, or a combination of all three. Like most conditions, the therapy of breast cancer must be individualized.

Follow-up of Therapy

Patients with diffuse tenderness and no dominant mass may be safely rechecked at a different time in the menstrual cycle. Patients who have undergone aspiration of a cyst (with clear fluid and disappearance of the palpable mass) should be rechecked in 2 weeks. Any reoccurrence of the cyst should prompt biopsy or additional evaluation. Some authors advocate a follow-up mammogram after cyst aspiration to delve for other lesions, although this is best individualized based on the needs and history of each patient.

Patients treated for breast cancer require frequent follow-up. Not only are these patients at higher risk for developing a new cancer on the opposite side but two-thirds of these patients will eventually develop distant metastasis. Any patient who has had breast cancer must be closely followed by physical examination and mammography (where appropriate). No biological markers yet exist to allow for either detection or monitoring of those with breast cancer.

CASE STUDIES

Case 21A

A 24-year-old G0 on triphasic oral contraceptives comes to your office with a complaint of a "lump" in her right breast. She reluctantly admits that she did not find the mass and that she would not have known that it was there had it not been for her husband. She has not had

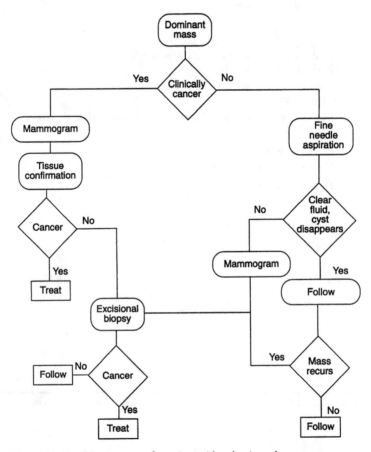

Figure 21.11. Management of a patient with a dominant breast mass.

any nipple discharge and does do breast self-examination "most months." She is very worried, as her mother died of breast carcinoma.

On your examination you find no change in the contour of either breast. No skin changes or nipple discharge can be found. There is a 1-cm, firm, smooth, round, mobile, nontender mass located in the upper outer quadrant of the right breast, approximately 5 cm from the areola.

Questions Case 21A

Based on the history and physical examination, you tell the patient that the most likely diagnosis is

A. Fibrocystic change
B. Fibroadenoma
C. Hematoma
D. Intraductal papilloma
E. Fat necrosis

Answer: B

Even though this patient may have fat necrosis or a hematoma, these conditions are less likely than fibroadenomas, based on the patient's age and findings. Fibrocystic change would be expected to demonstrate a longer history and cyclic changes. Intraductal papillomas are seldom felt as a mass but rather present with bleeding from the nipple.

The most appropriate next step would be

A. Reexamination in 3 weeks
B. Mammography
C. Needle aspiration or drainage
D. Needle biopsy
E. Excisional biopsy

Answer: B, D, or E

Given the patient's family history and level of concern, mammography followed by histological evaluation by needle biopsy or excision is appropriate. Some clinicians would argue that mammography is not required if excision is performed.

Case 21B

A 25-year-old G1 P1001 who delivered a son 8 weeks earlier presents with a complaint of a swollen, red, tender area on the left side of her right breast. She is breast-feeding, has no history of breast problems, and has no family history of breast cancer. On examination she is afebrile and her breasts are engorged, as she is soon scheduled to feed. There is a slightly reddened, swollen cystic area as described.

Questions Case 21B

The most likely diagnosis is

A. Duct ectasia
B. Galactocele
C. Fat necrosis
D. Fibrocystic change
E. Carcinoma

Answer: B

A localized, tender cystic swelling in a breast-feeding woman without evidence of infection is most consistent with a blocked excretory duct, a galactocele. Duct ectasia is the same problem in a nonlacting woman.

The best management is

A. Drainage by needle
B. Incision and drainage
C. Excision
D. Placement of word catheter
E. Radiation

Answer: A

Simple drainage is usually sufficient, with incision rarely required.

Case 21C

A worried 26-year-old G0 nurse taking oral contraceptives presents complaining of long-standing breast pain, now so bad that it keeps her from working 3 to 6 days per month. The pain is worse with movement and before her menses. She tearfully relates that her mother died of breast cancer at the age of 42 and her 28-year-old sister has metastatic breast cancer and is taking chemotherapy. On examination, her breasts are symmetrical and dense, with multiple tender cystic areas and sheets of dense tissue.

Questions Case 21C

The most likely diagnosis is

A. Mastitis
B. Fat necrosis
C. Carcinoma
D. Fibrocystic changes
E. None of the above

Answer: D

The prolonged time course, the complaint of cystic nodularity and pain, and the breast examination are consistent with fibrocystic changes. Unfortunately, this patient is at great risk for developing breast carcinoma given her family history.

Your best management is

A. Mammography

B.   A triphasic oral contraceptive
C.   Excision of all masses for histologic evaluation
D.   Bilateral mastectomies
E.   None of the above

Answer: A

Mammography, however, may be of little value if there are the usual profusion of radiodense areas in the pa-tient's breast. Needle aspiration of cysts may be helpful, as may treatment with progesterone. One of the most difficult decisions is when to biopsy the patient who has multiple lesions, has new ones developing all the time, and is also at high risk for cancer. Some patients in this situation will choose bilateral mastectomy rather than live with the continuing risk and fear of cancer.

chapter 22

CONTRACEPTION

The ability to control fertility has had more wide-ranging impact on society than almost any other aspect of medical practice, past or present. Since the subject of contraception has personal, religious, and political overtones, it can often lead to conflict, emotionality, and confusion. Helping the patient and her partner sort through their options is both important and rewarding. Before the physician can advise a couple on their contraceptive options, he or she must understand the physiologic or pharmacologic basis of action, the effectiveness, the indications and contraindications, complications, and advantages and disadvantages of the contraceptive methods available.

There are many methods of contraception considered reliable as well as numerous methods of dubious or no value arising from superstition or ignorance. Since no method is 100% reliable, failures are reflected in the descriptive measures of *method failure* (the failure rate inherent in the method if the patient uses it correctly 100% of the time) and *patient failure* (the failure rate seen when patients actually use the method, i.e., make mistakes in usage). Approximate pregnancy rates for various methods of contraception are shown in Table 22.1.

HOW CONTRACEPTIVES WORK

All contraceptive methods currently available act to prevent sperm and egg from uniting or to prevent implantation and growth of the embryo. These goals are accomplished by (*a*) inhibiting the development and release of the egg (oral contraceptives, implantable rods, long acting progesterone injection); (*b*) imposing a mechanical, chemical, or temporal barrier between sperm and egg (condom, diaphragm, foam, rhythm, and implantable rods); or (*c*) altering the ability of the fertilized egg to implant and grow (intrauterine devices,

diethylstilbestrol, postcoital oral contraceptives, and inducing menstruation or abortion (RU 486)). Each approach may be used successfully, individually or in combination, to prevent pregnancy, and each method has its own unique advantages and disadvantages.

FACTORS AFFECTING CHOICE OF CONTRACEPTIVE METHOD

While efficacy is important in the choice of contraceptive methods, it is not the only factor on which the final decision is based. Factors such as safety, availability, cost, degree to which method relies on or interferes with coitus (coital dependence), and personal acceptability to patient and partner all have a role to play in the decision. Although we tend to think of safety in terms of significant health risks, for many patients this also includes the possibilities of side effects. For a couple to use a method, it must be accessible, i.e., immediately available (especially in coitally dependent or use-oriented methods) and affordable for the patient. The effects of a method on spontaneity or modes of sexual expression may be important in some cases. The ability of a contraceptive method to provide some protection against sexually transmitted diseases may also be relevant. Furthermore, cultural, religious, or social considerations may influence a couple's choice of contraceptive method. Career or other life choices as well as plans for future fertility may influence the type and duration of the method chosen. Finally, the couple's feelings about which partner should take responsibility for contraception may be important. The clinician must be sensitive to all these factors that might influence the decision and provide factual information that fits the needs of the patient and her partner. A decision tree based on this concept is presented in Figure 22.1.

Table 22.1.
Failure Rates for Various Contraceptive Methods

Method	Estimated Pregnancy Rates[a] (%)
Oral contraceptives	<1–2
Implantable rod (Norplant)	<1
Long-acting injectable (progesterone, Depo-Provera)	<1
Intrauterine device	2–4
Diaphragm (with spermicide)	10–20
Condom	5–15
Spermicide	
Foam	15–30
Jelly, cream	15–35
Rhythm	
Calendar	15–45
Temperature	1–20
Temperature plus intercourse only after ovulation	1–10
Cervical mucus	1–25
Withdrawal	20–25
Postcoital douche	40
No method	90

[a] Rates are those during the 1st year of use, assuming variations in consistency of use.

HORMONAL CONTRACEPTIVES

For many women, *"birth control"* is synonymous with the oral contraceptive pill, which in turn is synonymous with hormonal contraception. Recently, their choices have expanded to injectable hormonal preparations (injectable medroxyprogesterone; Depo-Provera) and an implantable progestin mechanism (Norplant).

More than 150 million women worldwide have used oral contraceptives, and roughly one-third of sexually active, fertile women in the United States currently use these agents. It is estimated that about one-half of women in the United States 20 to 24 years old use oral contraceptives. Despite this widespread use, "the Pill" is often mistrusted or misunderstood. In a 1985 Gallup pole, two-thirds of the respondents said that they thought the Pill was more dangerous than pregnancy, and up to one-third thought that the Pill caused cancer. This lack of knowledge about such a commonly used contraceptive

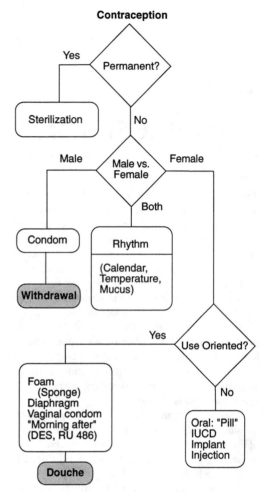

Figure 22.1. One of many possible decision-tree approaches to the choice of contraceptive methods. Methods shown in gray have a relatively higher failure rate and should not be used if pregnancy prevention is a high priority.

method makes patient education a high priority for those who care for these women.

Hormone-based contraceptives provide the most effective reversible pregnancy prevention available. Failure rates for oral contraceptives are in the range of 1% or less. Long-acting hormonal methods (injections and implantable capsules) have effectiveness rates that equal or even surpass sterilization. Because failures are generally related to missed pills, injectable or implantable long-acting agents share the same advantage that they provide reliable contraception without concern for daily compliance.

Table 22.2.
Estrogen and Progestin Content and Potency in Common Oral Contraceptives

Preparation	Estrogen	μg	Progestin	Days	mg	Progestin Potency
Demulen	Ethinyl estradiol	50	Ethynodiol diacetate		1	High
Ovral	Ethinyl estradiol	50	Norgestrel		0.5	High
Norlestrin 2.5/50	Ethinyl estradiol	50	Norethindrone acetate		2.5	Medium
Norlestrin 1/50	Ethinyl estradiol	50	Norethindrone acetate		1	Medium
Norinyl 1 + 50	Mestranol	50	Norethindrone		1	Low
Ortho-Novum 1/50	Mestranol	50	Norethindrone		1	Low
Demulen 1/35	Ethinyl estradiol	35	Ethynodiol diacetate		1	High
Norinyl 1 + 35	Ethinyl estradiol	35	Norethindrone		1	Low
Ortho-Novum 1/35	Ethinyl estradiol	35	Norethindrone		1	Low
Ortho-Novum 10/11	Ethinyl estradiol	35	Norethindrone		0.5	Low
followed by	Ethinyl estradiol	35	Norethindrone		1	Low
Brevicon	Ethinyl estradiol	35	Norethindrone		0.5	Low
Ovicon 35	Ethinyl estradiol	35	Norethindrone		0.4	Low
Modicon	Ethinyl estradiol	35	Norethindrone		0.5	Low
Lo/Ovral	Ethinyl estradiol	30	Norgestrel		0.3	Medium
Loestrin 1.5/30	Ethinyl estradiol	30	Norethindrone acetate		1.5	Medium
Nordette	Ethinyl estradiol	30	Levonorgestrel		0.15	Medium
Loestrin 1/20	Ethinyl estradiol	20	Norethindrone		1	Medium
Ovrette			Norgestrel		0.075	Low
Micronor			Norethindrone		0.35	Low
Nor-Q D			Norethindrone		0.35	Low
Ortho Tri-cyclen	Ethinyl estradiol	35	Norgestimate	1–7 8–14 15–21	0.18 0.215 0.25	Low
Ortho-Novum 7/7/7	Ethinyl estradiol	35	Norethindrone	1–7 8–14 15–21	0.5 0.75 1.0	Medium
Tri-Norinyl			Norethindrone	1–7 8–16 17–21	0.5 1.0 0.5	Medium
Tri-Levlen	Ethinyl estradiol	30×6	Levonorgestrel	1–6 7–11 12–21	0.05 0.075 0.125	Medium
Triphasil	Ethinyl estradiol	40×5	Levonorgestrel	1–6 7–11 12–21	0.05 0.075 0.125	Medium

Biochemistry and Methods of Action

Most of the oral contraceptive formulations available are *combinations of an estrogen and a progestin.* Currently, there are many estrogen-progesterone and progesterone-only products, with varying formulations, on the market in the United States (Table 22.2). The most frequently used synthetic estrogen is *ethinyl estradiol*, although a few products contain *mestranol*. Based on human endometrial response and selected biochemical markers, ethinyl estradiol is thought to be about 1.7 times as potent as the same weight of mestranol. Ethinyl estradiol is absorbed by the stomach; peak serum levels are reached within 1 hr of ingestion, with mestranol peaking somewhat later.

The *progestins* used in oral contraceptives are all androgens of varying potency, and all lack the methyl group on carbon 19 of the steroid molecule. Common examples of these progestins — in descending order of biologic progestin activity — are *norgestrel, ethynodiol diacetate, norethindrone acetate, norethynodrel, and norethindrone.* Oral contraceptives using the less-androgenic agents *desogestrel* and *gestodene* have recently been introduced.

Most oral contraceptives contain a fixed ratio of estrogen and progestin. *"Phasic" formulations* have been introduced that vary this ratio during the course of the month. This leads to a slight decrease in the total dose of hormone used per month but is also associated with a slightly higher rate of bleeding between periods. *Progestin-only oral contraceptives* have higher failure and complication rates and, as a result, are not widely used.

Hormonal contraceptives agents act to prevent pregnancy through several routes. These agents *block ovulation* by interfering with the pulsatile release of follicle-stimulating hormone (FSH) and luteinizing hormone (LH) from the pituitary. This appears to be the main effect that confers protection from pregnancy. The estrogenic components seem to preferentially inhibit FSH and are dose dependent, whereas the progestational agents preferentially inhibit the preovulatory LH surge with a lesser effect on FSH. Hormonal agents also *alter cervical mucus*, making it thicker and more difficult for sperm to penetrate. It has been postulated that the combined estrogenic and progestational influences on the endometrium result in a thinned, unstimulated, *atrophic change in the endometrium*, inhibiting implantation. This latter effect sometimes results in scant or missed menses. For most patients the establishing of regular, highly predictable, scant, and relatively painless menses is an added benefit of oral contraceptives.

Effects of Hormonal Contraceptives

Hormonal contraception affects more than just the reproductive system. Estrogens cause alterations in glucose tolerance, affect lipid metabolism, potentiate sodium and water retention, increase renin substrate, and can reduce antithrombin III.

Progestins increase sebum, facial and body hair, induce smooth muscle relaxation, and increase the risk of cholestatic jaundice. The newer progestational agents, desogestrel and gestodene, have less metabolic impact.

Oral contraceptives have many beneficial effects. As many as 1 in 750 women, or some 50,000 women a year in the United States, will avoid hospitalization because of the beneficial effects of oral contraceptives. Oral contraceptive users have a lower incidence of endometrial and ovarian cancer, benign breast and ovarian disease, and pelvic infection. Ectopic pregnancy is prevented along with the complications of intrauterine pregnancies. Menstrual periods are predictable, shorter, and less painful, and as a result, the risk of iron deficiency anemia is reduced. Fewer cases of toxic shock are reported. There even appears to be a protective effect against rheumatoid arthritis.

High-dose oral contraceptives are associated with a greater risk of serious complications, whereas low-dose products have a greater likelihood of *breakthrough bleeding and pregnancy.* Breakthrough bleeding is spotting that occurs in midcycle and usually disappears with continued use of the same preparation or with the use of preparations with more estrogen. *Serious complications* such as venous thrombosis, pulmonary embolism, cholestasis and gallbladder disease, stroke, and myocardial infarction were more likely for women using the high-dose early formulations of oral contraceptives. Hepatic tumors have also been associated with the use of oral contraceptives. These tumors are rare and have been most closely associated with high-dose mestranol-containing drugs. Although all of these complications are from 2 to 10 times more likely in pill users, they are still rare. Factors such as age, weight, and especially smoking also represent significant risk factors.

Less serious but more common side effects also depend on the dosage and type of hormones used. Estrogens may cause a feeling of bloating and weight gain, breast tenderness, nausea, fatigue, or headache. Progestins are often blamed for symptoms such as acne or depression. Most of these minor side effects may be treated by altering the dose or composition of the agent used.

The appearance of some symptoms in a patient using oral contraceptives mandates immediate evaluation of the patient with discontinuation of the oral contraceptive and initiation of a nonhormonal contraceptive method. Other symptoms do not require discontinuation of the oral contraceptive but do require immediate evaluation (Table 22.3).

A better understanding of steroid biochemistry has led to a continuing decrease in the dosage of hormones needed to provide effective contraception, which has also decreased complications and breakthrough bleeding. Every effort should be made to take advantage of lower-dosage products, while balancing the need for reliability and freedom from menstrual disturbances.

Patient Evaluation for Oral Contraceptive Use

Before considering oral contraceptives for a patient, a careful evaluation is required. Not only is *the Pill relatively or absolutely contraindicated in some patients* (Table 22.4) but even factors such as previous menstrual history may have an impact on the choice of these agents.

As an example, approximately 3% of patients may experience problems with resumption of their periods after prolonged oral contraceptive use (*postpill amenorrhea*). Younger women and those with *irregular periods* before the use of oral contraceptives are more likely to experience this problem after discontinuing their use, either because of the pills or a resumption of their previous menstrual pattern. These patients deserve counseling about this potential complication or a consideration of alternative methods.

Oral contraceptives may interact with other medications that the patient is taking. This interaction may reduce the efficacy of either the oral contraceptive or the other medications. Examples of drugs that decrease the effectiveness of oral contraceptives include penicillin-based antibiotics, tetracycline, barbiturates, ibuprofen, phenytoin, and the sulfonamides. Drugs that may show retarded biotransformation when oral contraceptives are also used include anticoagulants, insulin, methyldopa, hypoglycemics, phenothiazines, and tricyclic antidepressants. Before prescribing medications to women using oral contraceptives, the clinician should pay attention to possible drug interactions.

Injectable and Implantable Hormonal Contraceptives

Long-acting hormonal contraception is possible through the use of injectable or implantable progestins. Injectable medroxyprogesterone acetate (DMPA; Depo-Provera) and a device to implant levonorgestrel for slow release (Norplant) are both approved for use in the United States. These methods offer long-term reversible contraception (3 months for Depo-Provera; 5 years for Norplant) without the adverse effects of estrogen or the necessity of daily patient compliance. Both progestin methods act to suppress ovulation; thicken cervical mucus, impeding sperm transport; create an endometrium unsuitable for implantation; and alter the rate of ovum transport, all of which combine to prevent pregnancy.

Norplant, Depo-Provera, and other long-acting progestins are associated with a moderate in-

Table 22.3.
Symptoms That Require Intervention in a Patient Taking Oral Contraceptives

Symptom	Possible Etiology
Discontinue OCP,[a] start nonhormonal contraceptive method, immediate evaluation	
Loss of vision, diplopia	Retinal artery thrombosis
Unilateral numbness, weakness	Stroke
Chest/neck pain	Myocardial infarction
Slurring of speech	Stroke
Severe leg pain, tenderness	Thrombophlebitis
Hemoptysis, acute SOB,[b] chest pain	Pulmonary embolism
Hepatic mass, tenderness	Hepatic neoplasm, adenoma
Continue OCP, immediate evaluation	
Amenorrhea	Pregnancy
Breast mass	Breast cancer
Right upper quadrant pain	Cholecystitis, cholelithiasis
Severe headache	Pain preceding stroke
Galactorrhea	Pituitary adenoma

[a] Oral contraceptive pill.
[b] Shortness of breath.

cidence of menstrual disturbance and progesterone-related side effects. During the early stages of use, as many as one-third of women using these methods will experience breakthrough bleeding or amenorrhea. Women using long-acting injections generally will become amenorrheic, while many women using implantable rods return to cyclic menstrual bleeding while using the method.

Depo-Provera is given as a 150 mg injection every 3 months. As this dosage provides a contraceptive effect for 4 months, there is margin of error for repeat injection. Norplant rods are inserted subcutaneously in a short office procedure using local anesthesia. Presently available 6-rod preparations provide contraceptive effect for 5 years, at which time they must be replaced if continued contraception is desired (Fig. 22.2). Although these methods may not be reversed as simply as merely discontinuing a daily tablet, they are a convenient and attractive alternative for many women. Most women who discontinue Depo-Provera injection do not become fertile for 4 to 5 months thereafter, although 80% who are trying will become pregnant within 12 months.

BARRIER CONTRACEPTIVES

Among the oldest and most widely used contraceptive methods are those that *provide a barrier between sperm and egg* and include condoms (for one or both partners), diaphragms, and cervical caps. Each of these methods *depends on proper use before or at the time of intercourse and, as such, are subject to a higher failure rate than oral contraceptives, because of inconsistent or incorrect use as well as actual damage to the barrier material itself.* Despite this, *these methods provide relatively good protection* from

unwanted pregnancy; are inexpensive; may provide varying degrees of protection from sexually transmitted diseases; and in the case of condoms, do not require medical consultation.

Condoms

Condoms are sheaths usually worn over the erect penis or inside the vagina to prevent sperm from reaching the cervix and upper genital tract. Although almost one-half of all condoms are sold to women, the condom is the only reliable, nonpermanent method of contraception available to males. Condoms are widely available and inexpensive. They may be made of latex or, less commonly, animal membrane (usually sheep cecum). They are available with or without lubricants or spermicides, plain or with reservoir tips, in colors, flavors, and with ridges. There are even those that glow in the dark. Although most of these choices are of personal preference only, both lubrication and a reservoir tip reduce the likelihood of breakage.

The condom is well tolerated with only rare reports of skin irritation or allergic reaction. Some men complain of reduced sensation with the use of condoms, but this may actually be an advantage for those with rapid or premature ejaculation. The slippage and breakage rate in normal use is estimated at 5 to 8%.

The recent introduction of the *female condom* provides another option for some couples. This is a sheath, or vaginal liner, that fits into the vagina before intercourse. Like the traditional male condom, this contraceptive relies on patient motivation to ensure proper use with each episode of intercourse. Three devices are presently available: a condom that looks like a G-string panty with a

Table 22.4.
Contraindications to the Use of Oral Contraceptives

Absolute contraindications	Relative contraindications
Cardiovascular disease (severe)	Age 35+ with smoking
Cerebrovascular disease (stroke)	Diabetes mellitus
Congenital hyperlipidemia	Epilepsy
Hepatic disease (with abnormal liver function)	Galactorrhea (of unknown cause)
Hepatic tumor	Gallbladder disease
Malignancy (current): breast, endometrium, ovary	History of anovulation or oligoovulation
Obstructive jaundice of pregnancy (history)	Lactation
Ongoing pregnancy	Moderate uterine fibroids
Pulmonary embolism	Obesity
Vaginal bleeding (of unknown source)	Sickle-cell disease
Venous thrombosis	Vaginal adenosis
	Varicose veins (severe)
	Vascular headaches (migraine, cluster)

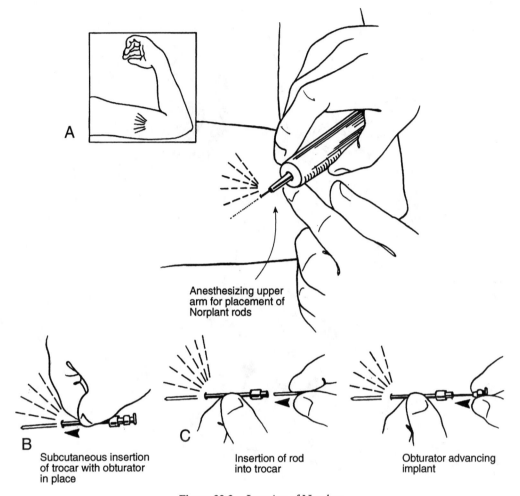

A Anesthesizing upper
arm for placement of
Norplant rods

B Subcutaneous insertion
of trocar with obturator
in place

C Insertion of rod
into trocar

Obturator advancing
implant

Figure 22.2.   Insertion of Norplant.

condom rolled within the crotch to be unrolled by
the penis; the Women's Choice condom, similar to
a male condom, with a 2 inch flexible ring that
hangs from the vaginal opening and a thickened
upper domed end that is inserted into the vagina
with a tampon-like applicator; and the Reality
condom, a polyurethane sheath with an open
ringed end to the outside and a closed internal
ring placed over the cervix, much like a diaphragm
(Fig. 22.3). All have slippage/breakage rates of
about 3%.

Both male and female latex condoms are
thought to provide *some protection against sexually
transmitted diseases.* Neither method provides complete protection, and couples should still be cautioned about high-risk behaviors.

Diaphragms and Cervical Caps

The diaphragm is a springy ring with a dome of
rubber. Proper use of a diaphragm includes apply-
ing a contraceptive jelly or cream containing spermicide to the center and rim of the device, which
is then inserted into the vagina, over the cervix,
and behind the pubic symphysis. In this position,
the diaphragm covers the anterior vaginal wall and
cervix.

There are three types of diaphragms made in
sizes from 50 to 105 mm in 2.5- and 5-mm increments. Most women use 60- to 85-mm diaphragms. The *flat or coil spring type* is suitable for
women with good vaginal tone; it forms a straight
line when pinched for insertion. The *arcing spring*

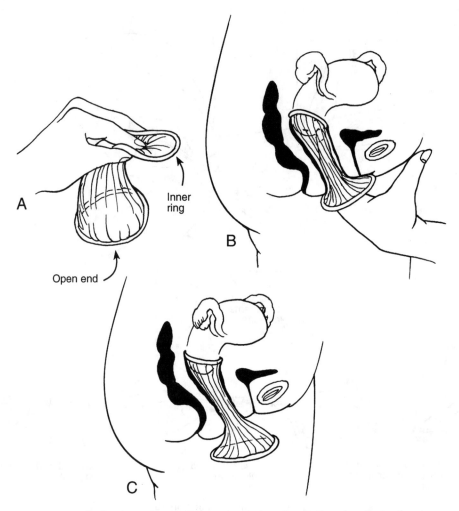

Figure 22.3. The female condom. **A,** Preparation for insertion. **B,** Insertion. **C,** Condom in proper position.

diaphragm comes in two types: the All Flex and the hinged types. These are easier for most women to insert and are more useful for women with poor vaginal tone, cystoceles, rectoceles, a long cervix, or an anterior cervix with a retroverted uterus. The diaphragm must be inserted before intercourse (up to 1 hr before) and be left in place for 6 to 8 hr after. It may then be removed, washed, and stored. Should additional intercourse be desired during the 6- to 8-hr waiting time, additional spermicide should be applied without removing the diaphragm and the waiting time restarted.

Diaphragms must be fitted to the individual patient. Fit may change with significant weight change, vaginal birth, or pelvic surgery. The diaphragm should be the largest that can be comfortably inserted, worn, and removed. If the diaphragm is too small, it may slip out during coitus because of vaginal elongation; if it is too large, it may buckle, causing discomfort, irritation, and leakage. The patient must be initially instructed in the proper positioning of the diaphragm, with the correct position subsequently verified by the patient each time it is used. If the cervix can be felt through the dome of the diaphragm, the positioning is correct. If a diaphragm is fitted in the postpartum period, its sizing should be reevaluated in 2 to 3 months because vaginal dimensions and support may change in the interval. The three

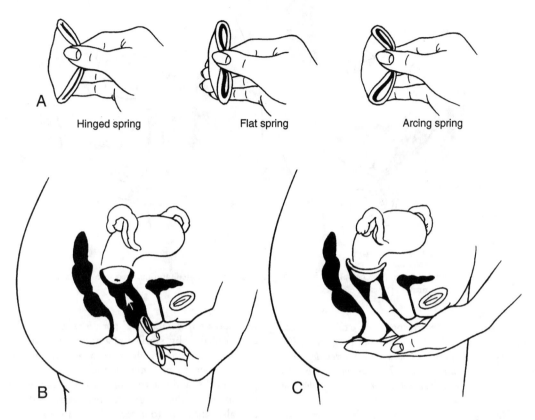

A Hinged spring   Flat spring   Arcing spring

B   C

Figure 22.4. Diaphragms. **A,** The three types of diaphragms. **B,** Insertion of the diaphragm. **C,** Checking to ensure that the diaphragm covers the cervix.

types of diaphragms and correct positioning of a diaphragm are shown in Figure 22.4.

Women who use diaphragms are slightly more susceptible to urinary tract infection, presumably because of pressure against the urethra and a relative urinary stasis.

Fitting a diaphragm involves two steps. The first step is a pelvic examination followed by trial-and-error fitting of various sizes of diaphragms until one meets the criteria noted above. The second step is to allow the patient to practice insertion, check for proper position, and remove the device, with supervision, until she is comfortable with the process and both she and the physician know that she is placing the diaphragm properly. Much of the failure associated with diaphragms may be traced to the patient not using the device because of discomfort with the method and/or improper placement.

The *cervical cap* is a smaller version of the diaphragm that is applied to the cervix itself. This method is associated with a relatively high degree of displacement and, therefore, of failure as well as association with cervicitis and toxic shock syndrome. It also requires considerable effort to fit.

Spermicides and the Vaginal Sponge

Although many "spermicidal" chemicals have been tried over the years, today's spermicides rely on one of two agents to immobilize or kill sperm: *nonoxynol-9 and octoxynol-3*. These compounds are inserted into the vagina before intercourse and are delivered in a variety of ways: creams, jellies, foams, films, suppositories, and sponges. They should be applied high into the vagina against the cervix, from 15 to 60 min before each act of intercourse, as the duration of maximal spermicidal effectiveness is usually no more than 1 hr. Douching should be avoided for at least 8 hr after use. There is no known association between spermicide use and congenital malformation.

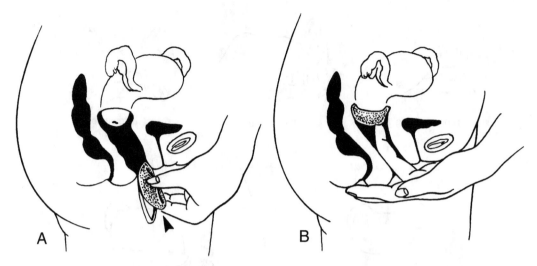

Figure 22.5 Vaginal sponge. **A,** The sponge is thoroughly moistened, folded, and inserted into the vagina. **B,** The sponge is placed firmly against the cervix.

Spermicides are inexpensive, well tolerated, and provide good protection from pregnancy. *For a well-motivated couple who wish a greater degree of protection, spermicides are often combined with condoms to achieve failure rates that approach those of hormonal methods.*

The *vaginal sponge* is a polyurethane device impregnated with the spermicide nonoxynol-9. It offers some protection as a barrier, but primarily it is a means to deliver spermicide. Its failure rate approaches that of the diaphragm and spermicide, and it has the advantage of over-the-counter purchase without physician evaluation. Its use has been associated with an increased incidence of vaginitis, increased risk of infection with chlamydia and gonorrhea, and toxic shock syndrome. Because of the latter risk, the vaginal sponge should not be used during menstruation. The vaginal sponge is inserted in the vagina before intercourse and left in place from 6 to 25 hr afterward. The spermicidal sponge was introduced to allow up to 24 hr of protection with a single application. However, a failure rate slightly higher than that of other spermicides, combined with reports of toxic shock, have tempered enthusiasm for this delivery system.

INTRAUTERINE DEVICES

Intrauterine contraceptive devices (IUCDs or IUDs) are inserted into the endometrial cavity and can remain for up to several years. This long-term contraception following a simple insertion is a main advantage of IUCDs. They act to *prevent implantation and growth of the fertilized egg,* probably by sterile inflammatory response of the endometrium along with an increase in the number of polymorphonuclear leukocytes, plasma cells, and macrophages, with sperm being consumed in the phagocytic processes. IUCDs are also thought to alter tubal transport and thereby changes of fertilization.

These devices have been made of various materials, but are generally plastic. Two kinds commonly used in the United States were the Lippes Loop, a serpentine-shaped device composed of inert polypropylene plastic, and the Saf-T-Coil, a T-configuration of polypropylene with helically shaped arms. Currently available IUCDs have increased efficacy through the addition of progesterone (Progestasert) or copper (ParaGard).

Intrauterine devices are usually inserted during menses, to avoid the disruption of a pregnancy. Known cervicovaginal infection, a history of pelvic inflammatory disease (PID), infertility, or unevaluated cervical or uterine disease are contraindications to IUCD insertion. Intrauterine devices have one or two filaments (strings), which protrude from the cervix. These serve to facilitate removal and allow confirmation of the IUCD's presence, minimizing the chance of undetected expulsion or migration. Should the IUCD become "lost," x-ray, ultrasound, laparoscopy, or hysteroscopy may be required to locate and retrieve the device.

Intrauterine contraceptive devices are associated with a *relatively low failure rate* but do suffer

Lippes Loop   Saf-T-Coil   Copper-7   Copp-T (Gravigard)   Progestasert

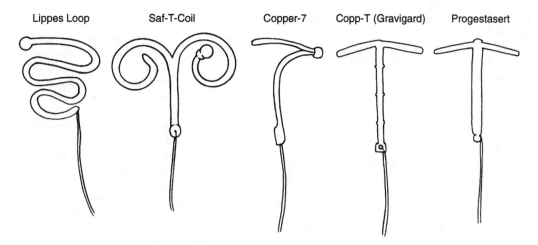

Figure 22.6.   Common IUCDs.

from a *higher rate of complications. Uterine perfora-tion* at the time of IUCD insertion is a relatively infrequent but serious complication. There is a 10% *spontaneous expulsion* rate during the 1st year following insertion. *Intermenstrual bleeding, men-orrhagia, and menstrual pain* are more common in IUCD wearers. The prevalence of this may range as high as 20% for nulliparous women.

Ectopic pregnancies are up to 10 times more common for women who wear IUCDs. This is thought to be because of the higher rate of *pelvic (tubal and ovarian) infections* also seen in IUCD us-ers. Because of concerns about ectopic pregnan-cies and sepsis, any possible pregnancy should be aggressively investigated in women with an IUCD in place. Concerns about pelvic infections and subsequent fertility often limit the use of IUCDs to women who are at low risk for sexually trans-mitted disease and to those less likely to desire further children, i.e., monogamous, multigravid patients.

NATURAL FAMILY PLANNING

So-called natural family planning (also called "the rhythm method") usually refers to methods that seek to *prevent pregnancy by either avoiding inter-course around the time of ovulation or using knowledge of the time of ovulation to augment other methods* such as barriers or spermicides. These methods are safe, cost little, and are more acceptable for religious reasons or for those couples who wish a more natural method. For couples who are highly motivated and for women with a regular men-

strual cycle, these methods may provide accept-able contraception.

The *estimation of the woman's "fertile" period* is based on calendar calculations, variations in basal body temperature, changes in cervical mucus, or a combination (sometimes called symptothermic method) of these methods. When the calendar is used, the fertile period would last from days 10 through 17 for a woman with an absolutely regu-lar 28-day cycle. Additional days are added to the fertile period based on the time of shortest and longest menstrual interval. Thus a woman with periods every 28 ± 3 days would be considered to be fertile from days 7 (10 − 3) to 20 (17 + 3). Basal body temperatures (BBTs) and changes in cervical mucus are used to detect ovulation. A rise in BBT of 0.5 to 1°F or the presence of thin, "stretchy" clear cervical mucus indicates ovula-tion.

Couples using these methods avoid intercourse until a suitable period after ovulation, i.e., from the start of menses until 2 to 3 days after tempera-ture rise or from the first awareness of the clear, copious mucous associated with ovulation until 4 to 5 days thereafter, indicated by the return of the milky or opaque mucus seen in the nonovulatory, or "safe," interval. These methods are especially difficult to use in the postpartum time, when men-strual regularity has not yet resumed and cervical secretions are varied in appearance. Resumption of normal pituitary function and ovulation usually occurs sometime in the 4th to 6th week post-partum but can vary with individuals, especially with breast-feeding. Ovulation has been reported as early as the 5th week postpartum, however, in a lactating patient.

These methods are less attractive to many couples because of the high level of motivation and cycle regularity required, along with the restrictions and loss of spontaneity placed on sexual relations.

POSTCOITAL INTERVENTION

Postcoital prevention of pregnancy is a poor substitute for planning and effective contraception. However, in instances of rape, unintended intercourse, IUCD expulsion, or barrier failure (such as condom breakage or diaphragm displacement), postcoital contraceptions are the only options immediately available. The use of *high-dose estrogen*, such as diethylstilbestrol (25 to 50 mg/day for 5 days) or oral contraceptives (Ovral, 2 tablets plus 2 tables 12 hr later), *may be effective if begun within 72 hr of exposure*. After this time or with multiple episodes of intercourse, efficacy is markedly reduced. Insertion of an IUCD up to 5 days after unprotected intercourse is often successful. Each of these methods is associated with numerous side effects and the risk of failure. When failure occurs, exposure to intrauterine steroids or an IUCD can have significant effects on the developing embryo. For this reason, these approaches are often reserved for those who would undergo a pregnancy termination should failure ensue.

The use of the antiprogesterone RU 486 (mifepristone) holds promise as an effective menstrual induction agent and abortifacient. Studies of this new agent indicate that it is safe and effective in inducing menstruation either when taken at the time of anticipated bleeding or in the case of documented early pregnancy. Social and ethical considerations will affect the availability and use of this and other postcoital agents.

INEFFECTIVE METHODS

Just as the clinician must provide information about effective contraception to those who request it, he or she must also counsel against routine use of less-than-effective techniques. *Folk lore–based techniques* such as postcoital douching, withdrawal before ejaculation (coitus interruptus), makeshift barriers (such as food wrap), and various coital positions should all be discouraged if pregnancy is to be avoided.

EXPERIMENTAL METHODS

Although there is very little new contraception research under way in the United States, there are several options that may have a role in the future. Hormonal manipulations using gonadotropin-releasing hormone (GnRH) analogs to prevent ovulation or sperm formation may be possible. The use of implantable steroids to provide an effective male contraceptive may be perfected. Vaginal steroids in the form of vaginal rings, or pessaries, show some promise. Oral antisperm agents have shown promise as well. One, *Gossypol*, a disesquiterpene aldehyde derived from the cotton plant, has shown some promise as an oral agent (20 mg daily for 4 months followed by a maintenance dose of 20 mg every other day) in decreasing spermatogenesis and sperm motility. However, concerns about its reversibility and consistent side effects (including fatigue, changes in appetite, gastrointestinal complaints, loss of libido, and weakness) have prevented approval of use in the United States. Even such modalities as testicular heating hold possibilities. It is certain that the drive to control fertility will continue to demand much from our technology.

CASE STUDIES

Case 22A

An 18-year-old nulligravid patient wants to know what is "the best method of birth control." She is not yet sexually active, although she and her boyfriend have been "close" on several occasions. The patient plans further education and correctly realizes that an unwanted pregnancy would spell disaster for her. She would not consider a pregnancy termination and the fear of pregnancy has become a problem for her and her boyfriend. Her history reveals that her periods are regular with cramping, for which she takes over-the-counter medications with some relief. She is currently taking no medications and knows of no allergies.

Questions Case 22A

In listing possible options, all of the following might be appropriate *except:*

A. Oral contraceptives
B. Vaginal spermicides
C. Diaphragm
D. IUCD
E. Rhythm

Answer: D

All of the methods listed might be possible for the couple to use. Given the patient's nulligravid status and history of dysmenorrhea, IUCDs are likely to be unsatisfactory.

The patient tells you that because of her fear of pregnancy, oral stimulation has become an important part of her and her boyfriend's sexual expression. Because they may not always have control over when they might have the opportunity for intercourse, they would also like to avoid methods that interfere with spontaneity. Based on this information, your best recommendation might be

A. Oral contraceptives
B. Vaginal spermicides
C. Diaphragm
D. IUCD
E. Rhythm

Answer: A

Oral contraceptive pills do not interfere with spontaneity and are effective anytime the opportunity of intercourse presents itself. A diaphragm would not be a good method because it does interfere with spontaneity. The couple's preference for oral stimulation makes vaginal spermicides and diaphragms (which also use spermicides) less desirable. (These agents are not toxic, per se, but do provide an objectionable taste for most couples.) Oral contraceptives are also likely to provide relief from the patient's menstrual discomfort.

Case 22B

A 22-year-old G1 P1001 patient had 6 progestin-containing rods implanted following the birth of her child 3 months ago. At the time of her 6-week postpartum check she was normal, but since that time she has developed slight random vaginal bleeding. The blood is light in amount and variable in color. She has no cramps, fever, or chills, and she is bottle feeding her infant.

Question Case 22B

The most likely cause of this condition is

A. Subinvolution of the uterus
B. Retained placental products
C. Progesterone-induced endometrial atrophy
D. Progesterone-induced endometrial hyperplasia
E. Irregular ovulation

Answer: C

Both answers A and B are unlikely to be found in an asymptomatic patient 3 months after delivery. Patients using implantable progestin-containing rods are generally anovulatory and develop a thin, atrophic endometrium. Patients should be reassured that the bleeding is expected to be self-limiting.

Case 22C

A 38-year-old G3 P2012 recently divorced business executive is taking a low-dose monophasic oral contraceptive, which she has taken since the birth of her last child 6 years ago. She has had no particular problems and does not smoke. She is not currently dating but wishes to continue effective contraception. Her pelvic examination is normal with the exception of 10-week fibroids.

Question Case 22C

Acceptable methods of contraception for this patient include

A. Tubal cautery
B. Rhythm
C. Oral contraceptives
D. Condom/foam
E. IUCD

Answer: All

For a patient who is sexually active on a sporadic basis, a use-oriented method may provide excellent protection from pregnancy without the possible problems of an ongoing method. She is an educated, potentially motivated patient who could use foam/condom, a diaphragm, or even rhythm quite effectively. The patient's age and finding of fibroids make oral contraceptives less desirable, although not unreasonable as long as close follow-up is maintained. The decision to undergo sterilization is an option that can be discussed, but is a decision that only the patient can make. The history suggests that this option has not been chosen, although it may also not have received consideration. An IUCD is less desirable because of possible expulsion by the uterus with fibroids and the fact that she is not necessarily going to be monogamous. This case is a good example of how contraception choices must be individualized for each patient and the relative risks of all alternatives discussed.

chapter 23

STERILIZATION

Sterilization offers highly effective birth control without continuing expense, effort, or motivation. *It is the most frequent method of controlling fertility used in the United States, with close to a million procedures performed annually.* About one in three married couples have chosen surgical sterilization as their method of contraception. Sterilization is the leading contraceptive method for couples when the wife is over 30 and for those who have been married more than 10 years.

Although it is possible to reverse some forms of sterilization, the difficulty of doing so, combined with the generally poor rate of success, demands that patients understand the permanent nature of the decision. The physician must be able to accurately counsel couples considering surgical sterilization and assist in determining the best method from those available. Surprisingly, twice as many women as men choose sterilization, despite the greater operative hazards involved, underscoring the need for accurate counseling of both members of the couple.

Changes in operative techniques; anesthesia methods; and attitudes of the public, insurance providers, and physicians have contributed to the rapid increase in the number of sterilization procedures performed each year. Modern methods of surgical sterilization are less invasive, less expensive, safer, and as effective — if not more effective — than those used 20 years ago. These factors have combined to decrease concern about the invasive nature of these procedures. *Counseling of patients must include the permanent nature of the procedures, the operative risks, and the chance of pregnancy (less than 1%). Despite careful counseling, approximately 1% of patients undergoing sterilization subsequently request reversal* of the procedure because of a change in marital status, loss of a child, or desire for more children. *Successful reversal occurs in only 40 to 60% of cases.*

All currently available surgical methods of sterilization prevent the union of sperm and egg, either by preventing the passage of sperm into the ejaculate (vasectomy) or by permanently occluding the fallopian tube (tubal ligation). The choice of which partner will undergo sterilization is generally a personal one. Although considerations of individual medical factors may affect this choice, the decision is most often based on the motivation of the individuals involved.

STERILIZATION IN MEN

About one-third of all surgical sterilization procedures are performed on men. Because the vas deferens is located outside the abdominal cavity, vasectomy is safer and generally less expensive than procedures done on women. Vasectomy is also more easily reversed than most female sterilization procedures. Vasectomy is routinely performed as an outpatient procedure, under local anesthesia. The procedure takes 15 to 20 min and consists of mobilizing the vas through a small incision in the scrotum; excision of a short segment of vas; and sealing the ends of the vas with suture, cautery, or clips (Fig. 23.1). Postoperative complications include bleeding, hematomas, and local skin infections, but these occur in less than 3% of cases. Some authors report a greater incidence of depression and change in body image following vasectomy than after female sterilization. This risk may be minimized with preoperative counseling and education. Concern has been raised about the formation of sperm antibodies in approximately 50% of patients, but no adverse long-term effects of vasectomy have been identified.

Pregnancy after vasectomy occurs in about 1% of cases. Many of these pregnancies result from intercourse too soon after the procedure, rather than from recanalization. Vasectomy is not immediately

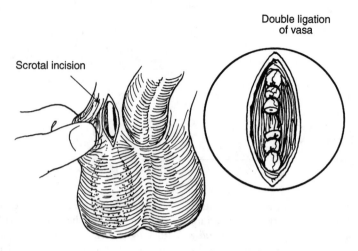

Double ligation
of vasa

Scrotal incision

Figure 23.1. Vasectomy.

effective. Multiple ejaculations are required before the proximal collecting system is emptied of sperm. For this reason, couples should use another method of contraception for 4 to 6 weeks or until azoospermia can be confirmed by semen analysis. Similar follow-up confirmation of efficacy is not routinely performed with female sterilization methods.

STERILIZATION IN WOMEN

Surgical sterilization techniques for women may be broadly divided into *postpartum* and *interval* (between pregnancies) *procedures*, although most techniques may be performed at either time. Factors such as parity, obesity, previous surgery or pelvic infections, and medical conditions (such as hypertension or respiratory diseases) may affect the timing and method chosen.

Laparoscopy

The development of efficient light sources, fiberoptic light guides, and smaller instruments has led to a dramatic increase in the use of laparoscopy for female sterilization. Performed as an outpatient interval procedure, laparoscopic techniques may be carried out under either local, regional, or general anesthesia. Small incisions, a relatively low rate of complications, and a degree of flexibility in the procedures possible have led to high physician and patient acceptability.

In laparoscopic procedures, a small infraumbilical incision is made in the skin and a trocar and sheath are placed into the abdominal cavity. Although most operators prefer to create a pneumo-

peritoneum before trocar placement, safe placement may also be accomplished without this step. The trocar is withdrawn and a laparoscope passed through the sheath into the abdominal cavity. For many procedures, two or more smaller trocars are passed (under direct vision) through the lower abdominal wall. A cannula or uterine manipulator is often employed to aid in visualizing pelvic structures and moving them into position for surgery. At the close of the procedure, the pneumoperitoneum is evacuated and the skin closed with one or two buried absorbable sutures and/or skin tapes. Closure of the facial defect is becoming more commonplace as the incidence of hernias at the trocar sites becomes more bothersome.

Occlusion of the fallopian tubes may be accomplished through the use of electrocautery (unipolar or bipolar), the application of a plastic and spring clip (the Hulka clip), or Silastic band (Yoon or Falope ring) (Fig. 23.2). The choice among laparoscopic methods is often based on operator experience and training, even though there are some theoretical differences that could guide in the decision-making process.

Electrocautery-based methods are fast and carry the lowest failure rates, but they carry a greater risk of inadvertent electrical damage to other structures, poorer reversibility, and a greater incidence of ectopic pregnancies when failure does occur (up to 25% of failures). Most operators agree that coagulation at two sites is preferable, with care being taken that the coagulation forceps is placed over the entire fallopian tube and onto the mesosalpinx so that the entire tube and its lu-

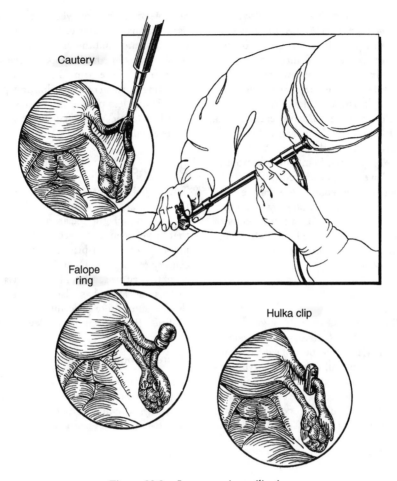

Cautery

Falope
ring

Hulka clip

Figure 23.2. Laparoscopic sterilization.

men are coagulated over a centimeter or so of the tube. Most operators also prefer bipolar cautery, because it has less risk of spark injury to adjacent tissue as the current is passed directly between the blades of the coagulation forceps.

The Hulka clip is the most readily reversed method because of its minimal tissue damage, but it also carries the greatest failure rate (up to 1%) for the same reason. As in coagulation, care must be taken to place the jaws of the Hulka clip over the entire breadth of the fallopian tube.

The Falope ring falls between the other two methods in both reversibility and failure rates but may have a higher incidence of postoperative pain, requiring strong analgesics. Care must be taken to draw a sufficient "knuckle" of fallopian tube into the Falope ring applicator so that the band is placed below the outer and inner borders

of the fallopian tube, thus occluding the lumen completely.

Laparotomy

The oldest methods of female sterilization have utilized laparotomy. Whether it is a small infra-umbilical incision made in the postpartum period or a small lower abdominal suprapubic incision (minilaparotomy) used as an interval procedure, laparotomy provides ready access to the uterine tubes. Permanent obstruction or interruption of the fallopian tubes may be then accomplished by a variety of means such as excision of all or part of the fallopian tube or the use of clips, rings, or cautery. Laparotomy techniques do not require the special tools or training needed for laparoscopy, which makes them attractive for many more physicians or smaller hospitals.

The most common method of tubal interruption done by laparotomy is the Pomeroy tubal ligation (Fig. 23.3). In this procedure, a segment of tube from the midportion is elevated and an absorbable ligature is placed across the base, forming a loop, or knuckle, of tube. This is then excised and sent for histologic confirmation. When healing is complete, the ends of the tube will have sealed closed, and there will be a 1- to 2-cm gap between the ends. Failure using this method is generally *in the range of 1 in 500 procedures.* Many modifications of this technique have been described (Table 23.1). These methods have acceptably low failure rates but are not as popular as the Pomeroy technique. Electrocoagulation or the application of clips or bands may also be accomplished through a laparotomy incision, although these are more widely used via laparoscopy.

Colpotomy

The thin wall of tissue between the vaginal canal and the posterior cul-de-sac also offers a convenient port of entry into the peritoneal cavity for sterilization procedures. All of the occlusive techniques used in laparoscopy, and many used with laparotomy, may be applied to the fallopian tubes via this route. Vaginal tubal procedures carry a high rate of vaginal incision site ("cuff") and ovar-

ian infections if prophylactic antibiotics are not used. Vaginal tubal procedures require restrictions on intercourse and the use of tampons or douches for 2 weeks while healing takes place. Some physicians place these same restrictions on patients following laparoscopic sterilization procedures as well. While less popular nowadays, this approach may have some advantage in the retroflexed and retroverted uterus.

Hysteroscopy

The possibility of transcervical obstruction of the fallopian tube avoids the inherent risks in penetration of the peritoneal cavity. Methods that have been proposed include the development of formed-in-place silicon plugs, chemical cautery (e.g., phenol), and occlusive agents such as methyl cyanoacrylate. Endometrial ablation by cautery or laser has also been suggested. Although all of these procedures offer exciting possibilities, they remain in the developmental stage.

Hysterectomy

Vaginal hysterectomy was once a preferred means of permanent sterilization for the multigravida. Nowadays, the morbidity of this procedure is felt to outweigh the benefits, especially with less ag-

Table 23.1.
Techniques of Tubal Ligation at Laparotomy

Technique	Procedure
Madlener	Tube elevated, base crushed in clamp, crushed area ligated with nonabsorbable suture
Pomeroy	Loop of tube from middle third of tube elevated, ligated with plain gut, and excised
Irving	Tube divided, proximal stump buried in uterine wall, distal stump buried in leaves of broad ligament
Cook	Tube divided, proximal stump buried in round ligament, distal stump buried in leaves of broad ligament
Kroener	Fimbriated end of tube excised
Aldridge	Fimbriated end of tube buried in broad ligament
Uchida	Mesosalpinx injected with saline-epinephrine solution and excised to expose tube, serosa of proximal end stripped off and majority of proximal segment removed, stump ligated with nonabsorbable suture and placed in broad ligament, distal end ligated, broad ligament closed with distal stump left outside the broad ligament
Partial salpingectomy	Part of tube removed
Total salpingectomy	All of tube removed
Cornual resection	Tube ligated 1 cm from cornua and excised with cornua, distal end buried in broad ligament, proximal wound covered with round ligament and broad ligament

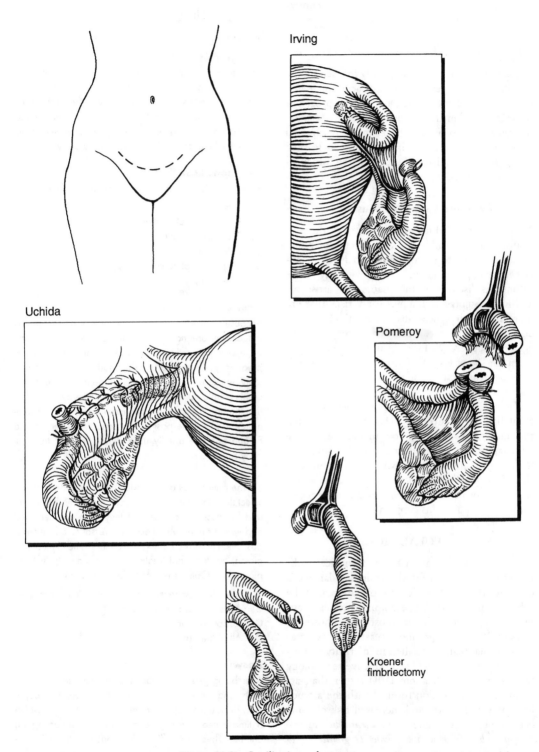

Figure 23.3.   Sterilization at laparotomy.

gressive surgical and nonsurgical means of contraception available.

Nonsurgical Methods

A great deal of interest is currently focused on the development of permanent contraception based on nonsurgical methods. One such approach is the creation of an antipregnancy vaccine. Based on immunization to progesterone, this experimental technique appears promising. As more is learned about the biochemistry of reproduction, other alternatives may become available.

Side Effects and Complications

No surgically based technology is free of the possibility of complications or side effects. Infection, bleeding, injury to surrounding structures, or anesthetic complications may occur with any of the techniques discussed in this chapter. Laparoscopic and hysteroscopic techniques carry risks that are unique to their special instrumentation, such as complications of trocar insertion or cervical damage, respectively. Failure of surgical sterilization occurs in 1% or less of all procedures and depends to some extent on the method chosen and operator experience.

Debate continues about the existence of a post-tubal ligation syndrome. It has been postulated that disruption of blood flow in the area of the fallopian tubes may influence ovarian function, leading to menstrual dysfunction and dysmenorrhea. Efforts to document or quantify such an effect have not been successful and the existence of this syndrome remains conjectural.

REVERSAL OF TUBAL LIGATION

Reversal of tubal ligation by microsurgical techniques is most successful when minimal damage is done to the smallest length of fallopian tube (Hulka clip, Falope ring, etc.), in some series approaching 50 to 75%. In most cases, however, rates of 25 to 50% are more reasonable expectations, so that many specialists in infertility recommend the use of assisted reproductive technology (e.g., in vitro fertilization; IVF) rather than attempts at tubal ligation reversal with the attendant low success rates and increased risk of tubal ectopic pregnancy. Indeed, *a patient who has undergone tubal reversal and becomes pregnant is presumed to have an ectopic pregnancy until intrauterine pregnancy is established.*

CASE STUDIES

Case 23A
A 26-year-old G3 P2002 patient is in your office for a routine prenatal visit at 34 weeks gestation. She tells you that she and her husband of 8 years have decided that their family will be complete with the birth of this next child, and they would like to know about sterilization options. Upon questioning, she says that she would like something done "Right away, if the baby is okay."

Questions Case 23A
Possible options for this couple include all of the following except:

A. Pomeroy tubal ligation
B. Tubal electrocautery
C. Falope ring
D. Vaginal tubal cautery
E. Vasectomy

Answer: D
Because of uterine size and the rich vascular supply induced by pregnancy, vaginal tubal sterilization techniques are generally not employed within 3 months of a pregnancy. Any of the other methods, including vasectomy, would be reasonable to include in the counseling of this couple. Of the choices listed, Pomeroy tubal ligation through a small infraumbilical incision is most commonly used for the postpartum patient. Cautery or the Falope ring are usually used during interval laparoscopy procedures.

The patient has a postpartum tubal ligation and you select the Pomeroy method. Three years later the patient and her husband decide that they wish another child and would prefer tubal ligation reversal to adoption, if possible. Hysterosalpingogram confirms the clinical suspicion that the tubal ligation has occluded both fallopian tubes. Options you can offer this couple include

A. Tubal ligation reversal by microsurgical techniques
B. Assisted reproductive technology
C. Adoption counseling
D. All of the above

Answer: D
After being given information about the risks, benefits, costs, and success rates of each alternative, this couple must decide their appropriate path, which may involve a time-limited trial of one path before embarking on another. These are difficult decisions and times for the couple, who require flexibility, compassion, and understanding by their physicians and friends.

Case 23B

A 23-year-old G2 P2002 patient asks your advice in choosing a method of sterilization. She has read about the options, and she presents you with a list of things she wants from her method: It should be reliable, safe, unlikely to cause future problems, quick and inexpensive, not affect libido, and not show.

Questions Case 23B

Which of the following should be included in your discussions with this patient? (Select all that apply.)

A. Reversibility
B. Operative techniques
C. Anesthetic options
D. Complications
E. Reversible alternatives (temporary methods)

Answer: All

Even though a patient has "read all about" a topic, it is imperative that a full discussion be undertaken. The likelihood of disappointment, regret, hostility, and even lawsuits can be greatly reduced by ensuring that the patient does, indeed, understand the ramifications of elective sterilization procedures and all her options. Each of the answers represents an important part of this counseling process, but by itself each is not sufficient to make an informed choice or provide an informed consent.

chapter 24

DYSMENORRHEA AND CHRONIC PELVIC PAIN

Millions of hours each year are lost from school and work because of symptoms of dysmenorrhea and chronic pelvic pain. With single-parent families and two-income households common today, the ability to diagnose and treat dysmenorrhea and chronic pelvic pain may be critical to a woman's and a family's economic status as well as to the patient's well-being.

Painful menstruation (*dysmenorrhea*) may be caused by clinically identifiable causes (*secondary dysmenorrhea*) or by an excess of prostaglandins, leading to painful uterine muscle activity (*primary dysmenorrhea*). The term *chronic pelvic pain* is generally applied to pelvic discomfort (not solely associated with menstruation), of more than 6 months duration.

Successful treatment of either dysmenorrhea or chronic pelvic pain requires a correct diagnosis. For most patients, this can be accomplished by a careful evaluation through history and physical examination. In some instances, evaluation using other modalities, including laparoscopy, may be needed. Once the diagnosis is established, specific and usually successful therapy may be instituted.

DYSMENORRHEA

Primary and secondary dysmenorrhea represent a source of recurrent disability for about 10 to 15% of women in their early reproductive years. It is uncommon for primary dysmenorrhea to occur during the first three to six menstrual cycles, when ovulation is not yet well established. The incidence of primary dysmenorrhea is greatest in women in their late teens to early twenties and declines with age. Secondary dysmenorrhea becomes more common as a woman ages, as it accompanies the rising prevalence of causal factors. The occurrence of either primary or secondary dysmenorrhea is not affected by childbearing.

Secondary Dysmenorrhea

The *causes of secondary dysmenorrhea* may be conveniently categorized into those processes that are outside the uterus, those that are within the wall of the uterus, and those that are internal or within the uterine cavity (Table 24.1). The mechanism by which these processes bring about menstrual pain is generally apparent when one considers that pain anywhere in the body occurs when there is inflammation, ischemia, stretch or distention, hemorrhage, or perforation. Pain results when these processes alter pressure in or around the pelvic structures, change or restrict blood flow, or cause irritation of the pelvic peritoneum. This may occur in combination with the normal physiology of menstruation, creating discomfort, or it may arise independently with symptoms becoming more noticeable during menstruation. *When symptoms continue between menstrual periods, these processes may be the source of chronic pelvic pain.*

Primary Dysmenorrhea

In patients with *primary dysmenorrhea*, no clinically identifiable cause of pain exists. Instead, there is *an excess of prostaglandin $F_2\alpha$ produced in the endometrium*. This potent smooth-muscle stimulant causes intense uterine contractions, resulting in intrauterine pressures that can exceed 400 mm Hg and increases in the baseline intrauterine pressure in excess of 50 mm Hg. Prostaglandin $F_2\alpha$ also causes contractions in other smooth muscle, resulting in the nausea, vomit-

Table 24.1.
Secondary Dysmenorrhea

Extrauterine causes
  Endometriosis
  Tumors (benign, malignant)
  Inflammation
  Adhesions
  Psychogenic (rare)
  Nongynecologic causes

Intramural causes
  Adenomyosis
  Leiomyomata

Intrauterine causes
  Leiomyomata
  Polyps
  Intrauterine contraceptive devices
  Infection
  Cervical stenosis and cervical lesions
  Extreme retroversion and retroflexion of the uterus

Table 24.2.
Pain and Associated Systemic Symptoms in Primary Dysmenorrhea

Symptom	Estimated Incidence[a] (%)
Pain spasmodic, colicky, labor-like; sometimes described as an aching or heaviness in lower middle abdomen; may radiate to the back and down the thighs; starts at onset of menstruation; lasts hours to days	100
Associated symptoms	
Nausea and emesis	90
Tiredness	85
Nervousness	70
Dizziness	60
Diarrhea	60
Headache	45

[a] In women with primary dysmenorrhea.

ing, and diarrhea reported by many women (Table 24.2). Prostaglandin production in the uterus normally increases under the influence of progesterone, reaching a peak at, or soon after, the start of menstruation. With the onset of menstruation, formed prostaglandins are released from the shedding endometrium. In addition, the necrosis of endometrial cells provides increased substrate arachidonic acid from cell walls for prostaglandin synthesis. In addition to prostaglandin $F_2\alpha$, prostaglandin E_2 is also produced in the uterus. Prostaglandin E_2, a potent vasodilator and inhibitor of platelet aggregation, has been implicated as a cause of primary menorrhagia.

Clinical Evaluation

When *evaluating the patient with menstrual pain*, special attention should be paid to the patient's *history*. Patients with *primary dysmenorrhea* will present with recurrent, month-after-month, spasmodic lower abdominal pain, which occurs on the first 1 to 3 days of menstruation. The pain is often diffusely located in the lower abdomen and suprapubic area, with radiation around or through to the back. The pain is described as "coming and going," or labor-like. The patient will often illustrate their description with a fist opening and closing. This pain is frequently accompanied by moderate to severe nausea, vomiting, and/or diarrhea. Fatigue, low backache, and headache are also common. Patients often assume a fetal position in an effort to gain relief and many will report having used a heating pad or hot water bottle in an effort

to decrease their discomfort. Dyspareunia is generally not found in patients with primary dysmenorrhea and, if present, should suggest a secondary cause.

In patients with *secondary dysmenorrhea*, symptoms may be slightly milder and are often more general in nature. The specific complaint that an individual patient has will be determined by their underlying abnormality. Frequently, a careful history will suggest the possibility of an ongoing problem and help direct further evaluations. Complaints of heavy menstrual flow, combined with pain, suggest uterine changes such as adenomyosis, myomas, or polyps.

Adenomyosis is islands of endometrial tissue within the myometrium, resulting in a usually tender, symmetrically enlarged, "boggy" uterus. Menses are especially uncomfortable. The diagnosis is supported by exclusion of other causes of secondary dysmenorrhea but can be definitely made only by histologic examination of a hysterectomy specimen.

Pelvic heaviness or a change in abdominal contour should raise the possibility of large leiomyomata or intraabdominal neoplasia. Fever, chills, and malaise should suggest the presence of an inflammatory process. A coexisting complaint of infertility may suggest endometriosis or chronic pelvic inflammatory disease. If the patient reports that her symptoms started only after placement of an intrauterine contraceptive device (IUCD), the IUCD must be regarded as the probable cause.

Assessment

For patients with dysmenorrhea, the physical examination is directed toward uncovering possible causes of secondary dysmenorrhea. The presence of asymmetry or irregular enlargement of the uterus should suggest myomas or other tumors. Symmetrical enlargement of the uterus is often found in patients with adenomyosis. Painful nodules in the posterior cul-de-sac and restricted motion of the uterus should suggest endometriosis. Restricted motion of the uterus is also found in cases of pelvic scarring from adhesions or inflammation. Thickening and tenderness of the adnexal structures caused by inflammation may suggest this diagnosis as the cause of secondary dysmenorrhea. Cultures of the cervix for *Neisseria gonorrhoeae or Chlamydia trachomatis* should be obtained if infection is suspected.

Physical examination of patients with primary dysmenorrhea should be normal. There should be no palpable abnormalities of the uterus or adnexa, and no abnormalities should be found on speculum or abdominal examinations. Patients examined while experiencing symptoms will often appear pale and "shocky," but the abdomen will be soft and nontender, with a normal uterus.

In evaluating the patient thought to have primary dysmenorrhea, the most important differential diagnosis is that of secondary dysmenorrhea. Although the patient's history is often characteristic, a diagnosis of primary dysmenorrhea should not be made without a thorough evaluation to eliminate other possible causes. In patients with chronic pain, the clinician must always consider nongynecologic causes as a possibility. In some patients, a final diagnosis may not be established without invasive procedures, such as laparoscopy.

Therapy

In patients with dysmenorrhea in whom no clinically identifiable cause is apparent, it is appropriate to presume a diagnosis of primary dysmenorrhea. Therapy with nonsteroidal antiinflammatory agents is generally so successful that, if some response is not evident, the diagnosis of primary dysmenorrhea should be reevaluated. Other useful components of therapy for primary dysmenorrhea include the application of heat; exercise, psychotherapy, and reassurance; and on occasion, endocrine therapy, i.e., oral contraceptives to induce anovulation.

Patients with primary dysmenorrhea will generally experience exceptional pain relief through the use of nonsteroidal antiinflammatory drugs (NSAIDs), which are prostaglandin-synthetase inhibitors. Treatments include 500 mg of mefenamic acid (Ponstel) followed by 250 mg every 4 to 6 hr, 1200 to 1600 mg of ibuprofen (Motrin) followed by 600 to 800 mg three times a day, or 150 mg of diclofenac (Voltaren) followed by 75 mg three times a day (Table 24.3). Over-the-counter dosages of ibuprofen or other NSAIDs may be used in many patients with milder symptoms.

In the very rare patient who does not respond to these therapies and whose pain is so severe as to be incapacitating, *presacral neurectomy* may be a consideration. The procedure involves surgical disruption of the "presacral nerve," the superior hypogastric plexus, which is found in the retroperitoneal tissue from the fourth lumbar vertebra to the hollow over the sacrum. It is associated with considerable morbidity if the adjacent venous structures are disrupted.

As in other areas of medicine, the best therapy is one directed toward the cause of the patient's problems. Hence, when a specific diagnosis is possible, therapy tailored to that process will be the most likely to succeed. Specific treatments for many of these processes are discussed in their respective chapters. When definitive therapy cannot be employed (e.g., in the case of a patient with adenomyosis in whom fertility is to be preserved, thereby making hysterectomy inappropriate), symptomatic therapy in the form of analgesics and/or modification of the menstrual cycle may be effective. The dysmenorrhea may be improved with the use of low-dose oral contraceptives in those patients who desire contraception and have no contraindications to their use.

CHRONIC PELVIC PAIN

The *prevalence* of chronic pelvic pain is less than that of dysmenorrhea but still represents a source of significant disability. It is a problem that often demands a great deal of time and resources, from both physician and patient, to make a diagnosis and establish treatment. In these patients, the pathophysiology involved can be quite variable (Table 24.4). In many patients, the pain itself becomes the disease. Indeed, in approximately one-third of patients with chronic pelvic pain who undergo laparoscopic evaluation, no identifiable cause is found. However, two-thirds of these patients will have potential causes identified where none was apparent before laparoscopy. A wide-ranging, often multidisciplinary, approach to these patients will yield the best results.

The *history* reported in chronic pelvic pain can be varied. In general, it will relate to the underlying etiology. As with the evaluation of any pain, attention must be paid to the description and timing of the symptoms involved. The presence of gastrointestinal symptoms, urinary difficulties, or back problems should suggest the possibility of nongynecologic causes. The history must include a thorough medical, surgical, menstrual, and sexual history. Inquiries should be made into the patient's home and work status, social history, and family history (past and present). The patient should be questioned about sleep disturbances and other signs of depression.

Assessment Hx Patient Recognition

As in patients with dysmenorrhea, the *physical examination* of patients with chronic pain is directed toward uncovering possible causative pathologies.

The patient should be asked to indicate the location of the pain. This will act as a guide to further evaluation and provide some indication of the character of the pain by the way in which the patient points. For example, if the location of the pain is indicated with a single finger, you are probably dealing with a different process than when the patient uses a sweeping motion of the whole hand. Maneuvers that duplicate the patient's complaint should be noted, but undue discomfort should be avoided to minimize guarding, which would limit a thorough examination. Many of the same conditions that cause secondary dysmenorrhea may cause chronic pain states. As in the evaluation of patients with dysmenorrhea, cervical cultures should be obtained if infection is suspected.

For most patients, a reasonably accurate differential diagnosis can be established through the history and physical examination. *At times, the wide range of differential diagnoses possible in chronic pelvic pain lends itself to a multidisciplinary approach,* which

Table 24.3
Clinical Drug Usage for Primary Dysmenorrhea

Drug (Trade name)	Initial Dose (mg)	Following Dose
Acetic/Salicylic Acids		
Indomethacin (Indocin)	25	25 mg t.i.d.
Tolmetin (Tolectin)	400	400 mg t.i.d.
Sulindac (Clinoril)	200	200 mg b.i.d.
Diflunisal (Dolobid)	1000	500 mg q. 12h.
Diclofenac (Voltaren)	75–150	75 mg b.i.d.
Ketorolac (Toradol)	10	10 mg q. 4–6h. (40 mg/24 hr max.)
Propionic Acids		
Ibuprofen[a] (Motrin, Rufen)	400	400 mg q. 4h.
Naproxen (Naprosyn)	500	250 mg q. 6–8h.
Naproxen[a] sodium (Anaprox)	550	275 mg q. 6–8h.
Fenoprofen calcium (Nalfon)	200	200 mg q. 4–6h.
Ketoprofen (Orudis)	75	75 md t.i.d. q. 4–6h.
Fenimates		
Mefenamic acid[a] (Ponstel)	500	250 mg q. 4–6h.
Meclofenamate (Meclomen)	100	50–100 mg q. 6h.

[a] FDA approved for primary dysmenorrhea.

Table 24.4
Chronic Pelvic Pain

Gynecologic causes	Other
Adnexal	Neoplasia
Adhesive disease	Parasites
Chronic infection	Other causes
Chronic ectopic pregnancy	Aneurysm
Torsion of pelvic mass or organ (generally a cause of acute pain)	Musculoskeletal
Ovarian cyst (generally not painful without bleeding or growth)	Chronic back pain
Uterine	Radiculopathy
Fibroid tumors (uncommon cause of pain)	Spondylolisthesis
Infection	Ankylosing spondylitis
Retrodisplacement (rare)	Strains
Urologic causes	Rectus hematoma
Infection	Biochemical
Calculi	Sickle-cell crisis/disease
Tumors	Acute intermittent porphyria
	Heavy-metal poisoning
Gastrointestinal causes	Black widow spider bites
Inflammatory	Neurologic
Chronic appendicitis	Tabes
Gastroenteritis	Herpes zoster (shingles)
Ulcerative colitis	Psychosocial
Ulcer disease	Somatization
Irritable bowel syndrome	Sleep disorders
Diverticulitis	Substance abuse
Mesenteric adenitis	Physical or sexual abuse
Biliary disease	Family or economic stress
Mechanical	
Constipation	
Herniation	
Obstruction	
Torsion	
Intussusception	

might include psychiatric evaluation and/or testing. Consultation with social workers, physical therapists, gastroenterologists, anesthesiologists, orthopaedists, and others should be considered. The use of imaging technologies or laparoscopy may also be required to determine a diagnosis.

The evaluation should begin with the presumption that there is an organic cause for the pain. Even in patients with obvious psychosocial stress, organic pathology can and does occur. Only when other reasonable causes have been ruled out should psychiatric diagnoses such as somatization, depression, or sleep and personality disorders be entertained.

Therapy

Patients with chronic pelvic pain offer a therapeutic challenge. In these patients, care must be taken that the therapy offered does not potentiate the underlying problem. Analgesics may be used, but sparingly, and every effort must be made to reduce the

risk of both emotional and physical dependence. Suppression of ovulation may be useful as either a therapeutic modality or as a diagnostic tool to assist in ruling out ovarian or cyclic processes. Surgical therapies are appropriate only when specific surgically treatable pathologies are present and thought to be the specific cause of the patient's complaints. Alternate treatment modalities such as transcutaneous electrical nerve stimulation (TENS), biofeedback, nerve blocks, laser ablation of the uterosacral ligaments, and presacral neurectomy may be used in selected patients. *In some cases, the goal in treatment may not be a cure, i.e., elimination of chronic pain, but rather successful management of the symptoms to allow maximal function and quality of life.*

FOLLOW-UP

Patients begun on therapy for pelvic pain (dysmenorrhea or chronic pain states) should be carefully monitored for success and the possibility of complications from the therapy itself. Patients on oral contraceptives for the first time should be asked to return for follow-up after 2 months and again after 6 months. Once successful therapy is established, routine periodic health maintenance visits should continue. Patients with chronic pain should be encouraged to return for follow-up on a periodic basis, rather than only when pain is present, thus avoiding reinforcing pain behavior as a means to an end.

CASE STUDIES

Case 24A

An 18-year-old, virginal college student presents with the complaint of recurrent, severe menstrual distress, which begins a few hours after the onset of menstrual flow and lasts for the first 48 hr of menstruation. The pain is crampy, recurrent, and located in the lower abdomen, just above the symphysis. She occasionally experiences nausea with vomiting, but her pain is unchanged after she vomits. She has taken an over-the-counter pain reliever containing ibuprofen with only slight improvement. Her periods are regular, and she is taking no other medications. Pelvic examination is difficult, but normal.

Questions Case 24A

The most likely diagnosis in this patient is

A. Leiomyomata
B. Primary dysmenorrhea
C. Endometriosis
D. Irritable bowel syndrome
E. Recurrent pelvic inflammatory disease

Answer: B

In a young virginal woman, the chance of leiomyomata, pelvic infection, or endometriosis is small. The patient's history offers no hint of symptoms that might be associated with irritable bowel disease, and her physical examination does not offer evidence of other processes as a cause of secondary dysmenorrhea. This information, combined with her typical history of crampy pain, makes primary dysmenorrhea the most likely diagnosis.

The best therapy for this patient would be

A. Oral contraceptives
B. High-bulk diet
C. Tylenol (acetaminophen) with codeine, 60 mg q. 4h.
D. Ampicillin, 250 mg q.i.d. for 10 days

E. Ponstel, 250 mg, two at onset of pain and one q. 4–6h. p.r.n.

Answer: E

Although the patient might get some relief from the use of oral contraceptives, unless she needs contraception, this may not be the best course of therapy. Treatment with high-bulk diet or ampicillin does not appear to be supported by the patient's probable diagnosis. Even though the patient has tried NSAID therapy in the form of over-the-counter products, this is still the best option. The lack of complete response is most likely because of the low dose in over-the-counter products and not necessarily to product selection. It is probable that, in higher prescription dosages, she will obtain relief. If higher-dose NSAID therapy is unsuccessful, oral contraceptives should be considered, even though this patient is not sexually active.

Case 24B

A 23-year-old, divorced mother of three, on government assistance, seeks help for symptoms of lower abdominal pain, which began 8 months ago. This coincided with her divorce and the loss of her job at a textile mill. Her pain is located in her left lower quadrant, but spreads to the right lower quadrant and to her back. The pain is worse with menstruation, bowel movements, and intercourse. She has tried multiple medications without benefit. Past history reveals an abusive marriage and two previous laparotomies for "ovarian cysts."

Questions Case 24B

Based on the most likely working diagnosis, the first examination or procedure that should be performed is

A. Laparoscopy
B. Sigmoidoscopy
C. Pelvic ultrasound
D. Bimanual pelvic examination
E. Psychological profile and depression index

Answer: D

Although it is very likely that this patient has some degree of depression and multiple psychosocial stresses, a physical cause must always be considered. Sigmoidoscopy and pelvic ultrasound are not indicated based on the symptoms presented. Laparoscopy is invasive and potentially carries more risk because of the patient's previous surgeries. Although it may be needed at some point in the future, it would be premature at this point. A pelvic examination offers the most information with the least risk as an initial step in evaluation of this patient with chronic pelvic pain.

On physical examination no overt gynecologic etiology for the patient's discomfort is noted, although there is some decreased mobility of the uterus and fullness in the adnexae, which are tender to palpation. Her recto-vaginal examination is negative as is her guaiac test. Her pain persists over several visits in the next 6 months, interfering with her work and life. Narcotic analgesics are only moderately successful in alleviating her discomfort, and she does not like the way she feels when using them. A routine laboratory evaluation including complete blood count (CBC), erythrocyte sedimentation rate (ESR), Pap smear, and cultures are all negative. The patient's financial and social situations have improved, but the pain is interfering with further improvement with her pain. The next most appropriate step would be

A. Laparoscopy
B. Sigmoidoscopy
C. Pelvic ultrasound
D. Bimanual pelvic examination
E. Psychological profile and depression index

Answer: A

Pelvic ultrasound will add little information, and there are no indicators that there is a significant psychological component. Without more specific bowel symptoms, sigmoidoscopy is not warranted. Diagnostic laparosopy is appropriate, after which further therapy may be warranted, depending on the findings.

chapter 25

PREMENSTRUAL SYNDROME

Premenstrual syndrome (PMS) is a group of physical, mood, and behavioral changes that occur in a regular, cyclical relationship to the luteal phase of the menstrual cycle. In affected women, *these symptoms occur in most cycles, resolving near the onset of menses with a symptom-free interval of at least 1 week.* This cyclic symptom complex may be minimally to totally disruptive of the patient's normal daily activities and/or relationships. First described in 1931, premenstrual syndrome is still a poorly understood condition, because there is no consensus on critical issues such as its pathophysiology, its diagnostic criteria, and optimal therapies. In fact, it has been suggested that PMS is actually more than a single clinical entity. Despite these areas of confusion, it is clear that patients do present with symptoms that wax and wane in relationship to their menstrual cycles. Physicians must, therefore, be aware of potential causes for these changes, including the possibility of PMS.

INCIDENCE

Because of the wide variability in the signs and symptoms that are considered in making a diagnosis of PMS, the reported incidence of the syndrome is great, ranging between 10 and 90%. Severe, debilitating PMS is reported in less than 10% of patients, although 70% of all women have some physical or emotional premenstrual symptoms. PMS appears to be most prevalent in women in their 30s and 40s, with a greater incidence in women with a past history of postpartum depression or other affective disorders. Accurate diagnosis is further confused by the similarity between some PMS symptoms and some psychiatric conditions.

SYMPTOMS

There have been well over 150 symptoms attributed to PMS. Each patient presents with her own constellation of symptoms, thus making *specific*

symptomatology less important than the cyclic occurrence of the symptoms. Attempts have been made to classify PMS symptoms into subgroups, but none of these classification systems has been accepted universally. *Somatic symptoms* that are most common include breast swelling and pain (mastodynia), bloating, headache, constipation and/or diarrhea, and fatigue. The most common *emotional symptoms* include irritability, depression, anxiety, hostility, and changes in libido. Common *behavioral symptoms* include food cravings, poor concentration, sensitivity to noise, and loss of motor skills. *Situational depression* is associated with PMS in some cases and aggravates PMS in others. As a result, the recognition of coexisting situational depression is important by careful questioning of marital and relationship problems, occupational difficulties or change, recent childbirth or child-rearing difficulties, and family or personal problems.

ETIOLOGY

Although the etiology of PMS has not yet been determined, there are many theories related to its pathogenesis. Each theory is supported by some scientific data and also explains a portion of the symptoms seen in patients. Unfortunately, no single, unified explanation accounts for the variations of PMS seen in all patients. The theories of the basis of PMS include the following.

Psychiatric Basis

The high incidence of anxiety, depression, and other symptoms that simulate psychiatric disorders led to the theory that PMS is merely cyclic manifestations of underlying psychopathology.

Endocrinologic Basis

It was originally thought that PMS was related to abnormal luteal-phase steroid levels, predominantly higher estradiol levels relative to progesterone levels. Significant alterations in estradiol and/or progesterone levels have not been found. This theory remains viable, however, because of the cyclic nature of symptoms. It is known that progesterone does have a sedative effect on the central nervous system and that both estrogen and progesterone receptors exist in the brain.

Diet Basis

Some patients with PMS seem to have a high intake of salt and refined carbohydrates, resulting in premenstrual hypogylcemic episodes, sometimes associated with outbursts of crying and violent behavior. Diet and evaluation for glucose intolerance are advocated in this subset of patients.

Endorphin Basis

There is a relative decrease in the luteal-phase endorphin levels in some patients who suffer from PMS. Because these endogenous opiates are associated with a sense of well-being, a decline in their production is seen as a cause for some of the findings in these patients. In addition, PMS symptoms are mimicked by some symptoms of opiate withdrawal. A strong argument in favor of the endorphin basis of PMS comes from patients who describe alleviation of symptomatology when moderate exercise is undertaken, presumably because of an exercise-associated increase in endorphin production.

Serotonin Basis

Premenstrual serotonin levels in PMS patients have been reported to be lower than in control patients. Because lower serotonin levels have been associated with clinical depression, affective changes in PMS may be explained on this basis. In addition, anxiety has been described as a possible state of serotonin excess. Therefore, dysfunction in serotonin neurotransmission is an attractive explanation for many PMS symptoms.

Prostaglandin Basis

Because prostaglandins are produced in the breast, brain, gastrointestinal tract, kidney, and reproductive tract and because these are areas that often present with physical symptoms in patients with PMS, a prostaglandin-associated basis for PMS remains attractive.

Fluid Retention Basis

Many women both with and without PMS report some premenstrual weight gain and edema. Although studies do not demonstrate an increased body weight in these patients, alterations of the renin-angiotensin-aldosterone axis as well as antidiuretic hormone have been suggested as a basis for PMS.

Vitamin Basis

Particular focus has also been placed on deficiency of vitamins A, B, and E as possible causes of PMS. Of note, vitamin B_6 (pyridoxine) is a cofactor in the production of serotonin as well as prostaglandin.

Other Bases

Other suggested bases for PMS include thyroid disorders, prolactin disorders, endometrial infection, and hypoglycemia.

DIFFERENTIAL DIAGNOSIS

Virtually any condition that results in mood or physical changes in any cyclic fashion may be included in the differential diagnosis of PMS. As a result, the physician must remain open-minded at the outset in order not to prematurely exclude the primary problem. Table 25.1 outlines the possible alternatives.

DIAGNOSIS

Because the etiology of PMS is unknown, there are no definitive historical, physical examination, or laboratory markers to aid in diagnosis. At present, the diagnosis of PMS is based on documentation of the relationship of the patient's symptoms to the luteal

Table 25.1.
Differential Diagnosis of PMS

Psychiatric Conditions	Medical Conditions
Anxiety disorders	Dysmenorrhea
Major depression	Endometriosis
Bipolar disorders	Thyroid disorders
Personality disorders	Endocrinopathies
Life-circumstance disorders (marital discord, etc.)	Anemia
Substance abuse	Hypokalemia
Somatoform disorders (hypochondriasis, somatization disorders)	Lupus erythematosus
Eating disorders	

NAME _____   AGE: _____   HEIGHT: _____   WEIGHT: _____

GRADING OF MENSES

0 - None   3 - Heavy
1 - Slight   4 - Heavy and clots
2 - Moderate

GRADING OF SYMPTOMS (COMPLAINTS)

0 - None
1 - Mild, present but does not interfere with activities
2 - Moderate, present and interferes with activities
   but not disabling
3 - Severe, disabling, unable to function

MONTH

DAY	1 2 3 4 5 6 7 8 9 10 11 12 13 14 15 16 17 18 19 20 21 22 23 24 25 26 27 28 29 30 31
Treatment Day	
Menses	

Nervous tension
Mood swings
Irritability
Anxiety

Weight gain
Swelling of extremities
Breast tenderness
Abdominal bloating

Headache
Fever, chills
Increased appetite
Heart pounding
Fatigue
Dizziness/faintness

Depression
Forgetfulness
Crying
Confusion
Insomnia

DYSMENORRHEA - PAIN

Cramps (low abdominal)
Muscle ache
Joint ache

Basal Weight in lbs.

Basal Body
Temperature

NOTES:

SYMPTOM DIARY

Figure 25.1. Menstrual symptom diary.

phase. This is best done by prospective documentation of symptoms using a *menstrual diary* (Fig. 25.1). Since the patient's memory of daily symptoms cannot be depended on for accuracy given the wide variety of and sometimes subtle nature of the symptoms, she is asked to monitor and record key symptoms and their severity on a daily basis.

To confirm the diagnosis of PMS, the patient must demonstrate a symptom-free follicular phase in contrast to the problems seen in the luteal phase.

A thorough physical examination is necessary to rule out organic pathology that might explain some of the physical symptoms such as dysmenorrhea, cyclic pelvic pain, and breast tenderness.

Otherwise, there are no specific physical findings helpful in diagnosing premenstrual syndrome.

TREATMENT

Because of the diverse symptoms of patients with PMS, a multidisciplinary team of providers, including a gynecologist, psychiatrist, psychologist, endocrinologist, nutritionist, and social worker, is often advocated. In addition, because the underlying pathophysiology is yet to be determined, a wide range of treatment protocols has been recommended. A major portion of any management scheme should include *education of the patient as well as her family* to clarify what is known about PMS as well as what to expect from possible therapies that might be undertaken. Education can, in and of itself, be therapeutic for patients who are otherwise lacking insight into the possible causes of their symptoms.

As part of the educational process, prospective charting of symptoms not only documents the cyclic or noncyclic nature of the patient's symptoms but also allows the patient to become a part of the diagnostic effort, thus helping her to take an active part in the diagnosis and management of her condition. Because the existence of cyclic patient symptom complexes cannot be disputed, it remains of critical importance for the physician to address the patient's specific concerns in a supportive fashion. In some cases, giving the symptoms a diagnostic label helps relieve the patient's concern that she may be "going crazy." Often a patient's symptoms will become less unbearable as she begins to understand her condition.

In addition to patient education, the following interventions have been shown to be helpful in selected groups of patients. Patients should be advised that no one therapy works for all patients and that a logical sequence of therapeutic manipulations may have to be done to achieve resolution of symptoms.

Diet recommendations emphasize fresh rather than processed foods. The patient is encouraged to eat more fresh fruits and vegetables and minimize refined sugars and fats. Some patients benefit by eating frequent small meals during the day rather than having three large meals, thereby minimizing hypoglycemia symptoms. Minimizing salt intake may help with bloating, and eliminating caffeine from the diet can reduce nervousness and anxiety.

Exercise has been found to be helpful in some patients, possibly by increasing endogenous production of endorphins.

Medications to induce anovulation have been reported to be of benefit in PMS. Since premenstrual symptoms are typically associated with ovulatory cycles, inducing an anovulatory state in women should be beneficial in many patients. This can be accomplished by using oral contraceptives, danazol, or gonadotropin-releasing hormone (GnRH) agonist. Oral contraceptives are a logical first choice for patients who also require contraception. Some patients, however, find a worsening of their symptoms when taking oral contraceptives. The use of *danazol and GnRH* agonist have been demonstrated to be beneficial in short-term studies, but long-term effects of either drug for PMS have not been fully evaluated. The use of either constitutes a "medical oophorectomy" and may be used as a trial before oophorectomy is undertaken.

Progesterone has been described to be effective delivered either as a vaginal or rectal suppository or as oral micronized progesterone. Although well-designed studies have not demonstrated its effectiveness, progesterone suppositories are widely used by patients who describe beneficial results.

Nonsteroidal antiinflammatory agents have been found to be useful for symptoms other than dysmenorrhea. This is possibly related to prostaglandin production in various sites in the body.

Diuretics — such as *spironolactone* (25 mg p.o. b.i.d. or t.i.d.), an aldosterone antagonist; *hydrochlorothiazide* (25–50 mg p.o. q.i.d. with potassium supplementation); or *Dyazide* (hydrochlorothiazide 25 mg/triamterene 50 mg q.i.d. without the requirement for potassium supplementation) — have been found to help control weight gain as well as some psychological symptoms. Bloating is also minimized in patients taking diuretics.

Anxiolytic and antidepressant medications have been widely studied and found to be useful in some patients, especially those not responsive to other regimens. The use of these medications has often been done in consultation with a psychiatrist, especially when there is significant depression. *Buspirone* (BuSpar) is a nonsedating, nonaddictive anxiolytic found effective in some cases. It is given as an initial dosage of 5 mg p.o. t.i.d. with meals but does not demonstrate its effect for about 2 weeks. *Alprazolam* (Xanax) is also an efficacious anxiolytic given in an initial dosage of 0.25 mg p.o. b.i.d. or t.i.d.

Vitamin therapy, including administration of pyridoxine (vitamin B₆), a cofactor in the synthesis of serotonin, has been shown to be helpful in some patients. There are reported side effects, including reversible peripheral neuropathy when large doses of pyridoxine are taken. Evening primrose oil, rich in vitamin E, has also been helpful in relieving both breast tenderness and depressive symptoms associated with PMS.

CASE STUDIES

Case 25A

A 29-year-old G2 P2 complains of periodic anxiety, depression, and irritability for 2 years. Her gynecologic history includes regular menses with mild cramps. Her breasts are also mildly tender before each period. She is presently using a diaphragm for contraception. Physical examination is normal.

Question Case 25A

What initial evaluation(s) should be recommended?

A. Pelvic ultrasound
B. Psychiatric consult
C. Monthly symptom calendar
D. Mammogram
E. Glucose tolerance test

Answer: C

Because of the periodic nature of these emotional symptoms, they may or may not be temporally related to the menstrual cycle. A prospective documentation of symptoms will aid in determining whether this is PMS or not. Pelvic ultrasound is unnecessary given the normal examination. A psychiatric consult may be needed if the patient's symptoms are severe, refractory to care, or causing significant emotional or interpersonal distress. A mammogram in this age group has little to offer in a patient with cyclic mastalgia. A glucose tolerance test is sometimes used to identify a patient with hypoglycemic episodes who might present with PMS-like symptoms, but would not be appropriate here.

Case 25B

A 40-year-old G4 P4 has struggled with documented PMS for several years. Despite treatments including vaginal progesterone, tranquilizers, vitamin B, and diuretics, she continues to have 10 days of premenstrual bloating, headaches, and mood swings. She requests a hysterectomy as definitive treatment.

Question Case 25B

Which of the following medical therapies is most appropriate instead of hysterectomy?

A. Fluoxetine
B. Oral progesterone
C. Bromocriptine
D. GnRH agonist
E. Ibuprofen

Answer: D

GnRH agonist is the most appropriate of the drugs listed. The patient believes that removing the uterus will be a cure to her problems. Unfortunately, it is the ovaries, not the uterus, which may be linked with the symptoms. The uterus and monthly menses serve only as a reference point to which her symptoms are related. The GnRH can provide a temporary oophorectomy as a trial before any consideration for surgical oophorectomy. If the patient improves with GnRH agonist, then symptoms return when the medication is discontinued, bilateral oophorectomy might be a consideration. All the other therapies have been utilized for patients with PMS, but will not affect the physiologic changes she is seeking. Each may have a role, however, in treatment of specific symptoms of PMS.

chapter 26

HUMAN SEXUALITY

An estimated 40% of couples have a sexual problem at some time during their relationship. Individuals not in a steady relationship experience sexual problems as well. Illness and stress increase the frequency and often severity of these problems as well as engendering new ones. Physicians must be able to identify these problems and know whether to offer treatment or make referral to a specialist.

The first problem faced by the physician is to determine if there is a sexual problem and to specifically identify it. By demonstrating a supportive and nonjudgmental attitude, the physician creates a sense that it is permissible to discuss sexual matters and problems. To create this kind of comfortable environment, each physician must explore his or her own attitudes about the range of sexual expressions that may be encountered, his or her own sexuality, and how to address both in a manner conducive to good patient care.

DEVELOPMENT OF SEXUALITY

Human sexuality begins with the distribution of Y chromosomes, but thereafter the paths to an individual's present sexual status are complex. Various endocrinologic factors determine the expression of genetic sexual assignment. Overlaying this are the learned behaviors, first from parents, then siblings and peers, then by the individual's maturing evaluation of her own character. Most individuals are ultimately comfortable with a heterosexual identity, but others may follow gay/lesbian, bisexual, or asexual life-styles. Further, these sexual identities may change during the course of an individual's life. In addition, there are other sexual practices adding to the variety of situations encountered by the physician, including transvestism, sadomasochism, exhibitionism, voyeurism, and sexual experiences with animals. Whether any or all of these are considered "normal" is often as much a political, legal and theological question as it is a medical one.

HUMAN SEXUAL RESPONSE

Unlike the cycle-dependent estrus of lower animals, *the human sexual response is functionally volitional* and dependent on a complex interplay of emotional and physiological factors. This variability allows considerable variety in the kinds of human sexual response (e.g., alternate sexual preferences, changes based on life-style or age, changes caused by physical or emotional disturbances, etc.) and opportunity for sexual dysfunction (e.g., vaginismus, changes associated with disease, etc.). Whatever the kind of sexual response possible for an individual, it is dependent upon two factors. First, an emotional and physical system that is sufficiently functional to allow a sexual response of some kind. Second, given a system with enough function for some response, *a sustained and sufficient sexual stimulation* to initiate the cascade of responses comprising the human sexual response. *Sustained* in this context means a stimulation that occurs over a long enough interval to effect arousal. Sufficient stimulation includes two parameters: physically correct and comfortable stimulation and stimulation effective enough to initiate and sustain the human sexual response. Many of the sexual difficulties presenting to the clinician involve unsustained or insufficient stimulation.

With effective and sustained stimulation, the *human sexual response* may be initiated. Masters and Johnson, Kaplan, and others have demonstrated the value of considering the continuum of events comprising the human sexual response as consisting of "phases." Masters and Johnson have described four phases (excitement, plateau, orgasm, and resolution), whereas Kaplan has suggested a modification, combining the excitement and plateau phases and adding a desire phase at

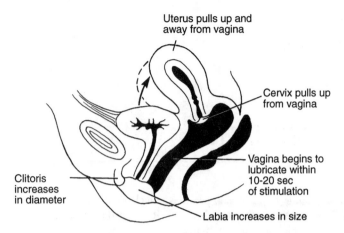

Figure 26.1. Excitement stage.

the start of the sexual response cycle. Both classifications are understood to be artificial in the sense that they describe highly variable components of a continuum of emotional and physiological events.

The *physiological components of the human sexual response* are mediated primarily by two processes: (*a*) changes in muscle tone, myotonic activity, and (*b*) changes in blood flow, especially vasocongestion. Figures 26.1 through 26.4 demonstrate some of the physiological changes seen in these phases. The duration of each phase varies with each individual and for a given individual at different times in their life. The human sexual response is a continuum of events with no clear boundaries between the described "phases." The value of these classifications lies in their use to understand the events comprising the human sexual response and to assist in the clinical classification of sexual problems and dysfunctions.

EVALUATING SEXUAL CONCERNS

Sexual History and Physical Examination

Some patients will present with a complaint involving a sexual issue or of a specific sexual dysfunction. Relatively detailed and focused questions are appropriate early on in the history taking, as these patients, by raising their issues, have indicated a willingness to discuss them. Other patients will have a medical problem that is known to be associated with sexual issues or problems, such as concerns about ability to enjoy sex after hysterectomy. Some of these patients will raise the related issues, whereas others will need to be carefully

questioned, guiding them to a discussion of the associated sexual topic.

Many patients, however, will neither express a sexually related complaint nor have a medical problem with a commonly associated sexual issue. These patients, however, often have sexually related problems, which need to be identified via the "sexual history" portion of the routine medical history. Introductory, nonobtrusive screening questions are useful. "How are things sexually?" "Do you have questions about sexual issues?" A question that gives much permission to discuss issues is: "Is there any way you would like your sex life to be different?"

The sexual history taken by the sex therapist is detailed and highly focused. For the most physicians, its purposes are less ambitious and two in content. First, it should convey to the patient a sense of comfort and trust that the physician regards sexuality and related issues as a legitimate part of health care. This is facilitated by the physician's general behavior, but also more specifically by care to listen carefully for hints of sexually related issues followed by nonobtrusive questions that give the patient "permission" to discuss her problems. If a patient perceives the physician as harboring prejudice toward her sexual values, communication is doomed to failure. Second, the physician should obtain enough information to determine if a sexual problem exists and whether it is appropriate to treat the patient or to refer her for more specialized care.

Physical examination for patients with sexual concerns is based on a thorough basic gynecologic examination. For example, dyspareunia in a young

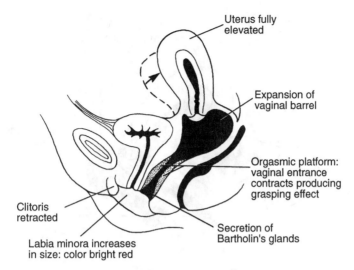

Figure 26.2. Plateau stage.

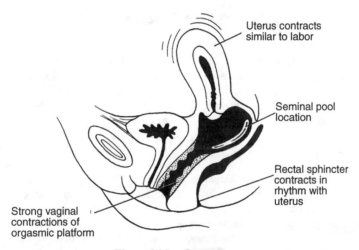

Figure 26.3. Orgasm stage.

woman might be associated with extensive endometriosis or adhesions following PID and, in an older woman not on hormone replacement therapy (HRT), with atrophic vaginitis. Detailed "sexiological" examinations involving sexual evaluation, education, and counseling are appropriately reserved for sex therapists.

Barriers to Evaluating Sexual Problems

There are many barriers between the patient with a sexuality-related problem and effective care. One of the less discussed but potentially difficult barriers occurs *when the physician is uncomfortable*

with his or her own sexuality and/or sexual issues, conveying this discomfort to the patient so that she, in turn, is unable to discuss her problems. A task for each physician is to review his or her own attitudes and feelings about sexual mattters, seeking help when needed to resolve them at least within the context of the professional relationship.

A related barrier occurs *when the physician feels inadequately prepared in knowledge or skills or has insufficient time* to deal appropriately with a sexual problem. In this situation, the physician may directly or indirectly avoid identification of such problems. This barrier can be overcome by obtaining sufficient information and evaluation/

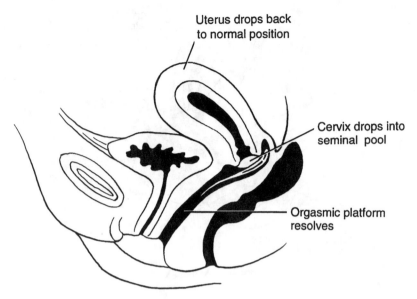

Uterus drops back
to normal position

Cervix drops into
seminal pool

Orgasmic platform
resolves

Figure 26.4.   Resolution stage.

management skills to identify a sexual problem, then treating the small number of problems amenable to limited care by a primary physician and referring the majority of problems to those with special training in sexual therapy.

Managing Sexual Problems

Some sexual problems/dysfunctions can be managed by the primary physician, whereas others are best referred immediately to a specialist in sex therapy. In general, single disorders of <1 year's duration in the context of a stable relationship are more likely to be amenable to simple interventions by a primary physician. Conversely, those patients whose dysfunction is comprised of multiple disorders, is of greater than a year's duration, and/or is in the context of a unstable relationship are usually best referred to a sex therapist. In addition, it is useful to determine whether a sexual complaint/dysfunction is primary (present throughout the patient's lifetime) or secondary (began after an interval of satisfactory sexuality) and whether it is constant (occurs in all situations, with all partners) or situational (occurs in some situations, with some partners).

In general, dysfunctions that are secondary and/or situational are more easily and successfully treated than those that are primary and/or constant. The former often involve simple problems causing sexual stimulation to not be effective or

sustained enough. Careful history taking to determine the problem and corrective counseling will often relieve the barrier to effective, sustained stimulation and return the couple to satisfactory sexuality.

It is also useful to determine where the dysfunction occurs in the human sexual response cycle. Sexual dysfunctions that occur in the later phases of the human sexual response cycle also tend to be easier to treat, with better outcomes expected, whereas in general those occurring in the desire or early excitement phases are often composed of emotional and physical factors complexly interrelated. Patients with complex problems are best referred to a qualified sex therapist.

The PLISSIT model for treatment of sexual problems is useful for the physician who chooses to treat a sexual problem along the guidelines noted. *P is permission,* giving the patient explicit or implicit permission to deal with sexual issues or problems. It also includes permission for normal behavior such as the normal exploration of sexuality via masturbation during the teen years. *LI is limited information,* providing the patient with pertinent limited amounts of useful information. In this example, learning that limited masturbation is normal and not harmful facilitates the permission. *SS is specific suggestion,* giving the patient one or two specific suggestions for action. For example, following childbirth some couples have less satisfaction with coitus because the woman's vaginal walls are less elastic or the muscles looser than previously. Teaching the patient Kegel exercises to strengthen these muscles may alleviate this complaint. *IT is intensive therapy*, which in the context of the primary care physician means referral to a specialist in sexual therapy. Examples would be therapy for orgasmic dysfunction, male sexual dysfunction, dyspareunia, etc.

CASE STUDIES

For each of the following situations, imagine yourself a primary care physician in a rural practice. You have been presented or discovered a sexual problem and taken a brief but reasonably complete history of the problem and a general sexual history. You must now decide whether to treat the patient yourself (A), perhaps using the PLISSIT model, or refer the patient to a specialist in the treatment of sexual problems (B).

For each case, choose one answer:

A. Treat
B. Refer

Case 26A

Your patient has been married for 6 months after a courtship of 2 years. At first, her marriage was fine, but now, with two new jobs and a new home, she and her husband just aren't enjoying sex like they did before marriage. They are worried that something is wrong with them or that perhaps they made a mistake in getting married.

Answer: A

It is reasonable to treat this couple using the PLISSIT model. The most likely problems are inappropriate expectations of each other and of marriage, exhaustion, and coping with new and worrisome responsibilities. For example, giving "permission" to feel as they do

may remove some underlying guilt that may be present. Providing "limited information" about the effects of their life on their sexual relationship may help explain their feelings. Making "specific suggestions" about how to set aside time for each other may aid the therapeutic process. If these steps are ineffective, referral would then be appropriate.

Case 26B

After 6 years of marriage to her policeman husband, your patient is worried about her femininity, i.e., whether she is normal. Despite a vigorous and previously quite satisfactory sex life, she is unable to have multiple orgasms with her husband during intercourse. Both she and her husband are worried. Their relationship is strained; sex is now a feared chore.

Answer: A

Limited information within the framework of the PLISSIT model will help this couple understand that multiple orgasm is a possibility but not a requirement for all people for every sexual encounter. Permission to continue their previously satisfactory sex life should be helpful.

Case 26C

Your patient has been at college for a year now, but has been unable to enjoy herself on a date, just as throughout high school. She "knows" that at her age she should enjoy sex, but it is simply repulsive to think about being touched by a man. She is afraid of her future, afraid she may actually be a lesbian, although she is aware of no more positive feelings about women then she has for men.

Answer: B

Whatever problems this young woman has, they are of long duration and by definition complex. The PLISSIT model helps in this case by allowing you to give her permission to be afraid, limited information that she can receive help, and referral for therapy.

VESTIBULE - NON KERATINIZED

Nerve Supply

Sup INTE Lymph
INNERVATION =

Sx BURNING ITCHING ODOR DISCHARGE

Hx SEXUAL ACTIVITY
NONOXYNOL 9 IS IRRITANT

CONTACT DERMATITIS

SEBORRHEIC DERMATITIS IN FAIRSKIN
                      RED HEADS

CRAB LOUSE   Tx KWELL
        IN PREGNANCY NIX or RID
SCABIES

TINEA CRURIS

VULVAR DYSTROPHY
    HYPERPLASTIC - WHITE E ACETIC ACID
        HYPER KERATOSIS   PRECANCEROUS
        2⁰ to IRRITATION
    LICHEN SCLEROSIS
        SYMMETRICAL
        THINNING of SKIN
        BIOPSY fr Dx
        Tx TESTOSTERONE CREAM
        NOT PRECANCEROUS
CANDIDA
    ↓ Cellular IMMUNITY

(PAGETS RED WHITE RED) PRECANCER
        Dont MISTAKE For CANDIDA
    KNICKERSON CULTURE of CANDIDA

chapter 27

VULVITIS AND VAGINITIS

Patients with vulvitis or vaginitis may present with acute, subacute, or indolent symptoms, ranging in intensity from minimal to incapacitating. Although generally nonspecific, the patient's history and symptoms may point to chemical, allergic, or other causes rather than infection. Irritation of the well-innervated tissues of the vulva often leads to intense pruritus. Edema, induration, and localized lesions, such as seen in herpes infection, may also be present (Table 27.1).

Vaginal secretions are always present to some extent; the amount and character of these secretions depend on the influence of chemical, mechanical, or pathologic conditions. Understanding the physiologic processes responsible for both normal and abnormal discharge will make the diagnosis of vulvitis and vaginitis more accurate.

History taking is especially important in patients with vulvar symptoms, including hygiene and sexual practices, use of deodorants and feminine products, changes in detergents, and other contact issues such as new or unusual clothes. Thorough physical examination by inspection and palpation is also important. Use of a hand magnifying lens may be useful in some instances. The physician must also be familiar with office and laboratory methods for establishing the diagnosis, especially the saline and KOH wet preparations for evaluations of vaginal secretions and discharges (Fig. 27.1). *Inaccurate diagnosis or overtreatment of a physiologic condition is doomed to fail and may even make the patient worse.*

The vulva and vagina are covered by stratified squamous epithelium. The vulva, but not the vagina, contains hair follicles and sebaceous, sweat, and apocrine glands. The epithelium of the vagina is nonkeratinized and lacks these specialized elements. The skin of the vulva is also vulnerable to secondary irritations from vaginal secretions, and both vulva and vagina are vulnerable to contact with external irritants (such as soap residue, perfumes, fabric softeners, or infestation by pinworms).

The vulva and vagina are sites of symptoms and lesions of several sexually transmitted diseases, such as herpes genitalis, human papilloma virus, syphilis, chancroid, granuloma inguinale, lymphogranuloma venereum, and molluscum contagiosum (see Chapter 28).

VULVITIS

Vulvar irritation and itching are the reasons for approximately 10% of all outpatient visits to gynecologists. Erythema, edema, and skin ulcers are all indications of possible *infection.* Ulcerative lesions should suggest the possibility of sexually transmitted disease such as *herpes or syphilis.* Other systemic diseases, such as *Crohn's disease,* may also present in this manner. Papillary lesions suggest *condyloma acuminatum or condyloma latum.* Screening should be done carefully for these and other sexually transmitted diseases. The vulvar skin is also subject to many common dermatoses, including intertrigo, seborrhea and seborrheic dermatitis, and psoriasis, as well as allergic reactions and infection with parasites such as *Pthirus pubis (the crab louse) and Sarcoptes scabiei (the itch mite).* Excoriation caused by the patient's scratching and fissuring of the skin of the vulva are often seen in vulvar irritation secondary to vaginal discharge. Chronic pruritus leads to itching and excoriation, and when chronic this is sometimes called neurodermatitis. In addition to treatment of the underlying cause of the pruritus, these patients may benefit from a time-limited treatment with a topical corticosteroid cream (hydrocortisone 1% twice or three times a day) to relieve inflammation and itching.

Diffuse reddening of the vulvar skin accompanied by itching and/or burning, but without

Table 27.1.
Clinical Aspects of Physiologic Vaginal Secretions and Common Vaginal Infections[a]

Characteristic	Physiologic	Gardnerella	Candidiasis	Trichomoniasis
Discharge				
Amount	Slight	Moderate	Variable	Moderate
Color	Yellow-white	Gray-white	White	Yellow-**green**
Odor	–	+++	–	+
Character	Thin	Thin	**Thick, curdy**	**Frothy**
pH	**3.5–4.5**	**5–5.5**	4–5	6–7
Symptoms				
Itching	–	–	++++	+
Burning	–	+	++	+
Findings				
Gross	Normal	Minimal erythema	Erythema, excoriation	**Petechiae**
Microscopic	**Few WBCs**	**Clue cells**	**Mycelia on KOH**	*Trichomonas*

[a] Items in boldface are of particular help in making a differential diagnosis.

obvious cause, should suggest a *secondary allergic vulvitis.* The list of possible local irritants can be quite extensive, including feminine hygiene sprays, deodorants, tampons or pads (especially those with deodorants or perfumes), tight-fitting synthetic undergarments, colored or scented toilet paper, and laundry soap or fabric softener residues. Even locally used contraceptives or sexual aids may be the source of irritation. A careful history, combined with the removal of the suspected cause, will usually both confirm the diagnosis and constitute the needed therapy. In rare cases, the use of hydrocortisone cream (1% cream applied twice a day to affected areas) may be needed to decrease the local inflammatory response.

Allergic *causes of vulvitis* are also frequently found in the occasional pediatric patient who presents with vulvovaginal itching. However, the investigation in these cases must also include sources of irritations such as foreign bodies (especially with an accompanying vaginitis or discharge), sexual abuse, and pinworms.

Local *Candida* infection is another cause of vulvar pruritus. This etiology must be considered in diabetes and others disposed to such infection and in situations where there has been a suboptimal response to treatment for another problem. The diagnosis and treatment are described later in this chapter.

In older patients, intense itching of the vulva may occur because of *atrophic changes* brought on by reduced estrogen levels. There will be a symmetrically reddened, smooth, and somewhat shiny look to the skin of the vulva and perineum. Biopsy will reflect the hypoplastic nature of this condition

and will help to differentiate this from lichen sclerosis, which has a similar appearance. When atrophic change is the cause, estrogen replacement, either locally or systemically, is the treatment of choice (see Chapter 37). In the case of *lichen sclerosis,* local application of 2% testosterone cream in a neutral base once or twice a day is generally effective.

Vulvar itching may be caused by infestation with *Pthirus pubis* or *Sarcoptes scabiei* (Fig. 27.2). This is especially true when itching of the mons is part of the patient's complaint. This itching is caused by an allergic sensitization from the parasite's bite. The crab louse is a different species from the body or head louse and is acquired by close contact or from bedding or towels. The crab louse is found exclusively in hairy areas, whereas the itch mite, while transmitted similarly, may be found anywhere in the skin surface. The diagnosis is generally made by looking for small black specks (excreta) on the skin, nits and eggs on hair shafts, or the parasites themselves. Local treatment with two applications of a γ-benzene hexachloride lotion (Kwell) is generally successful for infection from either parasite. Clothes, bedding, and those with whom close contact occurs must be disinfected/treated to break the infection cycle.

The vulva is subject to the same plethora of *dermatologic diseases* as other skin surfaces. *Contact dermatitis* is relatively common, with red, edematous skin surfaces and sometimes with vesicles and secondary infection. Treatment consists of removing the offending substance or material and wet compresses of Burrow's solution diluted 1 to 20, several times a day followed by drying. Hydrocor-

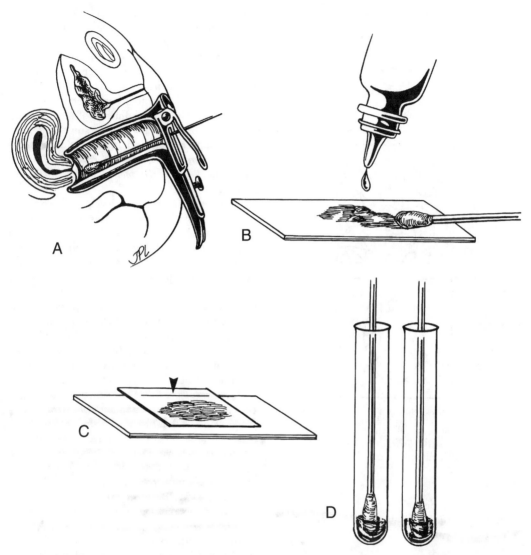

Figure 27.1. Saline and KOH preparations. A drop of physiologic saline and a drop of 10 to 20% potassium hydroxide (KOH) are placed on glass slides. **A,** Vaginal discharge is collected on a cotton-tipped applicator. **B,** The discharge is mixed in the droplets. **C,** The preparations are then covered with a cover slide for viewing. **D,** As an alternative, samples of discharge may be collected with two cotton-tipped applicators, which are then placed in small test tubes prepared with a few drops of NaCl and KOH solution. Material from these tubes are examined later in a similar manner.

tisone (0.5 to 1.0%) or fluorinated corticosteroids (Valisone, 0.1%) may be applied several times a day for symptom control. *Psoriasis* affects 1 to 3% of women and seems to have a familial pattern. This generalized pruritus skin disease of unknown cause is often refractory to simple fluorinated corticosteroids, and dermatologic consultation is required. *Seborrheic dermatitis* is another generalized

skin disease of unknown cause with rare vulvar manifestations, consisting of pale to yellow-red edematous lesions covered with a fine nonadherent scale. Treatment is also with hydrocortisone cream. *Hidradenitis suppurativa* is a chronic, unrelenting skin infection causing deep, painful scars and a foul discharge. Its differential diagnosis includes Crohn's disease of the vulva. Treatment

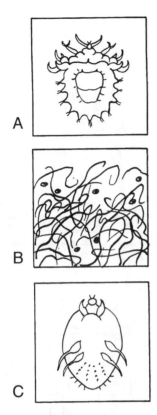

Figure 27.2. **A,** *Pthirus pubis* (the crab louse). **B,** Nits of the crab louse. **C,** *Sarcoptes scabiei* (the itch mite).

with local antibiotics and steroids is sometimes successful, but wide excision of the affected skin areas is often required.

VAGINITIS

The most common symptom associated with infections of the vagina is discharge. *Discharge from the vagina is normal physiologically; therefore, not all discharges from the vagina indicate infection.* This distinction is important to the diagnostic process but occasionally difficult for the patient to understand or accept.

Vaginal secretions arise from several sources. The majority of the liquid portion consists of mucus from the cervix. A very small amount of moisture is contributed by endometrial fluid, exudates from accessory glands such as the Skene's and Bartholin's glands, and from vaginal transudate. Exfoliated squamous cells from the vaginal wall give

the secretions a white to off-white color and provide some increase in consistency. The action of the indigenous vaginal flora also can contribute to the secretion. These components together constitute the normal vaginal secretions that provide the physiologic lubrication that prevents drying and irritation. The amount and character of this mixture vary under the influence of many factors, including hormonal and fluid status, pregnancy, immunosuppression, and inflammation. *Asymptomatic women produce, on the average, about 1.5 g of vaginal fluid per day. Normal vaginal secretions have no odor.*

After puberty, increased levels of glycogen in the vaginal tissues favor the growth of lactobacilli in the genital tract. These bacteria break down glycogen to lactic acid, lowering the pH from the 6 to 8 range, which is common before puberty (and after menopause), to the *normal menstrual vaginal pH range of 3.5 to 4.5.* In addition to the lactobacilli, a wide range of other aerobic and anaerobic bacteria may normally be found in the vagina at concentrations of 10^8 to 10^9 colonies per milliliter of vaginal fluid. Because the vagina is a potential space, not an open tube, a ratio of 5:1 anaerobic:aerobic bacteria is normal.

Increased vaginal discharge is associated with an identifiable microbiologic cause in 80 to 90% of cases. Hormonal or chemical causes account for most of the remaining cases. Most vaginal infections are caused by three infective agents: synergistic bacteria (bacteria vaginosis, nonspecific vaginitis), fungi (candidiasis), and protozoa, such as *Trichomonas* (trichomoniasis). Bacterial infections account for approximately 50% of infections, whereas fungi and *Trichomonas* account for roughly 25% each. Through gentle examination and simple microscopic investigation, the etiology of the patient's symptoms can be generally ascertained. *The value of microscopic examination of vaginal smears cannot be overstated. For this reason, any patient who complains of a vaginal discharge or irritation should be evaluated directly before therapy is suggested.*

Bacterial Vaginosis

Bacterial vaginosis is a diagnosis that has undergone a great deal of change and debate in the last few years. Once thought to be caused by the infection of *Gardnerella vaginalis* (formerly called *Haemophilus* or *Corynebacterium vaginale*), bacterial vaginosis is now felt to be a *symbiotic infection of anaerobic bacteria* (*Bacteroides* sp., *Peptococcus* sp., and

Mobiluncus sp.) and *Gardnerella*, both of which contribute to the clinical findings (Table 27.2).

Women with bacterial vaginosis generally complain of a *"musty" or "fishy" odor with an increased thin gray-white to yellow discharge*. The discharge may cause some mild vulvar irritation, but this is present in only about one-fifth of the cases. On examination, the vaginal discharge will be found to be mildly adherent to the vaginal wall and have a pH of 5.0 and 5.5. Mixing some of these secretions with KOH (10%) will liberate amines that may be detected by their fishy odor (positive "whiff test"). Microscopic examination made under saline wet mount will show a slight increase in white blood cells, clumps of bacteria, and characteristic *"clue cells,"* which are epithelial cells with numerous bacilli attached to their surface, making them appear to have indistinct borders and a "ground-glass" cytoplasm (Fig. 27.3).

Bacterial vaginosis may be treated with oral metronidazole (Flagyl, 500 mg twice a day for 7 days) or clindamycin (Cleocin, 300 mg p.o. b.i.d. for 7 days) or by intravaginal creams, using the same antibiotics (Metrogel or Cleocin cream) applied once or twice daily for 7 days. Because bacterial vaginosis may be transmitted sexually, treatment of the sexual partner(s) of patients with frequent recurrences should be considered.

Trichomonas Vaginitis

Trichomonas vaginalis is a flagellate protozoan that *lives only in the vagina, Skene's ducts, and male or female urethra* and may be freely transmitted by sexual intercourse. More than 60% of partners of women with *Trichomonas* infections will also be infected. Despite the large number of cases of symptomatic vaginitis caused by the organism, up to one-half of women with *Trichomonas* in the vaginal canal are asymptomatic. *Symptoms of Trichomonas infection* vary from mild to severe and may include vulvar itching or burning, copious *discharge* with rancid odor, dysuria, and dyspareunia. Although not present in all women, the discharge associated with *Trichomonas* infections is generally "frothy," thin, and yellow-green to gray in color, with a pH of 6 to 6.5 or above. *Examination* may reveal edema or erythema of the vulva. Characteristic petechia, or strawberry patches, in the upper vagina or on the cervix, are found in about 10% of patients.

The *diagnosis* is confirmed by *microscopic examination* of vaginal secretions suspended in normal saline. This wet smear will show large numbers of mature epithelial cells, white blood cells (WBCs),

Table 27.2.
Vaginitis — Altered Ecology

Finding	Normal	Bacterial Vaginosis
Organisms	10^8	10^{11}
Anaerobes:aerobes	5:1	1000:1
H_2O_2 production	High	Low
Lactobacillus	96%	35%
Gardnerella	5–60%	95%
Mobiluncus	0–5%	50–70%
Mycoplasma hominis	15–30%	60–70%

and the *Trichomonas* organism. *Trichomonas* is a fusiform protozoa just slightly larger than a white blood cell. The organism has three to five flagella extending from the narrow end. These flagella produce active movement that may facilitate identification of the organism (see Fig. 27.3).

Treatment of Trichomonas infections is by oral *metronidazole*. Because *Trichomonas* is very sensitive to metronidazole, 1-day therapy with 1 g in the morning and 1 g at bedtime will generally give a 90% cure rate. Treatment with 250 mg every 8 hours for 7 days or 2 g orally at one time will give comparable results. Many physicians prefer the single-day therapy because of its reduced cost and greater compliance. Debate continues with respect to treating asymptomatic partners of women with *Trichomonas* infections. If treatment is undertaken, the single-day therapy is usually adequate. Abstinence from alcohol use when taking metronidazole is necessary to avoid a possible disulfiram-like reaction. The use of metronidazole during pregnancy is not recommended because of reports of teratogenic effects. Many physicians, however, use the drug in the latter half of pregnancy for highly symptomatic patients.

Even though the pH generally associated with *Trichomonas* infections is different from that found with bacterial vaginosis, there are estimates of up to a *25% prevalence of bacterial vaginosis in those patients with Trichomonas*. Because of the overlap in metronidazole therapy for these two conditions, this debate is not significant for most patients. It may, however, be worthy of consideration in patients who receive alternative therapies or those with frequent recurrences of vaginal infections.

Although follow-up examination of patients with *Trichomonas* for test of cure is often advocated, they are usually not cost-effective, except

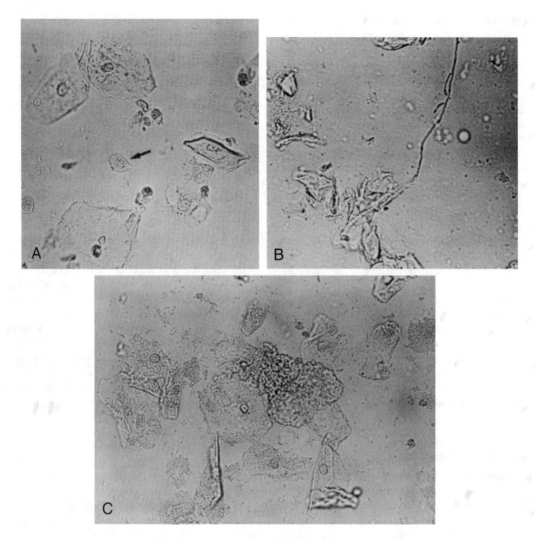

Figure 27.3. **A,** Trichomonads; a flagellated protozoan is easy to identify on NaCl wet mount because of its movement. **B,** Monilial infection; slide shows hyphae and budding yeast. **C,** Clue cells, which are epithelial cells with clumps of bacteria on their surfaces.

in the rare patient with a history of frequent recurrences. In these patients, reinfection or poor compliance must be considered as well as the possibility of infection with more than one agent or other underlying disease.

Candida (Monilial) Vaginitis

Monilial infections of the vagina are caused by ubiquitous *airborne fungi*. Approximately 90% of "yeast" infections are caused by *Candida albicans* with less than 10% caused by *C. glabrata, C. tropicalis,* or *Torulopsis glabrata. Candida* infections generally do not coexist with other infections and

are not considered to be sexually transmitted even though 10% of male partners have concomitant penile infections. Candidiasis is more likely to occur in women who are pregnant, diabetic, obese, immunosuppressed, on oral contraceptives or corticosteroids, or have had broad-spectrum antibiotic therapy. Practices that keep the vaginal area warm and moist, such as wearing tight clothing or the habitual use of panty liners, may also increase the risk of *Candida* infections.

The most common presenting complaint for women with candidiasis is *itching*, although up to 20% of women may be asymptomatic. Burning,

Table 27.3.
Topical Treatments for *Candida* Vaginitis

Medication	Regimen
Miconazole (Monistat)	Vaginal suppository: one 200-mg suppository inserted into vagina daily for 3 days
	Vaginal cream: applied intravaginally with applicator and on surface twice daily for 5–7 days
Clotrimazole (Gyne-Lotrimin)	Vaginal insert: 1 suppository inserted into vagina daily for 7 days
	Vaginal cream: applied intravaginally with applicator twice daily, once at bedtime for 7 days
Butoconazole (Femstat Prefill)	Vaginal cream: applied intravaginally with applicator at night for 3 days
Ketoconazole (Nizoral)	Vaginal cream: applied to affected areas nightly for 3 days
Terconazole (Terazol)	Vaginal cream: applied intravaginally at night for 3 days
	Vaginal suppositories: 1 suppository inserted at night for 3 days

external dysuria, and dyspareunia are also common. The vulva and vaginal tissues will often be bright red in color and excoriation is not uncommon in severe cases. *A thick, adherent "cottage cheese" discharge with a pH of 4 to 5 is generally found. This discharge is odorless.*

The *diagnosis* of candidiasis is based on history and physical findings, and confirmed by the identification of hyphae and buds in wet mounts of vaginal secretions made with 10% KOH solution, which lyses most epithelial and white cells (see Fig. 27.3). There is no direct correlation between the degree of symptoms and the number of organisms present. Because false-negative wet preps are not uncommon, culture confirmation may be obtained using Nickerson's or Sabouraud's media.

Treatment of Candida infections is primarily with the topical application of one of the synthetic imidazoles (Table 27.3). These agents will give good cure rates after 3 to 7 days of treatment. Despite greater than 90% relief of symptoms with these therapies, 20 to 30% of patients will experience *recurrences* after 1 month. Treatments based on nystatin or povidone-iodine have proven to be less effective than the imidazoles. Resistant strains of *C. tropicalis* or *Torulopsis glabrata* may respond to therapy with terconazole or gentian violet. Treatment with the oral agent fluconazole (Diflucan), 150 mg as a single dose, has been recently described. Patients with frequent recurrences should be carefully evaluated for possible risk factors such as diabetes or immune defects. Prophylactic local therapy with an antifungal agent should be considered when systemic antibiotics are prescribed.

Chronic Vaginitis

A problem for both physicians and patients is "chronic" or "recurrent vaginitis." Patients complain, often bitterly, of persistent vaginal discharge, odor, or both, without a readily identifiable cause or satisfactory response to treatment. These patients have frequently "tried everything" and visited several physicians without success. A careful history must be obtained, covering medical conditions and sexual and hygienic habits. A methodical physical examination and microscopic evaluation are also required.

In addition to the usual causes, one must evaluate alternative explanations for the patient's complaints. Victims of sexual assault (recent or quite far in the past) may present in this manner. A frank explanation of the possibility of reinfection must be carried out in individuals with true recurrent infections. The existence of additional sexual contacts for the patient or her partner should be explored in an appropriately nonjudgmental way. Alternate sources of excessive vaginal moisture, such as chronic cervical infections, must be evaluated. When the patient's complaints seem to exceed her physical and microscopic findings, the possibility of inappropriate expectations, inaccurate information, or psychologic dysfunction must be entertained.

CASE STUDIES

Case 27A

A 36-year-old G3 P2012 patient calls and states that she has one of her "yeast infections" again. She has just moved to the area, but her former physician would usually "just call something in," and she would like you to do so as well. Upon further questioning, you find that the patient is experiencing vulvar itching, mild dysuria, a thick discharge, and a mild vaginal odor.

Question Case 27A

The most appropriate initial action would be to

A. Prescribe miconazole suppositories for 3 days
B. Prescribe metronidazole 1 g b.i.d. for 1 day
C. Ask the patient to come in for an examination
D. Refer the patient to the local STD clinic
E. Prescribe oral nystatin therapy

Answer: C

Even though this patient may have a recurrent yeast infection, the symptoms of vaginal infections overlap to such a great extent that only a thorough evaluation (history, physical, and microscopic investigation) will reliably establish the diagnosis. Without a correct diagnosis, any therapy has the potential either to fail or to make the patient worse. Especially in a patient whom you have never examined, treatment based on examination is more appropriate than calling in a prescription.

Case 27B

A 54-year old patient comes to your office with the complaint of vaginal itching. The patient is in good health and on no medication, except for a diuretic for hypertension. Her last menstrual period was 3 years ago and she has recently begun experiencing mild hot flashes. On examination the patient's vulva is red but no edema is noted. The area of Bartholin's glands appears to be normal. The vaginal canal is also slightly reddened, and a small amount of slightly thickened discharge may be obtained from the vaginal apex.

Question Case 27B

Which of the following tests performed on the vaginal secretions would *not* be of assistance in this case:

A. Whiff test
B. 10% KOH wet prep
C. Culture on Nickerson's medium
D. Culture for bacteria
E. Saline wet prep

Answer: D

The vagina is normally populated by many species of bacteria; hence, culture of vaginal secretions for bacteria provides little useful information. Although it is likely that this patient is experiencing atrophic vulvitis and/or vaginitis, candidiasis or other infections are also possible and must be excluded by other means.

Case 27C

A 22-year-old newlywed comes to your office with the complaint of 3 days of vaginal "wetness" that stains her underwear yellow and an excessive odor. She notes some mild vulvar irritation but no dysuria or dyspareunia. Physical examination shows diffuse redness of the vulva and vagina, with copious amount of a yellow to gray discharge on the vaginal walls. Saline wet prep shows the following: 3+ epithelium, 2+ WBCs, 1+ motile sperm, moderate small rods, and occasional motile protozoa.

Question Case 27C

The most likely diagnosis is

A. Mechanical vulvitis
B. Contact dermatitis
C. Bacterial vaginosis
D. *Trichomonas* vaginitis
E. Monilial vaginitis

Answer: D

The finding of motile protozoa is virtually pathognominic for a *Trichomonas* infection. Although each of the other options had to be considered initially, the microscopic findings establish the diagnosis in this case.

chapter 28

SEXUALLY TRANSMITTED DISEASES

Sexually transmitted diseases run the gamut from vaginitis to life-threatening conditions such as acquired immunodeficiency syndrome (AIDS). The increasing prevalence of sexually transmitted disease has resulted in increased awareness among physicians and patients and, in some cases, changes in attitudes about acceptable behaviors and standards. The impact of sexually transmitted diseases for the individual and for society cannot be overlooked or overemphasized. Although some of these diseases can be acquired through nonsexual means, sexual transmission represents the major route by which most are spread.

The impact of changing sexuality has had far-reaching implications, not the least of which has been the explosive increase in the frequency and types of sexually transmitted diseases. For example, recently there has been an increase of approximately 30% in the reported number of cases of syphilis. The physician must be alert to the possibility of sexually transmitted disease in all patients, perform diagnostic evaluations and institute appropriate treatments promptly, and attempt to educate patients regarding the risks involved in today's sexually open society.

HISTORY AND PHYSICAL EXAMINATION

The sexual habits and modes of expression that individuals choose will affect their risk of infection as well as the site and presentation by which infection is manifest. For this reason, a detailed sexual history is important for all patients and invaluable for any in whom a sexually transmitted disease is either likely or suspected. Most of these infections require skin-to-skin contact or exchange of body fluids for transmission. Nonsexual activities that meet these criteria may also put the patient at risk.

All patients who are (or might be) sexually active should be examined with an awareness of the possibility of sexually transmitted disease. This is not a condemnation of the patient's lifestyle or personal choices, but rather a simple fact of life in today's society. The inguinal region should be inspected for rashes, lesions, and adenopathy. The vulva should be inspected for lesions, ulcerations, or abnormal discharge and palpated for thickening or swelling. The Bartholin's glands, Skene's ducts, and urethra cannot be overlooked because these are frequent sites of infection (e.g., gonorrhea). In patients with urinary symptoms, the urethra should be gently "milked" to express any discharge. The vagina and cervix must be inspected for lesions and abnormal discharge. When suspicion or risk is high, cultures of the urethra and cervix for gonorrhea, chlamydia, or other infections should be obtained. Last, the perineum and perianal areas must also be evaluated for signs of sexually transmitted diseases. Cultures of the rectum for gonorrhea should be obtained in those patients who engage in anal intercourse. For completeness, the oral cavity as well as cervical and other lymph nodes must be evaluated and cultures taken if indicated by the patient's modes of sexual expression. The findings obtained by this process, combined with the patient's history, will generally make the establishment of the proper diagnosis much easier. Furthermore, the sexual partner(s) of patients diagnosed with or suspected of having a sexually transmitted disease (STD) should receive their own evaluation. *It is vital to remember that 20 to 50% of patients with a sexually transmitted disease have one or more coexisting infections. When one venereal disease is found, others must be suspected.*

SPECIFIC INFECTIONS

Herpes Genitalis

Herpes simplex virus infection of the genital tract represents one of the most common sexually acquired diseases. Office visits for this infection have increased tenfold in the past 10 years. It is estimated that there are approximately 500,000 new cases each year. Herpes simplex infections are highly contagious. Roughly 75% of sexual partners of infected individuals will themselves contract the disease. About 85% of genital herpes lesions are caused by herpes simplex virus type 2 (HVS$_2$); this type differs slightly from the type 1 virus (HSV$_1$), which usually causes the "cold sore" lesions of the mouth but is also responsible for the balance of genital lesions.

The development of the classic vesicular lesions is often preceded by a prodromal phase of mild paresthesia and burning beginning approximately 2 to 5 days after infection in symptomatic patients. This will progress to very painful vesicular and ulcerated lesions 3 to 7 days after exposure (Fig. 28.1). Dysuria caused by vulvar lesions, or urethral and bladder involvement, may lead to urinary retention. Roughly 10% of patients with initial lesions will require hospitalization for pain control or management of urinary complications. Primary infections are also characterized by malaise, low-grade fever, and inguinal adenopathy in 40% of patients. Aseptic meningitis with fever, headache, and meningismus can be found in some

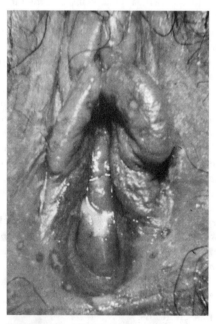

Figure 28.1. Herpes simplex virus infection. Note the small serpiginous, superficial lesions and edema of the vulva and urethral area.

patients 5 to 7 days after the appearance of the genital lesions. This generally resolves over the period of a week.

Physical findings consist of clear vesicles, which lyse and progress to shallow, painful ulcers with a red border. These may coalesce and frequently become secondarily infected and necrotic. These lesions may be found on the vulva, vagina, cervix, or perineal and perianal skin, often extending onto the buttocks. There are recurrent lesions in approximately 30% of patients, which are similar in character but milder in severity and shorter in duration than primary lesions, generally lasting 2 to 5 days.

The diagnosis of herpetic infections is made based on the characteristic history and physical findings. The diagnosis may be confirmed through the use of viral cultures taken by swab from the lesions. This is the most sensitive method of diagnosis and allows confirmation in as little as 48 hr. Scrapings from the base of vesicles may be stained by immunofluorescence techniques for the presence of viral particles. This technique provides results faster than cultures and carries approximately 80% agreement with culture results. Smears may also be stained with Wright's stain to visualize the characteristic giant multinucleated cells with eosinophilic intranuclear inclusions. The lesions of herpes simplex infections should be easily distinguishable from the ulcers found in chancroid, syphilis, or granuloma inguinale by their appearance and extreme tenderness.

The management of genital herpes infections is directed toward the management of local lesions and symptoms. When treating initial infections, the lesions should be kept clean and dry. Sitz baths, followed by drying with a heat lamp or hair dryer, work well for this purpose. Occasionally, the use of a topical anesthetic, such as 2% Xylocaine jelly, may be required. If secondary infections occur, therapy with a local antibacterial cream such as Neosporin may be of help. Acyclovir 5% ointment may be applied to the lesions every 3 hr and is recommended to decrease the duration of symptoms and viral shedding. Unfortunately, this therapy does not decrease the likelihood of recurrence, and the decrease in symptom duration is often minimal. For patients who have frequent recurrences, oral acyclovir (Zovirax, 200 mg t.i.d. increased to 5 times/day with lesions) is effective in decreasing both frequency and severity of flareups, but it should be limited to no more than 6 months of use. Hospitalization for intravenous acyclovir therapy (5 mg/kg infused at a constant rate over 1 hr, administered every 8 hr for 5 days in adult patients with normal renal function) may be required in cases of severe outbreak or in immunosuppressed or otherwise compromised patients. Until the vesicles are crusted over, the lesions are highly infectious, and intercourse should be avoided. Acyclovir ointment is useful in the treatment of men but not women.

In pregnant patients with active herpes infections and intact membranes, cesarean delivery should be considered. Vaginal delivery, when herpetic lesions are present, is associated with a 50% chance that the baby will acquire the infection, which is associated with significant morbidity and an almost 80% mortality rate.

Pelvic Inflammatory Disease

Pathogenesis

Infection of the upper female genital tract is predominantly by direct spread along the mucosal surfaces from initial infection of the cervix. The predominant organisms are *Chlamydia trachomatis* and *Neisseria gonorrhoeae.* A mucopurulent cervicitis is more common in *C. trachomatis* infection, as *N. gonorrhoeae* seems able to reside in the endocervical cells without always promoting a purulent inflammatory response. The endocervical mucus resists upward spread, especially during the progesterone-dominant part of the menstrual cycle. Oral contraceptives mimic this effect, which explains in part their action to limit pelvic inflammatory disease (PID). The cervical mucus may be penetrated by the bacteria, either directly or as riders on sperm or trichomonads or up an IUD string. When the cervicitis traverses the cervical barrier, endometrial infection occurs, followed rapidly in most cases by spread to the fallopian tube mucosa. Occasionally, an indolent endometritis will develop with further extension, more commonly with *Chlamydia* infection. Tubal ligation usually provides a barrier to spread, although in some cases small microchannels facilitate continued spread. The salpingitis that results may be localized, or it may spread causing peritonitis, adhesion formation, and abscess formation. The relative mobility of the fallopian tube probably contributes to the rapid and widespread extension of infection. In this anaerobic environment, anaerobes also thrive so that the infection in the upper portions of the genital tract is actually often polymicrobial, with a mixture of aerobic and anaerobic

organisms. However, as there is poor correlation between the diverse organisms cultured and the clinical patterns of disease, the models of *C. trachomatis* and *N. gonorrhoeae* serve well as disease models.

Chlamydia trachomatis

The second most common sexually transmitted disease is infection by *Chlamydia trachomatis.* Infection by this obligate intracellular parasite may manifest as cervicitis (mucopurulent cervicitis), acute urethritis, salpingitis, or pelvic inflammatory disease. *C. trachomatis* differs from those strains causing other chlamydial infections such as lymphogranuloma venereum (LGV). LGV has three stages: primary lesions, consisting of papules or ulcers; regional lymphadenopathy, the bubonic stage; and when the buboes suppurate, they develop draining fistulas and lymphatic obstruction, the third stage. More common than *N. gonorrhoeae* by as much as 10:1 in some studies, infections by *C. trachomatis* can be the source of significant morbidity, including chronic infection, chronic pelvic pain, and infertility. Infection rates are five times higher in women with three or more sexual partners and four times higher in women using no contraception or nonbarrier methods. In industrialized countries, series report asymptomatic cervical infection in 5 to 20% of women of childbearing age, with perhaps 5 to 10% of these developing ascending infection. Between 20 and 40% of sexually active women have antibodies to *Chlamydia.*

Clinically mild cases of cervicitis or pelvic infection by *Chlamydia* may be virtually asymptomatic yet culminate in infertility or ectopic pregnancy. Infection of the fallopian tubes causes a mild form of salpingitis with insidious symptoms. Once the infection is established, it may remain active for many months, with increasing tubal damage. Perihepatitis (Fitz-Hugh-Curtis syndrome), which consists of inflammation leading to localized fibrosis with scarring of the anterior surface of the liver and adjacent peritoneum, may be caused by chlamydial infections more often than by *N. gonorrhoeae* infection, with which it was originally described (Fig. 28.2). *Chlamydia* is also frequently found coexisting with or mimicking *N. gonorrhoeae* infection. Chlamydial infections are also responsible for nongonococcal urethritis and inclusion conjunctivitis.

Physical findings in infections caused by *Chlamydia* are often subtle and nonspecific. Eversion of the cervix with mucopurulent cervicitis may sug-

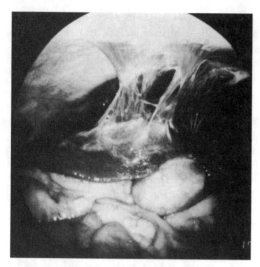

Figure 28.2. Fitz-Hugh-Curtis syndrome. Laparoscopic view of perihepatitis, showing scarring and string-like perihepatic adhesions associated with both gonococcal and chlamydial salphingitis.

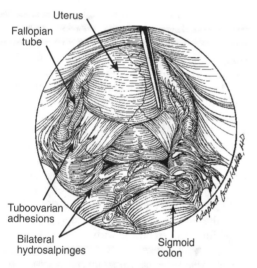

Uterus

Fallopian tube

Tuboovarian adhesions

Bilateral hydrosalpinges

Sigmoid colon

Figure 28.3. Sequelae of pelvic inflammatory disease. Laparoscopic view of multiple pelvic adhesions, including tuboovarian adhesions and bilateral hydrosalpinges.

gest the diagnosis. Any patient with acute PID or who is suspected of having gonorrhea should also be evaluated for *Chlamydia.*

The diagnosis of *Chlamydia* infection is suspected on clinical grounds. Cultures are generally used only to confirm the diagnosis, since it takes 48 to 72 hr to obtain culture results. Two screen-

ing tests have recently gained clinical popularity: an enzyme immunoassay (EIA) performed on cervical secretions and a monoclonal fluorescent antibody test carried out on dried specimens. The immunoassay technique is easy to do and has a 95% specificity. The monoclonal technique is faster, has a 85 to 90% sensitivity and 95% specificity, but requires precision in making the slide and using the fluorescent microscope for interpretation.

Outpatient treatment of suspected or confirmed infections with *Chlamydia* is with doxycycline (Doxycycline or Vibramycin, 100 mg p.o. b.i.d. for 7 days) or azithromycin (Zithromax, 1 g p.o.). Erythromycin (500 mg p.o. q.i.d. for 7 days) may be substituted for doxycycline in individuals unable to tolerate these medications or in pregnant patients. These treatments carry roughly 95% cure rates. Follow-up evaluation with culture or other tests as well as screening for other sexually transmitted diseases should be performed. Partners should either be treated or referred for immediate treatment.

Neisseria gonorrhoeae (Gonorrhea)

Infections with *N. gonorrhoeae*, a Gram-negative intracellular diplococcus, continue to be common, and the incidence is increasing. The emergence of penicillin-resistant strains, an increased frequency of asymptomatic infections, and changing patterns of sexual behavior have all contributed to the problem. The damage caused by *N. gonorrhoeae* infections and the anaerobic organisms that grow with them in the pelvic environment can lead to recurrent infection; chronic pelvic pain; or infertility caused by adhesion formation, tubal damage, and hydrosalpinx formation (Fig. 28.3). Infertility occurs in approximately 15% of patients after a single episode of salpingitis and rises to 75% after three or more episodes. The risk of ectopic pregnancy is increased 7 to 10 times in women with a history of salpingitis. It is estimated that PID results in $2.7 billion in direct medical costs and an additional $4 billion in indirect medical costs per year.

Infections with *N. gonorrhoeae* are easily acquired and can affect almost any part or organ of the body. For women, a single encounter with an infected partner will lead to infection 80 to 90% of the time. Most commonly, the first signs or symptoms of infection occur 3 to 5 days after exposure but are often mild enough to be overlooked. Infection in the lower genital tract is characterized by a malodorous, purulent discharge from the urethra, Skene's duct, cervix, vagina, or anus. Anal inter-

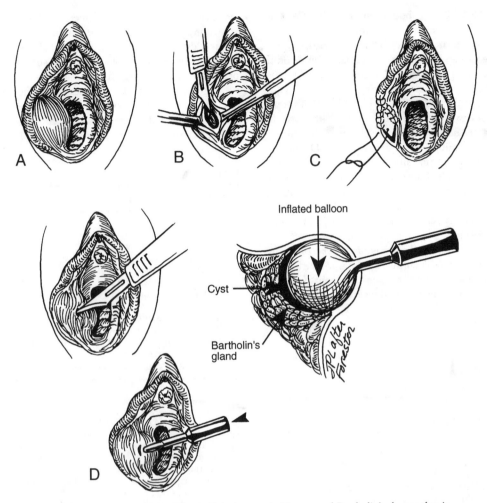

Figure 28.4. Surgical treatment of Bartholin's abscess. **A,** Unruptured Bartholin's abscess that is "pointing," i.e., there is a prominent area where there is only a very thin layer of tissue encapsulating the abscess. **B,** Incision of the abscess. **C,** The Marsuplization technique, where the edges of the cyst are sutured and the abscess is left to drain, sometimes packed with iodoform gauze, for the first 1 to 2 days. **D,** The Word catheter technique, where a special bulb-tipped catheter is placed into the cavity for 1 to 2 weeks to facilitate healing and reepitheliazation of the cavity wall.

course is not always a prerequisite to anal infection. The presence of greenish or yellow discharge from the cervix should alert the physician to the possibility of either *N. gonorrhoeae* or *C. trachomatis* infection. Infection of the Bartholin's glands is frequently encountered and can lead to secondary infections, abscesses, or cyst formation. When the gland becomes full and painful, incision and drainage can have excellent results (Fig. 28.4). Infection of the pharynx is found in 10 to 20% of heterosexual women with gonorrhea, and this site should not be overlooked when cultures are taken.

Approximately 15% of women with *N. gonorrhoeae* infections of the cervix will develop acute pelvic infections (PID). *N. gonorrhoeae* infection of the fallopian tubes, adnexa, or pelvic peritoneum generally results in pain and tenderness, fever or chills, and an elevated white blood count (Table 28.1). Peritoneal involvement can also include perihepatitis (Fitz-Hugh-Curtis syndrome). *N. gonorrhoeae* is the causative agent in roughly 50% of patients with salpingitis. Many patients require hospitalization for adequate care (Table 28.2). In severe cases or in patients with one or more prior episodes of PID, tuboovarian abscess (TOA) formation may occur. These patients are acutely ill, with fevers of up to 39.5°C, tachycardia, severe pelvic and abdominal pain, and nausea and vomiting. Findings in PID are often nonspecific (Fig. 28.5), and patients presenting with these symptoms must be differentiated from those with septic incomplete abortions, acute appendicitis, diverticular abscesses, and adnexal torsion (Table 28.3).

On examination, patients with PID may exhibit muscular guarding, and/or rebound tenderness. A purulent discharge is often seen at the cervix and should be sampled for Gram staining and culture. The adnexa are usually moderately to exquisitely tender and a mass or fullness may be palpable.

The laboratory diagnosis of *N. gonorrhoeae* infection is made by culture on Thayer-Martin agar plates kept in a CO_2-rich environment. Cultures should be obtained from the cervix, urethra, anus, and pharynx when appropriate. Cultures provide 80 to 95% diagnostic sensitivity. A solid-phase en-

zyme immunoassay for the detection of *N. gonorrhoeae* antigen is also available. Gram stain of any cervical discharge for the presence of this Gram-negative intracellular diplococcus may support the presumptive diagnosis.

Aggressive therapy for patients with either suspected or confirmed *N. gonorrhoeae* infection should be tailored to the site of infection and the individual patient. Initial treatment should not be

Table 28.2.
Factors Suggesting Hospitalization for Patients with Pelvic Inflammatory Disease

Nulliparity
Paralytic ileus
Peritonitis or toxicity
Pregnancy
Intrauterine contraceptive device use
Previous treatment failure
Significant gastrointestinal symptoms
Significant pain
Temperature >39°C
Tubo-ovarian abscess
Uncertain or complicated differential diagnosis
Unreliable patient
White blood count >20,000 or <4,000

Table 28.1.
Clinical Criteria for Diagnosis of PID

Tenderness
   Direct (abdominal)
   Adnexal
   Cervical
	All 3

Gram stain positive Temperature >38°C WBC >10,000 Pus on culdocentesis or laparoscopy	At least 1

Table 28.3.
Correct Diagnosis in Cases of Misdiagnosis of PID

Acute appendicitis	28% of cases
Endometriosis	17% of cases
Corpus luteum bleeding	12% of cases
Ectopic pregnancy	11% of cases
Adhesions	7% of cases
"Other"	28% of cases

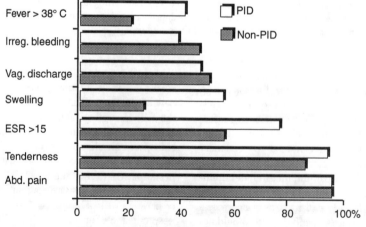

Figure 28.5. Frequency of symptoms in PID.

predicated on the results of cultures but rather on clinical suspicion. General guidelines for treatment are shown in Table 28.4. Hospitalized patients require high dose intravenous antibiotic therapy with an antimicrobial spectrum that covers aerobic and anaerobic organisms. Surgical drainage of an abscess or even hysterectomy may be warranted in patients who fail an aggressive course of parenteral antibiotics. Rupture of a tuboovarian abscess, with septic shock, is a life-threatening complication and should be treated surgically. After successful medical therapy, follow-up cultures and examination of the patient should be performed 3 to 5 days after completion of therapy.

Tuberculosis

Genital tuberculosis (TB) almost always results from miliary hematogenous or lymphatic spread from tuberculosis elsewhere, usually the lungs. Typically, the initial involvement is tubal, with spread to ovaries and endometrium occurring in about 30 to 50% of cases. Tuberculosis is a relatively uncommon infection in the United States, although its incidence is increasing in some immigrant and migrant groups, in those who are immunosuppressed, and in those who abuse drugs. The diagnosis is suspected on clinical grounds and confirmed by culture, with the endometrium being the most easily accessible tissue. The TB skin test indicates exposure but not location or current infection. Medical treatment is quite effective in most cases and consists of the use of one or more of five common agents: isoniazid (INH), rifampin, streptomycin, ethambutol, and pyrazinamide. Surgical treatment is sometimes required with persistent disease, abscess formation, and pelvic pain. The operation of choice in these circum-

stances is total abdominal hysterectomy with bilateral salpingo-oophrectomy after stringent medical therapy.

Human Papilloma Virus

Infection by the human papilloma virus (HPV) is responsible for almost as many cases of sexually transmitted disease as *N. gonorrhoeae*. This DNA virus is found in 2.5 to 4% of women. Over the past 15 years, the number of infected individuals has increased more than fivefold. Unlike other sexually transmitted diseases, sequelae of HPV infection may take years to develop. At least three subtypes (16, 18, and 31, primarily) have been associated with the development of cervical neoplasia.

Infection by HPV after a single contact with an infected partner, results in a 65% transmission rate. Following a 6-week to 3-month incubation period, infection by HPV causes soft, fleshy growths on the vulva, vagina, cervix, urethral meatus, perineum, and anus. They may occasionally also be found on the tongue or oral cavity. These growths are termed condyloma acuminata or venereal warts (Fig. 28.6). These distinctive lesions may be single or multiple and generally cause few symptoms. They are often accompanied by *Trichomonas* or *Gardnerella* vaginal infections. Since human papilloma virus is spread by direct skin-to-skin contact, symmetrical lesions across the midline are common (often called "kissing lesions").

The diagnosis of condyloma acuminata is made based on physical examination but may be confirmed through biopsy of the warts. Although cytologic changes typical of HPV can be found on Pap smears, Pap smears of the cervix will diagnose only about 5% of patients with the virus. Because the condyloma lata of syphilis may be confused

Table 28.4.
Gonorrhea and PID Therapy

Disease	Preferred Treatment	Alternative Treatment
Gonorrhea Urethral/cervical, rectal, pharyngeal	Ceftriaxone 250 mg i.m. + (doxycycline 100 mg b.i.d. × 7 days or tetracycline 500 mg p.o. q.i.d. × 7 days) or ceftriaxone 250 mg i.m. + azithromycin 1.0 g p.o.	Doxycycline 100 mg b.i.d. + (spectinomycin 2 g i.m. or ciprofloxacin 500 mg p.o. or cefixime 400 mg p.o. or ampicillin/ sulbactam 1.5 g i.m. + probenecid 1 g p.o.)
PID (outpatient)	(Cefloxitin 2 g i.m. + probenicid 1 g p.o. or ceftriaxone 250 mg i.m.) + doxycycline 100 mg p.o. b.i.d. × 14 days	Ofloxacin 400 mg p.o. b.i.d. × 14 days + (clindamycin 450 mg p.o. q.i.d. or metronidazole 500 mg p.o. b.i.d. × 14 days

HPV

with venereal warts, some care must be taken in making the diagnosis in patients at high risk for both infections. Venereal warts are usually characterized by their narrower base and more "heaped-up" appearance, whereas condyloma lata lesions have a flattened top.

Small, uncomplicated venereal warts are treated medically with either an application of a 25% solution of podophyllin in tincture of benzoin or trichloroacetic acid (TCA). One of these solutions is carefully applied to the warts and allowed to remain for 30 to 60 min. Vaseline or other protective medium may be applied to the surrounding skin so that a chemical burn does not occur. Treatment may be repeated every 7 to 10 days as needed. Podophyllin should not be used during pregnancy, because of potential fetal toxicity. If lesions persist or recur, cryosurgery, electrodesiccation, surgical excision, or laser vaporization may be required. Treatment with 5-fluorouracil cream is often used as an adjunct for cervical or vaginal lesions.

Lesions will be more resistant to therapy during pregnancy, in diabetic patients, in patients who smoke, or in patients who are immunosuppressed. In patients with extensive vaginal or vulvar lesions, delivery via cesarean section may be required to avoid extensive vaginal lacerations and

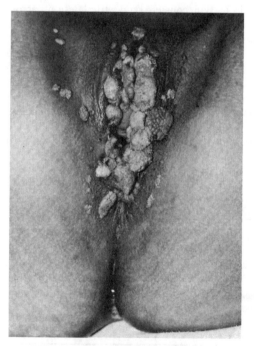

Figure 28.6. Condyloma acuminata.

problems suturing tissues with these lesions. Cesarean delivery also decreases the possibility of transmission to the infant, which can cause subsequent development of laryngeal papillomata, although the risk is small and in and of itself not an indication for cesarean section.

Any patient with a history of condyloma should have at least yearly Pap smear evaluations of the cervix. The sexual partners of patients with HPV should also be screened for the development of genital warts.

Syphilis

Since antiquity, syphilis has been the prototypic venereal disease. The incidence of syphilis has been rising in the past several years. Contributing to this rise is today's increased use of nonpenicillin antibiotics to treat resistant gonorrhea, whereas in the past, penicillin treatment of gonorrhea provided treatment for coexisting syphilis.

Treponema pallidum, the causative organism of syphilis, is one of a very small group of spirochetes that are virulent for humans. Since this motile anaerobic spirochete can rapidly invade intact moist mucosa, resulting in infection and chancre formation, the most common sites of entry for women are the vulva, vagina, and cervix. Chancres may also be found in or near the anus, rectum, pharynx, tongue, lips, fingers, or other areas. Transplacental spread may occur at any time during pregnancy and can result in congenital syphilis (see Chapter 6).

About 10 to 60 days after infection with *T. pallidum*, a painless ulcer will appear. This is the chancre of primary syphilis. The chancre has a firm, punched out appearance and has rolled edges (Fig. 28.7). Even though it is often accompanied by adenopathy, the chancre is commonly asymptomatic and missed. Serologic testing at this stage of syphilis will generally be negative. Healing of the chancre occurs spontaneously in 3 to 9 weeks.

At 4 to 8 weeks after the primary chancre appears, manifestations of secondary syphilis develop. This stage is characterized by low-grade fever, headache, malaise, sore throat, anorexia, generalized lymphadenopathy, and a diffuse, symmetric, asymptomatic maculopapular rash. This rash is often seen over the palm and soles and is sometimes referred to as "money spots." Highly infective secondary eruptions, called mucous patches, occur in 30% of patients during this stage. In moist areas of the body, flat-topped papules may coalesce, forming condyloma lata (Fig.

28.8). These may be distinguished from venereal warts by their broad base and flatter appearance. In untreated individuals, this stage, too, will pass spontaneously in 2 to 6 weeks as the disease enters into the latent phase.

In the late stages of the disease, transmission of the infection is unlikely, except via blood transfusion or placental transfer. However, crippling damage to the central nervous system, heart, or great vessels often develops. Destructive, necrotic, granulomatous lesions called gummas may develop 1 to 10 years after infection.

The diagnosis of syphilis may be made by identifying motile spirochetes on darkfield microscopic examination of material from primary or secondary lesions or lymph node aspirates. For most patients, the diagnosis will be established on the basis of serologic testing (Table 28.5). The VDRL and RPR are nonspecific tests that are rapid, inexpensive, and useful for screening. The FTA–ABS and MHA-TP tests are specific treponemal antibody tests that are confirmatory or diagnostic but are not used for routine screening. These latter tests are useful when assessing false-positive screening tests caused by such diverse conditions as atypical pneumonia, malaria, connective tissue disease, systemic lupus erythematosus, or some vaccinations (Table 28.6). When neurosyphilis is suspected, a lumbar puncture, with a VDRL performed on the spinal fluid, is required.

The treatment of choice for syphilis is penicillin G benzathine as outlined in Table 28.7. The patient should be followed by quantitative VDRL titers and examinations at 3, 6, and 12 months.

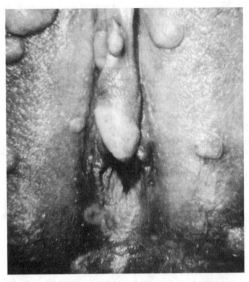

Figure 28.8. Condyloma lata of the vulva. The typical lesion of secondary syphilis, slightly raised, round or oval, plateau-like lesions of various sizes, often occurring in clusters. The edges are slightly indurated, and the surface is moist and covered with a grayish necrotic exudate. These lesions are highly infectious.

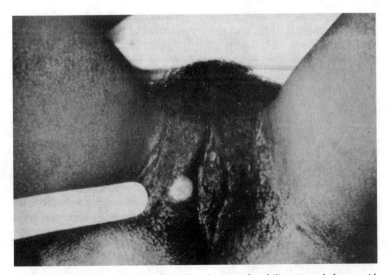

Figure 28.7. Chancre of the vulva. The chancre of syphilis, a rounded or ovoid raised lesion with indurated edges and a depressed center. The surface is reddish or reddish brown.

Acquired Immunodeficiency Syndrome

Acquired immunodeficiency syndrome (AIDS) is now one of the top five causes of death for young women. Although transmission of the human immunodeficiency virus (HIV) may be accomplished via blood transfusion, pregnancy, or the use of contaminated drug equipment such as needles, the exchange of body fluids during sexual activity represents a major mode of spread, making AIDS a sexually transmitted disease. This virtually uniformly fatal disease is generally diagnosed either through screening of individuals at high risk or suspicion when secondary infections or rare tumors, such as Kaposi's sarcoma, appear. Although women in heterosexual relationships are considered to be at somewhat lower risk than homosexual males and intravenous drug abusers, anyone with multiple sexual contacts risks exposure and infection. Women currently represent approximately 11% of AIDS cases (roughly 14,000 cases to date), and this rate is rising. Roughly 35% of women with AIDS have acquired their infection through heterosexual contact. While minority women represent the fastest growing subgroup to be infected, any sexually active woman may be at risk. Because the risk of transmission of AIDS to a fetus is approximately 50% and because maternal AIDS often worsens during pregnancy, pregnancy should be postponed until more is known or effective therapies become available.

The diagnosis of HIV infection is made on the basis of serum screening tests (immunoassay) and confirmed through the use of Western blot testing. Therapy with antimetabolities such as zidovudine (Retrovir) has been successful in delaying the progress of the disease for some patients. The results of long-term therapy and the

Table 28.5.
Types of Serologic Tests for Syphilis

Nontreponemal	Treponemal
Venereal disease research laboratory (VDRL)	Fluorescent treponemal–antibody absorption (FTA–ABS)
Rapid plasma reagin card test (RPR)	Microhemagglutination assay for antibodies to *T. pallidum* (MHA–TP)
Automated reagin test (ART)	

Table 28.6.
Sensitivity and Specificity of Serologic Tests for Syphilis

Test	Sensitivity			Latent Late	Specificity to Neurosyphilis
	Primary	Secondary	Early		
VDRL	78%	100%	96%	71%	98%
RPR	86%	100%	98%	73%	98%
FTA–ABS	84%	100%	100%	96%	97%
MHA-TP	76%	100%	97%	94%	99%

Table 28.7.
Treatment of Syphilis

Type	Preferred Treatment	Alternative Treatment
Primary, secondary, latent	Penicillin G benzathine, 2.4 MU i.m. **or** aqueous penicillin G procaine, 600,000 U i.m. every other day × 8 days; for latent: penicillin G benzathine, 2.4 MU i.m. weekly for 3 weeks	Tetracycline, 500 mg p.o. q.i.d. × 15 days Erythromycin 500 mg p.o. q.i.d. × 15 days in pregnant patients
Cardiovascular	Penicillin G benzathine, 2.4 MU i.m. weekly × 3 weeks **or** aqueous penicillin G procaine, 600,000 U i.m. every other day × 15 days	Tetracycline, 500 mg p.o. q.i.d. × 30 days Erythromycin 500 mg p.o. q.i.d. × 15 days in pregnant patients
Neurosyphilis	Crystalline penicillin G, 3–4 MU i.m. q. 4h. for at least 10 days	

Table 28.8.
Minor Sexually Transmitted Diseases

Disease	Causative Agent	Main Symptom	Diagnosis	Treatment
Chancroid	*Haemophilus ducreyi*	Painful "soft chancres," adenopathy	Clinical, smears, culture	Erythromycin, 500 mg q.i.d. for 10 days
Granuloma inguinale	*Calymmatobacterium granulomatis*	Raised, red lesions	Clinical, smears	Tetracycline, 500 mg q. 6h. for 3 weeks
Lymphogranuloma venereum (LGV)	*Chlamydia trachomatis*	Vesicle, progressing to bubo	Clinical, complement fixation test	Tetracycline, 500 mg q. 6h. for 3 weeks
Molluscum contagiosum	*Poxviridae* ·	Raised papule with waxy core	Clinical, inclusion bodies	Desiccation, cryotherapy, curettage
Parasites	*Pediculus, Sarcoptes scabiei*	Itching	Inspection	Lindane 1%
Enteric infections	*Neisseria gonorrhoeae, Chlamydia trachomatis, Shigella, Salmonella, protozoa*	Diarrhea	Culture	Based on agent
Vaginitis	*Trichomonas*	Odor, irritation	Microscopic examination of secretions	Metronidazole, 1 g A.M. and P.M. × 1 day or 500 mg b.i.d. for 7 days

development of improved treatment options have yet to become available.

Minor Sexually Transmitted Diseases

Chancroid, granuloma inguinale, lymphogranuloma venereum (LGV), molluscum contagiosum, parasite infections (such as pediculosis pubis or scabies), enteric infections, and some types of vaginitis (e.g., trichomoniasis) are infections that are spread through sexual activities. Pertinent information about these infections, some of which are seldom seen, is summarized in Tables 28.8 and 28.9.

CASE STUDIES

Case 28A

A 20-year-old college student comes to your office with the complaint of severe vulvar pain and itching, which has been present for 3 days. The patient first noted some "tingling" and irritation, followed by the development of open sores that are extremely painful. The patient also complains of extreme pain on urination. She reports a low-grade fever, but admits that she has not taken her temperature. When questioned, she concedes having broken up with her previous boyfriend and having become intimate with a new partner on one occasion about 1 week before the onset of symptoms. On examination, you find red, swollen labia with open ulcers that are painful to touch.

Questions Case 28A

To confirm your diagnostic suspicions, which of the following is most likely to be of help?

A. Microscopic examination of vaginal secretions mixed with 10% KOH
B. A "whiff" of vaginal secretions mixed with 10% KOH
C. Microscopic examination of material from the ulcerated lesions for giant cells
D. A cervical culture for gonorrhea
E. A serum test for syphilis (e.g., RPR)

Answer: C

The patient's history and physical findings suggest that this patient has a herpes vulvitis. If this is the case, screening for coexistent gonorrhea or syphilis is appropriate (answers D and E) but secondary to the diagnosis of the patient's complaint. Similarly, vaginal infections often oc-

Table 28.9.
Genital Lesions in Sexually Transmitted Diseases[a]

Characteristic	Herpes	Genital Warts	Syphilis	Chancroid	LGV	Granuloma Inguinale
Organism	Herpes simplex virus	Human papilloma virus	*Treponema pallidum*	*Haemophilus ducreyi*	*Chlamydia trachomatis*	*Calymmato- bacterium granulomatis*
Incubation	3–7 days	1–8 months	10–60 days	2–6 days	1–4 weeks	8–12 weeks
Primary lesion	**Vesicle**	Papule/ polypoid	Papule (chancre)	Papule/pustule	Papule/ pustule/ vesicle	Papule
Number	**Multiple coalesce**	Variable	1	1–3	Single	Single or multiple
Pain	**Yes**	No	**Rare**	**Often**	No	**Rare**
Shape	Regular	Irregular	Regular	Irregular	Regular	Regular
Margins	Flat	Raised	Raised	**Red, undermined**	Flat	**Rolled, elevated**
Depth	Superficial	Raised	Superficial	**Excavated**	Superficial	Elevated
Base	Red, smooth	Normal, pink, white	Red, smooth	**Yellow, gray**	Variable	Red, **rough**
Induration	None	None	**Firm**	Rare, soft	None	**Firm**
Secretions	Serous	None	Serous	**Purulent, hemorrhagic**	Variable	Rare, hemorrhagic
Lymph nodes	Firm, tender	**Normal**	Firm, nontender	Tender, suppurative	Tender, suppurative	Pseudo- adenopathy
Duration	5–10 days, **recurrent**	Months	Weeks	Weeks	Days	Weeks

[a] Scabies, molluscum contagiosum, *Candida*, and other dermatologic conditions (e.g., hidradenitis suppurativa) may also cause genital lesions. Items in boldface are of particular help in making a differential diagnosis.

cur as sexually transmitted diseases. Although *Trichomonas* infections are common in this group, they would not be tested for with the methods given in answers A and B. Screening for a vaginal infection is appropriate if history or physical findings suggest their presence.

The most reasonable therapy for this patient would be

A. Soap and water cleansing, air drying
B. Amoxicillin, 3 g, with probenecid, 1 g
C. Podophyllin 25% in benzoin
D. Metronidazole, 500 mg twice a day
E. Local steroid cream therapy

Answer: A

For initial infections with herpes, local cleansing to decrease the risk of secondary infection is the best therapy. Amoxicillin is an option for treating gonorrhea, whereas podophyllin is useful in treating condyloma, neither of which is likely in this patient. Similarly, metro-

nidazole is indicated for *Trichomonas*. Because of the viral nature of herpes, local steroids should be avoided. Acyclovir therapy for herpes is best started within 48 hr of the onset of lesions and is best carried out by either local cream or a oral dose of 200 mg five times per day. A three-times-a-day dosage is used for suppression of recurrences.

Case 28B

A 24-year-old married mother of three comes to the clinic with the complaint of "something growing down there." The patient first noted small growths on her labia 3 weeks previously, at the end of her menstrual period. These growths have persisted and enlarged. Several small growths have now appeared on the other side. The growths do not cause symptoms, but the patient had an aunt with breast cancer and so was concerned about what these might be. Past medical and surgical history are unremarkable. On physical examination, several small raised, shaggy lesions, ranging in size from 1 to 7 mm are noted on both labia and the perineum.

Question Case 28B

The most likely diagnosis in this patient is

A. Molluscum contagiosum
B. Genital herpes
C. Condyloma lata
D. Condyloma acuminata
E. Chancroid

Answer: D

The differential diagnosis of raised lesions must include molluscum contagiosum and condyloma lata, in addition to the more common condyloma acuminata. The lesions of molluscum contagiosum are more common over the lower abdomen and are distinguished by their central umbilication and yellowish cheesy appearance. Condyloma lata, found in syphilis, are usually flatter in appearance and have a broader base than venereal warts.

Case 28C

A 28-year-old unmarried nulligravid patient presents to you in the emergency room with a 6-hr history of diffuse lower abdominal pain. The pain was periumbilical but has now moved into the lower abdomen. She complains of a fever but has not taken her temperature. She notes mild nausea over the past hour. Past history reveals regular menstrual periods, with her last period occurring on schedule 1 week ago. She has had no previous surgeries or significant medical problems. She does note a similar episode 8 months previously for which she did not seek care. She is sexually active and has never used any contraception. On physical examination she has a pulse of 100, temperature of 38.10°C and a BP of 110/65. Examination of the abdomen finds diffuse tenderness in both lower quadrants. Pelvic examination is normal except for a yellowish discharge at the cervix, diffuse tenderness on motion of the uterus, and a tender fullness in both adnexa. You order a pregnancy test and a complete blood count (CBC) and perform cervical cultures.

Questions Case 28C

While you await the results of your laboratory tests, what is the most reasonable working diagnosis?

A. Ectopic pregnancy
B. Salpingitis (PID)
C. Appendicitis
D. Gastroenteritis
E. Threatened abortion

Answer: B

The results of the CBC return and you find a WBC of 14,000 with 82% segmented polys. The pregnancy test is negative and the culture will not be available for 48 hr. Based on this additional information, what is the most reasonable diagnosis?

A. Ectopic pregnancy
B. Salpingitis (PID)
C. Appendicitis
D. Gastroenteritis
E. Threatened abortion

Answer: B

Fever, lower abdominal pain, tachycardia, and cervical and bilateral adnexal tenderness all point to an inflammatory process in the pelvis. In a patient with infertility and a similar previous episode recurrent salpingitis (PID) is more likely than appendicitis. This is supported by the elevated white blood count and differential. Broad-spectrum therapy should be implemented based on clinical suspicion, even if the cultures should eventually return as "negative."

chapter 29

ABORTION

Abortion is the termination of a pregnancy prior to viability, typically defined as 20 weeks from the 1st day of the last normal menstrual period or a fetus weighing <500 g. Whether spontaneous or induced, there are profound medical as well as emotional implications associated with abortion. Because the lay expression for spontaneous abortion is "miscarriage," care should be taken to explain the terminology to the patient.

SPONTANEOUS ABORTION

The *incidence of spontaneous abortion* is estimated at 50% of all pregnancies, an estimate based on the assumption that many pregnancies spontaneously terminate without clinical recognition. An incidence of recognized spontaneous abortion of 15 to 25% is commonly cited, with approximately 80% occurring during the first 12 weeks of pregnancy.

Approximately 50% of early spontaneous abortions are attributed to chromosomal abnormalities, of which trisomy accounts for 40 to 50%, monosomy C for 15 to 25%, triploidy for about 15%, and tetraploidy for about 5%. If the first abortus is chromosomally abnormal, a second abortus will have a 80% chance of being abnormal as well. Risk factors associated with spontaneous abortion include increasing parity, increasing maternal age, increasing paternal age, and conception within 3 months of a live birth. Abnormal development of the early pregnancy (including the zygote, embryo, fetus, or placenta) is a common pathologic finding in spontaneous abortion. Expulsion of the pregnancy is typically preceded by death of the embryo or fetus.

The further that a pregnancy progresses before undergoing spontaneous abortion, the less likely that the fetus is chromosomally abnormal compared with first-trimester abortions. Second-trimester abortions are less likely to be chromo-

2nd Trimester Abortions

somal and more likely to be caused by maternal systemic disease, abnormal placentation, or other anatomic considerations. This difference is of great clinical significance, because these conditions can be treated and recurrent abortions can thereby potentially be prevented.

Maternal Factors

Infections Factors

Maternal systemic conditions that have been associated with spontaneous abortion include infections such as *Listeria monocytogenes, Mycoplasma hominis, Ureaplasma urealyticum,* and *toxoplasmosis* as well as viral infections such as rubella and cytomegalic inclusion disease.

Endocrine Factors

Insufficient secretion of progesterone by the corpus luteum or the placenta has been associated with spontaneous abortion. *Luteal phase inadequacy* occurs in about 3% of the general population but much more frequently in those suffering spontaneous pregnancy loss. Luteal phase defect is diagnosed by appropriately timed endometrial biopsy, not serum progesterone assay. Two non-specific drugs for improvement of luteal function are used: clomiphene, acting by increasing follicle-stimulating hormone (FSH), and human chorionic gonadotropin (hCG), which is the physiologic luteotropic stimulus. Although uncommon, uncorrected medical conditions such as *hyperthyroidism* and *diabetes* are also associated with an increased incidence of spontaneous abortion.

Environmental Factors

Spontaneous abortion has also been related to environmental toxins, radiation, and immunologic factors. Both *smoking and alcohol consumption* have been linked to miscarriages. Women who smoke more than one pack of cigarettes per day have an almost twofold increase in their rate of spontaneous abortion. Women who drink more than 2 days per week experience twice the abortion rate of those who do not.

Uterine Factors

Leiomyomata uteri, especially when located in a submucous position, have been associated with spontaneous abortion. It is uncommon for subserous or intramural leiomyomata of the uterus to be a causative factor of spontaneous abortion. Removal of the leiomyomata (myomectomy) is recommended only if it is determined that pregnancy wastage has been caused by this anatomic distortion.

Spontaneous abortion can also be caused by a *unicornuate or septate uterus*, with 20 to 30% of women with a unicornuate or septate uterus having reproductive difficulties, most frequently recurrent pregnancy loss. In utero exposure to *diethylstilbestrol (DES)* has been associated with abnormally shaped uteri as well as cervical incompetence.

Intrauterine synechiae (Asherman's syndrome) has been linked to spontaneous abortion, caused by an inadequate amount of endometrium to support implantation. This condition is typically a sequela of uterine curettage with subsequent destruction and scarring of the endometrium (Table 29.1).

Paternal Factors

Occasionally, a chromosomal abnormality in either parent may be a cause of spontaneous abortion. As a result, couples suffering recurrent abortions should have karyotyping of both parents. In addition, as with eggs, advanced age of sperm may also increase the rate of spontaneous abortion.

Fetal Factors

Genetic abnormalities of the conceptus is the most common cause of spontaneous abortion. More than 50% of abortions in the first trimester are caused by chromosomal anomalies, approximately half of which are autosomal trisomies. Whereas chromosomally abnormal pregnancies tend to terminate early, chromosomally normal pregnancies are usually lost later in gestation. Specifically, three-quarters of aneuploid abortions occur before 8 weeks, whereas the incidence of euploid abortions is highest at 13 weeks.

DIFFERENTIAL DIAGNOSIS OF ABORTION

Because the differential diagnosis of bleeding in the first trimester of pregnancy includes a wide range of possibilities such as ectopic pregnancy, hydatidiform mole, cervical polyps, and cervicitis, the patient should be examined whenever bleeding occurs. Any vaginal bleeding in the first half of an intrauterine pregnancy is presumptively called a *threatened abortion* unless another specific diagnosis can be made.

Threatened Abortion

Threatened abortion occurs in up to 25% of pregnancies with approximately half of these patients proceeding to spontaneous abortion. Those who carry a pregnancy complicated by threatened abortion to viability are at greater risk for preterm delivery, low birth weight, and a higher incidence of perinatal mortality. There does not, however, appear to be a higher incidence of congenital malformations in these newborns. Some patients describe bleeding at the time of their expected menses, sometimes referred to as the *placental sign or implantation bleeding*, which may be the result of ruptured blood vessels in the endometrium. The differential diagnosis includes a friable cervix without cervicitis, laceration, or polyp or even, on occasion, rectal or urethral bleeding.

Ultrasonography is especially useful to determine if an early pregnancy is intact. Lack of a gestational sac does not, however, rule out a very early viable pregnancy. Ultrasonography, in conjunction with quantitative human chorionic gonadotropin, has been used to identify viable pregnancies at various stages of gestation. Transabdominal ultrasonography can identify an intact gestation if the quantitative β-hCG exceeds 5000 to 6000 mIU/mL, whereas transvaginal ultrasonography can typically identify an early intact pregnancy when the β-hCG level exceeds 1500 mIU/mL.

Inevitable Abortion

An *inevitable abortion* is defined as rupture of the membranes and/or cervical dilation during the first half of pregnancy such that pregnancy loss is unavoidable. It is unusual for pregnancy to successfully reach viability in this circumstance. Uterine contractions typically follow and the products of conception are expelled. Conservative management of these patients significantly increases the risk of infection.

Table 29.1.
Causes of Spontaneous Abortion

Genetic factors (10–50%)	Infection
Nondisjunction	*Listeria monocytogenes*
Balanced translocation/carrier state	*Mycoplasma hominis*
	Ureaplasma urealyticum
Endocrine abnormalities (25–50%)	Toxoplasmosis
Luteal phase defect	Syphilis
Thyroid disease	
Hyperandrogenism	Systemic disease
In utero DES exposure	Diabetes mellitus
	Chronic renal disease
Reproductive tract abnormalities (6–12%)	Chronic cardiovascular disease
Leiomyomata uteri (submucous)	Systemic lupus/lupus anticoagulant
Septate uterus	
Bicornuate or unicornuate uterus	Environmental factors
Incompetent cervix	Toxins
Intrauterine adhesions	Radiation
Abnormality of placentation	Smoking
	Alcohol
	Anesthetic gases

Completed Abortion

Completed abortion refers to a documented pregnancy that spontaneously aborts all of the products of conception. Early in pregnancy, the fetus and placenta are generally expelled in toto.

Incomplete Abortion

In those cases of spontaneous abortions in which some tissue is retained, bleeding and pain result. Suction curettage of the uterus is usually necessary to remove the remaining products of conception and prevent further bleeding and infection (see Chapter 2). Postevacuation treatment with an oxytocic (methergine, 0.2 mg p.o. q. 8h. for 2 days) and an antibiotic (doxycycline, 100 mg p.o. b.i.d. for 3 days) reduces the risk of further bleeding and infection.

Missed Abortion

A *missed abortion* is the retention of a failed intrauterine pregnancy for an extended period, usually defined as more than two menstrual cycles. These patients present with an absence of uterine growth and may have lost some of the early symptoms of pregnancy. Although unusual, disseminated intravascular coagulopathy (DIC) can occur when an intrauterine fetal demise in the second trimester has been retained beyond 6 weeks after the death of the fetus. Evacuation of the uterus with suction curettage is recommended for pregnancy in the first trimester, while dilation and evacuation (D&E) or the use of prostaglandin suppositories is utilized for pregnancies that have advanced to the second trimester.

Recurrent Abortion

Recurrent abortion is a term used when a patient has had more than two consecutive or a total of three spontaneous abortions. In early abortions, there is a great likelihood of a chromosomal abnormality, whereas in later abortions, a maternal cause is more likely. Karyotyping is recommended for both parents when recurrent early abortion occurs, as there is a 3% chance of one parent being a symptomless carrier of a chromosomal abnormality after two fetal losses. The possibility of immunologic factors should also be explored. Correction of maternal medical conditions and/or anatomic deformities should be pursued for those patients with recurrent late abortions. These include surgical correction of uterine abnormalities, cerclage of the incompetent cervix, or lysis of intrauterine synechiae.

Recurrent abortion can be the result of *uterine anomalies*, especially septate uterus, although only about 25% of patients with septate uteri have problems with fetal wastage. Infertility is not usually a problem with these patients. Treatment is surgical, as seen in Figure 29.1.

The *incompetent cervix* is diagnosed mainly by its classic history of sudden expulsion of a normal sac and fetus between the 18th and 32nd week of pregnancy without prior pain or bleeding. Diagnosis is by history and observation of a lax, open cervical os. Treatment is surgical by the *cerclage*

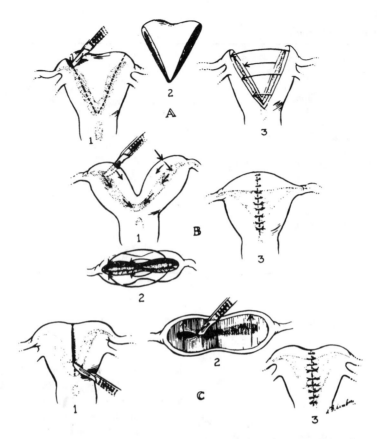

Figure 29.1. Surgical treatment of septate and bicornuate uterus. **A,** Septate Uterus. **B,** the Bicornuate Uterus. Techniques of surgical repair include [A] the wedge technique of Jones, [B] the transverse fundal incision of Strassman, and [C] the median bivalving technique of Tompkins.

procedures, which involve the placement of a "purse-string" suture about the cervix to close the incompetent cervix (Fig. 29.2). Such sutures are commonly placed during pregnancy when the cervix is found to be symptomlessly opening. The suture must be removed when labor ensues (or rupture of membranes occurs) or the patient must be delivered by cesarean birth. Allowing a patient to labor with a cerclage in place risks extensive laceration of the cervix and/or uterine rupture.

Intrauterine synechiae are usually associated with *Asherman's syndrome,* where a too vigorous curettage denudes the endometrium past the layer of the basalis so that webs of myometrium develop across the uterine cavity (the synechiae). Asherman's syndrome is associated with pelvic pain, amenorrhea or irregular menses, infertility, and recurrent pregnancy loss. The diagnosis is sus-

pected by history and confirmed by a hysterogram that shows the characteristic webbed pattern or by hysteroscopy. Treatment involves lysis of the synechiae and postoperative treatment with large doses of estrogen (conjugated estrogen, Premarin, 1.25 mg p.o. two to four times per day for several weeks) to facilitate endometrial proliferation, leading to the reestablishment of a normal endometrial layer.

TREATMENT OF SPONTANEOUS ABORTION

No intervention is necessary for patients with threatened abortion even if the bleeding is accompanied by low abdominal pain and cramping. If there is no evidence of significant pathology, and the pregnancy is found to be intact, the patient can be reassured and allowed to continue normal activ-

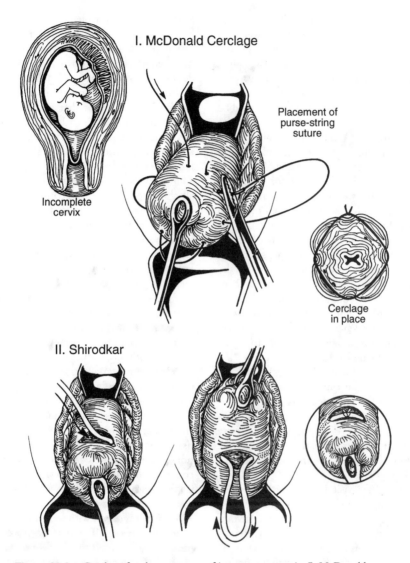

I. McDonald Cerclage

Placement of
purse-string
suture

Incomplete
cervix

Cerclage
in place

II. Shirodkar

Figure 29.2. Cerclage for the treatment of incompetent cervix. **I,** McDonald cerclage. Identification of incompetent cervix; **II,** placement of the purse-string suture about the cervix and tightening the purse-string; after cerclage is in place. II. Shirodkar cerclage.

ities. Intercourse is usually proscribed for 2 to 3 weeks, or longer, depending on the etiology of bleeding. Although commonly recommended, a short period of bedrest has no documented benefit.

If pain and bleeding persist, especially with significant hemodynamic alterations, or if ultrasound and hormonal evaluation identify a nonviable pregnancy, evacuation of the uterus should be carried out. Immediate considerations include control of bleeding, prevention of infection, pain relief (if needed), and emotional support.

Bleeding is controlled by ensuring that all the products of the conception have been expelled or removed from the uterus. This may be presumed in cases of complete abortion or may be accomplished through curettage in cases of incomplete, inevitable, missed, or septic abortions. Hemostasis is enhanced through uterine contraction stimulated by intravenous oxytocin or intramuscular Methergine (methylergonovine maleate). Removal of the products of conception also decreases the risk of infection, and this, combined with vaginal rest (no tampons, douches, or intercourse), provides adequate infection protection in most cases.

A mild analgesic may be required and should be offered. Rh– mothers should receive Rh immune globulin (RhoGAM). Chromosomal evaluation of spontaneous abortions is not recommended unless there is a history of recurrent abortion.

Emotional support is important for both the short- and long-term well-being of the patient as well as her partner. No matter how well prepared for the possibility of pregnancy loss a couple is, the event is a significant disappointment and cause of stress. When appropriate, the couple should be reassured that the loss was not precipitated by anything that they did or did not do and that there was nothing that they could have done to prevent the loss. Although a potentially sensitive issue, there is a natural tendency to try to find a reason for this type of letdown. This can lead to thoughts of "If we hadn't made love 2 weeks ago" or "if I hadn't let her pick up the grocery bag." These are clearly unrelated to the cause of most abortions and can easily lead to further stress in a relationship at a time when both partners need support the most. Couples are often reluctant to raise these issues in this situation, further increasing the risk of friction. These issues are best raised directly by the physician.

A follow-up office visit is generally scheduled for 2 to 6 weeks after the loss of a pregnancy. This is an appropriate time to evaluate uterine involution, assess the return of menses, and discuss reproductive plans. The causes (or lack of causes) of the pregnancy loss should also be reiterated. The impact of this loss on future childbearing should be discussed. A single pregnancy loss does not significantly increase the risk of future losses. Multiple pregnancy losses carry an increased risk for future pregnancies based, in part, on the higher likelihood of a continuing causative condition such as fibroids, immune diseases, or genetic disorders.

INDUCED ABORTION

Termination of an intact pregnancy before the time of viability can be done to safeguard the health of the mother or on a purely elective, i.e., voluntary, basis. Elective abortion has been legal since the Supreme Court decision of *Roe v. Wade.*

Since that time, various local and state laws have been proposed to significantly limit access to elective abortion. These laws will continue to undergo many court challenges as our society struggles to define a consistent national policy.

Before embarking on an elective abortion, patients must be aware that choices are available. These include continuation of pregnancy with subsequent adoption, continuation of pregnancy and keeping the child, and elective abortion during either the first or second trimester. Medical and/or surgical complications are associated with all choices, with the least complications related to elective abortion in the first trimester. Although there are complications associated with pregnancy termination, they are significantly less than those associated with carrying a pregnancy. First-trimester pregnancies are typically terminated by means of suction curettage, i.e., vacuum aspiration performed through the cervix. Second-trimester abortions are most commonly performed through the cervix, using suction or destructive forceps, or by the use of prostaglandins, as in the form of intraamniotic injections or vaginal suppositories.

The most common complication following an induced abortion is infection. The patient usually presents with fever, pain, a tender uterus, and mild bleeding. Oral antibiotics and antipyretics are usually sufficient to manage these mild infections. If tissue remains in the uterus, (incomplete abortion), suction curettage is also necessary. The third common complication following induced abortion is bleeding. Risk of death from abortion during the first 2 months of pregnancy is less than 1 per 100,000 procedures, with increasing rates as pregnancy progresses. There is no apparent risk to future pregnancies if the first- or second-trimester abortion has been free of complications. There appears to be a slight increased risk of premature delivery if more than three first-trimester pregnancies are terminated by elective abortion.

Other techniques used to perform abortions include hysterotomy, hysterectomy, intrauterine infusion of hypertonic solutions such as saline and urea, and the not-yet approved antiprogesterone medication RU 486 (mifepristone).

SEPTIC ABORTION

Occasionally, patients may present with a *septic abortion*, an infected complete or incomplete abortion in which the patient presents with sepsis, shock, hemorrhage, and possibly renal failure. It

ILLEGAL PAST 24 WKS

rarely occurs as a complication of a legal abortion but is more commonly associated with criminal abortions, those done illegally, under unsterile conditions, by persons who may have little or no knowledge of medicine or anatomy. Broad-spectrum parenteral antibiotics, fluid therapy, and prompt evacuation of the uterus are indicated. A careful evaluation for trauma, including perforation of the uterus or vagina, should also be carried out.

CASE STUDIES

Case 29A

A 20-year-old college student (G1 P1) presents with the complaint of 2 days of vaginal bleeding, 6 weeks after her last menstrual period. She has regular menstrual periods and uses condoms alone for contraception. She has had a positive home pregnancy test. The bleeding has been dark in color, painless, and began after intercourse.

Examination shows a small amount of dark blood in the vagina and at the cervical os. The cervix is closed and no tissue is visible. Bimanual examination reveals a slightly softened, normal size uterus and normal adnexa without masses or tenderness.

Questions Case 29A

Based on your assessment, your best course of management is

A. Perform a culdocentesis
B. Order a transvaginal ultrasound examination
C. Prescribe medroxyprogesterone (Provera) 10 mg/day
D. Recommend pelvic rest and light activity
E. Advise evacuation of the uterus by suction curettage
F. Order a serum quantitative β-hCG

Answer: F

While a home pregnancy test is probably reliable, confirmation is indicated, which will also provide additional quantitative information. Therapeutic maneuvers are premature, although pelvic rest and light activity would probably be included in any situation. Invasive procedures and expensive imaging procedures are not indicated.

The quantitative β-hCG is reported as 846 mIU/mL. You indeed recommend pelvic rest and only light activity, with the likely diagnosis being threatened abortion. She returns in 48 hr; she still has bleeding, although now more like a menstrual period, and a repeat β-hCG is

146 mIU/mL. On examination her uterus is firm; the cervix closed; there is no uterine, cervical, or adnexal tenderness; and she is afebrile. Your working diagnosis is

A. Intrauterine pregnancy
B. Threatened abortion
C. Incomplete abortion
D. Complete abortion
E. Missed abortion
F. Ectopic pregnancy

Answer: D

The evidence suggests a failed pregnancy with expulsion of the intrauterine contents. There is no clinical evidence of ectopic pregnancy or infection.

Your best management is

A. Continued clinical observation for a few more days
B. Discussion of contraception
C. RhoGAM if she is Rh–
D. Transvaginal ultrasonography to rule out the life-threatening possibility of ectopic pregnancy

Answer: A, B, C

Case 29B

A 32-year-old G2 P1001 presents with intense right lower-quadrant pain of 2 hr duration that is so severe she has difficulty walking. She tells you she had a positive urine pregnancy test in her doctor's office earlier in the week and that she was told she was about 6 weeks pregnant based on her last menstrual period and a pelvic examination.

In the last 2 weeks she has had some nausea and occasional emesis in the mornings and is not hungry. She has no history of sexually transmitted diseases. Her review of systems negative.

On examination she has a temperature of 99.2°F, her blood pressure is 120/65, her pulse 90 and firm. Her abdomen is tender to palpation without masses or rebound, although bowel sounds are diminished. On pelvic examination, her cervix is slightly tender, her uterus is at a 6- to 8-week size and retroverted, and there is an indistinct tender fullness in the right adnexa.

Questions Case 29B

Your differential diagnosis includes

A. Intrauterine pregnancy
B. Threatened abortion
C. Incomplete abortion
D. Ectopic pregnancy
E. Corpus luteum cyst
F. Pelvic inflammatory disease
G. Appendicitis

H. Diverticulitis

Answer: A, D, E, G

Pregnancy inside and outside the uterus, a pregnancy-related corpus luteum cyst, and appendicitis are all consistent with the data. Incomplete abortion is not, as there is no bleeding. PID is unlikely, because she is pregnant and her fever is low, although this can be a presentation of *Chlamydia*-associated infection. Diverticulitis is uncommon in her age group.

Your best management is

A. Quantitative β-hCG
B. Quantitative serum progesterone
C. Transvaginal ultrasound
D. Culdocentesis
E. Diagnostic laparoscopy

Answer: A, B, C, D

The serum β-hCG will help define the pregnancy and assist in the interpretation of ultrasound findings. Serum progesterone is advocated by many to identify a pregnancy that is unlikely to be viable. Transvaginal ultrasound is indicated, because there is the question of an adnexal mass and the location of the pregnancy has not been determined. Invasive procedures are not indicated at this time.

The β-hCG is 2,345 mIU/mL, and the serum progesterone is pending. Transvaginal ultrasound reveals a viable intrauterine pregnancy and a cystic right adnexal mass, $2 \times 3 \times 4$ cm. There is a small amount of fluid in the cul-de-sac of Douglas. Your most likely diagnosis is intrauterine pregnancy and a symptomatic corpus luteum cyst. You can reassure the patient and follow her clinically.

chapter 30

ECTOPIC PREGNANCY

INCIDENCE

Implantation outside of the uterine cavity is termed *ectopic pregnancy*, a condition that significantly jeopardizes the mother and is incompatible with continuing the pregnancy. In most cases the pregnancy is in the fallopian tube, i.e., *tubal ectopic pregnancy*. Catastrophic bleeding may occur when the implanting pregnancy erodes into blood vessels or ruptures through structures (typically the fallopian tubes) not suited to accommodate the growing conceptus.

Primarily because of an increasing prevalence of pelvic inflammatory disease (PID), the incidence of ectopic pregnancy has been increasing over the past few years: 1 ectopic pregnancy now occurs for every 66 intrauterine pregnancies. Despite this increase in the number of cases of ectopic pregnancy, maternal mortality has decreased markedly. In 1970, there were 3.5 maternal deaths per 1000 cases of ectopic pregnancy; now the rate is less than 1 per 1000. This improvement is primarily the result of better detection, allowing early intervention before massive bleeding occurs.

Pregnancies may implant in many locations in the genital tract and pelvis (Fig. 30.1). The vast majority of ectopic gestations (95%) occur in the fallopian tube (*tubal pregnancy*). Four of five tubal pregnancies occur in the ampullary portion of the fallopian tube. Infrequent locations include the cervix, ovary, and peritoneal cavity (respectively, *cervical, ovarian, and abdominal pregnancy*).

Patients with ectopic pregnancy not only are at risk for immediate morbidity and mortality from acute blood loss and risk of anatomic damage but have a significantly reduced fertility rate, with fewer than one-half of patients subsequently having a live full-term birth. As the *second leading cause of maternal mortality in the United States, ectopic pregnancy should be high in the differential diagnosis for any woman of reproductive age with acute pelvic or lower abdominal pain, with or without abnormal vaginal bleeding*. Pain early in pregnancy should also raise the possibility of ectopic pregnancy.

CAUSES OF ECTOPIC PREGNANCY

Knowing which patients are at higher risk can aid the physician in making an early diagnosis. The primary risk factor for ectopic pregnancy is a prior history of *salpingitis*. Damage from such infection may retard the passage of the fertilized ovum through the tube to the endometrial cavity, facilitating extrauterine implantation. Women with a history of salpingitis have a 6-fold increase in their risk of ectopic pregnancy. A previous ectopic pregnancy also increases the risk of future ectopic implantations by approximately 10-fold.

Age is an important risk factor. Women 35 to 44 years old have a threefold increase in the rate of ectopic pregnancy compared with women 15 to 24 years old. More than half of all ectopic pregnancies occur in women who have had *three or more pregnancies*. Finally, *Black and Hispanic women* also have a significantly higher risk of ectopic pregnancy.

Contrary to some reports, *sterilization, contraception, and abortion do not increase ectopic pregnancy frequency*. Oral contraceptives prevent ovulation, thereby significantly reducing pregnancies in all locations. Intrauterine contraception devices (IUCDs) prevent all types of pregnancies, although ectopic pregnancies may be reduced relatively less than intrauterine pregnancies, thereby giving the false impression that they are a risk factor. The higher prevalence of pelvic inflammatory disease in IUCD users, however, may increase the patient's risk even after the removal of the IUCD.

In patients with previous sterilization, the chance of ectopic pregnancy is increased, but because sterilization failures are so uncommon, the

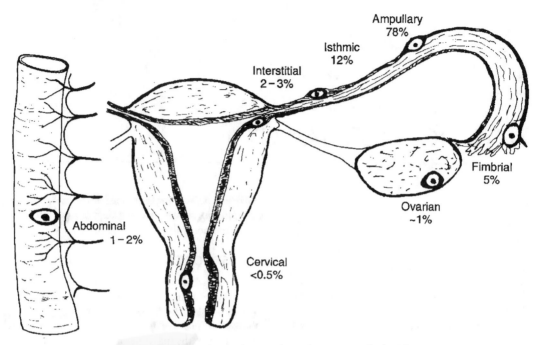

Figure 30.1. Incidence of types of ectopic pregnancy by location.

net effect of sterilization is to protect against ectopic pregnancies. Although 85% of sterilization failures are associated with intrauterine pregnancies, the possibility of an ectopic pregnancy should always be considered in patients with sterilization failures. Abortion itself does not predispose to ectopic pregnancy, although associated infection may do so. There has been a reported effect of ovulation induction in increasing the risk of ectopic pregnancy. This has been difficult to determine, because there is the potential for subclinical tubal disease in some infertile patients, which may itself be the primary cause of the ectopic pregnancy.

CLINICAL EVALUATION OF POSSIBLE ECTOPIC PREGNANCY

Symptoms of Tubal Pregnancy

The classic presentation of a patient with an ectopic pregnancy includes *abdominal pain, amenorrhea, and vaginal bleeding*, although all of these symptoms are not always present. The frequency of symptoms in patients with ectopic pregnancy is presented in Table 30.1.

The mechanism of *implantation* in ectopic pregnancies is similar to that of an intrauterine gestation. Symptoms arise from the development of he-

moperitoneum or the distention of a hollow viscus, such as the fallopian tube, or both. Early ectopic pregnancies are asymptomatic. As the pregnancy grows, the most common symptom is abdominal or pelvic pain, which is present in nearly all patients. The pain is generally described as colicky in character and may be unilateral (not necessarily on the same side as the ectopic) or bilateral, intermittent or constant, located in the lower or even upper abdomen. The proximal portions of the fallopian tube are not as able to adapt to the growing pregnancy, so an ectopic pregnancy in this area is likely to become symptomatic earlier in gestation.

In up to one-fifth of patients with extensive intraabdominal bleeding, irritation of the diaphragm causes referred pain to the shoulder. Irritation of the posterior cul-de-sac may cause an urge to defecate. These patients may present with a history of feeling faint or passing out while straining to have a bowel movement. Syncope occurs in approximately one-third of patients with ruptured tubal pregnancies, less frequently in unruptured cases.

Although patients with ectopic pregnancy typically have missed their normal menses, this history is often not given. By the time symptoms have developed, it has usually been 6 weeks since the last normal menstrual period. At this early stage, symptoms of pregnancy are not always present and cannot be used to rule in or rule out ectopic pregnancy.

As long as placental hormones are produced, there is usually no vaginal bleeding. Irregular vaginal bleeding results from the sloughing of the decidua from the endometrial lining. Vaginal bleeding in patients with an ectopic gestation may range from little or none to heavy, menstrual-like flow. In some patients, the entire "decidual cast" is passed intact, simulating a spontaneous abortion. (Fig. 30.2). Histologic evaluation of this tissue will confirm whether placental villi are present. In any patient with a positive pregnancy test, whenever evaluation of tissue passed spontaneously or obtained by curettage does not demonstrate villi, an ectopic implantation should be assumed to be present until proven otherwise.

Physical Findings in Tubal Pregnancy

Physical examination findings range from a totally normal examination in early unruptured ectopic pregnancy to hypovolemic shock and an acute abdomen in cases of ruptured ectopic pregnancy. Most healthy reproductive-age women are able to compensate for mild to moderate degrees of blood loss so that extensive blood loss is usually required to cause a fall in blood pressure and a rise in pulse. Only about 5% of patients present in hypovolemic shock, although blood loss is the major factor in 85% of ectopic pregnancy deaths. A summary of physical examination findings is presented in Table 30.2.

Fever is not expected, although a mild elevation in temperature in response to intraperitoneal blood may occur. A temperature of greater than 38°C may suggest an infectious etiology to a patient's symptoms. Abdominal distention and tenderness, with or without rebound, rigidity, or decreased bowel sounds, may be seen in cases of intraabdominal bleeding. Abdominal tenderness is present in 50 to 90% of patients with ectopic pregnancies, depending on the series cited. Cervical motion tenderness caused by intraperitoneal irritation and adnexal tenderness are commonly found. An adnexal mass is present in roughly one-third of cases, but its absence does not rule out the possibility of an ectopic implantation. The uterus may enlarge and soften throughout the first trimester, thus simulating an intrauterine pregnancy. A slightly open cervix with blood or decidual tissue may be found and mistaken for a threatened and/or spontaneous abortion.

Differential Diagnosis

The rapid and accurate diagnosis of ectopic pregnancy is imperative to reduce the risk of serious complications or death. Up to one-half of ectopic pregnancy–related maternal deaths have had a lag in treatment because of delayed or inaccurate

Table 30.1.
Symptoms of Ectopic Pregnancy

Symptoms	Prevalence, %
Abdominal pain	95–100
Generalized	50
Unilateral	35
Shoulder	20
Back	5–10
Abnormal uterine bleeding	65–85
Amenorrhea	75–95
<2 weeks	45
<6 weeks	35
Syncope ↑ c̄ ruptured tubal	10–18
Dizziness	20–35
Pregnancy symptoms	10–20
Nausea	15
Urge to defecate – irritation of posterior cul-de-sac	5–15

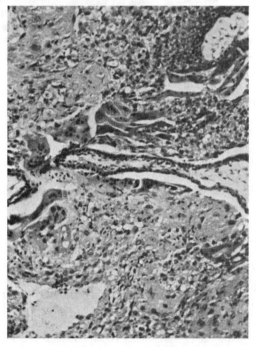

Figure 30.2. Decidual cast.

Table 30.2.
Physical Examination in Ectopic Pregnancy

Finding	Prevalence, %
Abdominal tenderness	80–90
Peritoneal signs	
Ruptured	50
Unruptured	5
Adnexal tenderness	75–90
Unilateral	40–75
Bilateral	50–75
Cervical motion tenderness	50–75
Adnexal mass	30–50
Contralateral	20
Uterus	
Normal size	70
Enlarged	15–30
Orthostatic changes	10–15
Temperature >37°C	5–10
Vomiting	15

diagnoses. *Any sexually active woman in the reproductive age group who presents with pain, irregular bleeding, and/or amenorrhea should have ectopic pregnancy as a part of the initial differential diagnosis.* Other elements of the differential diagnosis include complications of an intrauterine pregnancy (threatened, missed, complete, or incomplete abortion), nonpregnancy-related gynecologic conditions (acute and chronic salpingitis, follicular or corpus luteum cyst rupture, endometriosis, or adnexal torsion) and nongynecologic conditions (e.g., gastroenteritis and appendicitis).

DIAGNOSTIC PROCEDURES

The initial assessment in the otherwise hemodynamically stable patient must include a *pregnancy test*. With the sensitive assays available today, a negative pregnancy test excludes the possibility of ectopic pregnancy. Urinary pregnancy tests, which detect hCG levels to 50 mIU/mL, are now commonly available. They detect hCG as early as 14 days after conception and are positive in more than 90% of cases of ectopic pregnancy. Serum assays can detect the presence of hCG as early as 5 days after conception, but because they require additional time and expertise to perform, they are often not used in a potentially emergent clinical setting.

If a positive pregnancy test is obtained in association with a clinical scene consistent with ec-

topic pregnancy, the remainder of the workup will focus on evaluation of the viability and location of the pregnancy. *Quantitative β-hCG levels* can be followed at 2-day intervals. Early in pregnancy, these levels should increase by at least 66% in 48 hr. Failure to meet this criterion indicates a pregnancy not growing appropriately, thus increasing the suspicion of ectopic pregnancy. An inappropriate rise in hCG identifies a potentially abnormal pregnancy but does not identify its location. No single hCG result can be used to rule in or rule out ectopic pregnancy, unless it is negative.

A useful adjunct to serial quantitative levels of hCG is pelvic *ultrasonography* (Fig. 30.3). Ultrasonography cannot be relied on to routinely image a pregnancy outside the uterine cavity, but it can identify an intrauterine pregnancy with considerable accuracy, thus effectively ruling out ectopic pregnancy with the very rare possibility of a combined (heterotropic) pregnancy as the exception. Transabdominal ultrasonography should be able to identify an intrauterine gestation by the time the hCG level reaches 5000–6000 mIU/mL. The more sensitive transvaginal ultrasonography should show the pregnancy by the time the hCG level is 1500 mIU/mL. Failure to do so should further increase the suspicion that an ectopic pregnancy exists.

Although a low hematocrit is unusual, a complete blood count can document possible blood loss anemia and identify leukocytosis. If the white blood count (WBC) is >20,000 (WBC/dL), infection may be more likely than an ectopic pregnancy.

Serum progesterone concentration has also been used as a screening test for ectopic pregnancy. A progesterone of <5.0 ng/mL indicates a nonviable pregnancy, raising the suspicion of an ectopic pregnancy, Serum progesterone levels >25 ng/mL help in cases of suspected ectopic gestation, as only 2.5% of all abnormal pregnancies (ectopic or intrauterine) have serum progesterone levels above this level.

Curettage of the uterine cavity can also help rule out ectopic pregnancy. Although intrauterine and ectopic pregnancy can exist simultaneously in rare cases, identification of chorionic villi in curettings identifies an intrauterine location of the pregnancy and essentially rules out ectopic pregnancy. The Arias-Stella reaction, a hypersecretory endometrium of pregnancy seen on histologic examination is compatible not only with ectopic pregnancy but also with intrauterine pregnancy and is, therefore, not useful in identifying an ectopic

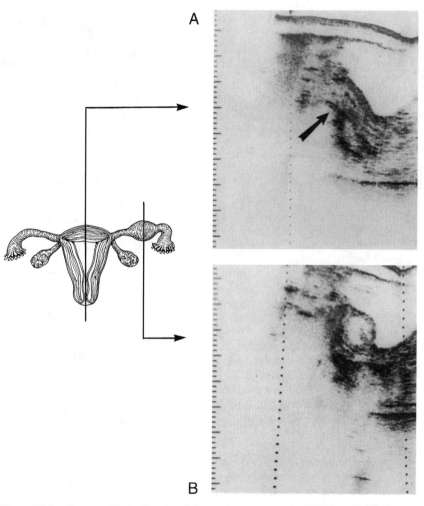

Figure 30.3. Sonographic findings in tubal ectopic pregnancy. **A,** Midline view through empty uterus. **B,** Paramidline view showing cystic mass in area of fallopian tube.

pregnancy. Instrumentation of the uterine cavity should be undertaken only after thorough consideration of the likelihood that an ongoing pregnancy might be interrupted.

Culdocentesis can aid in the identification of a hemoperitoneum, which in turn, may indicate a ruptured ectopic pregnancy, although other conditions such as a ruptured corpus luteum cyst can also cause a hemoperitoneum. An 18-gauge needle is inserted posterior to the cervix, between the uterosacral ligaments, and into the cul-de-sac of the peritoneal cavity (Fig. 30.4). Aspiration of clear peritoneal fluid (negative culdocentesis) indicates no hemorrhage into the abdominal cavity but does not rule out an unruptured ectopic

pregnancy. Aspiration of blood that clots can indicate either penetration of a vessel or rapid blood loss into the peritoneal cavity in which case the blood clot has not had time to undergo fibrinolysis. Nonclotting blood is evidence of hemoperitoneum (positive culdocentesis) in which the blood clot has undergone fibrinolysis. If nothing is aspirated (equivocal or nondiagnostic culdocentesis), no information is obtained. Unfortunately, no finding on culdocentesis can definitively rule in or rule out ectopic pregnancy, although a positive culdocentesis identifies blood in the peritoneal cavity and confirms the need for further evaluation to identify the source of the bleeding.

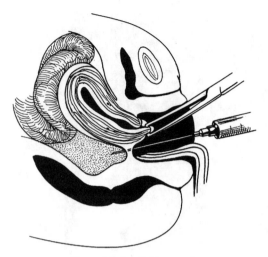

Figure 30.4. Culdocentesis.

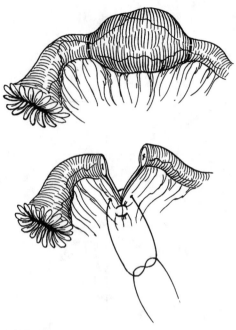

Figure 30.6. Surgical management of ectopic pregnancy: segmental resection and tubal reanastomosis.

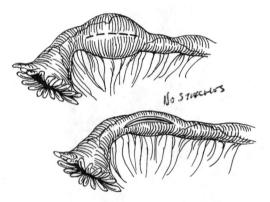

Figure 30.5. Surgical management of ectopic pregnancy: linear salpingostomy.

The most accurate technique of identifying an ectopic pregnancy is by direct visualization, done most commonly via laparoscopy or laparotomy. Even laparoscopy, however, carries a 2 to 5% misdiagnosis rate, because an extremely early tubal gestation may not be identified as it may not distend the fallopian tube sufficiently to be recognized as an abnormality. False-positive diagnoses may occur as a hematosalpinx may be interpreted as an unruptured ectopic pregnancy.

MANAGEMENT OF ECTOPIC PREGNANCY

The traditional management of a tubal pregnancy is surgical removal. Conservative surgical techniques have been developed that maximize preservation of reproductive organs. If done through the laparoscope, definitive diagnosis and treatment can be accomplished at the same operation with minimal morbidity, cost, and hospitalization. In a *linear salpingostomy* (Fig. 30.5), the surgeon makes an incision of the fallopian tube over the site of implantation, removes the pregnancy, and allows the incision to heal by secondary intention. A *segmental resection* is the removal of a portion of the affected tube with the potential of reanastomosing the tube at a later time (Fig. 30.6). *Salpingectomy* is removal of the entire tube, a procedure reserved for those cases in which little or no normal tube remains.

In selected cases, nonsurgical therapy may be advocated for the small, unruptured ectopic pregnancy. Expectant management involves no surgery and no medical therapy but allows the pregnancy to spontaneously regress as documented by serial hCG levels. *Methotrexate*, a folinic acid antagonist, has been successfully used to treat ectopic pregnancy via the oral or intramuscular routes, as well as by direct injection into the ectopic gestational sac. Table 30.3 shows the prototype management using methotrexate as a single-dose intramuscular treatment for unruptured ectopic gestations. This therapy is usually reserved for cases in which the

Table 30.3.

Single-dose Methotrexate Protocol for Ectopic Pregnancy Treatment *if < 3.5 cm + No √BSA?*

Day	Therapy[a]
0	hCG, D&C, CBC, SGOT, BUN, creatinine, blood type + Rh
1	MTX, hCG[b]
4	hCG[c]
7	hCG

[a] *hCG*, quantitative β-human chorionic gonadrotropin; *D&C*, = dilation and curettage; *CBC*, complete blood count; *SGOT*, serum glutamic oxaloacetic transaminase; *BUN*, blood urea nitrogen; *MTX*, intramuscular methotrexate, 50 mg/m^2.
[b] In those patients not requiring D&C before MTX initiation (hCG < 2000 mIU/mL and no gestational sac on transvaginal ultrasound), day 0 and day 1 are combined.
[c] With a <15% decline in hCG titer between days 4 and 7, give a second dose of methotrexate, 50 mg/m^2 on day 7. With a >15% decline in hCG titer between days 4 and 7, follow weekly until hCG is <10 mIU/mL.

ectopic gestation is less than 3.5 cm. in diameter and no cardiac activity is seen on ultrasound.

When conservative surgery or nonsurgical treatment is used, the patient must be followed posttherapy with serial quantitative β-hCG levels to monitor regression of the pregnancy. Surgery or Methotrexate therapy needs to then be considered if trophoblastic function persists as evidenced by persistent or rising levels of hCG.

Rh-negative mothers with ectopic pregnancy should receive *Rh immune globulin* (Rho-GAM) to prevent Rh sensitization.

Although traditionally diagnosed at the time of surgery, ectopic pregnancies are increasingly suspected and treated without either laparoscopy or laparotomy, thereby avoiding the inherent morbidity and cost of surgery. The algorithm shown in Figure 30.7 is an example of the nonsurgical diagnosis and treatment of ectopic pregnancy. Figure 30.8 demonstrates how this may be accomplished with minimal use of surgery.

Combined Pregnancy

Combined pregnancy (coincident or heterotropic pregnancy) occurs in approximately 1 in 30,000 pregnancies with simultaneous intrauterine and extrauterine gestations. Associated with abnormal development of one twin or superfetation, the treatment of the intrauterine pregnancy is individualized depending on the maternal status and wishes and the gestational age and clinical status

of the pregnancy. Management of the extrauterine pregnancy must account for the possible effect on the intrauterine gestation. Approximately 1 in 3 of the intrauterine pregnancies are reported as surviving in the limited number of cases reported.

Nontubal Ectopic Pregnancy

Ectopic implantations outside of the fallopian tube may present in a variety of ways and at different times in gestation, primarily related to the site of implantation. All are uncommon, deriving part of their morbidity from their locations and the remainder from delayed diagnosis.

Abdominal pregnancy occurs in 1 in 3000 to 4000 pregnancies, involving implantation on peritoneal surfaces — in order of frequency, on the adnexae, broad ligaments, sigmoid colon, uterine fundus, and elsewhere in the abdominopelvic cavity. There are two types of abdominal pregnancy. *Primary abdominal pregnancy* is primary implantation of the fertilized ovum, occurring in association with müllerian tract anomalies, delayed ovulation, endometriosis, PID, and fallopian tube dysfunction. *Secondary abdominal pregnancy*, which is more common, involves reimplantation somewhere in the abdominal cavity after the pregnancy has been separated from its primary site of implantation such as in tubal abortion (expulsion of a tubal pregnancy out the fimbriated end), tubal pregnancy rupture, or uterine rupture. Physical findings and symptoms are widely variable, depending on gestational age and site of implantation. Diagnosis is confirmed primarily by ultrasonography.

Abdominal pregnancy is usually discovered long before fetal viability, with treatment being removal of the pregnancy, but not the placenta if it is well developed and attached to vascular, vital structures because of the often uncontrollable hemorrhage that frequently ensues. The management of abdominal pregnancy with a viable or near viable pregnancy is extremely uncommon and best performed by a maternal-fetal medicine expert on a case-by-case basis. Survival of the fetus occurs in only 10 to 20% of cases, with up to one-half having significant deformity. The patient is given the option of continuing the pregnancy to fetal viability and operative delivery or operative termination of the pregnancy at the time of diagnosis. In either case, removal of the placenta is usually not attempted because of the risk of uncontrollable hemorrhage. Treatment with Methotrexate is commonly used to deal with the retained placenta.

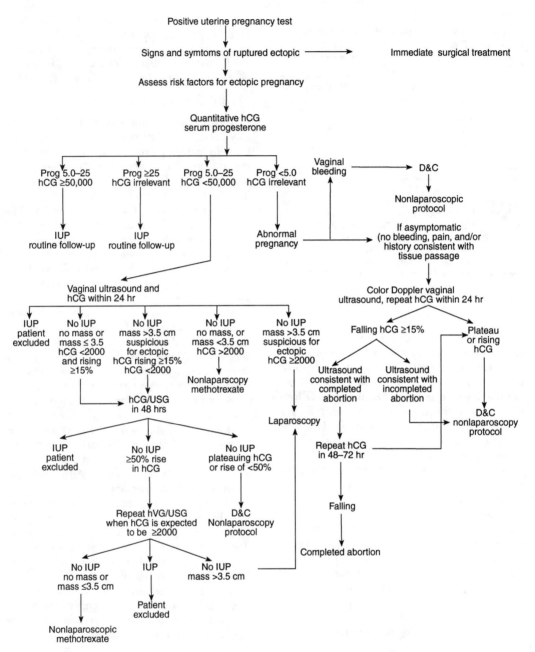

Figure 30.7. Nonsurgical diagnosis and treatment of ectopic pregnancy.

Cervical pregnancy occurs in 1 in 10,000 to 20,000 pregnancies, when the ovum implants in the cervical mucosa below the level of the histologic cervical internal os (Table 30.4). Cervical pregnancy often presents as an incomplete or threatened abortion, with uncontrollable hemorrhage as removal of the pregnancy tissue is attempted. Both conservative surgical treatments and arterial embolization have deen described for definitive management of cervical pregnancy. Hysterectomy is often needed to control the bleeding, especially when the pregnancy is 12 weeks gestational age or more. Methotrexate has been used when the diagnosis is made earlier, thereby avoiding the need for surgical intervention.

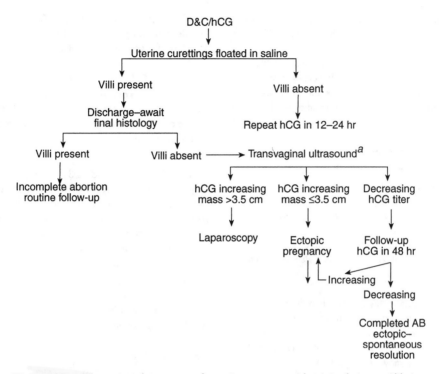

Figure 30.8. Diagnosis and treatment of ectopic pregnancy with minimal surgery (dilation and curettage). *a*, Repeat transvaginal ultrasound if performed >48 hr earlier; *AB*, abortion.

Table 30.4.
Rubins Criteria for Cervical Pregnancy

Cervical glands opposite placental attachment, chorionic villi in cervical canal, no chorionic villi in corpus

Intimate attachment of placenta to cervix

All or part of placental must be situated below entrance of uterine vessels and anterior/posterior uteroperitoneal reflections

No fetal elements in corpus uteri

Internal cervical os closed, external cervical os open or closed

Table 30.5.
Spiegelberg's Criteria for Ovarian Pregnancy

Fallopian tube	must be intact, including fimbria must be clearly separate from ovary must be microscopically free of gestational tissue
Ovary	must occupy normal position must be connected to uterus by ovarian ligament must be unquestioned ovarian tissue in wall of gestational sac

Ovarian pregnancy occurs uncommonly as well, with an incidence estimated from 1 in 7,000 to 1 in 50,000 pregnancies. The types of ovarian pregnancy are primary and reimplantation, or secondary, as with abdominal pregnancy. The criteria of Spiegelberg define the requirements for ovarian pregnancy (Table 30.5), which has a low morbidity, as it is often diagnosed as a tubal pregnancy and successfully treated by surgery, either wedge

resection of the pregnancy or oophorectomy, depending on the extent of ovarian damage.

CASE STUDIES

Case 30A

A 20-year-old college student (G1 P1) presents with the complaint of 2 days of vaginal bleeding, 6 weeks after her last menstrual period. She has had a positive urinary pregnancy test. The bleeding has been dark in color, painless, and began after intercourse. She has had no prior surgeries. She has had one episode of "a pelvic infection" in the past.

Examination shows a small amount of dark blood in the vagina and at the cervical os. The cervix is closed and no tissue is visible. Bimanual examination reveals a slightly softened uterus and an unremarkable adnexal examination.

Questions Case 30A

Your best course of management is

A. Advise an immediate culdocentesis
B. Request a transvaginal ultrasound examination
C. Prescribe medroxyprogesterone (Provera), 10 mg/day
D. Recommend pelvic rest and light activity
E. Advise evacuation of the uterus by suction curettage

Answer: D

A likely diagnosis in this situation is a threatened abortion, but a history of a "pelvic infection" is present in up to 70% of patients with ectopic pregnancies and should increase the clinician's suspicion that an unruptured ectopic pregnancy may be present. A transvaginal ultrasound examination may help to identify the presence of an intrauterine pregnancy, making the diagnosis of threatened abortion more probable. However, a β-hCG of greater than 1500 to 2500 mIU/mL is generally required before an intrauterine pregnancy is routinely visualized on transvaginal sonogram. Culdocentesis is a useful test to identify intraabdominal bleeding, but the patient's history is not suggestive of rupture or leakage from an ectopic implantation site. Because culdocentesis is invasive, it should be reserved for those cases where the possibility of intraabdominal bleeding is greater and the need for diagnostic information is more acute. Recommendations of therapy must be reserved until the possibility of an ectopic pregnancy has been addressed. If there is a delay before obtaining the ultrasound, treating the condition as a presumed threatened abortion is appropriate.

The patient returns the following day with continued spotting and the passage of a "glob of tissue," which she has brought in a jar. She is still without pain, although vaguely uncomfortable. The rush pathology report on the tissue is "necrotic debris and blood clot, unable to make histologic diagnosis, specifically, cannot discern whether or not there are chorionic villi present." Your best course of management is

A. Advise an immediate culdocentesis
B. Request a transvaginal ultrasound examination

C. Obtain serum quantitative β-hCG
D. Recommend pelvic rest and light activity
E. Advise evacuation of the uterus by suction curettage

Answer: B, C

Now the concern of passage of a decidual cast and an associated ectopic pregnancy is raised. β-hCG level will help in the interpretation of the transvaginal ultrasound examination.

The β-hCG is reported as 3100 mIU/mL. The transvaginal ultrasound is reported as a uterine cavity with indistinct, disorganized echoes and a cystic left adnexal mass, distinct from the ovary, which contains a cyst as well. There is some fluid in the cul-de-sac of Douglas. Your working diagnosis is now:

A. Intrauterine pregnancy
B. Threatened abortion
C. Incomplete abortion
D. Complete abortion
E. Ectopic pregnancy

Answer: D or E

Intrauterine pregnancy and threatened abortion have been effectively eliminated by the transvaginal sonogram. Incomplete abortion is likewise unlikely given the scant tissue seen on ultrasound. The tissue passed may have been a decidual cast and the cystic mass on the left, an ectopic pregnancy. Or the patient may have a benign cyst and passed her pregnancy completely.

Your best course of management is

A. Advise an immediate culdocentesis
B. Request a transvaginal ultrasound examination in 48 hr
C. Obtain serum quantitative β-hCG in 48 hr
D. Recommend pelvic rest and light activity
E. Advise evacuation of the uterus by suction curettage and diagnostic laparoscopy

Answer: B, C, D, or E

Given the lack of symptoms, observation with careful patient instruction and a repeat evaluation would be an acceptable management in a cooperative patient. Given the history of PID and the presence of a cyst consistent with a corpus luteum and another extrauterine and extraovarian cystic structure, ectopic pregnancy is a distinct possibility so that surgical evaluation at this time would also be an acceptable management. What would be unacceptable would be to assume a completed abortion and dismiss the patient from follow-up.

Case 30B

A 25-year-old G1 P0 patient begins to cramp and passes a clump of spongy tissue, which she brings to the office. A transvaginal ultrasound examination 1 week ago revealed an intrauterine gestational sac. On examination, her uterus is small and firm and her cervical os is closed with minimal bleeding.

Questions Case 30B

The best course of management is

A. Observe only
B. Observe and send specimen for pathologic evaluation
C. D&C
D. Diagnostic laparoscopy
E. Methotrexate therapy

Answer: B

The specimen may represent a completed abortion or it may be a decidual cast associated with an ectopic pregnancy. The latter is much less likely in this case, because of the ultrasound documented intrauterine pregnancy 1 week ago. In general, any tissue must be sent for histologic evaluation. A D&C would be appropriate if bleeding is persistent and incomplete abortion was suspected. Diagnostic laparoscopy would be used only if ectopic pregnancy were more likely, and treatment such as methotrexate is inappropriate unless ectopic pregnancy is diagnosed.

The specimen is reported as "products of conception." You continue to follow the patient who continues to complain of lower abdominal pain. Her initial β-hCG was 4700 mIU/mL, and now, 4 days later, it is 4000 mIU/mL. Your most likely diagnoses include

A. Missed abortion
B. Molar pregnancy
C. Choriocarcinoma
D. Combined pregnancy
E. Retained placental tissue

Answer: E then D, in order of likelihood

Retained placental tissue is the most common cause of this situation, and suction-curettage is indicated. A transvaginal ultrasound will help in evaluation of the differential diagnoses, which should include the rare combined pregnancy. Gestational trophoblastic disease is unlikely given the relatively low β-hCG level.

Case 30C

A 32-year-old G2 P2002 status who has had tubal ligation presents with 7 weeks of amenorrhea and vaginal spotting. Pelvic examination reveals a 6-week-size ante-verted uterus, a closed cervical os with minimal dark blood in the vaginal vault, and no palpable findings on adnexal examination. A urine pregnancy test is positive.

Questions Case 30C

Appropriate next steps in this patient's management include

A. Quantitative serum β-hCG
B. Quantitative serum progesterone
C. Transvaginal pelvic ultrasound
D. D&C
E. Diagnostic laparoscopy

Answer: C; possibly A and/or B

At 6 weeks gestational age with a positive urinary pregnancy test, transvaginal ultrasound should be able to identify an intrauterine pregnancy in virtually all cases. However, serum progesterone and β-hCG measurement would be helpful if no gestational sac were seen. Serum progesterone may help identify the viability of the pregnancy. Invasive procedures are not indicated absent a diagnosis.

The serum β-hCG is 3650 mIU/mL, the progesterone is 12 ng/mL. The transvaginal ultrasound is reported as no definite intrauterine pregnancy and no definitive extrauterine gestation or fluid in the cul-de-sac of Douglas. The patient's spotting has subsided somewhat, but she now complains of left lower quadrant crampy pain. Your most likely diagnosis is

A. Intrauterine pregnancy
B. Threatened abortion
C. Incomplete abortion
D. Complete abortion
E. Ectopic pregnancy

Answer: E

Your best course(s) of management is

A. Observation
B. D&C
C. Operative laparoscopy
D. Exploratory laparotomy
E. Methotrexate therapy

Answer: C or D, or B with E

Operative evaluation, either by operative laparoscopy or open laparotomy, is appropriate. Alternatively, a D&C would exclude the diagnosis of intrauterine pregnancy, thereby confirming the diagnosis of an extrauterine pregnancy allowing medical management, with methotrexate.

chapter 31

PELVIC RELAXATION, URINARY INCONTINENCE, AND URINARY TRACT INFECTION

Patients with pelvic relaxation present in many different and often subtle ways. To identify patients who would benefit from therapy, the physician should be familiar with the types of pelvic relaxation and the approach to the patient with symptoms suggestive of this problem. The physician must also be aware of common urinary tract conditions that affect women. Although pelvic relaxation and urinary tract disorders are frequently symptomatic, patients are often reluctant to voice their complaints. The physician must be sensitive to these complaints as well as to the physical findings that suggest a problem. Once a problem is identified, a logical and complete approach to evaluation and treatment can return the patient to normal health.

PELVIC RELAXATION AND URINARY INCONTINENCE

Our population is aging. Although not exclusively the province of old age, pelvic relaxation is more common as tissues become less resilient and the accumulated stresses of life have their effects. As a greater proportion of our patients move into their later years, more and more women will be at risk for pelvic relaxation and its attendant problems. Pelvic pressure and pain, dyspareunia, bowel and bladder dysfunction, and urinary incontinence may all result from loss of support for the pelvic organs. Almost half of all women have had the involuntary loss of a few drops of urine at some time in their life; 10 to 15% of women suffer significant, recurrent loss. Loss of pelvic support can have both medical and social implications that necessitate evaluation and intervention.

Causes of Pelvic Relaxation

The pelvic organs are supported by a complex interaction of muscles (e.g., levator muscles), fasciae (urogenital diaphragm, endopelvic fascia), and ligaments (such as the uterosacral and cardinal ligaments). Each of these structures can lose its ability to provide support through birth trauma, chronic elevations of intraabdominal pressure (e.g., obesity, chronic cough, or heavy lifting), intrinsic weaknesses, or atrophic changes caused by aging or estrogen loss. Loss of adequate support for the pelvic organs may be manifest by descent or prolapse of the urethra (urethral detachment or urethrocele), bladder (cystocele), or rectum (rectocele). True herniation at the top of the vagina (enterocele) can also occur. These anatomic defects are illustrated in Figure 31.1. Loss of support for the uterus can lead to varying degrees of descent of the uterus (uterine prolapse). When the uterus descends beyond the vulva it is termed procidentia. Loss of tissue support can also result in prolapse of the vaginal vault in patients who have had a hysterectomy. Although such loss of support (pelvic relaxation) may affect any of the pelvic organs individually, multiple organ involvement is most common.

Causes of Urinary Incontinence

A common complaint of patients with a cystocele or urethrocele is urinary incontinence. This does not occur in all patients, and the degree of incontinence is often not commensurate with the degree of pelvic relaxation. There is urine flow anytime the pressure inside the bladder exceeds the pressure in the urethra. This happens physio-

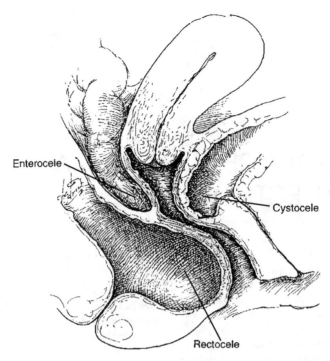

Enterocele

Cystocele

Rectocele

Figure 31.1. Loss of pelvic support.

logically during voluntary voiding when the muscles surrounding the urethra relax and the bladder contracts. It may also take place involuntarily when there is unequal transmission of intra-abdominal pressure to the bladder and urethra, as seen with the loss of pelvic support. When urethral support is lost, the urethra descends outside the influence of abdominal pressure. As a result, the bladder pressure exceeds urethral pressure briefly at times of strain or stress, resulting in stress incontinence.

If there is loss of normal innervation and control of bladder function, involuntary bladder contraction or bladder atony may result, leading to urgency and overflow incontinence, respectively. In addition, loss of urine may ensue anytime there is a breakdown of the social or emotional competence of the patient (e.g., psychosis or neurosis) or when the normal continence mechanism is bypassed, such as with fistulous openings.

Clinical Presentation

The symptoms caused by loss of pelvic support will vary based on the structure or structures involved and the degree of prolapse. The most common symptoms are those characterized as "pres-sure" or "heaviness." These symptoms are diffuse, low in the abdomen or pelvis, and are often worse late in the day, after lifting, or when standing for long periods. Backache and dyspareunia are also common complaints. When support for the bladder and urethra fails, urinary (stress) incontinence, frequency, hesitancy, incomplete voiding, or recurrent infections may result. A careful history that notes the associated symptoms and events, amount and duration of urine loss, and the position in which urine losses occur is important in establishing the correct diagnosis (Table 31.1).

Loss of rectal support may lead to problems such as constipation and painful or incomplete defecation. The patient with a symptomatic rectocele may need to press down on the posterior vagina with her fingers to promote bowel movements. When there is complete descent, the patient may be paradoxically asymptomatic and only note the protrusion of tissue from the vagina. Vaginal ulceration, bleeding, infection, or pain frequently accompanies complete descent. Symptoms of chronic constipation and difficulty passing stool are also compatible with obstructive lesions. Anoscopy or sigmoidoscopy should be considered, based on the needs of the individual patient.

Table 31.1.
Characteristics of Urinary Incontinence

Characteristic	Stress Incontinence	Urge Incontinence	Overflow Incontinence
Associated symptoms	None (occasional pelvic pressure)	Urgency, nocturia	Fullness, pressure frequency
Amount of loss	Small, spurt	Large, complete emptying	Small, dribbling
Duration of loss	Brief, corresponds to stress	Moderate, several seconds	Often continuous
Associated event	Cough, laugh, sneeze, physical activity	None, change in position, running water	None
Position	Upright, sitting; rare supine or asleep	Any	Any
Cause	Structural (cystocele, urethrocele)	Loss of bladder inhibition	Obstruction, loss of neurologic control

Evaluation

The evaluation of patients with pelvic relaxation rests primarily on the history and physical examination. Pelvic relaxation is best demonstrated by observing the vaginal area while having the patient strain. This may be done in either or both the supine and standing positions. A urethrocele or cystocele may be demonstrated by separating the labia and asking the patient to "strain down" or cough. When a urethrocele or cystocele is present, a downward movement and rotation of the anterior vaginal wall toward the introitus will be seen. To more fully evaluate the presence of a cystocele, rectocele, or enterocele, inspection should be carried out using a Sims or the lower half of a Graves speculum to retract the posterior vaginal wall. This facilitates the separate inspection of the anterior and posterior vaginal walls and allows differentiation of the structures involved. Descent of the uterus may be demonstrated either in this way or through palpation.

The degree of pelvic relaxation is often rated on a 1 to 3 scale based on the descent of the structure involved (Fig. 31.2). When descent is limited to the upper two-thirds of the vagina, it is said to be first degree. Second-degree prolapse is present when the structure approaches the vaginal introitus. Descent of the structure to outside the vaginal opening (such as the body of the uterus in the case of procidentia) is classified as a third-degree defect. The extent of urethral detachment, commonly referred to as urethrocele, may be quantified using the Q-tip test. This is done by placing a cotton swab in the urethra and measuring the an-

gle of upward motion caused by the patient straining. Upward rotation of greater than 30° from the starting point is generally associated with urinary stress incontinence because of loss of support of the critical urethrovesical junction.

When a significant cystocele or urethrocele is found, evaluation of urinary function is advisable. Compromise of ureteral drainage may occur in cases of significant downward displacement of the trigone as is seen in some cases of second- or third-degree descent. Urinary retention and subsequent infection may also occur and should be evaluated. Because of the frequent association of more than one cause of urinary incontinence, patients with incontinence should be considered for urodynamics testing.

Urodynamics testing refers to a group of procedures that evaluate bladder structure and functions. Although these procedures vary based on the needs of the patient and the preferences of the physician, they generally include cystometrics, cystoscopy, and provocative tests such as coughing or straining. Most centers include sophisticated evaluation of bladder compliance and contractility via cystometrics as well as evaluation of the voiding process itself. Pressure profiles of the bladder and urethra as well as fluoroscopic examinations may also be included. This battery of tests is very important in the objective reproducible evaluation of proposed therapies. Clinically, these tests are useful in the evaluation of patients where "mixed" etiologies are suspected before invasive intervention.

The Q-tip test is useful in documenting the degree of cystourethrocele present. The functional significance of a cystourethrocele may be

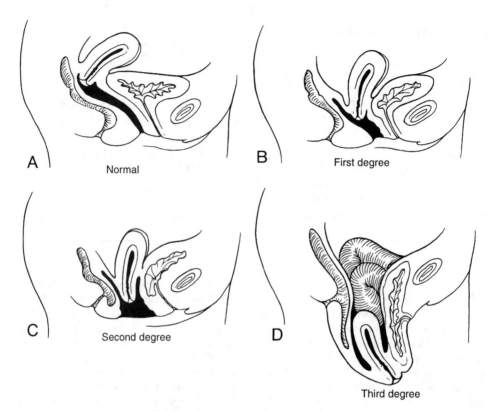

Figure 31.2.   Degrees of pelvic relaxation.

gauged by elevating the bladder neck (using fin-gers or an instrument) and asking the patient to strain (the Bonney test). If continence is achieved, these tests help to anticipate the effect of pessaries or surgery. Care must be taken that the test accu-rately reflects elevation of the structures and not merely obstruction of the urethra. Because of this uncertainty, these tests have been accorded less significance and should not provide the sole means of evaluation.

Differential Diagnosis

The presumptive diagnosis of pelvic relaxation is based on the evaluation of the structural integrity of pelvic support. Often the characteristics of the patient's complaint may suggest a diagnosis. Even though the differential diagnosis of pelvic relax-ation is generally simple, other processes must be considered. Urethral diverticulum or Skene's gland abscesses may mimic a cystourethrocele and, in the case of diverticula, may be a source of inconti-nence. These can be identified through symptoms, careful "milking" of the urethra, or cystoscopy.

The complaint of urinary loss may stem from me-chanical factors (such as a cystourethrocele), irrita-tion (mechanical or inflammatory trigonitis), neu-rologic causes (such as diabetes or detrusor instability), the effects of medications, or mental and psychosocial conditions. A vesicovaginal or ureterovaginal fistula must also be considered in the differential diagnosis. It is occasionally difficult to differentiate between a high rectocele and an enterocele. This distinction may be facilitated through rectal examination or the identification of small bowel in the hernia sac. It is common for the diagnosis of an enterocele not to be established un-til surgical repair is undertaken.

Most pelvic relaxation is the result of structural failure of the tissues involved, but other contribut-ing factors should be considered in the complete care of the patient. Has there been a change in intraabdominal pressure and why? Why does the patient have a chronic cough that has precipitated her symptoms? Is a neurologic process (such as diabetic neuropathy) complicating the patient's presenting complaint? Each of these issues should

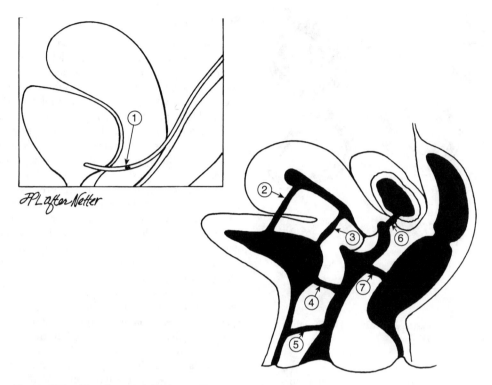

Figure 31.3. Female genital fistulae. *1*, Ureterovaginal; *2*, vesicouterovaginal; *3*, vesicocervicovaginal; *4*, vesicovaginal; *5*, urethrovaginal; *6*, enterovaginal; *7*, rectovaginal.

be considered prior to the selection of a diagnostic or therapeutic plan.

In the evaluation of involuntary loss of urine, the physician must also consider the possibility of fistulae. Fistulae between the vagina and the bladder (vesicovaginal), urethra (urethrovaginal), or the ureter (ureterovaginal) are generally the result of surgical trauma, irradiation, or malignancy. A communication between the bladder and the uterus (vesicouterine) may also be found on rare occasions. In addition, fistulae may occur between the rectum and vagina (rectovaginal fistulae), resulting in the passage of flatus or feces from the vagina (Fig. 31.3).

Nonsurgical Treatment Options

Because pelvic relaxation is a structural problem, the ultimate solutions are structural as well. These range from mechanical support (through pessaries) and exercises to strengthen the pelvic muscles, to surgical repair of the tissue defects. Estrogen replacement is also an important adjunct to other therapies in the postmenopausal woman.

In patients with urgency incontinence, effective therapy may include bladder training, biofeedback, or medical therapy. Bladder training programs are directed toward increasing the patient's bladder control and capacity by gradually increasing the amount of time between voidings. Often successful by itself, this may be augmented in difficult cases by biofeedback when available. Treatment with anticholinergic drugs (Pro-Banthine [propantheline bromide] and Ditropan [oxybutynin chloride]), β-sympathomimetic agonists (Alupent [metaproterenol sulfate]), musculotrophic drugs (Urispas [flavoxate hydrochloride] and Valium [diazepam]), antidepressants (Tofranil [imipramine hydrochloride]), or dopamine agonists (Parlodel [bromocriptine mesylate]) has had some success based on the character of the patient's problem.

The pelvic musculature may be strengthened through the use of Kegel exercises. This exercise program consists of the repetitive contraction of the pelvic floor muscles as if trying to stop the bladder from emptying. This is repeated many times throughout the day. Kegel exercises may be

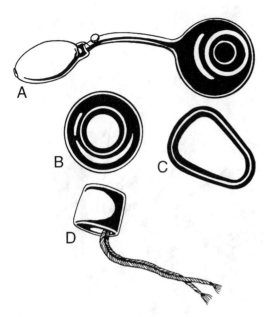

Figure 31.4.   Pessaries. **A,** Inflatable. **B,** Doughnut. **C,** Smith-Hodge. **D,** Cube.

helpful for some patients with mild incontinence. They may also help to provide better tissues should surgical repair be attempted.

A mechanical buttress for the pelvic organs may be provided through the use of pessaries. These are devices worn in the vagina to furnish support. Pessaries come in a variety of types and sizes, all designed to replace the missing structural integrity of the pelvis or to diffuse the forces of descent over a wide area. The most common forms of pessary are the Smith-Hodge, the ring (or doughnut), the ball, and the cube (Fig. 31.4). They are placed in the vagina in much the same way as a diaphragm. They occlude the vagina and hold the pelvic organs in a relatively normal position. Pessary therapy requires the cooperation and involvement of the patient but offers a good alternative to surgical repair for properly selected, well-motivated patients.

Patients who are fitted with a pessary for the control of pelvic relaxation need careful initial monitoring. Reexamination in 5 to 7 days to confirm proper placement, hygiene, and the absence of pressure-related problems (vaginal trauma or necrosis) is required. Evaluation in 24 hr may be advisable in patients who are debilitated or require additional assistance.

Surgical Therapy

Surgical repair of pelvic relaxation takes many forms, depending on the specific defect, ranging from hysterectomy for uterine prolapse to the creation of supportive slings for stress incontinence to occlusion of the vagina for vaginal vault prolapse in the elderly to plastic repairs to restore prolapsing structures to their original anatomic position (Table 31.2). These procedures may be carried out from either the vaginal or abdominal approach, and each has its own set of indications, advantages, disadvantages, complications, and failures. No one procedure is best, and each surgical approach must be individualized. Success is based not only on the procedure chosen but also on the skill of the surgeon, the degree of pelvic relaxation, and patient risk factors such as quality of tissues, obesity, and lifestyle (e.g., smoking). (Fig. 31.5)

Failure of rectovaginal support may be treated by reconstructing or reinforcing the rectovaginal space (posterior colporrhaphy). Prolapse of the vagina may be treated by suspending the vaginal vault to either the sacrospinous ligament (sacrospinous vaginal vault suspension) or to the sacrum itself (sacral colpopexy). Obliteration of the rectovaginal space (Moskowitz procedure) is also used to treat or prevent vaginal prolapse and enterocele formation. Enteroceles are treated like other hernias, with dissection and high ligation of the hernia sac.

Because of the frequent concurrence of defects in pelvic support and uterine descent, vaginal hysterectomy is often performed simultaneously with the reconstruction procedure. This corrects any symptoms referable to the descensus, provides access to the uterine support mechanisms to reinforce other repairs, and prevents the uterus from tearing down anterior and posterior repairs should further descent occur.

For patients whose medical conditions preclude long surgical procedures and who are not sexually active, partial or complete obliteration of the vaginal canal (LeFort procedure, colpocleisis) may be done to provide support to the pelvic structures.

Therapy for fistulae is primarily surgical. Occasionally fistulae that occur following surgery will spontaneously heal when adequate drainage or diversion of the urinary or fecal flow is provided. In all other cases, the only successful therapy consists of meticulous dissection of the fistulous tract and careful reapproximation of tissues. Recurrence is a common problem, especially in patients who have had radiation therapy for malignancies.

URINARY TRACT INFECTIONS

Women suffer urinary tract infection roughly 10 times more often than men. Approximately 15% of women will experience at least one urinary tract infection in their lifetime. This necessitates the physician having a familiarity with the diagnosis and treatment of a number of urologic disorders common to women.

Most urinary tract infections in women ascend from bacterial contamination of the urethra. Except in the case of tuberculosis or immunosuppressed patients, infections will rarely be acquired by hematogenous or lymphatic spread. The relatively short female urethra, exposure of the meatus to vestibular and rectal pathogens, and sexual activity that may induce trauma or introduce other organisms all increase the potential for infection. With estrogen deficiency, there is also a decrease in urethral resistance to infection, which contributes to ascending contamination. This increased susceptibility explains the almost 10% prevalence of asymptomatic bacteriuria found in postmenopausal women.

Clinical Aspects of Urinary Tract Infections

Approximately 95% of urinary tract infections are symptomatic, uncomplicated, do not ascend to the kidneys, and produce no permanent damage. Of first infections, 90% are caused by *Escherichia coli*, and these respond readily to antibiotic therapy. Anaerobic bacteria and yeasts are rare causes of infections, except in diabetic or immunosuppressed patients or those with chronic indwelling catheters.

Patients with urinary tract infections will typically present with symptoms of frequency, urgency, nocturia, or dysuria. The symptoms found will vary somewhat with the site of the infection. When there is irritation of the bladder or trigone, symptoms include urgency, frequency, and nocturia. Irritation of the urethra leads to frequency and dysuria. The physical examination will generally be nonspecific, although some patients may report suprapubic tenderness.

Evaluation

The evaluation of the patient suspected of having a urinary tract infection should include a urinalysis and a urine culture and sensitivity. These are generally obtained through a "clean-catch midstream" urine sample, which involves cleansing the vulva and catching a portion of urine passed during the middle of uninterrupted voiding. Urine obtained from catheters or suprapubic aspiration may also be used.

Laboratory analysis of the urine may be conducted or the sample examined microscopically by the clinician. This microscopic evaluation is carried out using a drop of urine or the precipitate from a centrifuged specimen. For uncentrifuged samples, the presence of more than one white blood cell per high power field carries a 90% accuracy in detecting infection. Centrifuged specimens may be scanned with low power for the presence of large numbers of white cells. Pyuria is defined as the presence of more than five white cells per high power field in the centrifuged specimen. Gram stain of urine samples or sediments may also be helpful in establishing the diagnosis of

Table 31.2.
Surgical Therapy for Urinary Incontinence

Type	Intent	Approach
Anterior vaginal repair (colporrhaphy, Kelly plication)	Provide support to the bladder and urethra by reinforcing the endopelvic fascia and vaginal epithelium	Vaginal
Retropubic suspension (Marshall-Marchetti-Krantz, Burch, paravaginal repair)	Repair defects in the endopelvic fascia and its attachments	Abdominal
Sling procedure (Pereyra, Stamey)	Supplement or replace the support of the bladder neck and urethra using suture or fascial slings	Combined abdominal and vaginal

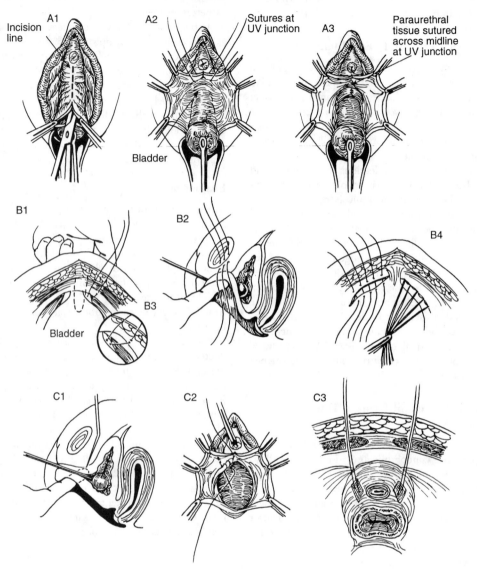

Figure 31.5. Surgical therapy for urinary incontinence. **A1–A3,** Anterior vaginal wall repair, the Kelly-Kennedy procedure. **A1,** Anterior vaginal wall is opened and undermined. **A2,** Paraurethral tissue lateral to the urethrovesical (UV) junction is sutured. **A3,** This creates a firm bar of tissue that supports the UV junction. **B1–B4,** Retropubic suspension procedures, the Marshall-Marchetti-Krantz procedure. **B1,** The suture is placed in the periurethral tissue and then into the pubic periosteum so that (**B2**) the urethra may be advanced upward into an intraabdominal position. **B3,** The Burch procedure, by which the tissue adjacent to the UV angle is sutured to the iliopectinal (Coopers) ligament. **B4,** The Richardson paravaginal repair, by which the sutures are placed between the superior sulcus of the vagina and lateral pelvic side wall at the level of the iliopectineal line. **C1–C3,** Sling procedures. **C1,** The Pereyra procedure, by which a needle is guided transabdominally into the paraurethral tissue and back through (**C2**) to be tied suprapubically, thus supporting the UV angle. **C3,** The Stamey procedure, by which a Dacron support material is used in the paraurethral tissue to buttress the tissue.

infection. "Dipstick" tests for infection based on the presence of leukocyte esterase are also useful.

Cultures of urine samples that show colony counts of >100,000 for a single organism generally indicate infection. Colony counts as low as 10,000 for *E. coli* are associated with infection when symptoms are present. When a culture report indicates the presence of multiple organisms, contamination of the specimen should be suspected.

Recurrent urinary tract infections should prompt a reevaluation. Possible causes that must be considered include incorrect or incomplete (i.e., noncompliant) therapy, mechanical factors such as obstruction, or compromised host defenses.

Therapy

The selection of therapy for patients with urinary tract infections is simple and generally successful. Hydration, urinary acidification (with ascorbic acid, ammonium chloride, or acidic fruit juices), and urinary analgesics (Pyridium [phenazopyridine hydrochloride]) are helpful in most cases. Once confirmation by urinalysis or culture has been obtained, antibiotic therapy should be instituted. Nitrofurantoin (Macrodantin) produces good urinary antibiosis without undue alteration of other flora, although it is not effective against *Proteus* infections. Antibiotics such as ampicillin, tetracycline, and trimethoprim-sulfamethoxazole (Septra, Bactrim) provide good coverage in the urinary tract but risk more alteration of vaginal or intestinal flora. Vaginal yeast infections may result from these antibiotic treatments. When pyelonephritis is suspected, aggressive antibiotic therapy with cephalosporins such as Keflex (cephalexin) or Duricef (cefadroxil) is indicated.

Patients who have been treated for urinary tract infections should have follow-up urinalysis and culture done 10 to 14 days after the initial diagnosis. This will document cure in most patients and identify those at risk for recurrence because of incomplete or ineffective therapy.

CASE STUDIES

Case 31A

An 18-year-old nulligravid patient presents to your office with the complaint of 3 days of urinary frequency, urgency, and dysuria. She was married 2 weeks ago and the symptoms first appeared following a weekend getaway with her husband. She is using condom and foam for contraception. She reports no fever or chills, and she is aware of no vaginal discharge. Your physical examination reveals no abnormal findings. You obtain a clean-catch urine and centrifuge the specimen. You examine the sediment under the microscope and find 20 to 30 white cells, a moderate number of epithelial cells, and some bacteria in each low power field.

Questions Case 31A

The best working diagnosis at this point is

A. Cystitis
B. Pyuria
C. Traumatic urethritis/trigonitis
D. Pyelonephritis
E. Vaginitis

Answer: C

The finding of a large number of white blood cells in the centrifuged urine specimen would normally be diagnostic of pyuria. This, combined with the patient's symptoms, supports the diagnosis of cystitis. In this case, however, the microscopic examination also showed a large number of epithelial cells, which means the specimen had had moderate contamination from vaginal secretions. Without symptoms of vaginal discharge or irritation, you cannot make the diagnosis of vaginitis, but you also cannot rely on the present urine sample to make the diagnosis of urinary tract infection. Trauma to the urethra and bladder trigone ("honeymoon cystitis") may imitate infection. The patient's recent marriage and the use of spermicides could support the possibility of mechanical or chemical irritation. Although you have not ruled out the possibility of infection, the circumstances suggest that infection may be less likely than traumatic urethritis.

To confirm your suspicions you might

A. Obtain a catheterized urine for examination
B. Request a culture and sensitivity on the specimen you have
C. Obtain a wet prep of vaginal secretions
D. Obtain a more detailed sexual history
E. Perform an intravenous pyelogram

Answer: D

Both a further exploration of the patient's sexual history and a better evaluation of the possibility of infection are indicated, but the invasive nature of urinary catheterization makes the evaluation of history a better choice. Based on the history, the need for a catheterized specimen may be better determined. You know from the presence of epithelial cells in the centrifuged specimen that the sample is contaminated and thus culture is compromised. Although a microscopic examination of vaginal secretions is easy to accomplish, there is no evidence for vaginitis in the patient's history or physical examination. Intravenous pyelography is invasive, expensive, and would not contribute to the diagnostic possibilities in this case.

Case 31B

A 64-year-old G5 P4 widowed patient comes to your office for her annual physical examination. She had a total hysterectomy 20 years ago for tumors. When you take your gynecologic history, the patient somewhat shyly admits that she is not sexually active but that she has recently met someone whom she likes. She also admits that she has begun experiencing a loss of urine when she coughs, laughs, or sneezes. This has made her self-conscious, and she is considering giving up her seniors' aerobics class.

Your physical examination shows her to be an 87-kg woman with a blood pressure of 138/92 and a pulse of 84. Her abdomen is protuberant, but no masses or tenderness is noted. Pelvic examination reveals atrophic changes in the vulva and vagina, a second-degree cystocele, slight descensus of the vaginal vault, and no palpable adnexa.

Question Case 31B

Which of the following is probably not indicated at this time:

A. Weight reduction
B. Estrogen therapy
C. Kegel exercises
D. Anterior colporrhaphy
E. Low-impact exercise program

Answer: D

The history and physical examination presented are consistent with stress incontinence caused by a cystourethrocele. The patient's symptoms are mild and do not warrant surgical intervention at this time. Should the symptoms become worse, urodynamic evaluation should also be considered before scheduling a surgical repair. Estrogen therapy (systemic or vaginal) and Kegel exercises may both help to improve the patient's symptoms. Weight reduction is a worthwhile goal for general health and to decrease the possibility of progression of her pelvic relaxation. The addition of a low-impact exercise program may help the weight reduction program and support the patient's self-esteem. Reassurance is always indicated.

chapter 32

ENDOMETRIOSIS

The clinical impact of endometriosis relates to its association with complaints such as infertility, dysmenorrhea, dyspareunia, and chronic pelvic pain. Endometriosis is characterized by the presence of endometrial tissue in extrauterine locations, most commonly the ovaries, uterosacral ligaments, rectovaginal septum, and pelvic peritoneum. The term *endometrioma* has been used to described an isolated collection of endometriosis involving an ovary that is large enough to be considered a tumor. The term *adenomyosis* refers to endometrial implants found deep within the uterine wall. Endometriosis and adenomyosis are benign conditions that have different clinical courses. Endometriosis is progressive, leading to ever-increasing symptoms and damage. When diagnosed early, surgical and medical therapies are available to relieve the symptoms, slow the progression, or ablate the disease. Adenomyosis is confined to the uterus and presents as progessive dysmenorrhea and menorrhagia (see Chapter 24).

INCIDENCE AND PREVALENCE

The diagnosis of endometriosis may be suspected clinically and strongly supported by findings at laparoscopy or laparotomy, but histologic confirmation of endometriosis is required to make a definitive diagnosis. Therefore, the true incidence of endometriosis is difficult to establish. Since laparotomy and/or endoscopy is required to confirm the clinical diagnosis, there are patients who have asymptomatic endometriosis who will be undiagnosed and patients who undergo surgery for unrelated reasons who are only then found to have incidental endometriosis.

It is estimated that 1 to 2% of women in the general population have endometriosis and that this rate increases to 30 to 50% in infertile women. Endometriosis occurs primarily in women in their 20s and 30s, although this may be a function of the frequency of evaluation of women in this age range for infertility and pelvic pain. Endometriosis is less frequently described in postmenopausal women. In adolescents, congenital anomalies that promote retrograde menstruation may be a common associated finding.

It has been thought that certain patient groups are at higher risk for developing endometriosis such as those who delay childbearing. Middle-class white patients who are described as high achieving and perfectionist were once considered at higher risk. This stereotypical description has not been proven valid. There is evidence, however, that there is a genetic predisposition in women whose first-degree relatives have had endometriosis.

PATHOGENESIS

The exact mechanism by which endometriosis develops is unknown. Three major theories are commonly cited.

1. Direct implantation of endometrial cells (Sampson's theory) has been postulated, typically by means of retrograde menstruation. This appears consistent with the occurrence of pelvic endometriosis and its predilection for the ovaries and pelvic peritoneum. This is also consistent with finding endometriosis in sites such as an abdominal incision or episiotomy scar. Direct implantation is commonly referred to as Sampson's theory because of his work that showed the possibility of such a mechanism.
2. Vascular and lymphatic dissemination (Halban's theory) of endometrial cells has been postulated. Distant sites of endometriosis can be explained by this process, i.e., the presence of endometriosis in locations such as lymph nodes, the pleural cavity, and kidney.
3. Coelomic metaplasia of multipotential cells in the peritoneal cavity (Meyer's theory) states that, under certain conditions, these cells can develop into functional endometrial tissue.

Each of these major theories has evidence to support it. It is probable that more than one theory is necessary to explain the diverse nature and locations of endometriosis. Underlying all of these possibilities is the yet-undiscovered immunologic factor that would explain why some women develop endometriosis while others with similar characteristics do not.

PATHOLOGY

Endometriosis is most commonly found on the ovary in 60% of patients and is typically bilateral. Other common pelvic structures involved include the pouch of Douglas (particularly the uterosacral ligaments and rectovaginal septum), the round ligament, the fallopian tube, and the sigmoid colon (Table 32.1). On rare occasion, endometriosis will be found in abdominal surgical scars, the umbilicus, and various organs outside of the pelvic cavity.

The gross appearance of endometriosis varies considerably. Subtle, minimal findings that have been biopsy proven to be endometriosis include 1-mm vascular hemorrhagic areas, white-opaque plaques on the peritoneal surfaces, and more classically, spots that have been described as "mulberry" or "raspberry" in appearance. These small areas may also be rust colored, dark brown, or like "powder burns" in appearance. Frequently, there is reactive fibrosis surrounding these lesions, which gives a puckered appearance. More advanced, disseminated disease causes further fibrosis and results in the typically dense adhesions found in patients whose pelvic anatomy may be obscured by the disease.

The ovary can develop large collections of endometriosis, which form cysts on the ovary. These are filled with thick, chocolate-appearing fluid, which is primarily old blood. These "chocolate cysts" are associated with endometriosis although hemorrhagic cysts of the ovary may also have this gross appearance. Endometriomas may reach 15 to 20 cm in size.

The microscopic diagnosis of endometriosis is made when there are endometrial glands, stroma, and a presence of hemosiderin-laden macrophages. The glands and stroma do function histologically and physiologically like uterine mucosa, and cyclic changes in response to hormones are noted. It is not, however, as well ordered as that which occurs in the endometrial cavity. In as many as one-third of cases, the microscopic diagnosis is not conclusive, despite a "classic" clinical appearance.

CLINICAL FEATURES   Small lesions missed By section of lg biopsy

Symptoms

Women with endometriosis demonstrate an exceptionally wide variation of symptomatology, the nature and severity of which may be surprisingly independent of both the location and extent of the disease. Women with extensive endometriosis may have few symptoms, whereas, paradoxically, those with minimal gross endometriosis may have severe pain. The classic symptoms of endometriosis include dysmenorrhea, deep thrust dyspareunia, infertility, abnormal bleeding, and pelvic pain.

The dysmenorrhea associated with endometriosis is not directly related to the amount of visible disease. Patients who present with dysmenorrhea that does not respond to oral contraceptives or nonsteroidal antiinflammatory agents should have endometriosis considered as a possible etiology. The dyspareunia is often associated

Table 32.1.
Sites of Endometriosis

Site	Frequency (Percent of Patients)	Site	Frequency (Percent of Patients)
Most common		Other gastrointestinal tract sites	5
Ovary (frequently bilateral)	60	Vagina	
Pelvic peritoneum over the uterus			
Anterior and posterior cul-de-sacs		Rare	
Uterosacral ligaments		Umbilicus	
Fallopian tubes		Episiotomy or surgical scars	
Pelvic lymph nodes	30	Kidney	
Infrequent		Lungs	
Rectosigmoid	10–15	Arms	
		Legs	
		Nasal mucosa	

with uterosacral or vaginal involvement with endometriosis. In addition, the uterus may be retroverted and fixed in the cul-de-sac because of the extensive adhesions. The dyspareunia is typically reported on deep penetration. There is, however, no correlation between dyspareunia and the extent of endometriosis.

Infertility is more frequent in women with endometriosis than in the general population. With extensive disease, pelvic scarring and adhesions may be responsible, but the exact mechanism for the infertility is unclear in patients with minimal endometriosis. Prostaglandins and autoantibodies have been implicated, but these relations remain unproven. Infertility may, in some cases, be the only complaint. In these cases, endometriosis is discovered at the time of laparoscopic evaluation as part of the infertility workup.

Abnormal bleeding occurs in approximately one-third of women with endometriosis. Sometimes, irregular menstrual periods are caused by anovulation. In many cases, there is premenstrual spotting, possibly the result of an associated luteal phase inadequacy.

Pelvic pain is a common finding in patients with endometriosis. In some cases, the patient's pain is not solely associated with the menstrual period (dysmenorrhea) or to coital activity (dyspareunia) but, rather, is a chronic, unremitting low pelvic discomfort. Chronic pelvic pain may be related to the adhesions and pelvic scarring found in association with endometriosis.

Other, less common symptoms of endometriosis include gastrointestinal symptoms such as rectal bleeding and dyschezia in patients with endometrial implants on the bowel, and urinary symptoms such as hematuria in patients with endometrial implants on the bladder or ureters. Occasionally, patients may present with an acute abdominal emergency, which may be associated with the rupture or torsion of an endometrioma.

Signs

The classic description of uterosacral nodularity on rectovaginal examination is consistent with significant gross disease involving that area, but it is not universally present. The uterus is often relatively fixed and retroflexed in the pelvis. Ovarian endometriomas may be tender, palpable, and freely mobile in the pelvis or adhered to the posterior leaf of the broad ligament or in the posterior cul-de-sac.

Physical findings in early endometriosis may be very subtle or even nonexistent. In cases of unexplained pelvic pain or infertility, the diagnosis of endometriosis should be entertained and diagnostic laparoscopy considered. It is recommended that visual and, ideally, histologic confirmation of endometriosis be obtained before institution of medical therapy for endometriosis. Typical clinical features of endometriosis are shown in Figure 32.1.

DIFFERENTIAL DIAGNOSIS

Depending on the symptoms, the differential diagnosis will change. In patients who present with chronic abdominal pain, consideration should be given to diagnoses such as chronic pelvic inflammatory disease, pelvic adhesions, gastrointestinal dysfunction, and other etiologies of chronic pelvic pain. In patients who present primarily with dysmenorrhea, both primary dysmenorrhea and etiologies for secondary dysmenorrhea should be considered. In patients who present with dyspareunia, other considerations should include chronic pelvic inflammatory disease, ovarian cysts, and symptomatic uterine retroversion. If abnormal bleeding is the primary presentation, investigation should rule out conditions such as

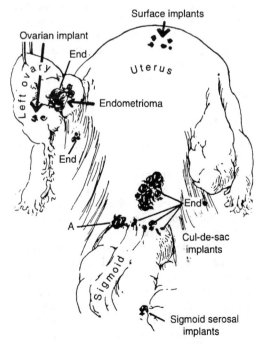

Figure 32.1. Clinical features of endometriosis. *End*, endometriosis; *A*, uterosacral implants.

anovulation, hypothyroidism, and hyperprolactinemia. If premenstrual spotting is the primary symptom, luteal phase defect, polyps, or cervical lesions should be considered. If the patient presents with sudden abdominal pain, considerations other than a ruptured endometrioma include ectopic pregnancy, acute pelvic inflammatory disease, adnexal torsion, and rupture of a corpus luteum cyst or ovarian neoplasm.

DIAGNOSIS

Because of the diverse ways in which patients with endometriosis present, history taking and physical examination can be considered only preliminary in nature. Establishing a diagnosis requires direct visualization at the time of diagnostic laparoscopy or laparotomy. Ideally, histologic confirmation of "endometriosis-appearing" lesions or implants should be obtained. Should rectal bleeding occur, barium enema and colonoscopy should be undertaken to exclude other primary gastrointestinal disorders and to evaluate for endometriosis involving these structures. Pelvic ultrasound cannot definitively make the diagnosis of endometriosis, nor are there any laboratory studies that are of value except to help rule out other conditions.

Once the diagnosis is made, the extent of the endometriosis should be properly documented. The most widely accepted classification system has been established by the American Fertility Society (Fig. 32.2). This system standardizes the extent of the disease and aids in tracking progression or regression of endometriosis after therapy has been instituted.

PREVENTION

There is no known method to prevent endometriosis. Instead, the prevention of the spread of this disease should be the goal once the diagnosis has been established. A high index of suspicion can lead to early diagnosis, resulting in treatment before the endometriosis has progressed extensively. For example, conditions of the lower genital tract that may predispose to retrograde menstruation should be corrected as soon as they are found. Diagnostic procedures that require retrograde insufflation of dye or gas through the fallopian tubes, e.g., hysterosalpingography, should not be done while the patient is menstruating. Because endometriosis appears to be suppressed by the prolonged progestational effect of pregnancy, conception has traditionally been recommended as a way

to prevent or minimize the effects of endometriosis. Unfortunately, there are no scientific data to support this latter recommendation. Furthermore, this recommendation potentially causes its own dilemma, since patients with endometriosis already are at greater risk for infertility.

TREATMENT

The diagnosis should be firmly established before instituting either medical or surgical therapy. The choice of therapy depends on the patient's individual circumstances, which include (a) presenting symptoms and their severity, (b) location and severity of endometriosis, and (c) desire for future childbearing. All of the medical treatments for endometriosis are temporizing measures to some extent. None can be expected to provide a permanent cure until extirpative surgery is undertaken or the hormonal stimulation is permanently removed.

Observation

There are selected cases in which patients can be treated expectantly, i.e., without either medical or surgical therapy. These include patients with very limited disease whose symptoms are minimal or nonexistent and/or those who are trying to get pregnant. In the occasional patient in her mid to late 40s with mild symptoms, consideration may be given to withholding therapy with the expectation that the decrease in menstrual hormones associated with menopause may not stimulate growth of disease.

Medical Therapy

All forms of medical therapy are aimed at inducing relative inactivity of the endometrial tissue. Because the glands and stroma of endometriosis respond to both exogenous and endogenous hormones, suppression of endometriosis is based on a medication's potential ability to induce atrophy of the endometrial tissue. This is optimal for patients who are currently symptomatic, have documented endometriosis beyond minimal disease, and/or desire pregnancy sometime in the future. The patient should be aware that recurrence after the completion of medical therapy is common and that medical therapy does not have an effect on adhesions and fibrosis caused by the endometriosis.

Beneficial effects have been obtained using combined estrogen and progestin oral contraceptive agents. Commonly referred to as "pseudopregnancy," the use of oral contraceptives in-

THE AMERICAN FERTILITY SOCIETY
REVISED CLASSIFICATION OF ENDOMETRIOSIS

Patient's Name _____ Date_____

Stage I   (Minimal)   · 1-5
Stage II (Mild)   · 6-15
Stage III (Moderate) · 16-40
Stage IV (Severe)   · >40

Laparoscopy_____ Laparotomy_____ Photography_____

Recommended Treatment_____

Total_____

Prognosis_____

	ENDOMETRIOSIS	<1cm	1-3cm	>3cm
PERITONEUM	Superficial	1	2	4
	Deep	2	4	6
OVARY	R Superficial	1	2	4
	Deep	4	16	20
	L Superficial	1	2	4
	Deep	4	16	20

	POSTERIOR CULDESAC OBLITERATION	Partial	Complete
		4	40

	ADHESIONS	<1/3 Enclosure	1/3-2/3 Enclosure	>2/3 Enclosure
OVARY	R Filmy	1	2	4
	Dense	4	8	16
	L Filmy	1	2	4
	Dense	4	8	16
TUBE	R Filmy	1	2	4
	Dense	4*	8*	16
	L Filmy	1	2	4
	Dense	4*	8*	16

*If the fimbriated end of the fallopian tube is completely enclosed, change the point assignment to 16.

Additional Endometriosis: _____   Associated Pathology: _____

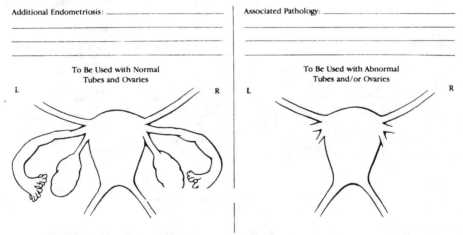

To Be Used with Normal
Tubes and Ovaries

To Be Used with Abnormal
Tubes and/or Ovaries

For additional supply write to: The American Fertility Society, 2131 Magnolia Avenue, Suite 201, Birmingham, Alabama 35256

Figure 32.2. Continued next page.

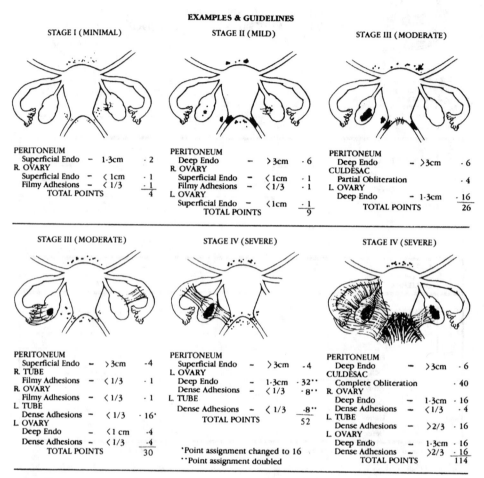

EXAMPLES & GUIDELINES

STAGE I (MINIMAL)

PERITONEUM
  Superficial Endo – 1-3cm   - 2
R. OVARY
  Superficial Endo – < 1cm   - 1
  Filmy Adhesions   – < 1/3   - 1
             TOTAL POINTS   4

STAGE II (MILD)

PERITONEUM
  Deep Endo   – > 3cm   - 6
R. OVARY
  Superficial Endo – < 1cm   - 1
  Filmy Adhesions   – < 1/3   - 1
L. OVARY
  Superficial Endo – < 1cm   - 1
             TOTAL POINTS   9

STAGE III (MODERATE)

PERITONEUM
  Deep Endo   – > 3cm   - 6
CULDESAC
  Partial Obliteration   - 4
L. OVARY
  Deep Endo   – 1-3cm   - 16
             TOTAL POINTS   26

STAGE III (MODERATE)

PERITONEUM
  Superficial Endo – > 3cm   -4
R. TUBE
  Filmy Adhesions   – < 1/3   - 1
R. OVARY
  Filmy Adhesions   – < 1/3   - 1
L. TUBE
  Dense Adhesions   – < 1/3   - 16*
L. OVARY
  Deep Endo   – < 1 cm   -4
  Dense Adhesions   – < 1/3   -4
             TOTAL POINTS   30

STAGE IV (SEVERE)

PERITONEUM
  Superficial Endo – > 3cm   - 4
L. OVARY
  Deep Endo   – 1-3cm   - 32**
  Dense Adhesions   – < 1/3   - 8**
L. TUBE
  Dense Adhesions   – < 1/3   - 8**
             TOTAL POINTS   52

*Point assignment changed to 16
**Point assignment doubled

STAGE IV (SEVERE)

PERITONEUM
  Deep Endo   – > 3cm   - 6
CULDESAC
  Complete Obliteration   - 40
R. OVARY
  Deep Endo   – 1-3cm   - 16
  Dense Adhesions   – < 1/3   - 4
L. TUBE
  Dense Adhesions   – > 2/3   - 16
L. OVARY
  Deep Endo   – 1-3cm   - 16
  Dense Adhesions   – > 2/3   - 16
             TOTAL POINTS   114

Determination of the stage or degree of endometrial involvement is based on a weighted point system. Distribution of points has been arbitrarily determined and may require further revision or refinement as knowledge of the disease increases.

To ensure complete evaluation, inspection of the pelvis in a clockwise or counterclockwise fashion is encouraged. Number, size and location of endometrial implants, plaques, endometriomas and/or adhesions are noted. For example, five separate 0.5cm superficial implants on the peritoneum (2.5 cm total) would be assigned 2 points. (The surface of the uterus should be considered peritoneum.) The severity of the endometriosis or adhesions should be assigned the highest score only for peritoneum, ovary, tube or culdesac. For example, a 4cm superficial and a 2cm deep implant of the peritoneum should be given a score of 6 (not 8). A 4cm deep endometrioma of the ovary associated with more than 3cm of superficial disease should be scored 20 (not 24).

In those patients with only one adnexa, points applied to disease of the remaining tube and ovary should be multipled by two. **Points assigned may be circled and totaled. Aggregation of points indicates stage of disease (minimal, mild, moderate, or severe).

The presence of endometriosis of the bowel, urinary tract, fallopian tube, vagina, cervix, skin etc., should be documented under "additional endometriosis." Other pathology such as tubal occlusion, leiomyomata, uterine anomaly, etc., should be documented under "associated pathology." All pathology should be depicted as specifically as possible on the sketch of pelvic organs, and means of observation (laparoscopy or laparotomy) should be noted.

Figure 32.2.   The American Fertility Society Revised Classification of Endometriosis.

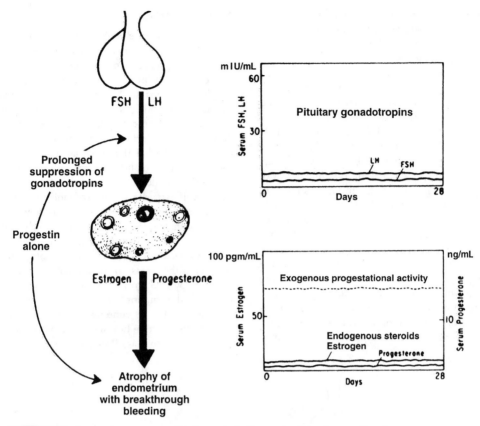

Figure 32.3. Progestin treatment of endometriosis. Progestin alone therapy directly suppresses gonadotropin release and thus ovarian steroidogenesis. It also directly affects the uterine endometrium and endometrial implants.

duces a decidual reaction in the functioning endometriotic tissue. Patients can also be maintained on oral contraceptive agents without intermittent withdrawal bleeding, thus avoiding secondary dysmenorrhea.

Progestins alone have also been administered by both the oral and parenteral routes (e.g., Provera [medroxyprogesterone acetate] 20 to 40 mg/day; Depo-Provera [depomedroxyprogesterone acetate], 100 mg i.m. every 2 weeks, then 200 mg monthly after 8 weeks). Progestins suppress gonadotropin release and, in turn, ovarian steroidogenesis; they also directly affect the uterine endometrium and endometrial implants (Fig. 32.3).

A state of "pseudomenopause" can also be induced with danazol, a 17 α-ethinyl testosterone derivative. Danazol suppresses both luteinizing hormone (LH) and follicle-stimulating hormone (FSH) midcycle surges so the ovary no longer produces estrogen and progesterone, which stim-

ulate endometriosis. At a dosage of 800 mg/day, amenorrhea occurs within 4 to 8 weeks after the onset of therapy. The desired endometrial atrophy results, but the patient also experiences vasomotor symptoms and other hypoestrogenic symptoms.

In spite of the term *pseudomenopause*, FSH and LH levels are suppressed rather than elevated as they would be in the physiologic menopausal state (Fig. 32.4). Side effects of danazol are related to its hypoestrogenic and androgenic properties, including acne in 15 to 20% of patients; spotting and bleeding in 10% of patients; hot flushes in 15% of patients; oily skin, growth of facial hair, decreased libido, and atrophic vaginitis in about 5% of patients, and deepening of the voice. Marked alterations of lipoprotein metabolism are induced, including a 60% decrease in serum high-density lipoprotein (HDL) cholesterol level and a 40% decrease in low-density lipoprotein (LDL).

Danazol provides relief from symptoms in approximately 80% of patients, with symptoms recurring in 5 to 20% of patients within one year after discontinuing the medication.

Gonadotropin-releasing hormone (GnRH) agonists such as leuprolide acetate, nafarelin acetate, and goserelin acetate have also been successfully used in treating endometriosis. Marked suppression of LH and FSH are noted, and the side effects are somewhat less troublesome than danazol for many patients. However, the therapy is quite expensive and parenteral administration is required. Daily injections, monthly shots, and nasal spray have all been shown to be effective by "down-regulating" the pituitary. Standard regimens include leuprolide acetate, 0.5 to 1.0 mg/ day administered subcutaneously for 6 months or as depot every 28 days; nafarelin acetate, one 200-mg spray into one nostril in the morning and one spray into the other nostril in the evening for 6 months; goserelin acetate, 3.6 mg i.m. every 28 days for 6 months. Efficacy for each of these agents appears comparable with that of danazol.

Surgical Therapy

The surgical management of endometriosis can be classified as either conservative or extirpative. Conservative surgery includes excision, cauterization or ablation (by laser or electrocoagulation) of visible endometriotic lesions, and preservation of the uterus and other reproductive organs to allow for a possible future pregnancy. Conservative surgery is often undertaken at the time of the initial diagnosis. Whether the initial laparoscopy is performed for pain or infertility, attempts to remove the existent endometriosis are undertaken by the surgeon. If extensive disease is found, conservative surgery involves lysis of adhesions, removal of active endometriotic lesions, and possibly reconstruction of reproductive organs. Success rates of conservative surgery appear to correlate with the severity of the disease at the time of surgery. Medical therapy is often added either before surgery, to reduce the amount of endometriosis with which the surgeon has to contend, or after surgery, to attempt to facilitate healing and avoid recurrence of the endometriosis. Pregnancy is also possible

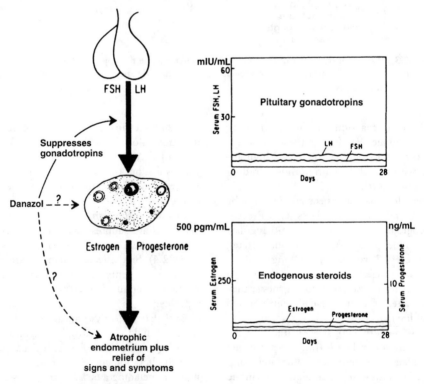

Figure 32.4. Danazol treatment of endometriosis. Danazol suppresses gonadotropin release and thus ovarian steroidogenesis.

after conservative surgical therapy, with 60% pregnancy rates being seen in patients with moderate disease.

Extirpative surgery for endometriosis is reserved only for cases where the disease is so extensive that conservative medical or surgical therapy is not feasible or when the patient has completed her family and wishes definitive therapy. Definitive surgery includes total abdominal hysterectomy, bilateral salpingo-oophorectomy, lysis of adhesions, and removal of endometriotic implants. The ramifications of not being able to conceive in the future must be thoroughly explored with the patient. Assuming that all the ovarian tissue is removed at the time of surgery, it is unlikely that any residual endometriosis will be stimulated by further endogenous hormonal production. Occasionally, in younger patients, ovarian tissue may be left to avoid the need for long-term estrogen-replacement therapy. This should be done only with the understanding that further surgery may be necessary to remove the remaining ovary should endometriosis recur.

Estrogen replacement therapy after definitive extirpative surgery for endometriosis should not be avoided for fear of stimulating recurrent disease. Only rarely is reactivation of endometriosis noted, a far smaller risk than that associated with prolonged estrogen deficiency, i.e., osteoporosis and cardiovascular disease.

CASE STUDIES

Case 32A

A 22-year-old woman seeks treatment for infertility. She and her husband have been having intercourse without conception for 17 months. Her history includes an induced abortion at the age of 16 and two episodes of pelvic infection, which required hospitalization. She reports significant menstrual discomfort and pain "when he pushes deep" during intercourse. On your examination you find the uterus to be retroverted and somewhat fixed. The patient reports moderate discomfort to uterine and cervical motion. There is some enlargement of the adnexa bilaterally.

Questions Case 32A

The most likely diagnosis is

A. Acute pelvic inflammatory disease (PID)
B. Endometriosis
C. Primary dysmenorrhea
D. Pelvic scarring due to pelvic infections

Answer: D

By history, this patient is most likely to have inactive scarring from the pelvic inflammatory disease. The patient does not have any symptoms of an acute infection, decreasing the possibility of acute PID. The history and physical examination provide enough suspicion of pelvic pathology to make secondary rather than primary dysmenorrhea more likely. Although endometriosis might explain the retroversion of the uterus and the patient's dyspareunia, endometriosis has not been documented.

What is the best recommendation for this patient?

A. Abdominal hysterectomy
B. In vitro fertilization
C. Danazol treatment
D. Diagnostic laparoscopy
E. Observation

Answer: D

Although the patient's most likely diagnosis based on history and physical examination is pelvic adhesions, the diagnosis of that entity as well as endometriosis can be made only by direct observation. Only with a firm diagnosis can appropriate therapeutic options be presented to the patient for consideration. At diagnostic laparoscopy, endometriosis involving the uterosacral ligaments, adnexae, and surrounding tissues is discovered. Biopsy of one implant confirms the diagnosis.

The best treatment option for this patient is

A. Expirtative surgery
B. Observation
C. Medical therapy
D. Conservative surgery
E. None of the above

Answer: C, D

With a desire for children, medical therapy is appropriate. Conservative surgery is also an option, with the particular procedure depending on the extent and location of disease found at surgery.

Case 32B

A 38-year-old woman presents for a premarital examination. She has never been pregnant, and she uses a diaphragm for contraception. Over the past 3 to 4 years she has had increasing problems with dysmenorrhea. The cramps no longer respond to over-the-counter ibuprofen. Before her wedding she would also like you to check the fit of her diaphragm because "lately it has been causing some pelvic and rectal discomfort" when she uses it. On examination she has significant cervical motion tenderness and thickening of the uterosacral ligaments. Endometriosis is suspected.

Question Case 32B

The patient should be advised that

A. An immediate pregnancy is desirable
B. Switching to an oral contraceptive might be beneficial
C. No therapy should be undertaken until exploratory surgery is performed
D. Therapy with a GnRH agonist should be started before her wedding
E. No specific therapy is needed at this time

Answer:　B

Although this patient may experience problems conceiving, the decision to have a child is always up to the patient and her partner, not the physician. While the presumptive diagnosis of endometriosis may be correct, definitive diagnosis cannot be made unless endometriosis is visualized and, preferably, biopsy proven. Nevertheless, some suggestions based on this presumption are appropriate. Because the patient is symptomatic, suppression using oral contraceptives might be beneficial, although not without risk at this patient's age and, in fact, would be contraindicated if she were a smoker. Aggressive therapy with GnRH agonist or danazol is optimally deferred until the diagnosis is established by laparoscopy.

chapter 33

SEXUAL ASSAULT

Sexual assault is the nonconsensual performance of acts, which in a consensual setting would be sexual or which involve genital structures in such a manner that the victim perceives a sexual intrusion. An estimated one of every four women and children in the United States are sexual assault victims. Because of the stigmata associated with sexual assault, only 1 of 10 victims seeks help. Unfortunately, those victims who do seek help are often as traumatized by those from whom they seek help as by those who assaulted them. Because of the complex problems caused by sexual assault, treatment by a *multidisciplinary team* using prepared protocols is best. The health care team has three tasks: *(a) care for the victim's emotional needs, (b) evaluate and treat medically, and (c) collect forensic specimens.*

CARING FOR THE ADULT SEXUAL ASSAULT VICTIM

Rape Trauma Syndrome

During sexual assault, the victim realizes that she cannot escape the situation and has lost control. This *loss of control*, which is the most serious emotional problem faced by the victim, is based in fact, because *threatened or actual violence is always an integral part of sexual assault.* Victims of sexual assault may react to the experience in various ways. One recognized aftermath is the *rape trauma syndrome.* This syndrome has three phases. The *acute phase of rape trauma syndrome* begins with the assault, but may not be fully manifest until the time of initial disclosure, when the victim first tells someone of the assault. In this emotionally volatile time, the victim may appear calm, may be tearful and agitated, or may move from one extreme to another. *An inability to think clearly or remember things such as her past medical history, termed "cognitive dysfunction," is a particularly distressing aspect of the syndrome.* The involuntary loss of cognition

may raise fears of "being crazy" or of being perceived as "crazy" by others. It is also frustrating for the health team unless it realizes that this is an involuntary reaction to the assault and not a willful action.

After the assault and before seeking care, the victim may have performed routine tasks such as shopping or cleaning the house. This *retreat to routine activities* is an emotional attempt to regain control, the presence or absence of which is not related to the severity of the assault. *Safety and regaining control are the victim's main emotional needs during this time.* The patient should be reassured about her immediate safety and offered as much control over events as is reasonable for her clinical situation. Discussing the sexual assault within a supportive environment facilitates a sense of control, even if the topics of discussion are themselves unpleasant.

During the *middle or "readjustment" phase* the patient appears to resolve most issues about the assault. This resolution involves a rationalization that she should or could have prevented the assault, coupled with unrealistic plans to avoid another assault. The plans of this phase ultimately break down in the *late or "reorganization" phase*, as the victim begins to deal with the reality of her victimization.

The late phase, which may be quite lengthy, is a difficult and very painful time, often characterized by drastic changes in lifestyle, friends, and work. Ongoing counseling is important if the victim is to fully recover from the emotional traumas of the assault.

Initial Care

A team member should remain with the patient to help provide a sense of safety and security. The patient should be encouraged, in a supportive, nonjudgmental manner, to talk about the assault and her feelings. This starts the patient's emotional care and also provides historical data. Treatment for life-threatening trauma is, of course, begun immediately. Fortunately, such trauma is uncommon, although minor trauma is seen in one-quarter of victims. Even in life-threatening situations, any sense of control that can be given the patient is helpful. Obtaining consents for treatment is not only a legal requirement but also an important aspect of the emotional care of the victim. Although patients are often reticent to do so, they should be gently encouraged to work with the police, as such cooperation is clearly associated with improved emotional outcomes for victims.

History taking about a sexual assault is uncomfortable for victims and health care providers alike. History taking is not, however, an additional trauma. Instead, it is both a necessary activity to gain medical and forensic information and an important therapeutic activity. Recalling the details of the assault in the supportive environment of the health care setting allows the victim to begin to gain an understanding of what has happened and to see that she and others can deal with the events. Victims of sexual assault characteristically perceive themselves as guilty of causing the assault, especially in situations in which they used poor judgment (e.g., hitchhiking). To say that any activity was acceptable when it involved poor judgment is a falsehood that destroys the patient's ultimate trust and the care provider's credibility. Reminding the patient that "*poor judgment is not a rapable offense*" helps the patient begin to place blame where it truly belongs: on the rapist.

Victims of sexual assault should be given a *complete general physical examination*, including a pelvic examination. Forensic specimens should be collected, and cultures for sexually transmitted diseases should be obtained. When collecting *forensic specimens*, it is critical that the clinician follows the directions on the forensic specimens kit. These specimens are kept in a health professional's possession or control until turned over to an appropriate legal representative. This "protective custody" of the specimens ensures that the correct specimen reaches the forensic laboratory and is called the "chain of evidence."

Initial *laboratory tests* should include cultures from the vagina, the anus, and usually, also the pharynx for gonorrhea and *Chlamydia*, rapid plasma reagin (RPR) for syphilis, hepatitis antigens, HIV if indicated (usually), UA and C&S, and a pregnancy test for menstrual-aged women (regardless of contraceptive status).

Antibiotic prophylaxis should be offered to all adult victims. The risk of infection is unknown, but it is clearly higher than for a consensual sexual experience. Recommended regimens include oral *doxycycline* (100 mg p.o. b.i.d. for 7 days) or oral *amoxicillin* (3 g p.o. once) plus *probenecid* (1 g p.o. once) followed by oral *erythromycin* base (500 mg p.o. b.i.d. for 7 days) for pregnant victims or those allergic to tetracyclines. In areas with a prevalence rate greater than 1% for antibiotic-resistant strains of *Neisseria gonorrhoeae*, ceftriaxone (Rocephin; 250 mg i.m.) followed by oral doxycycline (100 mg p.o. b.i.d. for 7 days) is recommended. *Tetanus toxoid* should be administered if indicated.

Short courses of *Diethylstilbestrol* (DES; 25 mg p.o. b.i.d. for 5 days) with *Compazine* (prochlorperazine; 10 mg p.o. q.8h.) may be given as a *postcoital contraceptive medication*. Another popular postcoital regimen is Ovral (0.05 mg ethinyl estradiol and 0.5 mg norgestrel), two tablets p.o. b.i.d. for 3 days. If a postcoital contraception is chosen, the patient should be reminded that these medications may be teratogenic so that a therapeutic abortion is recommended if pregnancy does occur despite their use.

Within 24 to 48 hr, victims should be contacted by phone or seen for an *immediate posttreatment evaluation*. At this time, emotional or physical problems are managed and follow-up appointments arranged for 1 and 6 weeks. Potentially serious problems such as suicidal ideation, rectal bleeding, or evidence of pelvic infection may go unrecognized by the victim during this time because of fear or continued cognitive dysfunction. Gently stated but specific questions must be asked to ensure that such problems have not arisen.

Subsequent Care

At the 1-week visit, a general review of the patient's progress is made and any specific new problems addressed. The next routine visit is at 6 weeks, when a complete evaluation including physical examination, repeat cultures for sexually transmitted diseases, and a repeat RPR are performed. Another visit at 12–18 weeks may be indicated for repeat HIV titers, although the present understanding of HIV infection does not allow an estimate of the risk of exposure for sexual assault victims. Each victim should receive as much counseling and support as is necessary, with referral to a long-term counseling program if needed.

CARING FOR THE CHILD SEXUAL ASSAULT VICTIM

A total of 90% of child victimization is by parents, family members, or family friends; "stranger rape" is relatively uncommon in children. The assailants play on the child's need for love and her dependency on family. To get past this conflict, it is best to interview child victims apart from parents and other family members, if possible by interviewers skilled in child interview techniques. Although such interviewing and the interpretation of information gained is difficult, in general, a child who displays a knowledge of sexual matters, anatomy, or function beyond that expected for her years is very likely a victim of sexual abuse. Expert interviewers may use such specialized techniques as anatomically correct doll play and drawing interpretation to facilitate the process.

The physical examination of a small child requires patience and much experience. Sedation should be avoided, because it cannot be done to sufficiently allay anxiety in an outpatient setting. Instead it usually adds to the child's fear and sense of helplessness. Examination under anesthesia may be required, although nonobtrusive techniques have been developed to avoid this procedure.

Prophylactic antibiotic therapy should be offered children if there is evidence that the assailant is infected, if follow-up compliance is unlikely, or if the assailant is a stranger. Otherwise, prophylactic antibiotic therapy is generally not indicated. Of course, any diagnosed infection in the child is treated as appropriate. Recommended regimens include amoxicillin (50 mg/kg body weight once) plus probenecid (25 mg/kg body weight to a maximum dose of 1 g). For penicillin-allergic children or in geographic areas with a high prevalence of penicillinase-producing gonococci, spectinomycin (40 mg/kg body weight i.m.) or ceftriaxone (125 mg i.m. once) followed by erythromycin (50 mg/kg body weight p.o. for 7 days).

It is the responsibility of the care team to determine if the child may safely return home or if the risk of ongoing abuse requires foster home placement or hospitalization. *Since suspected child sexual abuse must be reported to police and child welfare authorities*, these agencies may officially help in this decision, although responsibility rests with the care team at the time of the initial disclosure.

CASE STUDIES

Case 33A

15-year-old G2 P2 presents to the emergency room accompanied by police to whom she has reported a sexual assault. She is quiet but seems disoriented, dressed in a see–through blouse and tight stretch pants. She tells the nurses that she was raped by a "friend." The police ask that you speed your evaluation, because they have other calls and need to be on their way.

Questions Case 33A

Which of the following should guide your initial evaluation of this patient?

A. Rapid conclusion of the evaluation to cooperate with the police

B. Dismissing the claim of rape because it was a friend, hence clearly consensual sex rather than rape

C. Concern that the historical information is incomplete, requiring a full evaluation regardless of pressure to proceed more rapidly

D. Since she is a minor, calling her parents to get permission to see the patient and obtaining further information

Answer: C

Your primary responsibilities are emotional and physical health care of the patient. Cooperation with police is important, especially in the initial phase to provide immediate information for pursuit of the assailant. Thereafter, police action is best left until after health care is completed. Knowing that sexual abuse in children is often performed by family members, you may contact parents but plan to pay special attention to the child's history. The patient's attire is irrelevant unless torn, stained, or otherwise presents information about what has happened.

Your sexual assault team completes its evaluation, and you discover that your patient lives with her mother and stepfather. She is afraid to tell your team about details of what has happened, but does indicate it has been going on for some time. She is frightened to return home. Her physical examination is unremarkable except that her uterus is about 14 weeks size and soft.

What laboratory tests are indicated?

A. UA

B. Urine hCG

C. Urine drug screen

D. Pap smear

E. hepatitis screen

Answer: B

By history and examination, pregnancy is likely and a pregnancy test is appropriate. The other tests listed may be useful in general but do not address the specific issue: Who is abusing this child?

Case 33B

A 35-year-old mother of three and wife of a heavy-equipment operator presents, complaining that her husband raped her earlier in the day after she refused him "his sex." She says he threatened to beat her if she didn't "lie down and take it," so she did. Physical examination reveals only motile sperm in the vagina. The patient has had a postpartum tubal ligation. She says she wishes medical care but does not want the police notified, as they will "cause too much trouble." Her husband arrives, demands that you "get out of his business" and let his wife go so that she can fix dinner.

Question Case 33B

Your appropriate response(s) to this situation include

A. Tell the patient to go home, that how and when she and her husband have sex is their business and not yours

B. Complete a sexual assault workup

C. Notify the police

D. Call psychiatry, as the patient is clearly not demonstrating an appropriate response to a sexual assault

Answer: B, C

In some states, a husband cannot by law rape his wife (in effect, she is in the eyes of the law his sexual property), whereas in other states, rape is defined as a nonconsensual experience. In either case, this legal decision is not properly made by you, but by the police, who should be notified. You may support the patient's decision not to talk to the police — although you should encourage her to do so — but you must call the police because a violent crime has been reported and because you do not know what the situation is at home, especially in relation to the safety of the children.

chapter 34

REPRODUCTIVE CYCLE

In the female reproductive cycle, ovulation is followed by menstrual bleeding in a recurring, predictable sequence, if conception does not occur. This recurring sequence is established at puberty (around age 13) and continues until the time of menopause at around age 50. A regular, predictable reproductive cycle is usually established by age 15 and continues until age 45. Thus a woman has approximately 30 years of optimal reproductive function. In healthy women, reproductive cycles occur at about 28-day intervals, and most women ovulate 13 to 14 times per year, unless ovulation is interrupted by pregnancy, lactation, or oral contraceptive use.

The reproductive cycle depends on the cyclic interaction between hypothalamic gonadotropin-releasing hormone (GnRH), the pituitary gonadotropins follicle-stimulating hormone (FSH) and luteinizing hormone (LH), and the ovarian sex steroid hormones estradiol and progesterone. Through positive- and negative-feedback loops, these hormones stimulate ovulation, facilitate implantation of the fertilized ovum, and bring about menstruation. Feedback loops between the hypothalamus, pituitary gland, and ovaries are depicted in Figure 34.1. If any one (or more) of the above hormones becomes tonically elevated or suppressed, the reproductive cycle becomes disrupted and ovulation and menstruation cease. In the case of female reproductive dysfunction, it is essential to identify which hormones are either elevated or reduced.

HYPOTHALAMIC GnRH SECRETION

Hypothalamic GnRH (a decapeptide) is secreted in a pulsatile manner from the arcuate nucleus of the hypothalamus. The hypothalamus serves as the mainspring or pulse generator of the reproductive clock. Surgical ablation of the arcuate nu-

cleus in animals disrupts ovarian function, as does continuous infusion of GnRH agonists. Ovarian function can be restored by the pulsatile infusion of GnRH at 70- to 90-min intervals. The mechanism for stimulation of GnRH secretion is unknown; however, GnRH secretion is influenced by estradiol and catecholamine neurotransmitters. The latter influence may help explain psychogenic influences on the reproductive cycle. GnRH reaches the anterior pituitary gland through the hypothalamic-pituitary portal plexus. Pituitary gonadotropin secretion is stimulated and modulated by the pulsatile secretion of GnRH. *FASTER or SLOWER → FAILURE*

PITUITARY GONADOTROPIN SECRETION

The pituitary gonadotropins *FSH* and *LH* are protein hormones secreted by the anterior pituitary gland. FSH and LH are also secreted in pulsatile fashion in concert with the pulsatile release of GnRH; the magnitude of secretion and the rates of secretion of FSH and/or LH are determined largely by the levels of ovarian steroid hormones and other ovarian factors. When a woman is in a state of relative estrogen deficiency, the principal gonadotropin secreted is FSH. As the ovary responds to FSH secretion with estradiol production, there is a negative feedback to the pituitary gland to inhibit FSH secretion and facilitate LH secretion. This is discussed in more detail in association with the phases of the reproductive cycle.

OVARIAN SEX STEROID HORMONE SECRETION

Ovarian follicles respond to pituitary gonadotropin secretion by synthesizing the principal ovarian hormones *estradiol* and *progesterone.* Increasing levels of estradiol feed back to the pituitary gland via a negative-feedback mechanism, resulting in

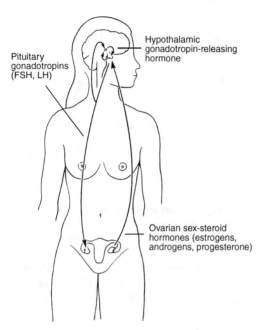

Figure 34.1. Cyclic interactions between the hypothalamus, pituitary gland, and ovaries.

decreased secretion of FSH and increased secretion of LH. This results in a marked increase in LH secretion, known as the LH surge, which triggers ovulation. With ovulation, the ovarian follicle is converted into a corpus luteum and begins secreting progesterone.

At birth, the human ovary is filled with *primordial follicles*. Each follicle contains an oocyte that is arrested in the prophase stage of meiosis. The oocyte is surrounded by a single layer of pregranulosa cells, which will become the granulosa cells. The pregranulosa cells are surrounded by a matrix of cells that will become the theca cells. Some primordial follicles respond to pituitary FSH during childhood, but ovulation does not occur until puberty, despite the stimulation and subsequent atresia of some follicles during childhood.

During a full reproductive cycle, one oocyte is brought to maturity before ovulation. In the process of bringing one oocyte to maturation, a number of oocytes are stimulated to partial maturation but subsequently undergo atresia before reaching ovulation. Why several oocytes are stimulated simultaneously but only one is ovulated is unknown.

During the process of follicular maturation, pregranulosa cells are stimulated by FSH to become *granulosa cells*, which begin secreting *estra-*

diol. Binding of FSH to receptors in the granulosa cells causes granulosa cell proliferation, increased binding of FSH, and increased production of estradiol. The follicle with the greatest number of granulosa cells, FSH receptors, and the highest estradiol production becomes the dominant follicle from which ovulation will occur.

As a primordial follicle is stimulated, the pretheca cells surrounding the granulosa cells become *theca cells*. The theca cells secrete *androgens*, which serve as the precursors for estradiol production by the granulosa cells. Current scientific theory holds that estradiol is secreted through a two-cell mechanism (Fig. 34.2). Androgens are first secreted by the theca cells. These androgens enter the granulosa cells by diffusion, where they are aromatized to estradiol.

After ovulation, the dominant follicle becomes the *corpus luteum*, which secretes *progesterone* to prepare the endometrium for implantation of a fertilized oocyte. If pregnancy does not occur, menstruation begins, and the cycle repeats. The

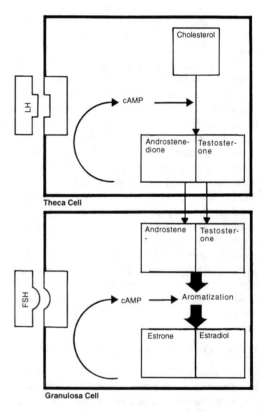

Figure 34.2. Two cell theories of estradiol production.

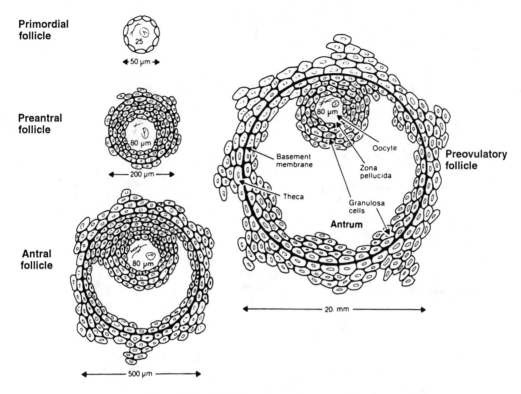

Figure 34.3. Follicular changes in menstrual cycle.

changes in the follicle during the follicular phase of the cycle are presented in Figure 34.3.

For purposes of discussion, *the reproductive cycle is divided into three phases: menstruation and the follicular phase, ovulation, and the luteal phase.* These three phases refer to the status of the ovary during the reproductive cycle.

REPRODUCTIVE CYCLE

Phase I: Menstruation and the Follicular Phase

When the oocyte ovulated in the previous cycle fails to become fertilized, the cyclic interaction between the hypothalamus, pituitary gland, and ovaries is reset, initiating a new reproductive cycle. The 1st day of menstruation is considered day 1 of the menstrual cycle. During menstruation, the endometrium is sloughed in response to progesterone withdrawal. This is followed by the follicular phase, during which a new endometrial lining of the uterus is formed in preparation for implantation of an embryo.

Women usually menstruate for 3 to 5 days. A woman will shed approximately 30 to 50 mL of dark, nonclotting menstrual blood during menstruation. Occasionally, tissue elements of endometrium can be identified in the menstrual effluent.

There may be uterine cramps during the first day or two of menstrual bleeding. These cramps are a result of the action of prostaglandins liberated from the endometrium at the beginning of menstruation. Prostaglandins are a group of endogenous 20-carbon hydroxy-unsaturated fatty acids, whose biosynthetic pathway begins with the precursor arachidonic acid (Fig. 34.4). The secretory endometrium synthesizes prostaglandins, especially $PGF_2\alpha$, under the influence of progesterone. The endometrial content of $PGF_2\alpha$ is higher during the secretory than follicular phase and is highest during early menstruation. At this time, prostaglandins are released and produce contractions of the uterine musculature and vasculature, causing contractile and ischemic pain (Fig. 34.5). These prostaglandin-associated uterine contractions also aid the expulsion of the menstrual effluent.

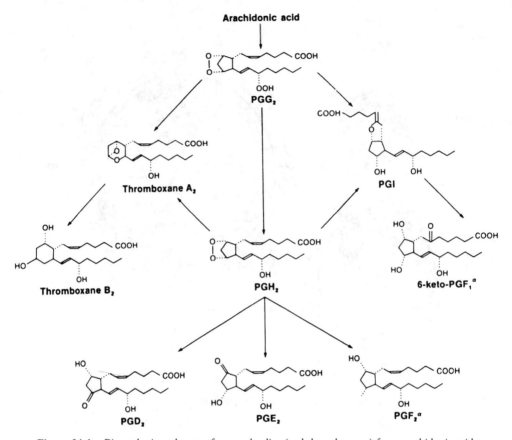

Figure 34.4. Biosynthetic pathways of prostaglandins (and thromboxanes) from arachidonic acid.

Menstruation also marks the beginning of the follicular phase of the cycle. With the beginning of menstruation, plasma concentrations of estradiol, progesterone, and LH reach their lowest point. Only FSH is increased at the beginning of menstruation. The increase in FSH begins about 2 days before the onset of menstruation and is involved in the maturation of another group of ovarian follicles and the selection of a dominant follicle for ovulation in the next cycle. FSH binds to receptors located in the granulosa cells of the primary oocyte. As FSH is bound to the granulosa cells, it stimulates their differentiation from a stratified squamous-type cell into a cuboidal cell. Moreover, FSH stimulates mitosis of the granulosa cells, thereby increasing the number of granulosa cells surrounding the oocyte. Under the influence of FSH, the granulosa cells begin to secrete estradiol.

Estradiol begins to rise in plasma by the 4th day of the cycle. Estradiol stimulates LH receptors on the theca cells, preparing them to increase

secretion of androgen precursors to estradiol and preparing the granulosa and theca cells for progesterone production after ovulation.

With rising estradiol, there is negative feedback on the pituitary gland to decrease the release of FSH and positive feedback on the pituitary gland to increase the release of LH. During the early follicular phase of the cycle, the FSH:LH ratio is >1; as the cycle progresses, the FSH:LH ratio becomes <1, demonstrating both positive and negative feedback effects of estradiol on the pituitary gland.

As follicles enlarge, they secrete both androgens and estrogens; however, if the estradiol:androgen ratio within the follicular fluid becomes <1, that follicle will become atretic and never become a dominant follicle. The dominant follicle is the one that has a follicular fluid estradiol:androgen ratio of >1.

As the dominant follicle secretes more and more estradiol, there is marked positive feedback

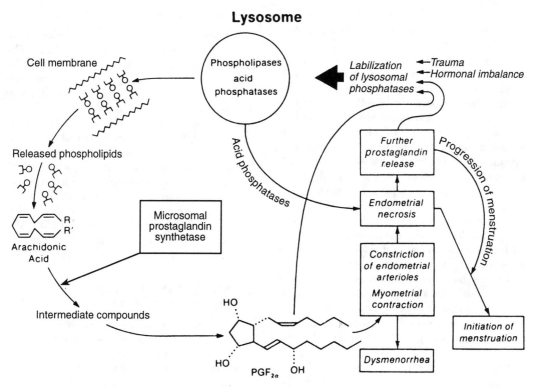

Figure 34.5. Menstrual-associated prostaglandin release and uterine contractions.

to the pituitary gland to secrete LH. By day 11 to 13 of the normal cycle, an LH surge occurs, which triggers ovulation. Ovulation occurs within 30 to 36 hr of the LH surge, causing the oocyte to be expelled from the follicle and the follicle to be converted into a corpus luteum to facilitate progesterone production during the remainder of the cycle. At the time of the LH surge just before ovulation, there is a concomitant rise in FSH. The mechanism for this FSH rise and its effect on the follicle are unknown.

Phase II: Ovulation

The mechanism for ovulation is poorly understood. As the dominant follicle enlarges and accumulates follicular fluid, it is said to "ripen" and become ready for release. Through animal studies, it has been demonstrated that intrafollicular prostaglandins play an essential role in release of the oocyte and that the administration of prostaglandin synthetase inhibitors will cause the oocyte to be retained within the follicle during the luteal phase of the cycle.

Many women experience a twinge of pain ("mittelschmerz") at the time of ovulation and can distinguish the time of ovulation with precision. Others will not experience pain but can appreciate the effects of changing hormone production that occur with ovulation.

The application of transvaginal ultrasound imaging has enabled physicians to follow the process of follicular growth and maturation and observe the collapse of the dominant follicle following ovulation. A condition of luteinized retained follicle has been recognized, in which the oocyte does not appear to be expelled from the follicle.

Phase III: Luteal Phase

The luteal phase of the cycle is characterized by a change in secretion of sex steroid hormones from estradiol predominance to progesterone predominance. As FSH rises early in the cycle and stimulates mitosis of granulosa cells and production of estradiol, additional LH receptors are created in the granulosa cells and theca cells. With the LH surge at the time of ovulation, these LH receptors bind LH and convert the enzymatic machinery of the granulosa and theca cells to facilitate production of progesterone.

Progesterone production depends on the initial FSH and LH signals from the pituitary gland. Adequate progesterone production is necessary to facilitate implantation of the fertilized oocyte into the endometrium and to sustain pregnancy into the early first trimester. If the initial rise in FSH is inadequate and if the LH surge does not achieve maximal amplitude, an "inadequate luteal phase," i.e., luteal phase defect, can occur. In the luteal phase defect, there is inadequate progesterone production to facilitate implantation of a fertilized oocyte or to sustain pregnancy.

The production of progesterone begins about 24 hr before ovulation and rises rapidly thereafter. A maximal production of progesterone occurs 3 to 4 days after ovulation and is maintained for approximately 11 days following ovulation. If fertilization and implantation do not occur, progesterone production diminishes rapidly, initiating events leading to the beginning of a new cycle.

The corpus luteum measures about 2.5 cm in diameter and has a characteristic deep yellow color. It can be seen on gross inspection of the ovary if laparoscopy or laparotomy are performed during the luteal phase of the cycle. As the corpus luteum fails, it decreases in volume and loses its yellow color. After a few months, the corpus luteum becomes a white fibrous streak within the ovary called the corpus albicans.

The corpus luteum has a fixed life span of 13 to 14 days unless pregnancy occurs. If the oocyte becomes fertilized and implants within the endometrium, the early pregnancy begins secreting human chorionic gonadotropin (hCG), which sustains the corpus luteum for another 6 to 7 weeks.

Progesterone has negative feedback on pituitary secretion of both FSH and LH. During the luteal phase of the cycle, both FSH and LH are suppressed to low levels. As the corpus luteum fails and progesterone secretion diminishes, FSH begins to rise to prepare a woman for the next reproductive cycle.

The cyclic changes in FSH, LH, estradiol, and progesterone along with the changes in the follicle, endometrium, vagina, and cervix are presented in Figure 34.6. Note the cyclic interaction between the four hormones during the course of a reproductive cycle.

Perimenopause

As a woman ages, the ovarian follicles diminish in number and become less sensitive to FSH. The process of ovulation becomes increasingly inefficient, less regular, and less predictable than in earlier years. A woman will begin to notice changes in her reproductive cycle at around age 38 to 42. Initially, she will notice a shortening of the cycle length. With increasing inefficiency of the reproductive cycle, the follicular phase shortens but the luteal phase is maintained at normal length. With the passing of time, some cycles become anovulatory so that the frequency of ovulation decreases.

As menopause approaches, the remaining follicles become almost totally resistant to FSH. The process of ovulation ceases entirely and cyclic hormone production ends with menopause.

CLINICAL MANIFESTATIONS OF HORMONAL CHANGES

The presence or absence of sex steroid hormones produce clinical manifestations that aid in establishing the phases of the reproductive cycle. The endometrium and endocervix, the breasts, the vagina, and the hypothalamic thermoregulating center all undergo cyclic changes in response to hormonal control. The changes in the endocervix and breasts can be directly observed, and the changes in the hypothalamic thermoregulatory center can be measured by recording the basal body temperature. The changes in the vagina can be identified by cytologic examination of the vaginal epithelium, and the changes in the endometrium can be evaluated by endometrial biopsy followed by histologic examination of the biopsy sample. Other changes can be ascertained through a careful history. Some of these changes include alteration of libido, abdominal bloating, fluid retention, mood changes, and uterine cramps at the onset of menstruation.

Endometrium

The endometrial lining of the uterus undergoes dramatic histologic changes during the reproductive cycle. During menstruation, the endometrium is sloughed to a basal level, consisting of compact stroma cells and short, narrow endometrial glands. Estrogen is a mitogenic hormone, which stimulates cell growth. With rising estradiol production during the follicular phase of the cycle, the endometrial stroma thickens and the

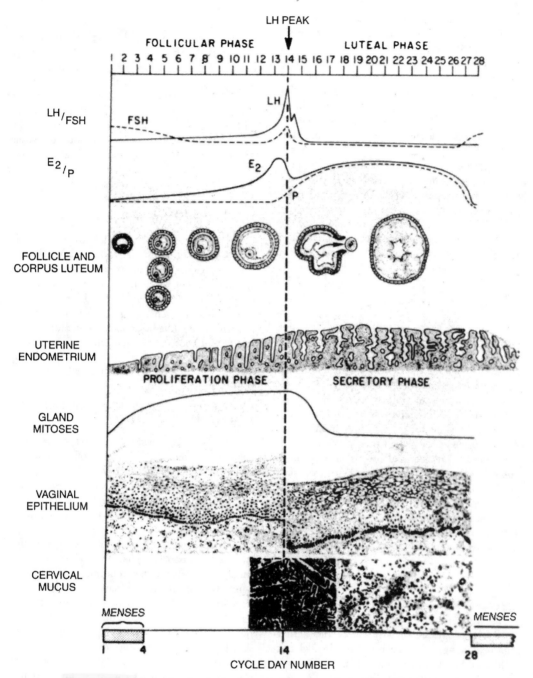

Figure 34.6. Composite changes in tissues and hormones during the reproductive cycle.

endometrial glands become elongated; this is a proliferative endometrium. The endometrium reaches a maximal thickness at the time of ovulation. If ovulation does not occur and a woman remains in an estrogenic state, the endometrium continues to thicken and the endometrial glands continue to elongate until the endometrium outgrows its blood supply and sloughs. This abnormal condition is the basis for dysfunctional uterine bleeding (see Chapter 36).

When ovulation occurs, the hormonal balance changes from an estrogenic state to a progestational state. Progesterone is not a mitogen, but causes differentiation of the tissues that contain progesterone receptors. Progesterone converts the proliferative endometrium into a secretory endometrium. The endometrial stroma becomes loose and edematous, and blood vessels entering the endometrium become thickened. The endometrial glands, which were straight and tubular in the proliferative phase of the endometrium, become tortuous and contain secretory material within the lumina. Following ovulation, distinct, recognizable changes occur within the endometrium at almost daily intervals. Therefore, the quality of the corpus luteum and stage of the reproductive cycle can be evaluated by histologic examination of a small sample of endometrium.

Endocervix

The endocervix contains glands that secrete endocervical mucus in response to hormonal changes. Under the influence of estradiol, the endocervical glands secrete large quantities of thin, clear, watery, endocervical mucus. This mucus facilitates sperm capture, sperm storage, and sperm transport. Sperm can be stored in the crypts of the endocervical glands for up to 7 days and then released into the upper genital tract for fertilization of an oocyte. Endocervical mucus production is maximal at the time of ovulation. With ovulation and the shift in hormone production from estradiol to progesterone, the endocervical mucus becomes thick, opaque, and tenacious. This type of mucus is an impediment to sperm capture, storage, and transport.

Breasts

The ductal elements of the breasts, nipples, and areolae respond to estradiol secretion. After ovulation, progesterone stimulates the acinar (milk producing) glands. Since the acinar glands are located in the tails of the breasts, this gives the breasts a more rounded configuration. Moreover, progesterone makes the venous pattern on the surface of the breasts appear more prominent and accentuates the small Montgomery glands contained within the areolae. These dynamic changes can be observed during the reproductive cycle and are seen in the development states of puberty.

Vagina

Estradiol stimulates vaginal thickening and maturation of the surface epithelial cells of the vaginal mucosa. Estradiol also facilitates vaginal transudation during sexual excitement, creating a moist, lubricated vagina for sexual intercourse. During the luteal phase of the cycle, the vaginal epithelium retains its thickness but the secretory changes are markedly diminished. Women report less sexual desire and sexual enjoyment during the luteal phase. This loss of sexual desire is even more marked during the early weeks of pregnancy.

Hypothalamic Thermoregulating Center

Progesterone shifts the basal body temperature upward by 0.6 to 1.0°F. This shift occurs abruptly with the beginning of the progesterone secretion and wanes abruptly with loss of progesterone secretion. The changes in the basal body temperature reflect the changing plasma progesterone concentration. The basal body temperature record is a useful tool for women and their physicians who want to evaluate the reproductive cycle in a dynamic and inexpensive way (see Fig. 38.3).

CLINICAL IMPLICATIONS OF THE REPRODUCTIVE CYCLE

Some women have exaggerated responses to the changing hormonal environment of the reproductive cycle and experience troublesome symptoms. The two conditions for which women seek medical attention as a result of the reproductive cycle are premenstrual syndrome (PMS) and primary dysmenorrhea.

The etiology and pathogenesis of *premenstrual syndrome* are poorly understood. There are many theories to explain this common condition, and a number of treatments have been devised for its correction. However, none of these theories has withstood scientific scrutiny. The emotional, physical, and behavioral symptoms of premenstrual syndrome occur during the luteal phase of the reproductive cycle, and these symptoms do not occur in anovulatory women. Thus premenstrual syndrome is directly associated with the reproductive cycle.

Primary dysmenorrhea is the occurrence of debilitating uterine cramps during the first 2 days of menstruation. Associated symptoms are diarrhea, nausea, vomiting, and headache. These symptoms are self-limiting and abate as menstruation ceases.

The etiology of primary dysmenorrhea is linked to the endometrial production and secretion of prostaglandins just before and during menstruation. Symptoms of primary dysmenorrhea can be directly alleviated by the administration of prostaglandin synthetase inhibitors and moderately alleviated by oral contraceptives to inhibit ovulation.

CASE STUDIES

Case 34A

A 24-year-old woman has regular, predictable menstrual cycles that began at age 13.

Questions Case 34A

Which of the following statements about the follicular phase of her cycle are correct?

A. Follicle-stimulating hormone initiates the development of a cohort of follicles, one of which will become the dominant follicle
B. Endometrial biopsy would reveal presence of a secretory endometrium
C. Endocervical mucus would be thin, clear, and watery during the late follicular phase
D. Estradiol is the predominant steroid hormone

Answer: A, C, D

The only incorrect statement is regarding the state of the endometrium, which would be proliferative. Secretory endometrium reflects a state of progesterone dominance and occurs in the luteal phase.

Which of the following statements about the luteal phase of the cycle are correct?

A. Progesterone is the predominant steroid hormone
B. Endocervical mucus is thick, sticky, and tenacious

C. Basal body temperature is elevated
D. It is during this phase of the reproductive cycle that some women develop cyclic emotional, physical, and behavioral symptoms

Answer: All

Each of the options is correct and each statement has clinical relevance in certain patients. A basic understanding of the underlying reproductive cycle physiology will facilitate diagnosis as well as treatment.

Case 34B

A 45-year-old woman notices a lengthening of her cycle from the usual 29 days to 50 to 60 days. She also experiences occasional hot flushes.

Question Case 34B

Which of the following statements are correct?

A. The number of ovarian follicles is still adequate for ovulation
B. Her FSH concentration is tonically elevated
C. Her FSH has altered, and the ovarian follicles are less responsive to the altered molecule
D. Her plasma estradiol concentration is zero

Answer: A

Although the total number of follicles continues to decrease with each cycle, the woman is apparently still having ovulatory cycles. The FSH concentration is not tonically elevated until the ovary no longer responds to FSH. Until then, it continues to fluctuate. The FSH molecule itself does not change in configuration during the perimenopausal period. The estradiol concentration is not zero, as the ovary continues to produce estradiol, albeit in less efficient fashion. The occasional vasomotor symptoms suggest waning of but not lack of ovarian function.

chapter 35

PUBERTY

Puberty is the physical, emotional, and sexual transition from childhood to adulthood. Although the transition occurs gradually, it contains a series of well-defined events and milestones. Few individuals have problems with this endocrine process. However, when puberty is delayed or advanced, an understanding of the hormonal events of puberty and the sequence of physical changes is essential for the physician to be able to evaluate the process and progress of sexual development. Moreover, an understanding of puberty is essential for an understanding of the process of reproduction.

The endocrine events that initiate the onset of secondary sexual maturation are unknown. The hypothalamic-pituitary-gonadal axis functions during fetal life and during the first few weeks following birth, after which the axis becomes quiescent. At about age 8 in boys and girls, the adrenal glands begin to secrete increasing quantities of dehydroepiandrosterone; approximately 2 years later, the gonads begin secreting gonadal sex steroid hormones. The process of secondary sexual maturation requires about 4 years from its beginning until full sexual maturation has been achieved; this process takes place in an orderly, predictable sequence. The events, age, and hormone(s) responsible for the sequence of *sexual maturation* in girls is presented in Table 35.1. The sequence of breast development (thelarche) is presented in Figure 35.1.

These events are predictable and reflect the secretion and action of hypothalamic peptide hormones and pituitary protein hormones, adrenal steroid hormones, and gonadal sex steroid hormones. An alteration in the sequence of these events suggests that there is an alteration in normal hormone secretion and action.

Three known critical elements play a role in the timing of *secondary sexual maturation.* These are adequate body fat, adequate sleep, and vision (optic exposure to sunlight).

Girls must attain a *critical body weight* — irrespective of height — before breast development begins. Moreover, a body weight of *106 pounds* must be achieved before menses begins, and a proportion of *body fat of 24%* is required to sustain ovulatory cycles. This theory of critical body weight has been challenged by a number of investigators but has held up well in clinical observations and practice. Girls who engage in strenuous exercise programs before puberty have delayed sexual development; girls who are obese as children have early menarche. The role of body weight in male secondary sexual maturation and in sustaining male reproductive function is not defined.

Sleep has varying effects on the gonadotropin secretory pattern in prepubertal children, intrapubertal children, and sexually mature adolescents. In prepubertal children, there is no correlation between sleep cycle and gonadotropin secretion. In intrapubertal adolescents — girls who have breast development and sexual hair growth but who have not menstruated and males who have penile and testicular enlargement but who have not ejaculated — there is a sleep-entrained gonadotropin secretory cycle. That is, during sleep, there is a marked increased in the secretion of follicle-stimulating hormone (FSH) and luteinizing hormone (LH). In sexually mature adolescents, the release of gonadotropins bears no relationship to the sleep cycle. Instead, gonadotropins are released at 6- to 8-hr intervals. This pattern is maintained for the remainder of a person's reproductive life, unless reproductive dysfunction occurs.

Optic exposure to sunlight is essential for timely secondary sexual development. Blind girls have delayed menarche and blind boys have delayed spermatogenesis and ejaculation. In hibernating animals who obviously have limited optic exposure, pituitary secretion of gonadotropins is suppressed during the period of hibernation. A similar mechanism is postulated for humans with decreased exposure to sunlight for any reason.

Abrupt *mood changes* occur during the period of secondary sexual maturation in girls and boys. Periods of depression, euphoria, and even violent behavior occur to some extent in many intrapubertal adolescents. Once full sexual maturation — with release of gametes — is completed, these mood changes disappear, so the physician can reassure

concerned, distraught parents that the mood changes will abate with time.

ABNORMALITIES OF PUBERTAL DEVELOPMENT

The abnormalities of puberty include delayed sexual maturation, incomplete sexual maturation, primary amenorrhea, and precocious puberty. The presence of any of these disorders requires investigation of the hypothalamic-pituitary-gonadal axis and the reproductive outflow tract. The initial investigation must begin with measurement of pituitary gonadotropins (FSH and LH). These hormones distinguish a hypothalamic-pituitary etiology from a gonadal etiology.

Delayed Sexual Maturation

The first step in sexual maturation is breast budding, which usually begins between 10 and 11 years in most girls. Some girls will begin breast budding by 8 years, and this falls within the range of normal. However, if breast budding does not begin by 13 years, puberty may be delayed or may not begin spontaneously. *Failure to establish a breast bud by age 13* should cause the physician to initiate an endocrine evaluation to elucidate the cause of

Table 35.1.
Sequence of Sexual Maturation in Girls

Event	Age (Years)	Hormone(s)
Breast budding	10–11	Estradiol
Sexual hair growth	10.5–11.5	Androgens
Growth spurt	11–12	Growth hormone
Menarche	11.5–13	Estradiol
Adult breast development	12.5–15	Progesterone
Adult sexual hair	13.5–16	Androgens

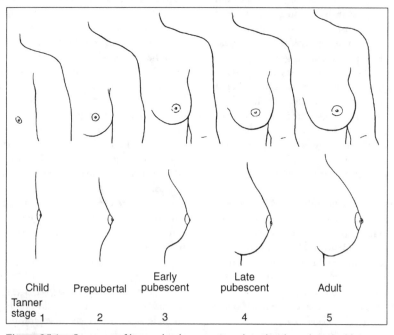

	Child	Prepubertal	Early pubescent	Late pubescent	Adult
Tanner stage	1	2	3	4	5

Figure 35.1. Sequence of breast development in pubertal girls as described by Tanner.

pubertal delay. Moreover, *if sexual hair growth precedes breast budding by more than 6 to 9 months* the physician should likewise initiate an endocrine evaluation. The most *common causes of delayed puberty* are presented in Table 35.2.

Premature Ovarian Failure

Ovarian failure can occur anytime prior to the expected time of menopause. *Ovarian failure is characterized by diminished or absent estrogen production in association with elevated gonadotropins.* The most common form of premature ovarian failure seen in prepubertal and pubertal girls is *Turner syndrome.* The features of Turner syndrome are failure to establish secondary sexual development along with somatic changes such as short stature, a webbed neck (pterygium colli), a shield chest with widely spaced nipples, and an increased carrying angle of the elbow (cubitus valgus).

The fundamental genetic defects in girls with Turner syndrome are absence of an X chromosome and no Barr bodies (Fig. 35.2). Genetic information that regulates the rate of ovarian follicular atresia is carried on the long arm of the X chromosome, whereas somatic information is carried on the short arm of the X chromosome. The absence of the entire X chromosome leads to loss of ovarian function and to the somatic features described above.

Partial deletions of the long arm of the X chromosome cause premature ovarian failure to occur at varying chronological ages. For example, complete loss of the long arm of the X chromosome results in premature ovarian failure before puberty, whereas a small fragmentary loss of the X-chromosome may not result in ovarian failure until many years after a normal puberty.

When breast development fails to occur at the expected age or when breast development begins and then fails to be completed, the physician should consider premature ovarian failure. This diagnosis is established easily by the finding of elevated gonadotropins. The diagnosis must be established promptly and estrogen administration initiated as soon as possible. Estrogen is necessary to stimulate breast development, genital tract maturation, and the beginning of menstruation. Administration of a low dose of estrogen is used to initiate secondary sexual maturation. Estradiol-17β (Estrace), 0.5 mg/day or conjugated equine estrogens (Premarin), 0.3 mg/day is an appropriate starting dose. Once breast budding begins, the dos-

Table 35.2.
Causes of Delayed Puberty

Premature ovarian failure
  Turner syndrome
  Long-arm X chromosomal deletion
  Alkylating chemotherapy

Inadequate gonadotropin-releasing hormone secretion
  Olfactory tract hypoplasia (Kallmann syndrome)
  Constitutional delayed puberty
  Craniopharyngioma
  Hypothalamic hamartoma
  Marijuana use

Inadequate gonadotropin secretion
  Isolated gonadotropin deficiency
  Prolactin-secreting pituitary adenoma

Inadequate body fat
  Anorexia nervosa
  Exercise-induced hypothalamic dysfunction

Genital tract abnormalities
  Imperforate hymen
  Vaginal and uterine agenesis (Rokitansky-Küster-
    Hauser syndrome)

age may be doubled. The usual dose of estrogen to initiate menarche is estradiol-17β, 2 mg/day or conjugated equine estrogens, 1.25 mg/day. Once menarche occurs, medroxyprogesterone (Provera), 5 to 10 mg for 10 to 12 days every month will complete breast development and produce cyclic uterine bleeding. If an excessive amount of estrogen is administered initially, long bone growth will be truncated and adult height compromised. A delay in estrogen administration can lead to the development of osteoporosis beginning during the teen years.

Hypothalamic Dysfunction

The arcuate nucleus of the hypothalamus secretes gonadotropin-releasing hormone (GnRH) in cyclic bursts, which stimulates release of gonadotropins from the anterior pituitary gland. Dysfunction of the arcuate nucleus disrupts the short hormonal loop between the hypothalamus and pituitary, resulting in no pituitary gland secretion of FSH or LH. In consequence, the ovaries are not stimulated to secrete estradiol and secondary sexual maturation is delayed.

An unusual cause of hypothalamic dysfunction is *Kallmann syndrome.* In this disorder, the olfactory tracts are hypoplastic and the arcuate nucleus does not secrete GnRH. Young women with Kallmann syndrome have no sense of smell and fail to have breast development and secondary sexual hair growth. The diagnosis of this condition can be made on initial physical examination by challenging olfactory function with known odors. Patients with this disorder will fail to recognize common odors such as coffee or rubbing alcohol. The prognosis for successful secondary sexual maturation and reproduction is excellent in Kallmann syndrome. Secondary sexual maturation can be stimulated by the administration of exogenous hormones or by the administration of pulsatile GnRH. When pregnancy is desired, ovulation can be induced by exogenous gonadotropin administration or by administration of pulsatile GnRH. Once pregnancy is established, the lack of pituitary secretions has no adverse effects.

Less common causes of hypothalamic dysfunction are *neoplasms and inflammatory disorders of the hypothalamic-pituitary axis.* Examples are craniopharyngioma, hamartoma of the pituitary stalk, and sarcoidosis of the hypothalamus. More than 70% of cases will be associated with calcifications in the suprasellar region on plain skull x-ray. If a suprasellar neoplasm is strongly suspected, a magnetic resonance image of the hypothalamic-pituitary area is indicated.

Use of marijuana by prepubertal and intrapubertal boys and girls will delay the onset of puberty. Marijuana blocks the release of GnRH from the hypothalamus; thus marijuana truncates gonadotropin secretion by the pituitary gland, which in turn delays gonadal function. With the increasing incidence of drug abuse by adolescents, this must be considered in the differential diagnosis of hypogonadotropic-hypogonadism.

Body Weight

Body weight seems to be a critical element for establishing full secondary sexual maturation, including the capacity for reproduction. Girls who are *underweight* have delayed puberty. Moreover, girls who participate in *strenuous athletics* such as gymnastics, ballet, and competitive running may

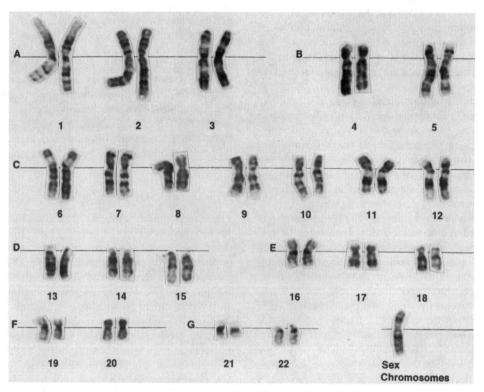

Figure 35.2. Karyotype of Turner syndrome: 45,X, one of the X chromosomes is missing. Approximately 50% of people with Turner syndrome have this 45,X karyotype; 15% have 46,X,i [Xq0]; 25% have 45,X/46,XX;46,XY;47,XXX; and 2 to 3% each have 46,X,Xp- and 46,X,r[X].

experience pubertal delay. Young female athletes who have pubertal delay will have the normal onset and sequence of secondary sexual maturation when they decrease their level of training. No residual harm results from this pubertal delay. Full reproductive function will be attained. However, there is risk of osteoporosis if ovarian estrogen secretion is delayed for many years.

Genital Tract Anomalies

During fetal life, müllerian ducts develop and fuse in the female fetus to form the upper reproductive tract, i.e., the fallopian tubes, uterus, and upper vagina. The lower and midportion of the vagina develop from the canalization of the genital plate. Approximately 1 in 10,000 females has a birth defect of the reproductive tract that presents as primary amenorrhea at the time of puberty. The simplest genital tract anomaly is *imperforate hymen.* In this condition, the genital plate canalization is incomplete and the hymen is, therefore, closed. In this simple defect, menarche occurs at the appropriate time, but because there is obstruction to the passage of menstrual blood, it is not apparent. This condition presents with pain in the area of the uterus and a bulging vaginal introitus. Hymenotomy is the definitive therapy.

In *müllerian agenesis (Rokitansky-Küster-Hauser syndrome),* the uterus is absent along with its cervical extremity and the vagina. All of the endocrine events of puberty occur at the proper time as the young woman establishes normal breast development, sexual hair growth, and ovulation. Yet, there is no menstruation. Physical examination leads to the diagnosis of müllerian agenesis. Renal anomalies (such as reduplication of the ureters, horseshoe kidney, or unilateral renal agenesis) occur in 25 to 35% of cases, and skeletal anomalies such as scoliosis occur in 15 to 25% of these women. Rokitansky-Küster-Hauser syndrome is generally sporadic in expression, although families displaying autosomal recessive inheritance are documented. If there is an affected child, the estimated risk of a second is about 4%; there is no way to determine whether the inheritance is familial or sporadic. There are several therapeutic approaches to this condition. An artificial vagina may be created by repetitive pressure to the perineum or by surgical construction followed by a split-thickness skin graft. After creation of a vagina, these women are able to enjoy sexual intercourse. With the advances in assisted reproductive technologies in-

cluding in vitro fertilization (IVF) and surrogacy, it is possible for women with this condition to have a genetic child.

Precocious Puberty

If physical signs of *secondary sexual development appear before the age of 8 years,* the physician should consider the diagnosis of precocious puberty. Precocious puberty occurs in girls more frequently than in boys. Most precocious puberty is isosexual, i.e., the sequence of pubertal events is appropriate for sexual development and leads to full sexual maturation. Idiopathic isosexual precocious puberty has no serious pathology. It causes only an advance in sexual maturation and carries the risk of short stature because of premature closure of the epiphyseal plates.

Occasionally, isosexual precocious puberty results from *tumors of the hypothalamic-pituitary stalk or transient inflammatory conditions of the hypothalamus.* In these situations, although sexual development begins early, the rate of sexual development is slower than the usual rate. In the case of inflammatory conditions, sexual development may begin and end abruptly. Laboratory studies show an appropriate rise in either gonadotropins or gonadotropins in the prepubertal range.

Precocious puberty may be the result of *inappropriate secretion of androgens or estrogens.* The most common cause of inappropriate hormone secretion is *congenital adrenal hyperplasia 21-hydroxylase type.* In this disorder, the adrenal glands are unable to produce adequate cortisol as a result of a partial block in the conversion of progesterone to desoxycorticosterone. Since this step is mediated by the enzymatic action of 21-hydroxylase, deficiency of the enzyme leads to an accumulation of adrenal androgens, which results in precocious adrenarche. In girls, there is premature development of pubic hair followed by axillary hair. Breast development either does not occur or is incomplete for the stage of sexual development. Measurement of adrenal androgens — such as dehydroepiandrosterone, dehyderoepiandrosterone sulfate, and androstenedione — leads to the diagnosis.

Medical therapy consists steroid replacement, a standard regimen being hydrocortisone (25 mg/m^2/day) in divided doses, with 9-α-fluorocortisone at a dosage of 15 to 75 mg twice a day for those with salt wasting. Therapy should be instituted as early as possible to achieve maximum benefit (Fig. 35.3). Surgical therapy is often also

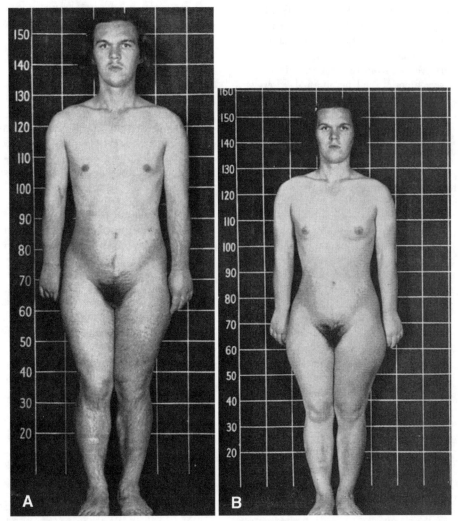

Figure 35.3. Medical treatment of congenital adrenal hyperplasia. **A,** Untreated 16-year-old with characteristic short stature, short arms and legs, absence of breast development, and growth of hair on body and face. **B,** Same patient after 3 months of cortisone therapy. Note alteration of body habitus to a more feminine configuration and reduction of hirsutism.

required, depending on the degree and nature of the effect, including removal of redundant erectile tissue, provision of an exteriorized vagina to allow for menstruation and sexual intercourse, and preservation of the sexually sensitive glans clitoris.

In males with this condition, there is premature enlargement of the phallus and the appearance of axillary and pubic hair. However, the testicles remain small because the source of androgens is of adrenal rather than of testicular origin. Again, adrenal hormones are elevated. Once the diagno-

sis is established, treatment should commence immediately. If not, short stature will result.

Rarely, there will be *inappropriate secretion of estrogens* in girls. This can result from ovarian neoplasms or from inappropriate secretion of chorionic gonadotropin by hepatic or gonadal neoplasms. In these conditions, there will be rapid breast development without sexual hair growth. Menarche may be established within a few months of thelarche. This deviation from the expected pattern of secondary sexual maturation suggests an abnormality.

Isosexual precocious puberty can be treated by the administration of an exogenous GnRH agonist. These agents block the periodic secretion of GnRH and suppress pituitary gonadotropin secretion. If precocious puberty is within a few months of the expected time of normal puberty, it is probably wise to allow puberty to progress. However, if puberty is advanced by several years, the process should be arrested. If the events of puberty do not progress in the expected way, an evaluation for hormonal abnormalities and/or hypothalamic-pituitary tumors is advised. If an abnormality is found, it should be treated specifically.

CASE STUDIES

Case 35A

A 15-year-old girl is brought by her mother for evaluation because she has never menstruated.

Questions Case 35A

Which of the following is the normal sequence in secondary sexual maturation?

A. Hair growth, growth spurt, thelarche, menarche
B. Growth spurt, hair growth, thelarche, menarche
C. Thelarche, hair growth, growth spurt, menarche
D. Thelarche, growth spurt, menarche, hair growth

Answer: C

Secondary sexual maturation should occur in an orderly sequence. Table 35.1 summarizes these events.

Which of the following laboratory studies would be indicated on *initial* evaluation on this patient?

A. Chromosomal karyotype
B. CT scan of the pituitary gland
C. FSH and LH
D. Progesterone

Answer: C

Although all the tests listed may be used as part of the evaluation in different situations, for the initial evaluation of the patient described, gonadotropin measurement is the most cost-effective.

Initial laboratory studies suggest premature ovarian failure. Which of the following would be the most useful diagnostic test for establishing this diagnosis?

A. Chromosomal karyotype
B. CT scan of the pituitary gland
C. Dehydroepiandrosterone, dehydroepiandrosterone sulfate
D. Progesterone

Answer: A

Premature ovarian failure is diagnosed by finding elevated (i.e., menopausal) gonadotropin levels. The most common etiology of this in prepubertal girls is Turner syndrome in which one X chromosome is absent. Chromosomal karyotype is, therefore, the most appropriate test.

Case 35B

A 16-year-old girl presents with primary amenorrhea. She has normal secondary sexual development including breast development, pubic and axillary hair growth, and adult height.

Questions Case 35B

The differential diagnosis would include all of the following *except:*

A. Müllerian agenesis
B. Pregnancy
C. Premature ovarian failure
D. Kallmann syndrome

Answer: D

Patients with Kallmann syndrome do not have spontaneous breast development or sexual hair growth and, therefore, would not fit this clinical presentation.

A physical examination reveals absence of the vagina. Based on this additional information, which management would you institute?

A. Creation of an artificial vagina
B. Administration of exogenous estrogen
C. Administration of pulsatile GnRH
D. Counseling to decrease strenuous physical activity

Answer: A

The patient described has müllerian agenesis (Rokitansky-Küster-Hauser syndrome). Because there is no uterus, the patient will never have menstrual periods. Once the vagina is developed, either by surgical construction or by a series of perineal pressure exercises, normal sexual activity can be anticipated.

chapter 36

AMENORRHEA AND DYSFUNCTIONAL UTERINE BLEEDING

Menstruation (cyclic uterine bleeding) is usually established by age 13 and continues until about age 45 to 50. Each menstrual cycle should follow ovulation. Once established at puberty, in most women menstrual cycles remain regular and predictable until menopause approaches.

Amenorrhea and dysfunctional uterine bleeding are the most common gynecologic disorders of reproductive age women. *Absence of menstruation is amenorrhea; irregular menstruation without anatomic lesions of the uterus is dysfunctional uterine bleeding.* Amenorrhea and dysfunctional uterine bleeding are discussed as separate topics in this chapter. However, the pathophysiology underlying amenorrhea and dysfunctional uterine bleeding may be the same.

AMENORRHEA

If a young woman has never menstruated, she is classified as having *primary amenorrhea*. If a woman has previously menstruated but has failed to menstruate within 6 months, she is classified as having *secondary amenorrhea*. The designation of primary or secondary amenorrhea has no bearing on the severity of the underlying disorder or on the prognosis for restoring cyclic ovulation. Terms often confused with these include *oligomenorrhea*, defined as a reduction of the frequency of menses, with the interval being >40 days but <6 months, and *hypomenorrhea*, defined as a reduction in the number of days or the amount of menstrual flow. Amenorrhea probably occurs in 5% or less of all women during their menstrual lives.

The physiology of ovulatory menstrual cycles is presented in Chapter 34. When there is disruption of hypothalamic-pituitary-ovarian endocrine function or alteration of the genital outflow tract (obstruction of the uterus, cervix, or vagina or

scarring of the endometrium) menstruation will cease. Causes of amenorrhea are divided into those arising from (*a*) pregnancy, (*b*) hypothalamic-pituitary dysfunction, (*c*) ovarian dysfunction, and (*d*) alteration of the genital outflow tract.

Pregnancy

Since the most common cause of amenorrhea is pregnancy, it is essential to exclude pregnancy in the evaluation of amenorrhea. Often, a history of breast fullness, weight gain, nausea, and a "feeling of being pregnant" suggests the diagnosis of pregnancy. The diagnosis can be confirmed by a pregnancy test. It is important to rule out pregnancy to allay the patient's anxiety and to avoid unnecessary testing. Also, some of the treatments for other causes of amenorrhea can be harmful to an ongoing pregnancy.

Hypothalamic-Pituitary Dysfunction

Release of hypothalamic gonadotropin-releasing hormone (GnRH) occurs in a pulsatile fashion. When this pulsatile secretion of GnRH is disrupted or altered, the anterior pituitary gland is not stimulated to secrete follicle-stimulating hormone (FSH) and luteinizing hormone (LH). The result is an absence of regular ovulation and menstruation.

GnRH release is modulated by catecholamine secretion from the central nervous system and by feedback of sex steroids from the ovaries. Alterations in catecholamine secretion and metabolism and in sex steroid hormone feedback disrupt ovulation and menstruation. In addition, alteration of blood flow from the hypothalamus to the pituitary gland through the hypothalamic-pituitary portal plexus can disrupt the signaling process that leads

Table 36.1.
Causes of Hypothalamic-Pituitary Amenorrhea

Functional causes	Psychogenic causes
Weight loss	Chronic anxiety
Excessive exercise	Pseudocyesis
Obesity	Anorexia nervosa
Drug-induced causes	Other causes
Marijuana	Head injury
Tranquilizers	Chronic medical illness
Neoplastic causes	
Prolactin-Secreting	
Pituitary Adenomas	
Craniopharyngioma	
Hypothalamic	
Hamartoma	

to ovulation. This alteration can be caused by tumors that alter blood flow.

The most common causes of hypothalamic-pituitary dysfunction are presented in Table 36.1. Most hypothalamic-pituitary amenorrhea is of functional origin and can be corrected by modifying causal behavior or by stimulating gonadotropin secretion.

In each of the disorders resulting in hypothalamic-pituitary amenorrhea, there is interference with the hypothalamic release of GnRH or interference with the pituitary secretion of FSH and LH. The physician cannot differentiate hypothalamic-pituitary causes of amenorrhea from ovarian or genital outflow causes by medical history or even physical examination alone. However, there are some clues in the medical history and physical examination that would suggest a hypothalamic-pituitary etiology for amenorrhea. A history of any condition listed in Table 36.1 should cause the physician to consider hypothalamic-pituitary dysfunction. Moreover, women with hypothalamic-pituitary dysfunction usually do not complain of hot flushes and sleep problems as do women who have ovarian failure.

The way to definitively identify hypothalamic-pituitary dysfunction is to measure FSH, LH, and prolactin in blood. In these conditions, FSH and LH are in the low range. Prolactin will be normal in most conditions but will be elevated in prolactin-secreting pituitary adenomas.

Ovarian Failure

In ovarian failure, the ovarian follicles are either exhausted or are resistant to stimulation by pituitary FSH and LH. As the ovaries fail, blood con-

centrations of FSH and LH increase. This is the basis for the chemical diagnosis of ovarian failure. Women with ovarian failure experience the symptoms and signs of estrogen deficiency that are listed in Table 36.2.

Women with estrogen deficiency caused by ovarian failure usually experience hot flushes, whereas those with estrogen deficiency caused by hypothalamic-pituitary dysfunction usually do not experience hot flushes. This is an important differential point in the medical history. A summary of causes is presented in Table 36.3. A detailed description of these causes is presented in Chapter 37.

Obstruction of the Genital Outflow Tract

Obstruction of the genital outflow tract will prevent menstrual bleeding even if ovulation occurs. Most cases of outflow obstruction result from congenital *abnormalities in the development and canalization of the müllerian ducts.* Imperforate hymen and absence of a uterus and/or vagina are the most common anomalies that result in primary amenorrhea. Even with attempted surgical correction, menstruation and fertility may not be restored.

Table 36.2.
Signs and Symptoms of Ovarian-associated Estrogen Deficiency

Symptoms	Signs
Hot flushes	Vaginal dryness
Mood changes	Thin vaginal epithelium
Sleep disturbances	Thinning of skin
Vaginal dryness	Hot flashes
Dyspareunia	

Table 36.3.
Causes of Ovarian Failure

Chromosomal causes of ovarian failure
 Turner syndrome (45,X gonadal dysgenesis)
 X chromosome long-arm deletion (46,XX q5)

Unknown causes
 Gonadotropin-resistant ovary syndrome (Savage syndrome)
 Premature natural menopause

Immunologic cause
 Autoimmune ovarian failure (Blizzard syndrome)

Iatrogenic cause
 Ovarian failure because of effects of alkylating chemotherapy

Scarring of the uterine cavity (Asherman syndrome) is the most frequent cause of secondary amenorrhea of anatomic origin. Women who undergo dilation and curettage (D&C) for retained products of pregnancy are at particular risk for developing scarring of the endometrium. Moreover, scarring may occur as the result of infection of the uterine cavity. Cases of mild scarring can be corrected by surgical lysis of the adhesions performed by D&C or hysteroscopy. However, severe cases are often refractory to therapy. Estrogen therapy should be added to the surgical treatment to stimulate endometrial regeneration to "cover" the uterine lesions.

Treatment of Amenorrhea

It is essential to first establish a cause for the amenorrhea. In hypothalamic amenorrhea, ovulation can usually be restored by changing behavior in women who have functional amenorrhea with potential restoration of ovulatory cycles. Women with central nervous system tumors should be considered on an individual basis for surgical therapy. Often, central nervous system tumors are benign and need not be removed. The *hyperprolactinemia associated with some pituitary adenomas* results in amenorrhea and galactorrhea. About 80% of all pituitary tumors secrete prolactin, causing galactorrhea, and these are treated with the dopamine agonist *bromocriptine (Parlodel)*. Ovulation can also be induced by the administration of gonadotropins (see Chapter 38). Women with genital tract obstruction require surgery to create a vagina or to restore genital tract integrity. In some, menstruation will never be established if the uterus is absent. Women with premature ovarian failure require exogenous estrogen replacement. Hormone replacement regimens are discussed in Chapter 37.

DYSFUNCTIONAL UTERINE BLEEDING

Failure to ovulate results in either amenorrhea or irregular uterine bleeding. *Irregular bleeding, unrelated to anatomic lesions of the uterus, is referred to as dysfunctional uterine bleeding.*

Patients with amenorrhea do not ovulate at all, and those with dysfunctional bleeding do so only periodically. However, although women with amenorrhea do not menstruate, women with dysfunctional uterine bleeding have irregular, often heavy, uterine bleeding. How can these two disparate conditions have the same cause? The answer relates to estrogen levels. *Women with amenorrhea and no genital tract obstruction are in a state of estrogen deficiency.* There is inadequate estrogen to stimulate growth and development of the endometrium. Therefore, there is inadequate endometrium for uterine bleeding to occur. In contrast, *women with dysfunctional uterine bleeding are in a state of chronic estrus.* They have constant, noncyclic blood estrogen concentrations that stimulate growth and development of the endometrium. Without the predictable effect of ovulation, there is an absence of progesterone-induced changes. Eventually, the endometrium outgrows its blood supply and sloughs from the uterus.

When there is chronic stimulation of the endometrium from low plasma concentrations of estrogens, the episodes of dysfunctional uterine bleeding will be infrequent and light. Alternatively, when there is chronic stimulation of the endometrium from increased plasma concentrations of estrogens, the episodes of dysfunctional uterine bleeding can be frequent and heavy. In this situation, the dysfunctional uterine bleeding can result in hemorrhage so heavy that it requires hospitalization for intense medical treatment or even minor surgical therapy (dilation of the cervix and curettage of the uterine cavity) if medical therapy is not successful.

Dysfunctional uterine bleeding is most likely to occur in association with polycystic ovarian disease, exogenous obesity, and adrenal hyperplasia.

Women who develop secondary amenorrhea may first experience a phase of dysfunctional uterine bleeding. This can occur becasue of weight loss, prolactin-secreting pituitary adenomas, premature ovarian failure, and other causes of amenorrhea. Since amenorrhea and dysfunctional uterine bleeding both result from anovulation, it is not surprising that they can occur at different times in the same patient.

Dysfunctional uterine bleeding can occasionally occur in association with ovulation. Although this may seem a contradiction, subtle alterations in the mechanisms of ovulation can produce abnormal cycles even when ovulation occurs, e.g., the luteal phase defect. In the *luteal phase defect*, ovulation does occur; however, the corpus luteum of the ovary is not fully developed to secrete adequate quantities of progesterone to support the endometrium for the usual 13 to 14 days and is not adequate to support a pregnancy if conception does occur. The menstrual cycle is shortened, and menstruation occurs earlier than expected. Although this is not classical dysfunctional uterine bleeding, it is considered to be in the same category.

Table 36.4.
Anatomical Causes of Irregular Bleeding

Uterine lesions	Cervicitis	Pessaries
Myomas	Cervical condyloma	
Polyps		Bleeding from other sites
Endometrial carcinoma	Vaginal lesions	Urethral caruncle
	Carcinoma, sarcoma, or adenosis	Infected urethral diverticulum
Cervical lesions	Laceration or trauma	Gastrointestinal bleeding
Neoplasia	Infections	Labial lesion
Polyps	Foreign bodies	(neoplasm, trauma, infection)
Cervical eversion	(diaphragm, tampons)	

Another example is midcycle spotting in which patients report bleeding at the time of ovulation. In the absence of demonstrable pathology, this self-limited bleeding can be attributed to the sudden drop in estrogen level at this time of the cycle.

Diagnosis of Dysfunctional Uterine Bleeding

Dysfunctional uterine bleeding should be suspected when menstrual cycles are not regular and predictable and when cycles are not associated with the premenstrual molimina associated with ovulatory cycles. These include breast fullness, abdominal bloating, mood changes, edema, weight gain, and menstrual cramps.

Before a diagnosis of dysfunctional uterine bleeding is made, anatomical causes of abnormal uterine bleeding must be excluded. These include uterine leiomyomata, inflammation/infection of the genital tract, carcinoma of the cervix or endometrium, cervical erosions, cervical polyps, and lesions of the vagina. Women with these organic causes for bleeding typically have regular, ovulatory cycles with superimposed irregular bleeding (Table 36.4).

If the diagnosis is uncertain from history and physical examination alone, a woman may keep a *basal body temperature chart* for 6 to 8 weeks to look for the shift in the basal temperature that occurs with ovulation. In the cases of anovulation and irregular bleeding, an *endometrial biopsy* may reveal endometrial hyperplasia. Since dysfunctional uterine bleeding results from chronic, unopposed estrogenic stimulation of the endometrium, the endometrium will appear proliferative or, with prolonged estrogenic stimulation, hyperplastic.

Treatment of Dysfunctional Uterine Bleeding

The risks to a woman with dysfunctional uterine bleeding are incapacitating blood loss and/or endometrial hyperplasia or carcinoma. Uterine bleeding can be severe enough to require hospitalization. Both hemorrhage and endometrial hyperplasia can be prevented by appropriate management.

The primary goal of treatment of dysfunctional uterine bleeding is to convert the proliferative endometrium into secretory endometrium, which results in predictable uterine withdrawal bleeding. This goal can be achieved by administration of a progestational agent for a minimum of 10 days, the most commonly used being medroxyprogesterone acetate (Provera) (Table 36.5). When the progestational agent is discontinued, uterine withdrawal bleeding will ensue, thereby mimicking physiologic withdrawal of progesterone.

As an alternative, administration of oral contraceptives will suppress the endometrium and establish regular, predictable withdrawal cycles. No particular oral contraceptive preparation is better than any of the others. Women who take oral contraceptives as treatment for dysfunctional uterine bleeding will often resume dysfunctional uterine bleeding after therapy is discontinued.

If a patient is being treated for a particularly heavy bleeding episode, once organic pathology has been ruled out, treatment should focus on two issues: (*a*) control of the acute episode and (*b*) prevention of future recurrences. Both high-dose estrogen and progestin therapy as well as combination treatment (oral contraceptive pills 4 per day) have been advocated for management of heavy dysfunctional bleeding in the acute phase. Long-term preventive management may include either intermittent progestin treatment or oral contraceptives.

CASE STUDIES

Case 36A

A 27-year-old woman complains of 6 months of amenorrhea.

Table 36.5.
Progestational Therapy for Anovulatory Uterine Bleeding

Drug	Dose
Norethindrone (Norlutin)	5–10 mg q.d. for the first 7–10 days of each month
Norethindrone acetate (Norlutate)	5–10 mg q.d. for the first 7–10 days of each month
Medroxyprogesterone acetate (Provera)	10–20 mg q.d. for the first 7–10 days of each month
Megestrol acetate (Megace)	40 mg q.d. for 3 months
Progesterone in oil (Lipolutin)	50–100 mg i.m. monthly
17-α-hydroxyprogesterone (Delalutin)	125 mg i.m. monthly

Questions Case 36A

All of the following could affect her menstrual cycles *except:*

A. Change in body weight
B. Marijuana use
C. Müllerian agenesis
D. Pregnancy

Answer: C

Patients with müllerian agenesis present with primary amenorrhea, not secondary amenorrhea as this patient does. In all patients of reproductive age, pregnancy should be ruled out as the first stage of evaluation.

If evaluation reveals elevated gonadotropins, which of the following statements are correct?

A. The patient may have a loss of chromosomal material on the long arm of the X chromosome
B. Her ovaries may be depleted of ovarian follicles
C. She may have numerous ovarian follicles that are resistant to FSH and LH
D. She may have hypothalamic dysfunction

Answer: A, B, C

A, B, and C are all clinical circumstances that can result in elevated gonodatropins. Each can be described as ovarian failure. The elevated gonadotropins are a result of the ovary not producing adequate amounts of hormones to feed back to the pituitary. Hypothalamus dysfunction would result in lower or normal gonadotropins.

If evaluation reveals low gonadotropins, which of the following statements are correct?

A. The patient has decreased hypothalamic release of gonadotropin-releasing hormone
B. Her ovaries are depleted of ovarian follicles
C. Ovulation can be induced by administration of exogenous FSH and LH

D. The examiner should inquire about changes in body weight, stress, and marijuana use

Answer: C, D

A low level of gonadotropins does not usually suggest decreased GnRH release, as any aberration in the normally delicate pulsatile release can result in loss of physiologic mechanisms. The importance of low gonadotropin levels is that it is not ovarian failure that has caused amenorrhea.

Case 36B

A 33-year-old woman gives a history of irregular menstrual cycles. She has basal body temperature records of 12 months duration that reveal ovulation occurring three times during that period.

Questions Case 36B

Which of the following statements are correct?

A. The patient has interruption of the cyclic interaction between gonadotropins and sex steroid hormones
B. The endometrium varies between a proliferative endometrium and a secretory endometrium every month
C. The patient is at high risk for endometrial hyperplasia
D. She does not need to use contraception to prevent pregnancy

Answer: A

This is a good example of intermittent ovulation resulting in dysfunctional bleeding. The patient's risk of endometrial hyperplasia is very low since the intermittent progestational effect of ovulatory cycles is protective. The endometium will become secretory only when ovulation has occurred, which in this patient was three times in 1 year. Contraception is still needed, as there is no way to predict when she will ovulate.

Further evaluation reveals tonic elevation of LH. Based on this additional data, which of the following statements are correct?

A. LH can be suppressed by administration of oral contraceptives
B. Ovulation can probably be induced by administration of clomiphene citrate
C. The patient may have elevated androgens
D. Obesity frequently coexists with dysfunctional uterine bleeding

Answer: All

This clinical picture is commonly seen in patients with oligoovulation and oligomenorrhea. If the patient wants to conceive, medical induction of ovulation can usually be accomplished. Otherwise, oral contraceptives are commonly used to regulate menstrual periods. Hyperandrogenism may be a contributory factor to the irregular ovulation (see Chapter 39). Obesity can also contribute, as peripheral fat stores convert androstenedione to estrone, thereby chemically increasing estrogen production and adversely affecting cyclic estrogen feedback.

chapter 37

MENOPAUSE

Ovarian function ceases by age 55 years in 95% of women, with the mean age being about 50 years. The cessation of menses is *menopause*. The *climacteric* is the period of waning ovarian function, i.e., the transition from the reproductive to the nonreproductive years. An increasing number of Americans are included in the latter group, because the female life expectancy has lengthened and the number of women in this age group is expanding (Fig. 37.1). If a woman reaches the age of 50 years today, she can expect to live another 30 to 35 years and will thus spend about one-third of her life after menopause. If for no other reasons than these, understanding the health issues of these women, including the evaluation and treatment of menopause, is important.

MENSTRUATION AND MENOPAUSE

Unlike the male who is able to renew gametes on a daily basis, the female has a fixed number of gametes for her reproductive life. In the fetus, approximately 8 million primordial oocytes migrate into the ovarian stroma at about 20 weeks of gestation. The process of follicular atresia begins before birth. At the time of birth, the female infant has approximately 1 to 2 million oocytes; by puberty, she has about 400,000 oocytes remaining. By age 30 to 35, the number of oocytes has decreased to about 100,000. For the remaining reproductive years, the process of oocyte maturation and ovulation becomes increasingly inefficient.

A woman will ovulate approximately 400 oocytes during her reproductive years. The process of *oocyte selection* is poorly understood. During the reproductive cycle, a cohort of oocytes is stimulated to begin maturation, but only 1 or 2 complete the process and are eventually ovulated.

It is unclear why one oocyte becomes atretic and degenerates while another oocyte achieves full maturation and ovulation.

Follicular maturation is induced and stimulated by the pituitary release of follicle-stimulating hormone (FSH) and luteinizing hormone (LH). FSH binds to its receptors in the follicular membrane of the oocyte and stimulates follicular maturation. LH stimulates the theca luteal cells surrounding the oocyte to produce androgens as well as estrogens and serves as the triggering mechanism to induce ovulation. With advancing reproductive age, the remaining oocytes become increasingly resistant to FSH. Thus plasma concentrations of FSH begin to increase several years in advance of actual menopause.

Menopause marks the end of a woman's reproductive life. The mean age of menopause throughout the world today is 50 years. Approximately 25% of women will experience menopause before age 45; 95% of women will be menopausal by age 55 years (Fig. 37.2). Menopause is a physiologic process. However, the consequences of ovarian failure can diminish a woman's quality of life and can predispose her to osteoporosis and an increased risk of cardiovascular disease.

The postmenopausal ovary is not quiescent. Under the stimulation of LH, theca cell islands in the ovarian stroma produce hormones, primarily the androgens androstenedione and testosterone. Testosterone appears to be the major product of the postmenopausal ovary. Testosterone concentrations decline after the menopause but remain two times higher in menopausal women with intact ovaries than in those whose ovaries have been removed or are premenopausal. Estrone is the predominant endogenous estrogen in postmenopausal women. The con-

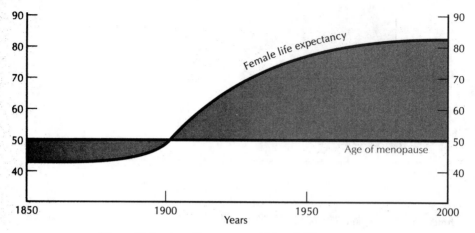

Figure 37.1. Age of menopause and female life expectancy.

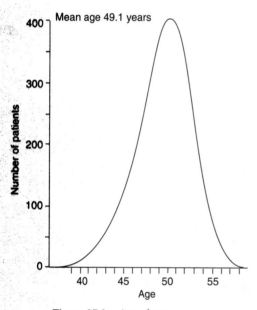

Figure 37.2. Age of menopause.

changes occur in the frequency and length of menstrual cycles. A woman may note shortening or lengthening of her cycles. The luteal phase of the cycle remains constant at 13 to 14 days, whereas the variation of cycle length is related to a change in the follicular phase. Women in their 20s and 30s will ovulate 13 to 14 times per year. Several years in advance of menopause, the frequency of ovulation decreases to 11 to 12 times per year and, with advancing reproductive age, will decrease to 3 to 4 times per year.

With the change in reproductive cycle length and frequency, there are concomitant changes in the plasma concentration of FSH and LH. More *FSH* is required to stimulate follicular maturation. Beginning in the late 30s and early 40s, the concentration of FSH begins to increase. This is the first chemical evidence of ovarian failure. The 5- to 10-year period before menopause is termed *perimenopause*. During the perimenopausal years, women begin to experience symptoms and signs of estrogen deficiency as reproductive function becomes increasingly inefficient. Relative changes in FSH as a function of stage of life is presented in Table 37.2.

Hot Flushes and Vasomotor Instability

Coincident with the change in reproductive cycle length and frequency, *the hot flush is the first physical manifestation of ovarian failure*. Occasional hot flushes begin several years before actual menopause. *The hot flush is the most common symptom of impending ovarian failure.* More than 95% of perimenopausal and menopausal women experience hot flushes.

centration is directly related to body weight, because androstenedione is converted to estrone in fatty tissue (Table 37.1).

SYMPTOMS AND SIGNS OF OVARIAN FAILURE

Menstrual Cycle Alterations

Soon after an adolescent woman has her first menstrual cycle, regular, predictable menstrual cycles are established that continue until about 40 years of age. Around 40 years, the number of ovarian follicles becomes substantially depleted and subtle

Table 37.1.
Steroid Hormone Serum Concentrations in Premenopausal Women, Postmenopausal Women, and Women Status Post Oophorectomy

Hormone	Premenopausal (Normal Ranges in Parentheses)	Postmenopausal	Postoophorectomy
Testosterone	325 (200–600)	230	110
Androstenedione	1500 (500–3000)	800–900	800–900
Estrone	30–200	25–30	30
Estradiol	35–500	10–15	15–20

Hot flushes have rapid onset and resolution. When a hot flush occurs, a woman experiences a sudden sensation of warmth. The skin of the face and the anterior chest wall become flushed for approximately 90 sec. With resolution of the hot flush, a woman feels cold and will break out into a "cold sweat." The entire phenomenon lasts less than 3 min. The hot flush is the result of declining estradiol-17β secretion by the ovarian follicles. As a woman approaches menopause, the frequency and intensity of hot flushes increase. Hot flushes may be disabling, producing *diaphoresis*, especially at night. When perimenopausal and postmenopausal women receive estrogen replacement, hot flushes usually resolve in 3 to 6 weeks. If a menopausal woman does not receive estrogen-replacement therapy, hot flushes will usually resolve spontaneously within 2 to 3 years.

Sleep Disturbances

Ovarian failure with consequent declining estradiol induces a change in a woman's sleep cycle so that restful sleep becomes difficult and for some, impossible. The latent phase of sleep, i.e., the time required to fall asleep, is lengthened; the actual period of sleep is shortened. Therefore, perimenopausal and postmenopausal women complain of having difficulty falling asleep and of waking up soon after going to sleep. This is one of the most disabling and least appreciated adverse effects of menopause. Women with marked sleep aberration are often tense and irritable and have difficulty with concentration and interpersonal relationships. The sleep cycle is restored to the premenopausal state by the administration of replacement estrogens.

Table 37.2.
Relative Changes in FSH as a Function of Life Stages

Life Stages	FSH (mIU/mL)
Childhood	<4
Prime reproductive years	6–10
Perimenopause	14–24
Menopause	>30

Vaginal Dryness and Genital Tract Atrophy

The vaginal mucosa, cervix, endocervix, endometrium, and myometrium are estrogen-dependent tissues. With decreasing estrogen production, these tissues become atrophic, resulting in various symptoms. The vaginal epithelium becomes thin and cervical secretions diminish. Women experience vaginal dryness while attempting or having sexual intercourse, leading to diminished sexual enjoyment. *Atrophic vaginitis* also may present with itching and burning related to sexual activity. The thinned epithelium is also more susceptible to becoming infected by local flora.

The endometrium also becomes atrophic, sometimes presenting with postmenopausal spottin. The paravaginal tissues that support the bladder and rectum become atrophic, resulting in possible bladder (cystocele) and rectal (rectocele) prolapse. In addition, uterine prolapse is more commom in the hypoestrogenic patient. Because of atrophy of the lining of the urinary tract, there may be symptoms of dysuria and urinary frequency. The *senile urethritis* often improves dramatically with estrogen-replacement therapy, leading to loss of the symptoms of urgency, frequency, and dysuria.

Loss of support to the urethrovesical junction may result in stress urinary incontinence.

Therapy with replacement estrogens restores the integrity of the vaginal epithelium, relieving symptoms of vaginal dryness and dyspareunia. Sexual pleasure is often restored. Estrogen-replacement therapy partially restores the integrity and support of the tissues surrounding the vagina. If a menopausal woman has symptomatic pelvic relaxation, estrogen-replacement therapy should be administered for several months before surgical correction is considered. In some cases, estrogen replacement plus pelvic muscle (Kegel) exercises will reverse the changes sufficiently to reestablish continence without surgery.

Mood Changes

Perimenopausal and postmenopausal women often complain of volatility of affect. Some women experience depression, apathy, and "crying spells." These may be caused directly by estrogen deficiency, by estrogen-deficiency associated sleep disturbance, or by both. Not only are these emotional symptoms disturbing to a woman but her inability to control these feelings is equally of concern. The physician should provide counseling and emotional support as well as medical therapy. The role of estrogens in central nervous system function is unknown. However, it is well established that sex steroid hormone receptors are protean in the central nervous system. Estrogen replacement in perimenopausal and postmenopausal women often diminishes these mood swings.

Skin, Hair, and Nail Changes

Estrogen influences *skin* thickness. With declining estrogen production, skin tends to become thin, less elastic, and eventually more susceptible to abrasion and trauma. Estrogen replacement helps restore the thickness and elasticity of skin.

Table 37.3.
Risk Factors for Osteoporosis

Reduced weight for height	Cigarette smoking
Family history of osteoporosis	Nulliparity
	High alcohol intake
Early menopause or oophorectomy	High caffeine intake
Low calcium intake	

Some women will notice *changes in their hair and nails* with the hormonal changes of menopause. Estrogen stimulates the production of sex hormone binding globulin, which binds androgens and estrogens. With declining estrogen production, there is less available sex hormone–binding globulin, which results in more free testosterone. This may result in *increased facial hair.* Moreover, changes in estrogen production affect the rate of hair shedding. Hair from the scalp is normally lost and replaced in an asynchronous way. With changes in estrogen production, hair is shed and replaced in a synchronous way, resulting in the appearance of increased scalp hair loss. This is a self-limiting condition and requires no therapy, but patients do require reassurance. *Nails become thin and brittle* with estrogen deprivation, but are restored to normal with estrogen replacement.

Osteoporosis

Bone demineralization is a natural consequence of aging. Diminishing bone density occurs in both men and women. However, the onset of bone demineralization occurs 15 to 20 years earlier in women than in men and is accelerated after ovarian function ceases. Bone demineralization not only occurs with natural menopause but has been reported in association with decreased estrogen production in certain groups of young women. Other factors contribute to the risk of osteoporosis (Table 37.3).

The role of estrogen in stimulating and maintaining *bone density* is unclear. Estrogen receptors have been demonstrated in osteoblasts. This finding suggests a permissive and perhaps even essential role for estrogen in bone formation. Bone density diminishes at the rate of approximately 1 to 2% per year in postmenopausal women compared with approximately 0.5% per year in perimenopausal women. Of all the therapies used for the prevention and treatment of osteoporosis, estrogen replacement seems to be most effective.

If a woman does not receive estrogen in the first 5 years following menopause, she will have a progressive, linear decrease in bone mineral mass. However, if estrogen replacement is initiated before or at the time of menopause, bone density is maintained at the premenopausal levels. Although it is somewhat controversial as to whether starting estrogen replacement in woman 5 or more years after menopause has an effect on bone density, it is generally recommended.

Table 37.4.
Signs and Symptoms Associated with Menopause in Women Not on Estrogen Replacement Therapy

Vulva and vagina	Dyspareunia (atrophic vaginitis) Blood: stained discharge (atrophic vaginitis) Pruritus vulvae	Cardiovascular system	Angina and coronary heart disease
		Skeleton	Fracture of hip or wrist Backache
Bladder and urethra	Frequency and/or urgency Stress incontinence	Breasts	Reduced size Softer consistency Reduced support
Uterus and pelvic floor	Uterovaginal prolapse	Emotional symptoms	Fatigue or diminished drive Irritability
Skin and mucous membranes	Dryness or pruritus Easily traumatized Loss of resilience and pliability Dry hair or loss of hair Minor hirsutism of face Dry mouth Voice changes: reduction in upper register		Apprehension Altered libido Insomnia Feelings of inadequacy or nonfulfillment Headache, tension
		Metabolic	Vasomotor symptoms: hot flashes Diaphoresis

Calcium supplementation is not a substitute for estrogen replacement. In several studies comparing estrogen with calcium, patients who received calcium alone had continued loss of bone mineral mass, whereas those who received estrogens had a stabilization of bone mineral mass. It is appropriate, however, to recommend 1000 to 1500 mg of daily calcium as a supplement for menopausal women.

Cardiovascular Lipid Changes

With approaching ovarian failure, changes occur in the cardiovascular lipid profile. Total cholesterol increases, high-density lipoprotein (HDL) cholesterol decreases, and low-density lipoprotein (LDL) cholesterol increases.

The administration of exogenous estrogens to perimenopausal and postmenopausal women promotes normalization of the cardiovascular lipid profile. Women who receive estrogen-replacement therapy have a lowered incidence of myocardial infarction and stroke than women who do not receive estrogen-replacement therapy (Table 37.4). Smoking markedly reduces the beneficial effect of estrogen-replacement therapy regardless of the cholesterol level (Table 37.5).

PREMATURE OVARIAN FAILURE

By definition, premature ovarian failure is menopause that occurs before age 42. Approximately 5% of women will experience premature menopause. The

Table 37.5.
The Effect of Smoking on the Beneficial Effect of Estrogen Replacement Therapy on Coronary Artery Disease via Cholesterol Levels

Smoking Status	Cholesterol (Percent Reduction)	
	<235	>235
Nonsmoker	65	90
Smoker	35	70

diagnosis should be suspected in a young woman with hot flashes and other symptoms of hypoestrogenism and secondary amenorrhea. The diagnosis is confirmed by the laboratory findings of menopausal FSH levels. Interestingly, hot flashes are not as common as might be expected in this group of patients. The diagnosis has profound emotional implications for most patients, especially if their desires for childbearing have not been fulfilled, as well as metabolic and constitutional implications. For some, premature ovarian failure may be the cause of infertility, and for others, the cause for the menopausal symptoms. There are many causes of premature loss of oocytes and premature menopause (Table 37.6), some of the more common of which are discussed below.

Genetic Factors

There are several factors that influence a woman's reproductive life span. Genetic information that

Table 37.6.
Causes of Premature Loss of Oocytes

Decreased number of germ cells
    Failure of germ cell migration
    Inherited reduction in germ cell number

Accelerated atresia
    Inherited tendencies
    Chromosomal abnormalities
        Gonadal dysgenesis
        With stigmata of Turner syndrome
        Pure (46,XX or 46,XY)
        Mixed disorder
        Trisomy X with or without chromosomal
          mosaicism
    Defects in gonadotropin secretion
        Secretion of biologically inactive forms
        Subunit α or β defects
    Congenital thymic aplasia
    Gonadotropin receptor and/or postreceptor defects
        (resistant ovary or Savage's syndrome)

Postnatal destruction of germ cells
    Physical causes
        Chemotherapeutic agents
        Viral agents
        Surgical extirpation
    Autoimmune disorders
        With associated endocrine disorders
        Isolated

determines the length of a woman's reproductive life is carried on the distal long arm of the X chromosome. Partial deletion of the long arm of one X chromosome results in premature ovarian failure. Total loss of the long arm of the X chromosome, as seen in Turner's syndrome, results in ovarian failure at birth or in early childhood. When suspected, these diagnoses can be established by careful mapping of the X chromosome.

Gonadotropin-resistant Ovary Syndrome (Savage Syndrome)

Some women with premature ovarian failure have an adequate number of ovarian follicles, yet these follicles are resistant to FSH and LH. A number of pregnancies have been reported in women with the gonadotropin-resistant ovary syndrome during the administration of exogenous estrogen. This fact suggests a role for estrogens in stimulating FSH receptors in the ovarian follicles.

Autoimmune Disorders

Some women develop autoantibodies against thyroid, adrenal, and ovarian endocrine tissues. These autoantibodies may cause ovarian failure. Some

women will respond to estrogen replacement therapy with subsequent resumption of ovulation.

Smoking

Women who smoke tobacco can undergo ovarian failure some 3 to 5 years earlier than the expected time of menopause. It is established that women who smoke metabolize estradiol primarily to 2-hydroxyestradiol. The 2-hydroxylated estrogens are termed *catecholestrogens* because of their structural similarity to catecholamines. The catecholestrogens act as antiestrogens and block estrogen action. The mechanism for premature ovarian failure in women smokers is unknown. However, the effects of smoking should be considered in smokers who are experiencing symptoms of estrogen deficiency.

Alkylating Cancer Chemotherapy

Alkylating cancer chemotherapeutic agents affect the membrane of ovarian follicles and hasten follicular atresia. One of the consequences of cancer chemotherapy in reproductive age women is loss of ovarian function. Young women being treated for malignant neoplasms should be counseled of this possibility.

Hysterectomy

Surgical removal of the uterus (hysterectomy) in reproductive-age women is associated with ovarian failure some 3 to 5 years earlier than the expected age. The mechanism for this occurrence is unknown. It is likely to be associated with alteration of ovarian blood flow resulting from the surgery.

Low Body Weight

Because adipocytes play a role in estrogen production and estrogen storage, slender women experience menopausal symptoms earlier than do women of normal body habitus and obese women. Moreover, slender women tend to be more difficult to normalize with exogenous estrogen replacement during the menopausal years. Women who are less than their ideal body weight at the time of menopause should be counseled regarding the clinical implications of their weight.

MANAGEMENT OF MENOPAUSE

All of the signs and symptoms of menopause result from declining estradiol-17β production by the ovarian follicles. *Exogenous estrogen administration* to the perimenopausal and postmenopausal woman will obviate most of these changes. In

Table 37.7.
Common Estrogren Preparations and Dose Equivalence of Estrogenic Components

Estrogen	Preparation	Dose Equivalency
Conjugated estrogen		
Premarin	Oral — 0.3, 0.625, 0.9, 1.25, and 2.5 mg	0.625
	Vaginal — 0.625 mg/g of cream	
Esterified Estrogen		
Estratab	Oral — 0.3, 0.625, 1.25, and 2.5 mg	
Estratest	Oral — 0.625 and 1.25 mg methyltestosterone	0.625
	1.25 and 2.5 mg methyltestosterone	
17β Estradiol		
Estraderm (transdermal patch)	0.05, 0.10	0.05
Micronized Estradiol		
Estrace	Oral 0.5, 1.0, and 2.0 mg	1.0
	Vaginal 0.1 mg/g	
Estropipate (piperazine estrone sulfate)		
Ogen, Ortho-est	Oral 0.3, 0.625, 1.25, 2.5, and 5.0 mg	0.75
Ogen	Vaginal 1.5 mg/g	

addition, estrone and estriol are metabolic by-products of estradiol-17β.

The *objective of estrogen-replacement therapy* should be to diminish the signs and symptoms of ovarian failure and restore estrogen homeostasis. There are several different estrogen preparations available through various routes of administration (Table 37.7). Conjugated estrogens (Premarin, Ogen) have been used as oral medication for decades as primary hormone preparations for estrogen replacement. Conjugated estrogens are unconjugated in the gastrointestinal tract and delivered to the target tissues as estrone. Conjugated estrogens are effective in diminishing the symptoms of estrogen deficiency, in maintaining bone mass, and restoring plasma lipids to more normal levels.

Estradiol-17β can be administered orally; however, it then is oxidized in the enterohepatic circulation to estrone. Estradiol-17β remains unaltered if it is administered transdermally, transbucally, transvaginally, intravenously, or intramuscularly. Unfortunately, intramuscular estradiol administration results in unpredictable fluctuations in plasma concentration. When estradiol is administered across the vaginal epithelium, absorption is poorly controlled and pharmacologic plasma concentrations of estradiol can result. The *transdermal administration* of estradiol results in steady, sustained estrogen blood levels and is the preferred alternative method (instead of oral dosing) of estrogen administration (Estraderm).

The administration of continuous *unopposed estrogens* can result in endometrial hyperplasia and possibly lead to endometrial adenocarcinoma. Therefore, it is essential to administer a progestin, most commonly medroxyprogesterone acetate (Provera), in conjunction with estrogens in women who have not undergone hysterectomy. To achieve this protective effect, the progestin chosen must be administered a minimum of 10 days each month (Table 37.8).

There are two principal *regimens for estrogen-replacement therapy*. Continuous estrogen replacement with cyclic progestin administration results in excellent resolution of symptoms and cyclic withdrawal bleeding from the endometrium. One of the difficulties of this method of therapy is that many postmenopausal women do not want to continue having menstrual cycles. As a result, many physicians and patients choose to avoid the problem of cyclic withdrawal bleeding by the daily administration of both an estrogen and a progestin.

There is a wide *variety of estrogen preparations available*. The following are comparable dosages: conjugated equine estrogens, 0.625 mg; estrone sulfate, 0.625 mg; estradiol-17β, 1 mg; and transdermal estradiol-17β, 50 μg. Most perimenopausal and menopausal women will respond to one of these preparations, all of which are adequate to prevent osteoporosis and to provide protection from cardiovascular disease. Most women will experience relief from hot flushes, vaginal dryness, sleep disturbances, and mood

Table 37.8.
Common Progestin Preparations and Dose Equivalence of Progestin Components

Progestin	Preparation	Dose Equivalency
Medroxyprogesterone		
Provera	Tablets in 2.5, 5.0, and 10.0	10.0
DepoProvera	Injectable, 100 and 400 mg/mL	
Norethindrone acetate		
Aygestin	Tablet, 5 mg	5.0
Norlutate	Tablet, 5 mg	

changes. The administration of 5 to 10 mg of *medroxyprogesterone acetate* (Provera) given for 10 to 12 days each month will convert the proliferative endometrium into a secretory endometrium, bring about endometrial sloughing, and prevent endometrial hyperplasia or cellular atypia. If continuous progestin therapy is used to produce endometrial atrophy, 2.5 mg of medroxyprogesterone acetate per day is used.

An annual pelvic examination with Pap smear and mammogram (after age 50) is advisable for all women who are taking hormone-replacement therapy.

CAUTIONS IN ESTROGEN REPLACEMENT

Patients with unexplained abnormal vaginal bleeding should not receive estrogen-replacement therapy until the cause of the bleeding is ascertained and treated appropriately. In addition, patients with active liver disease or chronically impaired liver function should generally not receive estrogen replacement.

Carcinoma of the Breast

Carcinoma of the breast has been a contraindication to estrogen replacement. In light of the benefits of estrogen replacement therapy in regard to osteoporosis and cardiovascular disease, selected patients may not be considered inappropriate for estrogen replacement therapy. It may be reasonable to administer estrogen replacement to women who have documented estrogen-receptor–negative breast tumors and negative axillary lymph nodes. Any such patients should be several years removed from their original diagnosis and treatment to minimize risks. As this is still controversial, extreme *caution must be exercised when making the decision to administer estrogen to women with a history of breast cancer.*

Thromboembolic Disease

Oral estrogens stimulate the production of clotting factors, but estradiol administered by the transdermal route has no effect on clotting. Therefore, women with a history of thromboembolic disease can safely receive transdermal estradiol therapy.

Endometrial Carcinoma

There is little evidence to suggest that estrogens should be withheld from women with a history of carcinoma of the endometrium if the tumor was limited to the endometrium and myometrium. Women with metastatic endometrial carcinoma should not receive exogenous estrogens.

CASE STUDIES

Case 37A

A 46-year-old woman complains of increasing irritability, hot flushes, and an increasingly irregular menstrual cycle over the last 12 months. Her mother died of breast cancer. She had three uncomplicated pregnancies and has been well, with no other problems other than varicose veins.

Questions Case 37A

Which of the following signs and symptoms would be expected?

A. Sleep disturbance
B. Dry skin
C. Loss of hair
D. Vaginal irritation after coitus
E. Oily skin

Answer:　A, B, C, D

The loss of estrogen can result in many physiologic changes. Of those listed, only oily skin is not caused by estrogen deprivation.

Which of the following findings would be expected?

A. Increased FSH
B. Decreased FSH
C. Increased LH
D. Decreased LH
E. Increased bone density

F. Decreased bone density
G. Increased total cholesterol
H. Decreased total cholesterol

Answer: A, C, G

If this patient is experiencing early menopause, FSH and LH will be elevated and total cholesterol may be increased. Untreated, bone density will decline over several years, but the findings now would most likely be normal.

Which are appropriate therapeutic steps?

A. Oral progestin
B. Oral estrogen
C. Oral calcium
D. Oral tranquilizers
E. Parenteral progesterone
F. Parenteral estrogen
G. Parenteral calcium
H. Parenteral tranquilizers

Answer: A, B, C

Oral estrogen replacement is appropriate for treatment of menopausal symptoms. Progestin therapy is indicated in addition to estrogen whenever the patient still has a uterus. Calcium supplementation is also a good idea as additional therapy to prevent osteoporosis. Parenteral preparations of any of these drugs are rarely needed. Tranquilizers are not routinely indicated, as estrogen-replacement therapy usually successfully treats the mood changes. Because of the first-degree relative with breast carcinoma, yearly breast examination by a physician and yearly screening mammography are indicated.

Case 37B

A 27-year-old woman presents with a history of amenorrhea and hot flushes for the last 6 months. Laboratory studies reveal elevated FSH and LH.

Questions Case 37B

The differential diagnosis would include all of the following *except:*

A. Gonadotropin-resistant ovary syndrome
B. 46,XX q-ovarian dysgenesis
C. Idiopathic ovarian failure
D. Pituitary prolactinoma

Answer: D

A pituitary prolactinoma would present with amenorrhea, but the gonadotropins would not be elevated as seen in this case. An elevated prolactin level would be expected if a prolactinoma were present.

Which of the following is not a potential therapy for this patient?

A. Estrogen and progestin replacement
B. Securing a donor oocyte
C. Biopsy of the ovaries
D. Maintaining ideal body weight

Answer: D

The vasomotor symptoms of premature ovarian failure should respond to estrogen replacement. Progestin is a part of the therapeutic regimen to prevent endometrial hyperplasia. The use of donor oocytes could be used if assisted reproductive technology were to be tried in the future. Biopsy of the ovary may be considered if ovarian dysgenesis is a possibility. Body weight is often associated with anovulation and amenorrhea but is not a factor in premature ovarian failure.

chapter 38

EVALUATION OF THE INFERTILE COUPLE

Infertility affects 15% of reproductive age couples in the United States. During the 20-year period from 1970 to 1990, the incidence of infertility appeared to increase; however, the incidence now appears stable. *Infertility is defined as a couple's failure to conceive following 1 year of unprotected sexual intercourse.* This definition is emphasized in the cumulative monthly pregnancy rates for couples engaging in unprotected coitus (Fig. 38.1). The reasons for increased incidence of infertility may be related in part to changes in lifestyle, e.g., such as maintaining low body weight, marijuana, deferred childbearing, and increased sexual contacts with an associated increased incidence of pelvic inflammatory diseases.

Reproductive age is synonymous with a woman's reproductive years (*generally defined as ages 15 to 44 years*, although menarche and pregnancy before age 15 is not uncommon and pregnancy after 44 is no longer rare). Since this 15- to 44-year-old cohort is the healthiest segment of the population, it is surprising that 15% of this group experiences reproductive dysfunction. With such a high incidence in an otherwise healthy population, one must look for causes of infertility resulting from environment and lifestyle. During the 20-year period when the incidence of infertility was rising, there was a corresponding increase in the knowledge of reproductive physiology and in the diagnosis and treatment of infertility. Formerly, there was little hope for the infertile couple; today, 85% of couples can expect to have a child with appropriate diagnosis and treatment for "infertility."

The inability to conceive a child or carry a pregnancy places a great emotional burden on infertile couples. The quest to have a child becomes the driving force in the infertile couple's life. Friends, family, and often occupation can be subordinated to this medical problem. Unlike dysfunction of other organ systems, dysfunction of the reproductive system does not directly produce physical or mental abnormalities. Yet, the mental anguish of infertility is nearly as incapacitating as the pain or life restrictions of other diseases. *The emotional needs of infertile couples must be recognized and fully addressed.*

CAUSES OF INFERTILITY

Infertility can be reduced to *three generic causes* that account for 95% of reproductive dysfunction. These causes are *(a) anovulation, (b) anatomical defects of the female genital tract, and (c) abnormal spermatogenesis.* The frequency of these causes is presented in Figure 38.2. Each of these categories can be investigated by a simple diagnostic procedure that gives a high probability of establishing a cause. In the initial investigation of the infertile couple, it is important for the physician to establish, as rapidly as possible, the major cause(s) of the infertility.

The *initial evaluation of the infertile couple* should include the following studies:

1. Basal body temperature recording of the female partner — evaluation of ovulation;
2. Hysterosalpingogram — evaluation of reproductive tract;
3. Semen analysis — evaluation of spermatogenesis.

The *basal body temperature* recording is an excellent screening test for ovulation. The characteristic biphasic temperature shift occurs in more than 90% of ovulating women (an example is shown in Fig. 38.3). Note the rise in temperature that coincides with ovulation. At 13 to 14 days after ovulation, the basal temperature drops and menstruation begins within 24 to 36 hr. A temperature elevation of longer than 16 days suggests pregnancy. Alternatively, a serum progesterone can be drawn during the luteal phase to document ovulation.

Analysis of a semen specimen obtained by masturbation provides immediate information about the quantity and quality of seminal fluid, the density of the sperm, the morphology of sperm, and the motility of sperm. The male partner is instructed to abstain from coitus for 2 to 3 days before the test, because coitus during this time interval lowers the sperm count in some cases. It is important to collect all the ejaculate, as the first part contains the greatest density of sperm. The analysis should be performed no more than 2 hr after the specimen is collected, preferably sooner, thus collection of the specimen at the site of analysis is preferable. A normal semen specimen should contain a con-

centration of <u>motile sperm</u> of <u>>20 million/mL</u> with at least 60% motile sperm (Table 38.1). A normal semen analysis excludes a male cause for infertility in more than 90% of couples. The causes of abnormal semen analyses are presented in Table 38.2.

The *hysterosalpingogram,* an x-ray study of the internal female genital tract, provides important information about the tract's architecture and integrity. A radiopaque dye is injected through the cervix into the uterine cavity and fallopian tubes

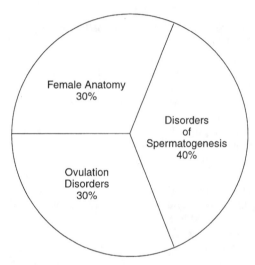

Figure 38.2. Pie graph presenting the distribution of common causes of infertilty.

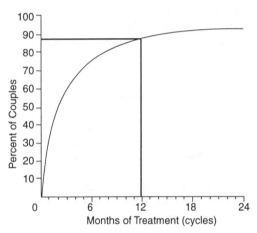

Figure 38.1. Conception rates for fertile couples.

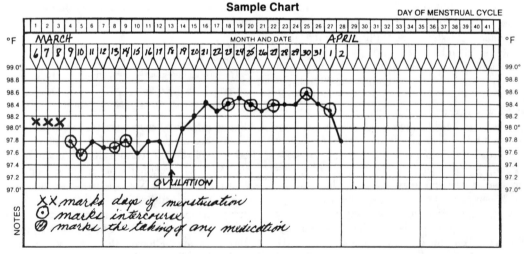

Figure 38.3. A basal body temperature record in an infertile woman receiving clomiphene citrate. Note the biphasic temperature shift on day 15. A temperature that remains elevated for more than 16 days may indicate pregnancy.

and then into the peritoneal cavity, assuming that the tubes are patent. The internal architecture of these structures is then outlined on x-ray. The hysterosalpingogram has a diagnostic accuracy of approximately 70% for detecting anatomic abnormalities of the genital tract. A diagnostic laparoscopy is another method of evaluating the genital tract but is complementary to the hysterosalpingogram (Table 38.3). The pelvic cavity, including visualization of the "external surfaces" of the uterus, ovaries, fallopian tubes, and support structures, is evaluated.

Anovulation

A healthy woman between age 18 and 36 ovulates 13 to 14 times per year. The typical menstrual cycle is 28 days long, with ovulation occurring on the 14th day. Menstruation begins on the 28th day and lasts approximately 5 days. *The ovulatory menstrual cycle* is divided into the follicular phase and the luteal phase. During the *follicular phase* of the menstrual cycle, estradiol-17 β is the predominant hormone. Its actions on its target tissues result in increased turgor of the ductal elements of the

Table 38.1.
Criteria that Define Normal Semen Analysis

Sperm count per milliliter	
Normal fertile	>20,000,000
Subfertile	between 5,000,000 and 20,000,000
Infertile	<5,000,000
Volume	≥2.5 mL
Viscosity	Full liquefaction within 60 min
Motility	60% motile within 4 hr of collection; higher motility suggests higher fertility
Differential	<25% abnormal forms

Table 38.2.
Causes of Abnormal Semen Analysis

Abnormal sperm count	
No sperm (azoospermia)	Klinefelter's syndrome or other genetic disorders
	Sertoli cell only syndrome
	Semniferous tuble or Leydig cell failure
	Hypogonadotrophic hypogonadism
	Ductal obstruction
	Varicocele
	Exogenous factors, including heat
Few sperm (oligospermia)	Genetic disorder
	Endocrinopathies, including androgen receptor defects
	Varicocele and other anatomic disorders
	Maturation arrest
	Hypospermatogenesis
	Exogenous factors (heat, etc.)
Abnormal sperm morphology	Varicocele
	Stress
	Infection (mumps)
Abnormal motility	Immunologic factors, male-female incompatibility
	Infection
	Defect in sperm structure or metabolism
	Poor liquefaction of semen
	Varicocele
Abnormal volume	
No ejaculate	Ductal obstruction
	Retrograde ejaculation
	Ejaculatory failure
	Hypogonadism
Low volume	Obstruction of ejaculatory ducts
	Absence of seminal vesicles and vas deferens
	Partial retrograde ejaculation
	Infection

Table 38.3.
Tests in the Infertility Workup

Possible Cause	Test	Comments
Anovulation	Basal body temperature	Patient must do each morning
	Endometrial biopsy	Office procedure in late luteal phase
	Serum progesterone	Blood test
	Urinary ovulation-detection kit	Home use at midcycle
Anatomic disorder	Hysterosalpingogram	X-ray in proliferative phase
	Diagnostic laparoscopy	View external surfaces of pelvic organs
	Hysteroscopy	Visualize endometrial cavity
Abnormal spermatogenesis	Semen analysis	Normal value 20 millon/mL, 2 mL volume, 60% motility
	Postcoital test	Midcycle timing
Immunologic disorder	Antisperm antibodies	Male and female tested

breasts; increased production of clear, watery endocervical mucus; and proliferation of the endometrium. The *luteal phase* of the menstrual cycle is dominated by the secretion of progesterone by the corpus luteum. Progesterone acts on the acinar elements of the breasts to produce rounding of the lateral quadrants and on the endocervix to convert the thin, clear endocervical mucus into a sticky mucoid material. Progesterone also converts the endometrium to a secretory pattern, which accepts the embryo for implantation and supports subsequent fetal growth and development.

Progesterone shifts the thermoregulatory center and increases the set point of the basal body temperature. Following ovulation, the basal body temperature increases by approximately 0.6°F and remains elevated until menstruation begins. With involution of the corpus luteum, progesterone production abruptly decreases and the basal body temperature shifts downward; menstruation ensues soon after.

The menstrual history helps the physician ascertain if a woman ovulates regularly. A history of regular menstrual periods strongly suggests regular ovulation. Characteristically, *following ovulation* and preceding menstruation, an ovulating woman will experience some fullness and heaviness of the breasts, decreased vaginal secretions, abdominal bloating, mild peripheral edema with slight increase in body weight, and occasional episodes of depression. In a minority of patients, the physical and emotional changes may be debilitating, the so-called *premenstrual syndrome*. These changes do not occur in anovulatory women. Therefore, *a history of these cyclic*

changes may be interpreted as presumptive evidence of ovulation.

Diagnostic studies to confirm ovulation, in addition to recording the basal body temperature, include the endometrial biopsy, measurement of serum progesterone and the urinary ovulation-detection kit. The *endometrium* undergoes specific histologic changes on an almost daily basis following ovulation. These changes can be detected from an endometrial biopsy. This is a useful procedure for evaluating certain causes of infertility, but it is expensive and provides only static information. *Progesterone* increases in plasma following ovulation and can be measured to confirm that ovulation has occurred. However, a single measurement provides little information that cannot be obtained by a well-kept basal body temperature chart. Ovulation detection kits are available that measure changes in urinary LH. As the LH surge begins, more LH will be excreted in the urine, which can be measured by qualitative detection kits. This is useful in helping to predict ovulation, but it does not confirm ovulation. Ovulation-detection kits should not be used routinely, but can be useful when ovulation prediction is needed, such as in the timing of artificial insemination.

Symptoms such as irregular unpredictable menstrual cycles and episodes of *amenorrhea* as well as signs of hirsutism, acne, galactorrhea, and increased or decreased vaginal secretions *suggest anovulation*. A woman with irregular menstrual cycles can be presumed to be anovulatory. In this case, maintaining a basal body temperature record is not necessary.

Given a history of irregular menstrual cycles the physician should look for signs of abnormal androgen, prolactin, and gonadotropin secretion. A woman who is anovulatory should have some or all of the following tests drawn, depending on individualized evaluation of the case: follicle-stimulating hormone (FSH), luteinizing hormone (LH), prolactin, androstenedione, total testosterone, and dehydroepiandrosterone sulfate (DHEAS). If thyroid dysfunction is suspected, thyroxin (T_4) and thyroid-stimulating hormone (TSH) should be measured as well. The results of these hormonal studies will help the physician understand the etiology of the chronic anovulation. Once the etiology of anovulation is established, a treatment regimen designed to induce ovulation can be developed for the patient. Any agent that will set in cyclical motion the secretion of gonadotropins or estradiol will stimulate ovulation.

Anatomic Disorders of the Female Genital Tract

Sperm Transport, Fertilization, and Implantation

The female genital tract facilitates the migration of sperm from the posterior vaginal fornix toward the unfertilized egg. *Cervical mucus* secreted by the endocervix traps the coagulated ejaculate, where the sperm are stored and capacitated for immediate or later migration into the endometrial cavity and fallopian tubes.

At the time of ovulation, the oocyte is either picked up directly by the fimbriated extremity of the fallopian tube or retrieved from the pelvic cul-de-sac. The oocyte is then transported to the proximal portion of the fallopian tube, where fertilization occurs. The fertilized oocyte cleaves and forms a zygote and then an embryo. At 3 to 5 days following fertilization, the embryo enters the *endometrial cavity*, where it implants into the secretory endometrium for subsequent growth and development. The cells of the cervix, endometrium, and endosalpinx respond to progesterone secretion from the ovarian follicle. *The internal anatomic genital tract serves as more than a simple conduit for sperm and eggs. Indeed, these are dynamic structures that are essential for normal transportation, fertilization, and implantation.*

Disorders

The most *common disorders* of the female genital tract are acquired during the early reproductive years. The most common cause of fallopian tube disease is *acute salpingitis.* Organisms that infect the fallopian tubes include *Neisseria gonorrhoeae* and *Chlamydia trachomatis.* These organisms alter the functional integrity of the fallopian tubes and can lead to fallopian tube obstruction.

Hysterosalpingography

Less common congenital anatomical abnormalities of the female genital tract can range from a simple septum of the upper uterine cavity to a complete reduplication of the genital tract with a double vagina, double cervix, and double uterus. Endometriosis, scarring and adhesions from pelvic inflammation or surgery, tumors of the uterus (e.g., leiomyoma) and ovary, and (rarely) sequelae of trauma may also distort the reproductive tract anatomy.

The hysterosalpingogram is an essential diagnostic tool for evaluation of the internal genital structures. The hysterosalpingogram should be performed between the 7th and 11th day of the menstrual cycle. If it were performed during menses, the risk of iatrogenic retrograde menstruation would be increased. If performed later, it could interfere with the possible ovum transport, fertilization, or implantation.

There are several important characteristics of the normal hysterosalpingogram (Fig. 38.4). The endometrial cavity should be smooth and symmetrical. Indentations and irregularities of the endometrial cavity suggest uterine leiomyomata or chronic scarring of the endometrium from previous surgery. The proximal two-thirds of the fallopian tubes should be slender, approximating the diameter of a pencil lead. The distal one-third of the fallopian tubes is the ampulla and should appear dilated compared with the proximal two-thirds. The fimbrial folds should appear as linear radiolucencies along the longitudinal axis of the tube. Examples of hysterosalpingograms, demonstrating two common abnormalities, are shown in Figure 38.5.

During the radiographic study, dye should *spill* promptly from the fallopian tubes into the peritoneal cavity. In a pelvis free of adhesions, dye will intersperse between loops of bowel, producing characteristic radiographic crescents throughout the pelvis. Moreover, dye should spill freely into the cul-de-sac and dispense throughout the pelvis. Failure to observe these late changes in the hysterosalpingogram suggests the possibility of peritubal adhesions or endometriosis, which restrict normal fallopian tube mobility.

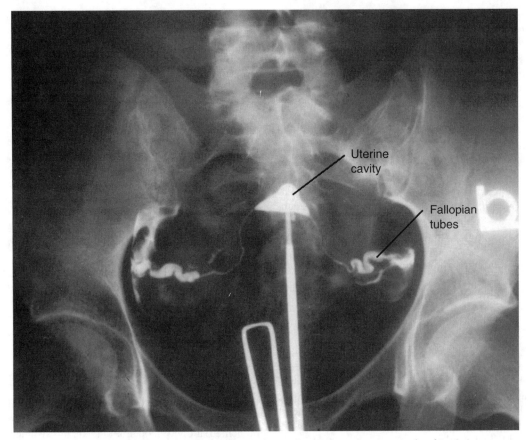

Figure 38.4. A hysterosalpingogram showing normal genital tract anatomy and architecture.

A hysterosalpingogram that shows an abnormality of the fallopian tubes should be followed with a *diagnostic laparoscopy. The hysterosalpingogram provides information about the surfaces of the genital tract organs, whereas diagnostic laparoscopy provides information about the external surfaces of these organs.* In addition, hysteroscopy can provide direct visualization of the endometrial cavity as well as access to possible correction of lesions found.

Abnormalities of Spermatogenesis

Problems of spermatogenesis account for *>40% of cases of infertility.* Unlike oocytes, which are ovulated periodically, sperm are being constantly produced by the germinal epithelium of the testicles. As sperm mature within the germinal epithelium, they are released into the epididymis where maturation occurs before ejaculation.

The *sperm generation time* is approximately 73 days. Thus an abnormal sperm count is a reflection of events that occurred 73 days before the collection of a semen specimen. Alternatively, a minimum of 73 days is required to observe the change in sperm production following therapy for oligospermia.

Sperm production is thermoregulated. Intratesticular temperature is regulated by contraction and relaxation of the scrotum. Sperm production occurs at a temperature of approximately 1°F less than body temperature. External thermal shock to the testicles can result in reduced sperm production. Examples include spending time in a hot tub, sitting on the testicles for long periods of time with poor heat dispersion, and wearing tight clothing that pulls the testicles against the body for extended periods of time. In many cases, one of these causes can be discovered from a carefully obtained history or from observation.

As the follicle of the ovary responds to FSH and LH, the Leydig cells and germinal epithelium

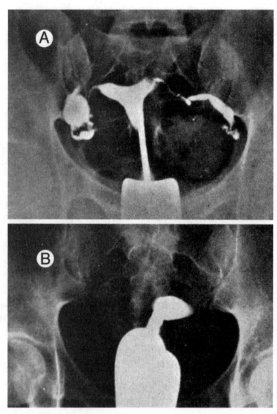

Figure 38.5. Abnormal hysterosalpingograms. **A,** Bilateral hydrosalpinx obstructing the fallopian tubes at the fimbriated ends. Arcuate uterus. **B,** Bilateral tubal occlusion at the cornu; uterus overdistended with radiopaque medium.

of the testicles also respond to gonadotropic stimulation. In some males, the germinal epithelium becomes fibrotic and sperm production is diminished. In others, testosterone production by Leydig cells is decreased. Men with oligospermia should have gonadotropin hormones measured to exclude testicular failure. Suspected testicular failure should be confirmed by testicular biopsy.

The man who has *poor sperm production* as a result of hormonal abnormalities does not respond well to induction of spermatogenesis. Some men with marginal testicular failure or poor gonadotropic production will respond to the administration of clomiphene citrate. This is appropriate therapy for a limited time.

Another method besides sperm analysis to evaluate sperm density and sperm motility is the *postcoital test (Sims-Huhner test)*. The test should be timed to take place during the late follicular phase of the menstrual cycle just before ovulation. At this time of the cycle, cervical mucus is abundant and facilitates sperm survival and transport. The couple should have intercourse approximately 8 hr before the test is scheduled. The female partner undergoes a speculum examination to expose the cervix. With a tuberculin syringe, a small sample of endocervical mucus is aspirated from the endocervical canal. This is placed on a glass side and examined under a microscope. Normally, 8 to 10 motile sperm are seen per high-powered field in the cervical mucus. This simple test provides important information about coitus, ejaculation, sperm pickup, sperm motility, and sperm storage within the endocervical canal. Preferably, this test is done with both partners in attendance. The male then has the opportunity to better understand his partner's reproductive system and both can view the cervical mucus under the microscope.

Recently, *immunologic causes of infertility* have received attention. Both men and women can produce *antisperm antibodies*. If the woman produces antisperm antibodies, sperm will be immobilized in the cervical mucus. If the male produces antisperm antibodies (3 to 20% of "infertile" men), sperm will agglutinate and will be unable to penetrate the cervical mucus. The diagnosis of antisperm antibodies is made by performing immunologic studies on both partners. If antisperm antibodies exist in the woman, timed intrauterine insemination of washed sperm into the endometrial cavity may produce a pregnancy. There is no known effective treatment for men with antisperm antibodies, although attempts at therapy include washing and concentration of sperm with either intracervical or intrauterine insemination and high-dose steroid therapy.

For some couples, there will be no biological explanation for their infertility. Physicians must look for men and women with low body weight, individuals or couples who use marijuana, or something else in their lifestyle that may compromise reproduction. These "normal" infertile couples may comprise up to 10% of those seeking treatment for infertility.

Table 38.3 summarizes the tests that may be included in the infertility work-up.

TREATMENT OF THE INFERTILE COUPLE

Anovulation

If *anovulation* is the cause of infertility, therapy should be directed to *restore ovulation by the administration of ovulation-inducing agents*. The most frequently used therapy is *clomiphene citrate*. Clomiphene citrate is an antiestrogen, which combines with and blocks estrogen receptors at the hypothalamic and pituitary level, thus inducing, by a negative-feedback effect, an increase in FSH release from the pituitary. FSH in turn is one of the major signals stimulating the development of follicles. Before therapy, the patient should be taking basal body temperature measurements, which are used to monitor therapy. Progesterone (50 to 100 mg) is given intramuscularly, and clomiphene is begun on the 5th day of menses. Depending on the hormonal milieu of the patient, 50 to 100 mg are given from day 5 to day 9. If the patient ovulates, it will occur approximately 14 days after the first day of clomiphene administration. In the absence of ovulation, the schedule of medication

may be altered by increasing the daily dosage of clomiphene, increasing the duration of administration, or administering hCG timed to substitute for the absent LH surge. This is commonly given as 5000 IU of hCG at the time of optimum cervical mucus. The maximum dosage of clomiphene is usually 150 mg/day.

If a woman fails to respond to clomiphene citrate, *follicle-stimulating hormone* can be administered directly to stimulate follicular growth. A purified preparation of gonadotropins from the urine of postmenopausal women (Pergonal [menotropins]) is usually used. Pergonal contains about 75 or 150 IU of both FSH and LH per dose and must be given parenterally, as it is inactivated if given orally. If exogenous follicle-stimulating hormone is administered, monitoring requires frequent measurement of estradiol-17 β and frequent ultrasound imaging of the ovarian follicles. The therapy is expensive and includes significant risk of three complications: hyperstimulation of the ovaries, multiple gestation, and fetal wastage.

Anatomic Abnormalities

In the event an anatomic abnormality of the genital tract is discovered, a *surgical treatment* is usually recommended. Lysis of pelvic adhesions will result in freeing of entrapped internal genital structures. In case of fallopian tube obstruction, the obstruction can be corrected surgically. However, for these operations to be successful, the endosalpinx must be healthy. If the endosalpinx has been altered such that ovum pickup and transport cannot occur, one of the assisted reproductive technologies — primarily in vitro fertilization — must be considered as an option. Correction of abnormalities of the endometrial cavity can also be accomplished, often at the time of hysteroscopic diagnosis.

Inadequate Spermatogenesis

Problems of spermatogenesis should be addressed by trying to eliminate alterations of thermoregulation. Attempts at induction of spermatogenesis can be made by the administration of clomiphene citrate. However, the response to this therapy is usually less than 20%.

If spermatogenesis cannot be improved, couples may choose to use *artificial insemination using donor sperm* (AID); several techniques are in common use (Fig. 38.6). Couples may also choose one of the

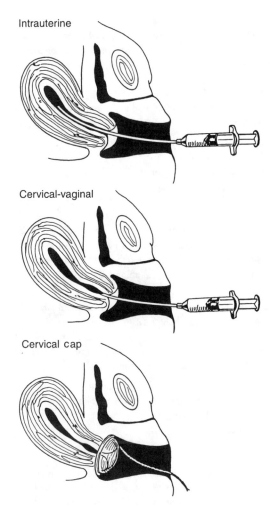

Intrauterine

Cervical-vaginal

Cervical cap

Figure 38.6. Techniques of artificial insemination.

assisted reproductive technologies such as gamete intrafallopian tube transfer (GIFT) or in vitro fertilization (IVF) to facilitate fertilization using the infertile partner's sperm.

Assisted Reproductive Technologies

An explosion of assisted reproductive technologies has occurred in the last decade. These include in vitro fertilization, gamete intrafallopian tube transfer, and zygote intrafallopian tube transfer (ZIFT). These technologies provide infertility specialists with tools to bypass the normal mechanisms of gamete transportation and fertilization. However, IVF, GIFT, and ZIFT are expensive and place infertile couples on an emotional roller coaster. The expected successful

outcome from IVF in properly selected couples is approximately 18 to 22% per cycle. The expected successful outcome for properly selected couples for GIFT and ZIFT is approximately 22 to 28% per cycle. Strict indications for the use of these procedures must be maintained to prevent misuse and exploitation of couples. The probability of pregnancy in a healthy couple is approximately 18 to 20% per cycle. Assisted reproductive technologies do not enhance the possibility of pregnancy in couples who do not have appropriate indications for their use and they should be used only in carefully selected cases.

With the array of imaging techniques, pharmacologic agents, and surgical procedures available to the physician, there are many treatment options for infertile couples. Thus the physician can be optimistic in counseling infertile couples about the prognosis for having a child. At the same time, while offering encouragement, the physician must be aware of the psychological impact that infertility has on both partners and their family. Appropriate therapy must include psychological support.

CASE STUDIES

Case 38A

A couple in their late 20s presents for evaluation of infertility. The woman is nulligravid and has regular menses. The husband has never fathered a child. They have had unprotected sexual intercourse for 18 months. Neither has a history of sexually transmitted disease or major illness. The male reports no difficulty with erection or ejaculation.

Questions Case 38A

Which of the following is the most likely cause of their infertility?

A. An ovulation disorder
B. An abnormality of spermatogenesis
C. An anatomic disorder of the female's reproductive tract
D. Immunologic disorder

Answer: B

Problems with spermatogenesis are found in about 40% of couples with infertility, whereas abnormalities of ovulation and anatomical disorders of the female reproductive tract each account for about 30% of infertility cases. An ovulation disorder is unlikely, given her regular menstrual history. There is no reason to expect an anatomic abnormality, but this will need to be evaluated along with the possibility of infertility of immunologic etiology.

Which of the following diagnostic studies would not be indicated as part of this couple's *initial* evaluation?

A. Basal body temperature record
B. Semen analysis
C. Hysterosalpingogram
D. Diagnostic laparoscopy

Answer: D

Basal body temperature records are an excellent method of confirmation of ovulation, and semen analysis, of confirmation of spermatogenesis. Hysterosalpingography should be a part of initial infertility evaluations to rule out possible endometrial or tubal pathology. Diagnostic laparoscopy is used to evaluate the external surfaces of the female reproductive tract but requires a hospital surgical procedure. It should, therefore, be reserved until other initial tests are completed. Hysteroscopy may also be used for detailed evaluation of the intrauterine cavity and is commonly performed in conjunction with laparoscopy.

The female partner is found to have anovulation, despite her history of regular menses. The next step in the evaluation is to:

A. Induce ovulation with clomiphene citrate
B. Perform artificial insemination
C. Induce ovulation with exogenous gonadotropins
D. Perform diagnostic laparoscopy to rule out other causes of infertility

Answer: A

Initial treatment with clomiphene citrate will often be sufficient to induce ovulation. Occasionally, other agents such as Pergonal and hCG may be necessary. If ovulation does not occur, evaluation as to the etiology is indicated. Artificial insemination is not yet indicated, since it does not address the identified dysfunction. Laparoscopy would also be premature at this point.

Case 38B

A 37-year-old woman with a history of gonococcal salpingitis presents with her husband and expresses a complaint of infertility.

Questions Case 38B

Which of the following studies is indicated on initial evaluation?

A. Basal body temperature record
B. Semen analysis
C. Hysterosalpingogram
D. Endometrial biopsy

Answer: A, B, C

Without evidence of anovulation, the endometrial biopsy is not indicated, whereas evaluation of the male (semen analysis) is routine and the hysterosalpingogram is performed to rule out fallopian tube obstruction.

The hysterosalpingogram reveals bilateral tubal obstruction. A consultant advises against corrective surgery because of the very poor prognosis for successful outcome from reconstructive pelvic surgery. Which of the following should be recommended?

A. Gamete intrafallopian tube transfer
B. Homologous intrauterine insemination
C. In vitro fertilization
D. Adoption

Answer: C

Because of the tubal obstruction, transfer of a gamete to the fallopian tube would not be appropriate. Similarly, intrauterine insemination would not overcome the anatomic block. IVF, if economically feasible for the couple, could provide a solution to the problem by bypassing the blocked fallopian tube. By obtaining the woman's eggs and fertilizing them with the man's sperm, then placing them into the prepared uterus, the couple has the opportunity of having a child that is genetically theirs. Adoption is always an option in cases when the couple is unable to conceive.

chapter 39

HIRSUTISM AND VIRILIZATION

A woman who complains of being too hairy or too masculine presents a diagnostic and therapeutic challenge for the physician. Hirsutism and virilization may be clinical clues to an underlying *androgen excess disorder*. The physician should consider the sites of androgen production and the mechanisms of androgen action when evaluating and treating hirsutism and virilization. *The most common cause of hirsutism is polycystic ovarian disease, the second most common cause is adrenal hyperplasia.* These conditions must be established by laboratory diagnosis. *Treatment of androgen excess should be directed at suppressing the source of androgen excess or blocking androgen action at the receptor site.*

Androgens play three essential roles in female reproductive function: (*a*) they are precursors for estrogen biosynthesis, (*b*) they stimulate and maintain sexual hair growth, and (*c*) they drive the female libido. However, exposure to excess androgens, through either excess production or increased action, results in increased body hair and acne.

Hirsutism is defined as excess body hair. It is manifested initially by the appearance of midline *terminal hair*. Terminal hair is darker, coarser, somewhat kinkier than vellus hair, which is soft, downy, and fine. When a woman is exposed to excess androgens, terminal hair will first appear on the lower abdomen and around the nipples, next around the chin and upper lip, and finally between the breasts and on the lower back. Usually a woman with hirsutism will also have *acne*. In Western cultures, terminal hair on the abdomen, breasts, and face is considered unsightly and presents a cosmetic problem for women. At the first sign of hirsutism, women often consult their physician to seek a cause for the excess hair growth and seek treatment to eliminate it.

Virilization is defined as masculinization of a woman. It is associated with marked increase in circulating *testosterone*. As a woman becomes virilized, she first notices enlargement of the clitoris followed by temporal balding, deepening of the voice, involution of the breasts, and a remodeling of the limb-shoulder girdle. Over time, she takes on a more masculine appearance, as shown in Figure 39.1.

ANDROGEN PRODUCTION AND ANDROGEN ACTION

In women, *androgens are produced in the adrenal glands, the ovaries, and adipose tissue* where there is extraglandular production of testosterone from androstenedione. The following three androgens may be measured in evaluating a woman with hirsutism and virilization.

1. *Dehydroepiandrosterone* (DHEA): a weak carbon-5 androgen secreted principally by the *adrenal glands*.
2. *Androstenedione* (A): a weak carbon-4 androgen secreted in equal amounts by the *adrenal glands and ovaries*.
3. *Testosterone* (T): a potent carbon-4 androgen secreted by the *adrenal glands and ovaries* and produced in *adipose tissue* from the conversion of androstenedione.

The sites of androgen production and proportions produced are presented in Table 39.1.

In addition, testosterone is also converted within the hair follicle and within genital skin to *dihydrotestosterone* (DHT), which is an androgen even more potent than testosterone. This metabolic conversion is the result of the local action of 5α-reductase on testosterone at these sites. This is the basis for constitutional hirsutism, which is discussed later.

Adrenal androgen production is regulated by pituitary secretion of adrenocorticotropic hormone (ACTH). ACTH stimulates the adrenal cortical production of cortisol. In the metabolic sequence of cortisol production, DHEA is one precursor hormone. In enzymatic deficiencies of adrenal steroidogenesis (21-hydroxylase deficiency and 11β-

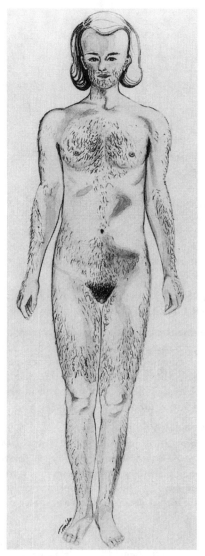

Table 39.1.
Sites of Androgen Production

Site	DHEA (Percent)	Andro-stenedione (Percent)	Testosterone (Percent)
Adrenal glands	90	50	25
Ovaries	10	50	25
Extraglandular	0	0	50

Figure 39.1. A woman with virilization. Note the clitoral enlargement, temporal balding, masculine body habitus, and hirsutism.

trogen production by granulosa cells of the ovarian follicles. In conditions of sustained or increased LH secretion, androstenedione and testosterone increase. The metabolic relationship between androgens and estrogens is shown in Figure 39.3.

Extraglandular testosterone production occurs in adipocytes (fat cells) and depends on the magnitude of adrenal and ovarian androstenedione production. When androstenedione production increases, there is a dependent increase in extraglandular testosterone production. When a woman becomes obese, the conversion of androstenedione to testosterone in adipocytes increases.

Testosterone is the primary androgen that causes increased hair growth, acne, and the physical changes associated with virilization. After testosterone is secreted from its site of production, it is bound to a carrier protein — *sex-hormone-binding globulin* (SHBG) — and circulates in plasma as a bound steroid hormone. Only a small fraction (1 to 3%) of testosterone is unbound (free). Bound testosterone is unable to attach to testosterone receptors and is, therefore, metabolically inactive. It is the small fraction of free hormone that exerts the effects. SHBG is produced by the liver. Estrogens stimulate hepatic production of SHBG. Greater estrogen production is associated with less free testosterone, whereas decreased estrogen production is associated with increased free testosterone. Therefore, measurement of total testosterone alone may not reflect the fraction of free testosterone.

Testosterone receptors are scattered throughout the body. For the purpose of this discussion, testosterone receptors will be considered only in hair follicles, sebaceous glands, and genital skin. Free testosterone enters the cytosol of testosterone-dependent cells. There it is bound to a testosterone receptor and carried into the nucleus of the cell to initiate its metabolic action. *When testosterone is excessive,* there is increased hair growth, acne, increased libido, and rugation of the genital skin.

hydroxylase deficiency), DHEA accumulates and is further metabolized to androstenedione and testosterone. The flow of adrenal hormone production is shown in Figure 39.2.

Ovarian androgen production is largely under the control of luteinizing hormone (LH) secretion from the pituitary gland. LH stimulates theca-lutein cells surrounding the ovarian follicles to secrete androstenedione and, to a lesser extent, testosterone. These androgens are precursors for es-

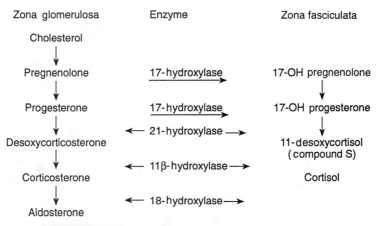

Figure 39.2. A schematic flow chart of adrenal steroidogenesis.

Moreover, some individuals have increased 5α-reductase within hair follicles, resulting in excessive production of DHT.

CONDITIONS CAUSED BY OVARIAN ANDROGEN EXCESS

Polycystic Ovarian Disease

Polycystic ovarian disease (PCOD) is the *most common cause of androgen excess and hirsutism.* The etiology of this disorder is unknown. Some cases appear to result from a genetic predisposition, whereas others seem to result from obesity or other causes of luteinizing hormone (LH) excess. One proposed mechanism for PCOD is shown in Figure 39.4.

The symptoms of polycystic ovarian disease include *oligomenorrhea, amenorrhea, anovulation, acne, hirsutism, and infertility.* The disorder is characterized by chronic anovulation or extended periods of anovulation.

PCOD is related to obesity by the following mechanism. LH stimulates the theca-lutein cells to increase androstenedione production. Androstenedione undergoes aromatization to estrone within adipocytes. Although estrone is a weak estrogen, it has a positive feedback action or stimulating effect on the pituitary secretion of LH. LH secretion is, therefore, stimulated by increased estrogen. With increasing obesity, there is increased conversion of androstenedione to estrone. In many women with PCOD, obesity seems to be the common factor, and the acquisition of body fat coincides with the onset of PCOD. With the increased rise in androstenedione, there is coinci-

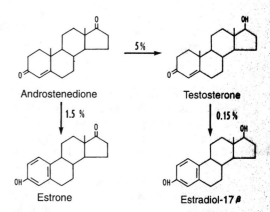

Figure 39.3. The metabolic interrelationships between androgens and estrogens. The percentages indicate the extent of metabolism in adipocytes.

dent increased testosterone production, which causes acne and hirsutism.

PCOD is a functional disorder whose treatment should be targeted to interrupt the disorder's positive feedback cycle. Hormonal studies in women with PCOD show the following: (*a*) increased LH:FSH ratio, (*b*) estrone in greater concentration than estradiol, (*c*) androstenedione at the upper limits of normal or increased, and (*d*) testosterone at the upper limits of normal or slightly increased.

The most common therapy for PCOD is the *administration of oral contraceptives,* which will suppress pituitary LH production. Oral contraceptives have several beneficial effects. By suppressing LH, there is decreased production of androstenedione and testosterone. The ovarian contribution to the total androgen pool is thereby decreased.

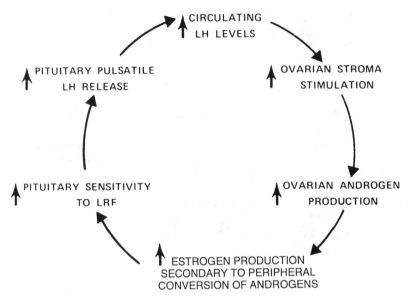

Figure 39.4.   A mechanism for polycystic ovarian disease proposed by Yen. *LRF*, luteinizing-releasing factor.

Acne clears, new hair growth is prevented, and there is decreased androgenic stimulation of existing hair follicles. By preventing estrogen excess, oral contraceptives also prevent endometrial hyperplasia. In addition, the women will have cyclic predictable withdrawal bleeding episodes.

If a woman with PCOD wishes to conceive, oral contraceptive therapy is not a suitable choice. If the patient is obese, a *weight reduction* diet designed to restore the patient to a normal weight should be instituted. With body weight reduction alone, many women resume regular ovulatory cycles and conceive spontaneously. With weight reduction, there is decreased aromatization, which interrupts PCOD at the level of the adipocyte. In some women who desire pregnancy, ovulation induction with clomiphene citrate is needed. Ovulation induction is facilitated by weight reduction in obese women.

Women undergoing ovulation induction may be given Provera, 10 mg/day for 10 days before beginning ovulation induction. Provera suppresses endogenous LH and induces a withdrawal cycle. Clomiphene citrate, 50 mg/day from cycle days 5 to 9 is administered to stimulate follicle-stimulating hormone (FSH) secretion. If ovulation does not occur with this dosage of clomiphene citrate, the dosage is increased the next cycle to 100 mg/day from days 5 to 9. The dosage of clomiphene citrate should not exceed 150 mg/day.

In some women, *a variation of PCOD occurs* in which *the patient also has insulin-resistant diabetes mellitus*. A common physical sign of this condition is acanthosis nigricans in the skin folds. *Acanthosis nigricans* is characterized by thickening of the skin on the back of the neck, under the breasts, and in the intertriginous areas of the thighs. This is found most often in obese patients, and with weight loss, the skin changes resolve spontaneously.

Hyperthecosis

Hyperthecosis is a *more severe form of polycystic ovarian disease.* In cases of hyperthecosis, *androstenedione* production may be so great that testosterone reaches concentrations such that early signs of *virilization* appear. Women with this condition may exhibit some temporal balding, clitoral enlargement, deepening of the voice, and remodeling at the limb-shoulder girdle. Hyperthecosis is refractory to oral contraceptive suppression. It is also more difficult to successfully induce ovulation in women with this condition.

Sertoli-Leydig Cell Tumors

Sertoli-Leydig cell tumors (also called androblastoma and arrhenoblastoma) are ovarian neoplasms that secrete testosterone. These tumors constitute less than 0.4% of ovarian tumors and usually occur in women between the ages of 20 and 40. The tumor is most often unilateral and may reach a size of 7 to 10 cm in diameter.

Women with a Sertoli-Leydig cell tumor will have a rapid onset of *acne, hirsutism* (three-fourths of patients), *amenorrhea* (one-third of patients), and *virilization.* In the short span of 6 months, a woman may cease having ovulatory menses and exhibit extensive body hair, temporal hair recession, clitoral enlargement, and deepening of the voice. A characteristic clinical course of two overlapping stages is described: first, the stage of *defeminization,* characterized by amenorrhea, breast atrophy, and loss of the subcutaneous fatty deposits responsible for the rounding of the feminine figure; second, the stage of *masculinization,* characterized by clitorial hypertrophy, hirsutism, and deepening of the voice.

Laboratory studies of this disorder show suppression of FSH and LH, a low plasma androstenedione, and a marked elevation of testosterone. An *ovarian mass* is usually palpable on pelvic examination and confirmed by sonography. Once the diagnosis is suspected, there should be no delay in *surgical removal* of the involved ovary. The contralateral ovary should be inspected, and if it is found to be enlarged should be bisected for gross inspection.

Following surgical removal of a Sertoli-Leydig cell tumor, ovulatory cycles return spontaneously and further progression of hirsutism is arrested. If the clitoris has become enlarged, it will not revert to its pretreatment size. However, temporal hair is restored, and the body habitus will become feminine once again. The 10-year survival rates for this low-grade malignant ovarian tumor approximate 90 to 95%. For recurrent metastatic tumors, combination chemotherapy has been recommended, but the experience is insufficient to provide meaningful outcome information.

Uncommon Virilizing and Masculinizing Ovarian Tumors

Gynandroblastoma is a very rare ovarian tumor, having both granulosa cell and arrhenoblastoma components. The predominant clinical feature is masculinization, although estrogen production may simultaneously produce endometrial hyperplasia and irregular uterine bleeding. Treatment is surgical as in Sertoli-Leydig cell tumors.

Lipid (Lipoid) cell tumors are usually small ovarian tumors, containing sheets of round, clear pale-staining cells with a differential histologic diagnosis of hilus cell tumors, stromal luteoma or pregnancy, and Sertoli-Leydig cell tumors. The clinical presentation is *masculinization or defeminization* associated with elevated 17-ketosteroids in many cases. Treatment is surgical as in Sertoli-Leydig cell tumors.

Hilus cell tumors arise from an overgrowth of mature hilar cells or from ovarian mesenchyme. They are characterized clinically by masculinization which supports the idea that hilar cells are the homologs of the interstitial or Leydig cells of the testis. Histologically, the tumors contain pathognomonic Reinke albuminoid crystals in most cases (Fig. 39.5), and grossly, they are always small, unilateral, and benign. Treatment is surgical removal.

ADRENAL ANDROGEN EXCESS DISORDERS

Congenital Adrenal Hyperplasia

In the sequence of adrenal steroidogenesis, *dehydroepiandrosterone (DHEA)* is a key hormone. DHEA is a precursor for androstenedione and testosterone. The most common cause of increased adrenal androgen production is adrenal hyperplasia as a result of *21-hydroxylase deficiency.* 21-hydroxylase catalyzes the conversion of progesterone and 17α-hydroxyprogesterone to desoxycorticosterone and compound S. When 21-hydroxylase is deficient, there is an accumulation of progesterone and 17α-hydroxyprogesterone, which are metabolized subsequently to dehydroepiandrosterone. This disorder affects approximately 2% of the population and is caused by an alteration in the gene for 21-hydroxylase, which is carried on chromosome 6. The genetic defect is autosomal recessive and has variable penetrance.

In the most severe form of 21-hydroxylase deficiency, the newly born female infant is virilized. However, milder forms are more common and can appear at puberty or even later in adult life. A mild deficiency of 21-hydroxylase is frequently associated with terminal body hair, acne, subtle alterations in menstrual cycles, and infertility. *When 21-hydroxylase deficiency is manifested at puberty,* adrenarche may precede thelarche. The history of pubic hair growth occurring before the onset of breast development may be a clinical clue to this disorder. The *diagnosis of 21-hydroxylase deficiency* is made by measuring *increased dehydroepiandrosterone sulfate (DS) and androstenedione* in plasma.

↑ DHEAS + ANDROSTENEDIONE

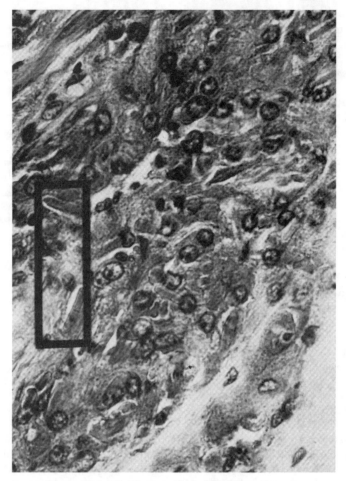

Figure 39.5. Reinke crystalloid of the hilus cell tumor.

The diagnosis of *late-onset adrenal hyperplasia* is suspected in a woman with hirsutism, acne, and menstrual irregularities. This diagnosis is established by measuring plasma concentrations of DS, androstenedione, and testosterone. In this condition, it is not unusual to find an increased plasma DS, increased androstenedione, and normal or slightly increased testosterone. When this hormone pattern is reported, the physician should follow up with an *ACTH stimulation test*.

A less common cause of adrenal hyperplasia is *11β-hydroxylase deficiency*. 11β-hydroxylase catalyzes the conversion of desoxycorticosterone to cortisol. A deficiency in this enzyme also results in increased androgen production. The clinical features of 11β-hydroxylase deficiency are mild hypertension and mild hirsutism. The *diagnosis* of 11β-hydroxylase deficiency is made by demonstrating increased plasma desoxycorticosterone.

Treatment of Adrenal Hyperplasia

In adrenal hyperplasia, the adrenal glands require increased ACTH secretion to stimulate adequate cortisol production. To maintain normal cortisol production, the adrenal glands oversecrete androgens.

This condition can be managed easily by *supplementing glucocorticoids*. Usually, prednisone, 2.5 mg daily, will suppress adrenal androgen production to within the normal range. When this therapy is instituted, facial acne usually clears promptly, ovulation is restored, and there is no new terminal hair growth.

Medical therapy for adrenal and ovarian disorders cannot resolve hirsutism; it can only suppress new hair growth. Hair that is present must be controlled by shaving, by use of depilatory agents, or by electrolysis.

Adrenal Neoplasms

An adrenal adenoma is a rare cause of hirsutism. In androgen-secreting adrenal adenomas, there is a rapid increase in hair growth associated with severe acne, amenorrhea, and sometimes virilization. In androgen-secreting adenomas, DS is usually elevated above 6 μg/mL. The diagnosis is established by computed axial tomography or magnetic resonance imaging of the adrenal glands, which shows the adrenal adenoma. Adrenal adenomas must be removed surgically.

CONSTITUTIONAL HIRSUTISM

Occasionally after a diagnostic evaluation for hirsutism, there will be no explanation for the cause of the disorder. By exclusion, this condition is often called *constitutional hirsutism*. Data support the hypothesis that women with constitutional hirsutism have *greater activity of 5α-reductase* than do unaffected women. These women ovulate regularly and have normal hormone concentrations. Women with constitutional hirsutism may respond to treatment with *spironolactone,* a mild diuretic designed to limit aldosterone production. This drug *binds androgen receptors,* thus blocking androgenic activity. A dosage of 50 to 100 mg/day will suffice for the treatment of constitutional hirsutism.

IATROGENIC ANDROGEN EXCESS

Danazol

Danazol is an *attenuated androgen designed for the suppression of pelvic endometriosis.* It has androgenic properties, and some women will develop hirsutism, acne, and deepening of the voice while taking the drug. If these symptoms develop, the value of the danazol should be weighed against the side effects before continuing therapy. Pregnancy should be ruled out before initiating a course of danazol therapy, as it can produce virilization of the female fetus.

Oral Contraceptives

The progestins in oral contraceptives are impeded androgens. Rarely, a woman taking oral contraceptives will develop acne and even hirsutism. If this occurs, another product with a less andro-

genic progestin should be selected or the Pill should be discontinued. Moreover, evaluation for the coincidental development of late-onset adrenal hyperplasia should be done.

CASE STUDIES

Case 39A

A 19-year-old unmarried woman presents with a complaint of being "too hairy." Her history includes severe irregular menstrual cycles, worsening acne; and hair growth on the face, breasts, and lower abdomen. She is on no medication, is sexually active, uses condoms for contraception, and otherwise feels well. She is depressed about the new hair growth.

Questions Case 39A

The most likely cause for this group of symptoms is

A. Congenital adrenal hyperplasia
B. Sertoli-Leydig cell tumor of the ovary
C. Polycystic ovarian disease
D. Constitutional hirsutism

Answer: C

PCOD is the most common cause of this patient's complaints. Although she was focused on the increase hair growth, further history revealed androgen excess in general, with symptoms comparable with PCOD. Which of the following laboratory studies should be performed?

A. DHEA
B. Progesterone
C. Androstenedione
D. Testosterone

Answer: A, C, D

LH stimulates androstenedione production, which is aromatized in the fat cells to estrone, which stimulates pituitary LH production: a positive feedback loop. Very high testosterone levels may suggest the need for a Gyn ultrasound examination of the ovaries, because such levels are associated with Sertoli-Leydig cell tumors. DHEA is the "key hormone" in adrenal hyperplasia. Progesterone levels are not helpful in the workup of hirsuitism.

A diagnosis of polycystic ovarian disease is made. An initial treatment plan should include

A. Clomiphene citrate
B. Oral contraceptives
C. Prednisone
D. Spironolactone

Answer: B

Because this patient does not wish to get pregnant, oral contraceptive therapy will be the best choice of therapy, as it provides effective contraception and also suppresses LH production.

Case 39B

A 27-year-old G0 complains of the gradual appearance of terminal hair on the face and lower abdomen. She has noted subtle changes in her menstrual cycle length. She has tried to conceive for 1 year but has been unsuccessful. Her blood pressure is normal.

Questions Case 39B

Of the following, which is the most likely cause for these symptoms?

A. Hyperthecosis
B. Constitutional hirsutism
C. Late-onset adrenal hyperplasia (21-hydroxylase type)
D. Late-onset adrenal hyperplasia (11α-hydroxylase type)

Answer: C

Late-onset adrenal hyperplasia should be suspected in women with hirsutism, acne, and menstrual irregularities. Infertility is also common.

Initial laboratory studies show an elevated dehydroepiandrosterone sulfate (DS). Which of the following is the most appropriate next diagnostic study?

A. Gonadotropin-releasing hormone (GnRH) stimulation test
B. ACTH stimulation test
C. FSH and LH measurement
D. Thyroid stimulation test

Answer: B

DS and androstenedione are elevated in 21-hydroxylase deficiency, the most common disorder causing adrenal hyperplasia. ACTH stimulation will confirm this diagnosis.

A diagnosis of late-onset adrenal hyperplasia (21-hydroxylase type) is made. Which of the following therapies should be initiated?

A. Clomiphene citrate
B. Oral contraceptive suppression
C. Prednisone
D. Thyroid-replacement therapy

Answer: C

Glucocorticoid supplementation will suppress adrenal androgen production. Facial acne usually clears, and ovulation resumes.

chapter 40

CELL BIOLOGY AND PRINCIPLES OF CANCER THERAPY

Treatment of cancers involving the breast and genital organs can involve surgery, chemotherapy, radiation therapy, and hormone therapy, used alone or in combination. The specific treatment plan depends on the type of cancer, the stage of the cancer, and the characteristics of the individual patient. Individualizing treatment is an important characteristic of cancer therapy.

THE CELL CYCLE AND CANCER THERAPY

Knowledge of the cell cycle is important in understanding cancer therapies. Many treatments are based on the fact that cancer cells are constantly dividing, making them more vulnerable to agents that interfere with the cell division process.

The cell cycle consists of four phases (Fig. 40.1). During the G_1 phase, there is synthesis of RNA and protein that prepares the cell for DNA synthesis, which occurs in the S phase. The G_2 phase is a period of additional RNA, protein, and specialized DNA synthesis. This leads to mitosis (M phase), where cell division occurs. After mitosis, cells can again enter the G_1 phase or can "drop out" of the cell cycle and enter a resting phase (G_0). Cells in G_0 do not engage in the synthetic activities characteristic of the cell cycle and, therefore, are not vulnerable to therapies aimed at actively growing and dividing cells. The *growth fraction* is the number of cells in a tumor that are actively involved in cell division (i.e., not in the G_0 phase). The growth fraction of tumors decreases as they enlarge, because vascular supply and oxygen levels are decreased. *Surgical removal of tumor tissue* (cytoreductive debulking surgery) *can result in G_0 cells* reentering the cell cycle, thus making them more vulnerable to chemotherapy and radiation therapy.

The *generation time* is the length of the cell cycle, from M phase to M phase. For a given cell type, the lengths of the S and M phases are relatively constant, whereas G_2 and, especially, G_1 vary. The variable length of G_1 can be explained by cells entering G_0 for a period and then reentering the cycle.

Chemotherapeutic agents and radiation kill cancer cells by first-order kinetics. This means that they kill a constant fraction of tumor cells, instead of a constant number. The implication of this is that a number of intermittent doses is more likely to be curative than a single large dose.

CHEMOTHERAPY

Chemotherapeutic agents can be (a) cell-cycle (phase) nonspecific, which means that they can kill in all phases of the cell cycle and are useful in tumors with a low growth index, or (b) *cell-cycle (phase) specific,* which kill in a specific phase of the cell cycle and are most useful in tumors that have a large proportion of cells actively dividing. Figure 40.1 contains examples of common drugs and their sites of action within the cycle.

There are several *classes of antineoplastic drugs* (Table 40.1). *Alkylating agents* primarily interact with DNA molecules to interfere with base pairing, produce cross-links, and cause single- and double-strand breaks. This interferes with DNA, RNA, and protein synthesis. Dividing cells are most sensitive to the effects of these drugs. The late G_1 and S phases are the times of maximum sensitivity. Dividing cells are most sensitive to the effects of these drugs. The late G_1 and S phases are the times of maximum sensitivity. Alkylating-like agents probably act, in part, through the formation of interstrand and intras-

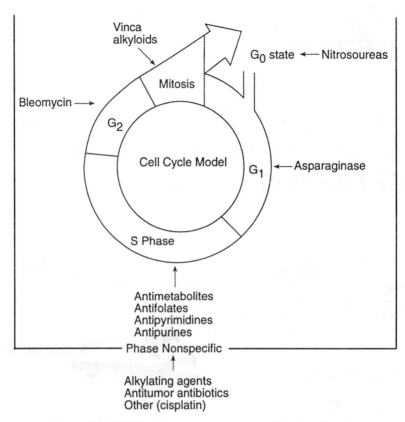

Figure 40.1.   Actions of antineoplastic agents within the cell cycle.

trand linkages in DNA. The major side effects of the alkylating agents are myelosuppression and immunosuppression. They also may result in amenorrhea.

The *antitumor antibiotics* intercalate between DNA base pairs to inhibit DNA-directed RNA synthesis and also are involved in the formation of free radicals, causing strand breakage. They are phase nonspecific, i.e., they are effective in all phases of the cell cycle. Their general side effects are similar to the alkylating agents. Other side effects are drug specific.

The *antimetabolites* are structural analogs of normal molecules necessary for cell function. They competitively interfere with the normal synthesis of nucleic acids and, therefore, are most active during the S phase of cell division. They may cause bone marrow suppression or in GI-mucositis when given in a bolus.

Plant (vinca) alkaloids primarily prevent the assembly of microtubules, thus interfering with the M phase of cell division. They may cause bone marrow suppression or an anaphylactoid reaction.

Cisplatin binds to DNA to cause interstrand and intrastrand cross-links. A major side effect is the impairment of renal tubular function.

Antineoplastic drugs are toxic because they act on normal as well as cancer cells. Rapidly dividing cell types are most sensitive. For example, the cells of the erythroid, myeloid, and megakaryocytic series are damaged by common neoplastic drugs. Granulocytopenia and thrombocytopenia are predictable side effects. Patients with low granulocyte counts are at high risk for fatal sepsis, and those with sustained thrombocytopenia are at risk for spontaneous gastrointestinal or acute intracranial hemorrhage. Prophylactic antibiotics are usually administered to febrile patients to prevent serious infection, and platelet transfusions are employed to decrease the risk of hemorrhage. Table 40.2 describes the major side effects of antineoplastic agents.

There are limitations in the use of single agents. These include the development of drug resistance and toxicity. As a consequence, combination chemotherapy has come into use.

Table 40.1.
Examples of Antineoplastic Drugs

Alkylating agents
  Nitrogen mustard (Mustargen, HN)
  Cyclophosphamide
  Chlorambucil (Leukeran)
  Busulfan (Myleran)
  Melphalan (Alkeran, L-PAM)
  Hexamethylmelamine

Antitumor antibiotics
  Doxorubicin (Adriamycin)
  Bleomycin (Blenoxane)
  Actinomycin D (dactinomycin, Cosmegen)
  Mitomycin C (Mutamycin)
  Mitoxantrone

Antimetabolites
  Methotrexate (MTX, amethopterin)
  6-mercaptopurine (6-MP, Purinethol)
  5-fluorouracil (fluorouracil, 5-FU)
  Hydroxyurea (Hydrea)

Plant alkaloids
  Vinblastine (Velban)
  Vincristine (Oncovin)

Other
  Cis-diamminedichloroplatinum (cisplatin)

Table 40.2.
Major Side Effects of Antineoplastic Drugs

Hematologic	Cardiac
Granulocytopenia	Cardiomyopathy
Thrombocytopenia	
	Urinary
Gastrointestinal	Chronic azotemia
Mucositis	Acute renal failure
Necrotizing	
enterocolitis	Neurologic
	Peripheral neuropathies
Immunosuppression	Ototoxicity
	Paresthesias
Dermatologic	
Alopecia	Reproductive
	Amenorrhea
Hepatic	
Pulmonary	
Interstitial pneumonitis	

The *interactions between drugs used in combination* are defined as *synergistic* (result in improved antitumor activity or decreased toxicity than with each agent alone), *additive* (result in enhanced antitumor activity equal to the sum of each individual agent), or *antagonistic* (result in less antitumor activity than each individual agent). Drugs used in combinations should (*a*) be effective when used singly, (*b*) have different mechanisms of action, and (*c*) be additive or, preferably, synergistic in action.

Chemotherapy is administered in a variety of regimens. *Adjuvant chemotherapy* is usually a short course of combination chemotherapy that is given in a high dose to patients with no evidence of residual cancer after radiotherapy or surgery. The purpose is to eliminate any residual cancer cells. *Induction chemotherapy* is usually a combination chemotherapy given in a high dose to cause a remission. *Maintenance chemotherapy* is a long-term and low dose regimen that is given to a patient in remission to maintain the remission by inhibiting the growth of remaining cancer cells.

RADIATION THERAPY

Ionizing radiation causes the production of free hydrogen ions and hydroxyl (OH^-) radicals. In the presence of sufficient oxygen, H_2O_2 is formed, which affects DNA and, eventually, the cell's ability to divide. As with chemotherapy, killing is by first-order kinetics. Since dividing cells are more sensitive to radiation damage and since not all cells in a given tumor are dividing at any one time, *fractionated doses of radiation are more likely to be effective than a single dose.* Providing multiple lower doses of radiation also reduces the deleterious effects on normal tissues.

The basis of fractionated dosage comes from the *"four Rs" of radiobiology.*

1. *Repair of sublethal injury.* When a dose is divided, the number of cells that survive is greater than if the dose were given at one time (higher total amounts of radiation can be tolerated in fractionated as opposed to single doses).
2. *Repopulation.* Reactivation of stem cells occurs when radiation is stopped; thus regenerative capacity depends on the number of available stem cells.
3. *Reoxygenation.* Cells are more vulnerable to radiation damage in the presence of oxygen; as tumor cells are killed, surviving cells will be brought into contact with capillaries, making them radiosensitive.
4. *Redistribution in the cell cycle.* Since tumor cells are in various phases of the cell cycle, fractionated doses make it more likely that a given cell will be irradiated when it is most vulnerable.

The rad has been used as a measure of the amount of energy absorbed per unit mass of tissue. A new standard measure of absorbed dose is the *Gray*, which is defined as 1 joule per kilogram; *1 Gray is equal to 100 rad.* Radiation is delivered in two general ways: external irradiation (teletherapy) and local irradiation (brachytherapy). *Tele-*

therapy now depends on the use of high-energy (>1 million eV) beams, because this spares the skin and delivers less toxic radiation to the bone. Tolerance for external radiation depends on the vulnerability of surrounding normal tissues. Teletherapy usually is used to shrink tumors before localized radiation.

Brachytherapy depends on the inverse square law: the dose of radiation at a given point is inversely proportional to the square of the distance from the radiation source. To put the radioactive material at the closest possible distance, brachytherapy uses encapsulated sources of ionizing radiation implanted directly into tissues (interstitial) or placed in natural body cavities (intracavity). *Intracavity devices* can be placed within the uterus or vagina and then afterloaded with radioactive sources (cesium-137). This method protects health personnel from radiation exposure. *Interstitial implants* use isotopes (iridium-192, iodine-125) formulated as wires or seeds. These implants are usually temporary.

Complications associated with radiation therapy can be acute or late (chronic). *Acute reactions* affect rapidly dividing tissues, such as epithelia (skin, gastrointestinal mucosa, bone marrow, and reproductive cells). Manifestations are cessation of mitotic activity, cellular swelling, tissue edema, and tissue necrosis. Early problems associated with irradiation of gynecologic cancers include enteritis, acute cystitis, vulvitis, proctosigmoiditis, and occasionally, bone marrow depression. *Chronic complications* occur months to years after completion of radiation therapy. These include obliteration of small blood vessels or thickening of the vessel wall, fibrosis, and reductions in epithelial and parenchymal cell populations. This results in chronic proctitis, hemorrhagic cystitis, formation of uterovaginal or vesicovaginal fistula, and rectal or sigmoid stenosis as well as gastrointestinal fistulae.

HORMONAL THERAPY

The therapeutic importance of the presence of cellular *estrogen receptors (ER)* has been well established in breast cancers. There is a good relationship between the presence of ER and the response of patients to endocrine therapy. Normally, estrogen enters cells and binds to ER in the cytoplasm. The complex is translocated to the nucleus, where it binds to acceptor sites on chromosomes, resulting in activation of RNA and protein synthesis. The drug tamoxifen acts as a competitive inhibitor of estrogen binding. The tamoxifen-ER complex also binds to chromosomes but does not activate cell metabolism. This decreases cellular activity and cell division, thus reducing tumor growth. Tamoxifen is used in the adjunct treatment of breast cancer.

There also are *progestin receptors (PR)*, which appear to be located in the nucleus of progestin-sensitive cells. The progestins appear to interfere with the actions of estrogens, androgens, and gonadotropins.

CASE STUDIES

Case 40A

A patient with a large ovarian tumor undergoes total abdominal hysterectomy with bilateral salpingo-oophorectomy for widespread disease. Most of the tumor mass is removed.

Question Case 40A

Which of the following is a likely result of this operation?

A. The proportion of tumor cells in G_0 will increase

B. The growth fraction of the remaining tumor will decrease

C. The proportion of tumor cells that are sensitive to antineoplastic agents will increase

D. A single dose of chemotherapy will be able to kill the remaining tumor cells

Answer: C

Removal of part of a tumor mass increases the growth fraction (the number of cells that are actively dividing). Therefore, the proportion of cells in G_0 (the nondividing phase) will decrease and the proportion of cells sensitive to antineoplastic agents will increase (since dividing cells are more sensitive). A single dose of chemotherapy will probably not be sufficient to kill the remaining tumor cells, because cells still will be killed by first-order kinetics.

chapter 41

VULVAR AND VAGINAL DISEASE AND NEOPLASIA

VULVAR DISEASE

Appreciation of vulvar symptoms and examination for vulvar dermatologic pathology and other lesions constitute a significant part of primary health care for women. Noninflammatory vulvar pathology is found in women of all ages, but is particularly significant in perimenopausal and postmenopausal women because of concern regarding the possibility of vulvar neoplasia. *The major symptoms of vulvar disease include pruritus, burning, nonspecific irritation, and/or appreciation of a mass.* Diagnostic aids for the assessment of noninflammatory conditions are likewise relatively limited in number and include, in addition to careful history, inspection and biopsy. *Because vulvar lesions are often difficult to diagnose, liberal use of vulvar biopsy is central to good care.*

The opening sections of this chapter discuss a range of vulvar pathologic conditions, including nonneoplastic dermatoses, white lesions (atrophic and hyperkeratotic lesions), benign vulvar mass lesions, vulvar intraepithelial neoplasia, and vulvar cancer. Inflammatory conditions of the vulva are discussed in Chapter 27. Table 41.1 outlines common vulvar diseases.

Common Vulvar Dermatoses

Lichen Simplex Chronicus

In contrast to many dermatologic conditions that may be described as "rashes that itch," lichen simplex chronicus (LSC) can be described as *"an itch that rashes."* Although oversimplified, this dermatologic maxim adequately describes the condition. It is thought that the majority of patients develop this disorder secondary to *an irritant dermatitis, which progresses to lichen simplex chronicus as a result of the effects of chronic mechanical irritation* from scratching and rubbing an already irritated area. The mechanical irritation contributes to epidermal hyperplasia, which, in turn, leads to heightened sensitivity that triggers more mechanical irritation.

Accordingly, the history of these patients is one of *progressive vulvar pruritus and/or burning*, which is temporarily relieved by scratching or rubbing with a washcloth or some similar material. *Etiologic factors* for the original pruritic symptoms often are unknown but may include sources of skin irritation such as laundry detergents, fabric softeners, scented hygienic preparations, and the use of colored or scented tissue. These potential sources of symptoms must be investigated. Any domestic or hygienic irritants must be removed, in combination with treatment, to break the cycle described above.

On *clinical inspection*, the skin of the labia majora, labia minora, and perineal body often shows diffusely reddened areas with occasional hyperplastic or hyperpigmented plaques of red to reddish brown. One may also find occasional areas of linear hyperplasia, which show the effect of grossly hyperkeratotic ridges of epidermis. Biopsy of patients who have these characteristics findings is usually not warranted.

Empiric *treatment* to include antipruritic *medications* such as Benadryl (diphenhydramine hydrochloride) or Atarax (hydroxyzine hydrochloride) that inhibit nighttime, unconscious scratching, combined with a mild to moderate topical steroid cream applied to the vulva, will usually provide relief. A *steroid cream* such as hydrocortisone (1 or 2%) or, for patients with significant areas of obvious hyperkeratosis, triamcinolone acetonide (0.1%; Kenalog) or betamethasone valerate (0.1%;

Table 41.1.
Common Vulvar Diseases

Common vulvar dermatoses
  Lichen simplex chronicus (LSC)
  Lichen planus
  Psoriasis
  Seborrheic dermatitis
  Vestibulitis

White lesions
  Hyperplastic vulvar dystrophy
  Lichen sclerosis (atrophic vulvar dystrophy)

Vulvar intraepithelial neoplasia (VIN)
  Without atypia
  With atypia, including carcinoma in situ

Vulvar carcinoma
  Paget's disease
  Squamous cell carcinoma

Valisone) may be used. *If significant relief is not obtained within 3 months, diagnostic vulvar biopsy is warranted.*

Lichen Planus

Although lichen planus is usually a desquamative lesion of the vagina, occasional patients will develop lesions on the vulva near the inner aspects of the labia minora and vulvar vestibule. Patients may have areas of whitish, lacy bands of keratosis near the reddish ulcerated-like lesions characteristic of the disease. Typically, complaints include *chronic vulvar burning and/or pruritus* and insertional (i.e., entrance) dyspareunia and a profuse vaginal discharge. Because of the patchiness of this lesion and the concern raised by atypical hyperplastic lesions, *biopsy may be warranted* to confirm the diagnosis in some patients. In lichen planus, biopsy shows an absence of atypia in the hyperplastic area. Examination of the vaginal discharge in these patients frequently reveals large numbers of acute inflammatory cells in the absence of significant numbers of bacteria. Accordingly, most often the diagnosis can be made by the typical history of vaginal/vulvar burning and/or insertional dyspareunia coupled with a physical examination that shows the bright red patchy distribution and a wet prep that shows large numbers of white cells.

Treatment for lichen planus is topical *steroid preparations* similar to those described above. In patients with marked degrees of hyperkeratosis, a stronger steroid preparation such as fluocinonide 0.05% (Lidex cream) or triamcinolone acetonide

(0.5%; Aristocort) may be used. Length of treatment for these patients is often shorter than that required to treat lichen simplex chronicus, although lichen planus is more likely to reoccur.

Psoriasis

Psoriasis may involve the vulvar skin as part of a generalized dermatologic process. With approximately 2% of the general population suffering from psoriasis, the physician should be alert to its prevalence and likelihood of vulvar manifestation. Moreover, because it may appear at menarche, pregnancy, and menopause, the physician may be consulted by the patient for what she perceives to be a gynecologic disorder.

The *lesions* are typically slightly raised round or ovoid patches with a silver scale appearance atop an erythematous base. These lesions most often measure approximately 1 × 1 to 1 × 2 cm. Most patients are concerned by the appearance of this lesion, as pruritus is usually not marked. *The diagnosis is generally known because of psoriasis found elsewhere on the body, obviating the need for vulvar biopsy to confirm the diagnosis.*

Treatment often occurs in conjunction with consultation by a dermatologist. Like lesions elsewhere, vulvar lesions usually respond to topical cold tar preparations, followed by exposure to ultraviolet light as well as corticosteroid medications, either topically or by intralesional injection. Since vulvar application of some of the photoactivated preparations can be somewhat awkward, topical steroids are most effective, using compounds such as betamethasone valerate 0.1% (Valisone).

Seborrheic Dermatitis

Isolated vulvar seborrheic dermatitis is rare. The diagnosis is usually made in patients complaining of vulvar pruritus who are known to have seborrheic dermatitis in the scalp or other hair-bearing areas of the body. The lesion my mimic other entities such as psoriasis, tinea cruris (jock itch), or lichen simplex chronicus. *The lesions are pale red to a yellowish pink and may be covered by an oily appearing, scaly crust.* Because this area of the body remains continually moist, occasional exudative lesions include raw "weeping" patches, caused by skin maceration, which are exacerbated by the patient's scratching. As with psoriasis, *vulvar biopsy is usually not needed* when the diagnosis is made in conjunction with known seborrheic dermatitis in other hair-bearing areas.

For patients with acute exudative variations of seborrheic dermatitis, initial perineal hygiene includes the use of *Burrow's solution soaks.* After remediation of the exudative phase, standard treatment includes *topical corticosteroid lotions or creams* containing a mixture of an agent that penetrates well such as betamethasone valerate in conjunction with Eurax (crotamiton) to control the intense pruritus. As with lichen simplex chronicus, the use of antipruritic agents such as Atarax or Benadryl as a bedtime dose in the first 10 days to 2 weeks of treatment will frequently help break the sleep/scratch cycle and allow the lesions to heal.

Vestibulitis

Vulvar vestibulitis is a condition without known etiology. It involves the acute and chronic inflammation of the vestibular glands, which lie just inside the vaginal introitus near the hymeneal ring. The involved glands may be circumferential to include areas near the urethra, but most commonly involves posterolateral vestibular glands in the 4 and 8 o'clock positions (Fig. 41.1). The diagnosis should be suspected in all patients who present with *new onset insertional dyspareunia.* Patients with this condition frequently complain of progressive insertional dyspareunia to the point where they are unable to have intercourse. The history may go on a few weeks but most typically involves progressive worsening over the course of 3 or 4 months. Patients also complain of pain upon tampon insertion and at times during washing or bathing the perineal area.

Physical examination is the key to diagnosis. Because the vestibular glands lie between the folds of the hymeneal ring and the medial aspect of the vulvar vestibule, diagnosis is frequently missed when inspection of the perineum does not include these areas. Once the speculum has been placed in the vagina, the vestibular gland area becomes impossible to identify. After carefully inspecting the proper anatomic area, light touch with a moistened cotton applicator will recreate the pain exactly for those patients who have vulvar vestibulitis. In addition, the regions affected are most often evident as small, reddened, patchy areas.

Because the cause of vestibulitis is unknown, treatments are varied and range from temporary sexual abstinence and application of cortisone ointments and topical xylocaine jelly to more radical treatments such as surgical excision of the vestibular glands. No single treatment has proved highly efficacious, and treatment must be individualized based on the severity of patient symptoms and the sexual disability that is present.

Recent limited data suggest that some patients may benefit from low-dose tricyclic medication (amitriptyline and imipramine) to help break the cycle of pain, while other limited reports suggest the use of calcium citrate to change the urine composition by removing oxalic acid crystals. Those advocating changing the urine chemistry cite evidence to suggest that oxalic acid crystals are particularly irritating when precipitated in the urine of patients with high urinary oxalic acid composition. The efficacy of calcium citrate use needs to be studied in prospective randomized trials but preliminary data look promising.

Benign Vulvar Lesions

Sebaceous or inclusion cysts are caused by inflammatory blockage of the sebaceous gland ducts and are small, smooth nodular masses, usually arising from the inner surfaces of the labia minora and majora, that contain cheesy, sebaceous material. They may be easily excised if their size or position is troublesome.

The round ligament inserts into the labium majora, carrying an investment of peritoneum. On occasion, peritoneal fluid may accumulate therein, causing a *cyst of the canal of Nuck or hydrocoele.* If

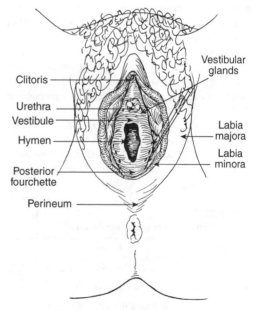

Figure 41.1. Vestibular glands.

such cysts reach symptomatic size, excision is usually required.

Fibromas arise from the fibrous tissue of the vulva and are usually small. If they are large, however, they may become pedunculated. Of historical interest is the almost unbelievable 268-lb pedunculated vulvar fibroma reported by Buckner in 1851. Treatment is, of course, surgical excision. *Lipomas* appear much like fibromas, are quite rare, and are also treated by excision.

Hidradenoma is a rare lesion arising from the sweat glands of the vulva. It is almost always benign, is usually found on the inner surface of the labia majora, and is treated with excision.

Nevi are benign, usually asymptomatic, pigmented lesions whose importance is that they must be distinguished from malignant melanoma, 3 to 4% of which in females occur on the external genitalia. Biopsy of pigmented vulvar lesions is important for this reason.

VULVAR NEOPLASIA

Historically, the classification of vulvar disease has used descriptive terminology based on gross morphologic appearance. Accordingly, such terms as leukoplakia, kraurosis vulvae, and vulvar dystrophy have been used. Standardization of nomenclature and classification by symptoms, gross appearance, and histology were lacking. To improve standardization and thus treatment of these disorders, the International Society for the Study of Vulvar Disease (ISSVD) established a modified classification in 1987. This classification has generally been accepted by different medical disciplines, including gynecology, dermatology, and pathology. The rationale for this description is based on both gross and microscopic morphology (Table 41.2).

Vulvar dermatoses have been described previously. The following discussion includes a description of squamous cell hyperplasia (formerly hyperplastic dystrophy) and lichen sclerosis.

Table 41.2.
ISSVD Classification of Vulvar Disease

	Description
I	Squamous cell hyperplasia
II	Lichen sclerosis
III	Other dermatoses

Squamous Cell Hyperplasia (Hyperplastic Dystrophy)

In considering the various types of vulvar neoplasia, the clinician should be aware that gross appearance may not be consistent with underlying cellular architecture and that often atrophic lesions, such as lichen sclerosis, may appear grossly to be hyperplastic. Furthermore, within the group of true hyperplasia lesions, there is a need to confirm whether the hyperplasia is accompanied by atypia. As a result, classification of intraepithelial vulvar disease becomes a matter of close cooperation between the clinician, who must first appreciate the need for thorough investigation, and the pathologist, who is called on to confirm the presence of lesions that may have premalignant or malignant potential. Because these distinctions cannot always be made on physical examination alone and because many of these lesions present with similar symptoms, *liberal use of vulvar biopsy is encouraged to provide definitive diagnosis and ensure rational treatment.*

Many hyperplastic lesions without atypia evolve from chronic irritation and secondary thickening of the vulvar skin and are classified under the LSC group (which were discussed earlier in this chapter). As with many of the other lesions, vulvar pruritus is the main presenting symptom. On gross inspection of the vulva, areas may be isolated and include obviously hyperkeratotic skin with secondary excoriation. These changes may diffusely involve the vulva or may occur as isolated ridges or patches. In the presence of gross abnormalities of the vulvar skin, directed biopsies of the lesions are warranted.

The microscopic appearance confirms the diagnosis. *Squamous cell hyperplasia without atypia* characteristically shows hyperkeratosis as well as acanthosis with an absence of mitotic figures. These lesions are usually treated as described in the previous discussion of lichen simplex chronicus, using various types of *topical, highly penetrating corticosteroid creams.* The patient can be reassured that these lesions usually respond to treatment with complete resolution and do not predispose to further premalignant or malignant vulvar disease.

Lichen Sclerosis

Lichen sclerosis, previously called lichen sclerosis et atrophicus, has confused clinicians and pathologists because of inconsistent terminology and because it is associated with other types of vulvar pathology, including those of the hyperplastic variety. As with the other disorders, *chronic vulvar pruritus* occurs in most patients. Typically, *the vulva is diffusely involved with very thin, whitish epithelial areas* termed "onion skin" epithelium. Most patients have involvement on both sides of the vulva, with the most common sites being the labia majora, labia minora, the clitoral and periclitoral epithelium, and the perineal body. The lesion may extend to include a perianal "halo" of atrophic, whitish epithelium. In severe cases, there is loss of many normal anatomic landmarks, including obliteration of labial and periclitoral architecture as well as severe stenosis of the vaginal introitus. Some patients will have areas of cracked skin, which are prone to bleeding with minimal trauma. Patients with these severe anatomic changes complain of difficulty in having normal coital function.

Microscopic confirmation of lichen sclerosis is mandatory. The histologic features are pathognomonic and include areas of hyperkeratosis, despite epithelial thinning; a zone of homogeneous, pink-staining collagenous-like material directly under the epithelial layer; and a band of chronic inflammatory cells, consisting mostly of lymphocytes.

It is important to remember that there may be associated areas of hyperplasia mixed throughout or adjacent to these typically atrophic-appearing areas. In patients with this so-called *mixed dystrophy*, there is a need to treat both components to effect resolution of symptoms. Patients with histologic confirmation of a large hyperplastic component should initially be treated with well-penetrating corticosteroid creams. With improvement of these areas (usually 2 to 3 weeks), therapy can then be directed to the lichen sclerosis component.

The treatment of choice for lichen sclerosis is topical testosterone propionate (2%) in white petrolatum. This is applied twice daily for 3 months and, with improvement in symptoms, may be used on a chronic basis once or twice a week, depending on the need. Patients need to be reassured that this disorder is not premalignant, but that the lesion is unlikely to resolve totally. Intermittent treatment may be needed indefinitely. This is in marked contrast to the hyperplastic lesions without atypia, which usually totally resolve within 6 months.

Neither lichen sclerosis nor hyperplastic dystrophy without atypia significantly increases the patient's risk of developing cancer. It has been estimated that this risk is in the 2 to 3% range when there is no pre-existing atypical hyperplasia. However, since patients who have had these disorders are more likely to eventually develop atypical hyperplasia, they need to be followed carefully and rebiopsied liberally if there is a return of vulvar symptoms or new lesions.

VULVAR INTRAEPITHELIAL NEOPLASIA

Vulvar intraepithelial neoplasia (VIN) may be classified as VIN-I, mild dysplasia; VIN-II, moderate dysplasia; or VIN-III, severe dysplasia, carcinoma in situ. Also included in the category of intraepithelial neoplasia lesions are vulvar condylomata. Other lesions represented include Paget's disease and level 1 melanomas. Condylomata are discussed in the section on inflammatory vulvar lesions, and Paget's disease and level I melanomas are mentioned briefly later in this section.

VIN-I and VIN-II

Early vulvar intraepithelial neoplasia (VIN-I and VIN-II) represents *true neoplastic lesions* that, as with their counterparts in the cervix, are thought to have a *high predilection for progression* to severe intraepithelial lesions and eventually carcinoma.

Presenting complaints include *vulvar pruritus, chronic irritation, and a development of raised mass lesions.* Normally, the lesions are localized and fairly well isolated and are raised above the normal epithelial surface to include a slightly rough texture. These lesions are usually found along the posterior vulva and in the perineal body, although they may occur anywhere on the vulva. They typically have a whitish cast or hue. As with other vulvar lesions, diagnosis by biopsy is mandatory.

Microscopically, these lesions mimic intraepithelial neoplasia elsewhere, including mitotic figures and nuclear pleomorphism, with loss of normal differentiation in the lower one-third to one-half of the epithelial layer. As with the cervix, the degree of dysplasia increases to a point where full-thickness change indicates severe intraepithelial neoplasia and/or carcinoma in situ. Changes consistent with human papilloma virus (HPV) infection are occasionally seen with these lesions and suggest an association between various types of HPV and the occurrence of vulvar intraepithelial neoplasia. Lesions that are typically condyloma in origin will not have features of attenuated maturation and have an absence of pleomorphism and atypical mitotic figures.

VIN-III (Carcinoma in Situ)

Full-thickness loss of maturation indicates lesions that are at least severely dysplastic, including areas that may represent true carcinoma in situ. Common presenting complaints include *intractable pruritus and nonspecific vulvar irritation with gross lesions that are similar to earlier grades of VIN* occurring in patchy, fairly well-isolated areas. Occasional patients may have extensive vulvar involvement. The color changes in these lesions range from white, hyperplastic areas to reddened or dusky patch-like involvement, depending on whether there is associated hyperkeratosis.

As with the other vulvar disorders, *diagnosis of vulvar intraepithelial neoplasia is made by biopsy*. In patients without obvious raised or isolated lesions, careful inspection of the vulva is warranted using a magnifying device such as a hand lens or visor. Washing the vulvar skin with a dilute solution of 3% acetic acid often accentuates the white lesions and may also help in revealing abnormal vascular patterns. When present, these areas should be selectively biopsied in multiple sites to thoroughly investigate the grade of vulvar intraepithelial neoplasia and reliably exclude the presence of invasive carcinoma.

The goal in treating VIN is to quickly and completely remove all involved areas of skin. A variety of treatments are available, depending on the extent of the lesion and the severity of the dysplasia. Most *isolated and limited VIN-I or VIN-II lesions* may be removed by local excision in the office or by *cryocautery, electrodesiccation, or laser cautery* with local anesthetic. Extended lesions showing VIN-I or VIN-II are usually treated with laser ablation in an ambulatory surgery area using a general anesthetic.

VIN-III, including carcinoma in situ, is best treated by wide *local excision with or without combination laser ablation,* depending on the area of involvement. This usually requires a general or regional anesthetic and often requires inpatient hospitalization, depending on the extent of the vulvar surgery. Occasionally, for diffuse or recurrent disease, simple vulvectomy is warranted.

Paget's Disease

Paget's disease is characterized by extensive intraepithelial disease, including characteristic intraepithelial pathologic findings. It is identical histologically to Paget's disease of the breast. Although not common, Paget's disease of the vulva may be associated with carcinoma of the skin. Similarly, patients with Paget's disease of the vulva have a higher incidence of underlying internal carcinoma, particularly of the colon and breast.

The treatment for vulvar Paget's disease is wide local excision or simple vulvectomy, depending on the amount of involvement. Recurrences are more common with this disorder than with vulvar intraepithelial neoplasia, necessitating wider margins when local excision or vulvectomy is performed.

Melanoma

Vulvar melanoma usually presents with *a raised, irritated, pruritic, pigmented lesion.* Melanoma accounts for only 5% of all vulvar malignancies, and when suspected, *wide local excision* is necessary for diagnosis and staging. For level 1 melanoma, wide local excision is usually adequate. An in-depth discussion of this entity is beyond the scope of this book; however, the clinician should be aware that irritated, pigmented, vulvar lesions mandate excisional biopsy for definitive diagnosis.

VULVAR CANCER

Vulvar carcinoma accounts for approximately 4% of all gynecologic malignancies, with 90% of these carcinomas being of the *squamous cell* variety. The typical clinical profile includes women in their *postmenopausal years,* most commonly between the ages of 65 and 70. *Vulvar pruritus* is the most common presenting complaint. In addition, patients may notice a red or white ulcerative or exophytic lesion arising most commonly on the posterior two-thirds of either labium majus. An exophytic ulcerative lesion need not be present, further underscoring the need for thorough biopsy in patients of the age group who complain of vulvar symptoms. There is *often a delay in treatment of these patients* because of reluctance of patients in this age group to present to their physicians and further reluctance on the physicians' part to investigate the symptoms and findings thoroughly via vulvar biopsy.

Although a *specific etiology* for vulvar cancer is not known, it has been shown that there may be progression from prior intraepithelial lesions, including those that are associated with certain types of human papilloma virus.

Natural History

Squamous cell carcinoma of the vulva generally *remains localized for long periods of time and then spreads in a predictable fashion to the regional lymph nodes,* including those of the inguinal and femoral chain. Lesions of greater than 2 cm in diameter and 0.5 cm in depth have an increased chance of nodal metastases. The overall incidence of lymph node metastasis is approximately 30%. Lesions arising in the anterior one-third of the vulva may spread to the deep pelvic nodes, bypassing regional inguinal and femoral lymphatics.

Evaluation

After suspicious lesions are biopsied and the diagnosis of invasive squamous cell carcinoma of the vulva confirmed, other studies that may be obtained include *chest x-ray and intravenous pyelogram*. For patients with lesions near the urethra and/or patients with lesions involving the anus or perineal area, preoperative *cystoscopy and proctoscopy*, respectively, are indicated.

The *staging classification* was altered by the Federation of Gynecology and Obstetrics (FIGO) in 1988 (Table 41.3). This staging convention uses the analysis of the removed vulvar tumor and microscopic assessment of the regional lymph nodes as its basis. The change from clinical staging to this surgical staging convention was necessitated by the observation that clinical assessment of this disease contained many errors, in particular, the assessment of inguinal and femoral adenopathy.

Treatment

Although the mainstay for the treatment of invasive vulvar cancer is surgical, a number of advances have been made to help individualize patients into treatment categories in an effort to reduce the amount of radical surgery while not compromising survival. Accordingly, not all patients undergo radical vulvectomy with bilateral nodal dissections. Individualized approaches include the following.

- Conservative vulvar operations for patients with unifocal lesions.
- Elimination of routine pelvic lymphadenectomy.
- Avoidance of groin dissection in patients with unilateral lesions less than 1 mm in depth.
- Elimination of contralateral groin dissection in patients with unilateral T1 lesions who have negative ipsilateral nodes.
- Separate groin incisions for those patients with indicated bilateral groin dissection.
- Use of postoperative radiation therapy to decrease incidence of groin recurrence in patients with 2 or more positive groin nodes.

Adjunctive treatment with chemotherapy in cases of recurrent vulvar cancer has only limited value.

Prognosis

The corrected 5-year survival rate for all vulvar carcinoma is approximately 70%, with cure rates approaching 90% if the patient has negative inguinal and femoral lymph nodes at the time of her first surgery. If metastatic disease is found in the regional nodes, survival falls off dramatically to as low as 20% if the deep pelvic nodes are involved.

Carcinoma of Bartholin's Gland

Carcinoma of Bartholin's gland is uncommon, arising from either the squamous epithelium of the ducts or the glandular epithelium of the greater vestibular glands. This cancer is usually diagnosed in the fifth decade or afterward upon presentation as an usually asymptomatic vulvar mass. Treatment is radical vulvectomy and bilateral lymphadenectomy and radiation therapy if the pelvic nodes are positive. Recurrence is a disappointingly common event and a 5-year overall survival rate of 50 to 60% is noted.

VAGINAL DISEASE

Benign Vaginal Masses

Gartner duct cysts arise from vestigial remnants of the wolffian or mesonephric system that course along the outer anterior aspect of the vaginal canal. These cystic structures are usually small and asymptomatic, but on occasion they may be larger and symptomatic so that excision is required.

Inclusion cysts are usually seen on the posterior lower vaginal surface, resulting from imperfect approximation of childbirth lacerations or episiotomy. They are lined with stratified squamous epithelium, their content is usually cheesy, and they may be excised if symptomatic.

VAGINAL NEOPLASIA

Carcinoma in situ of the vagina and invasive vaginal cancer are among the rarest of gynecologic neoplasms. They are often multifocal, associated with other lower genital tract intraepithelial or invasive neoplasms.

Carcinoma in Situ of the Vagina

Carcinoma in situ (CIS) appears to occur more commonly in the third decade of life onward, al-

Table 41.3.
FIGO Staging for Carcinoma of the Vulva

Stage 0	
Tis	Carcinoma in situ; intraepithelial carcinoma
Stage I	
T1 N0 M0	Tumor confined to the vulva and/or perineum; <2 cm in greatest dimension; nodes are not palpable
Stage II	
T2 N0 M0	Tumor confined to the vulva and/or perineum; >2 cm in greatest dimension, nodes are not palpable
Stage III	
T3 N0 M0	Tumor of any size with . . .
T3 N1 M0	1. Adjacent spread to the lower urethra and/or the vagina, or the anus, and/or . . .
T1 N1 M0	2. Unilateral regional lymph node metastasis
T2 N1 M0	
Stage IVA	
T1 N2 M0	Tumor invades any of the following:
T2 N2 M0	Upper urethra, bladder mucosa, rectal mucosa, pelvic and/or bilateral regional node metastasis
T3 N2 M0	
T4 any N M0	
Stage IVB	
Any T	Any distant metastasis including
Any N, M1	pelvic lymph nodes

Rules for Clinical Staging
The rules for staging are similar to those for carcinoma of the cervix

TNM Classification of Carcinoma of the Vulva

T	Primary tumor
Tis	Preinvasive carcinoma (carcinoma in situ)
T1	Tumor confined to the vulva and/or perineum; <2 cm in greatest dimension
T2	Tumor confined to the vulva and/or perineum; >2 cm in greatest dimension
T3	Tumor of any size with adjacent spread to the urethra and/or vagina and/or to the anus
T4	Tumor of any size infiltrating the bladder mucosa and/or the rectal mucosa, including the upper part of the urethral mucosa and/or fixed to the bone
N	Regional lymph nodes
N0	No lymph node metastasis
N1	Unilateral regional lymph node metastasis
N2	Bilateral regional lymph node metastasis
M	Distant metastasis
M0	No clinical metastasis
M1	Distant metastasis (including pelvic lymph node metastasis)

though its exact incidence is unknown. One-half to two-thirds of patients with vaginal CIS will have an antecedent or coexistent neoplasm of the lower genital tract. Approximately 1 to 2% of patients who undergo hysterectomy for cervical CIS and many patients who undergo radiation therapy for other gynecologic malignancy will ultimately develop CIS of the upper vagina. This is one of the arguments for yearly Pap smears after hysterectomy. The importance of vaginal CIS is its potential for progression to invasive vaginal carcinoma, as the lesions themselves are usually asymptomatic and have no intrinsic morbidity.

CIS of the vagina must be differentiated from other causes of red ulcerated or white hyperplastic lesions of the vagina such as herpes, traumatic lesions, hyperkeratosis associated with chronic irritation (e.g., from a poorly fitting diaphragm), or adenosis. Inspection and palpation of the vagina are the mainstays of diagnosis, but unfortunately, this is often done in a cursory fashion during the routine pelvic examination. Pap smears of the vaginal mucosa are sometimes rewarding, although

Table 41.4
Clinical Staging of Vaginal Carcinoma

Stage	Description
0	Carcinoma in situ
I	Carcinoma limited to the vaginal mucosa
II	Carcinoma involving the subvaginal tissue but not extending onto the pelvic wall
III	Carcinoma extending onto the pelvic wall
IV	Carcinoma extending into the mucosa of the bladder or rectum or distant metastases

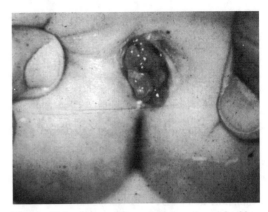

Figure 41.2. Sarcoma botryoides in a 6-month-old child. The grape-like polypoid tumors protruding through the vaginal introitus are asymptomatic, except for a slight bloody discharge.

colposcopy with directed biopsy is the definitive diagnostic maneuver, just as it is in cervical intraepithelial neoplasia.

The goals of treatment of CIS of the vagina are ablation of the intraepithelial lesion while preserving vaginal depth, caliber, and sexual function. Laser ablation, local excision, and chemical treatment with 5-fluorouracil cream (Efudex 5%) are all used for limited lesions; total or partial vaginectomy with application of a split thickness skin graft is usually reserved for failure of the previously described treatments. Cure rates of 80 to 95% may be expected.

Invasive Vaginal Cancer

Invasive vaginal cancer accounts for about 1 to 2% of gynecologic malignancies. *Squamous cell carcinoma* makes up about 95% of these malignancies, occurring primarily in women over 55 years old. The remainder of vaginal carcinomas consist of *adenocarcinoma of the vagina (clear cell adenocarcinoma, usually related to diethylstilbesterol [DES] exposure before 18 weeks gestation while in utero) and vaginal melanoma.*

The staging of vaginal carcinoma is nonsurgical (Table 41.4). Radiation therapy is the mainstay of treatment for squamous cell carcinoma of the vagina, with radical hysterectomy combined with upper vaginectomy and pelvic lymphadenectomy being used for selected patients with upper vaginal lesions and pelvic exenteration and radical vulvectomy being used for selected patients with lower vaginal lesions involving the vulva. Most young women with clear cell carcinoma have lesions located in the upper one-half of the vagina and wish to maintain ovarian and vaginal function. Radical hysterectomy with upper vaginectomy combined with pelvic lymphadenectomy is often the primary treatment for

these patients, with radiation therapy following. The overall 5-year survival rate for squamous cell carcinoma of the vagina is 50% and for clear cell adenocarcinoma of the vagina, 80%, with stage I and II patients having the best prognosis. Melanoma is treated with radical surgery; radiation and chemotherapy have little efficacy.

Sarcoma botryoides (or embryonal rhabdomyosarcoma) presents as a mass of grape-like polyps arising from the undifferentiated mesenchyme of the lamina propria of the anterior vaginal wall and protrudes from the introitus of very young girls and infants (Fig. 42.2). There is often an associated bloody discharge in these frightening tumors. The tumor spreads locally, although it may have distant hematogenous metastases. This tumor was treated in the past with pelvic exenteration, but because this procedure was so unpalatable in this age group, wide excision combined with chemotherapy is often used in an attempt to salvage as much bowel and bladder function as possible.

CASE STUDIES

Case 41A

A 72-year-old woman comes in with a complaint of vulvar itching for the past 8 months. This has become progressively worse over the last 2 months to the point where it awakens her two or three times at night as she finds herself scratching unconsciously. Her past gynecologic history is unremarkable. She underwent normal menopause in her early 50s and is on no chronic medication. Her general health is excellent.

Examination reveals external genitalia that are somewhat atrophic as appropriate for her age. Circumferentially around the inner aspect of the labia majora, the lateral aspect of the labia minora, and the skin over the clitoral hood there is a diffuse whitish epithelial change. This coalesces in the perineal body and extends to within a centimeter of the anal verge. Scattered throughout this area are patches of what appear to be hyperkeratotic skin in the perineal body and some isolated excoriation presumably secondary to her scratching. The remainder of the gynecologic examination is normal.

Question Case 41A

What is the next step in the management of this patient?

A. Administer topical testosterone propionate
B. Administer topical corticosteroid cream
C. Administer topical antifungal preparations
D. Administer Benadryl at bedtime
E. Perform directed vulvar biopsy(ies)

Answer: E

This case illustrates a postmenopausal patient with inflammation of the vulva secondary to one of the so-called vulvar dystrophies. Since the histologic variation is unclear and since intraepithelial neoplasia cannot be ruled out by gross examination, it is mandatory to perform a vulvar biopsy in this patient. If the entire lesion is homogeneous and a single biopsy would be representative, this is probably adequate. If on the other hand, as with this patient, there are areas of heterogeneity (hyperkeratosis and/or ulceration or excoriation), two or three biopsies may be warranted to make the diagnosis.

Application of the appropriate medication and/or surgical treatment can then be offered after histologic verification of the problem.

Case 41B

A 67-year-old patient presents to the office having noticed a "sore" on her vulva. She has been aware of this for approximately 8 months but has not come in hoping it would go away. Currently, it is bleeding slightly and is irritated by her underclothing. Vulvar examination reveals a 1 x 1 cm slightly raised but "cratered lesion" in the posterior left labium majus. There are no other apparent abnormalities. Examination of her groin reveals two "marble size" lymph nodes in her left inguinal ligament area.

Question Case 41B

The most likely diagnosis is

A. Epidermoid carcinoma of the vulva
B. Chancroid
C. Amelanotic melanoma
D. Granuloma inguinale
E. Lymphogranuloma venereum

Answer: A

Given the patient's age and physical findings, she most probably has squamous cell carcinoma of the vulva. This is suggested by an exophytic but cratered lesion in the posterior two-thirds of the vulva with a highly suspicious groin examination. It is mandatory in this patient to obtain one or two vulvar biopsies at the margin of the puckered epithelium to confirm the diagnosis.

chapter 42

CERVICAL NEOPLASIA AND CARCINOMA

Cervical carcinoma serves as the model of a "controllable" cancer, controllable in the sense that (*a*) there is an identifiable precursor lesion (cervical intraepithelial neoplasia; CIN) with a natural history of usually slow progression to frank cervical cancer, (*b*) there is a cheap and noninvasive screening test (Pap smear) and a follow-up diagnostic procedure (colposcopy) for diagnosis, and (*c*) there are simple and effective treatments of the precursor lesion (cryotherapy, laser ablation, LEEP excision, and cold knife cone biopsy) with high cure rates.

Because it is usually possible to identify and treat the asymptomatic precursor lesion, cervical cancer is now the second rather than the first most common malignancy in women. Furthermore, with improved treatment of cervical cancer when disease progression has gone beyond the precursor lesion, cure rates of up to 90% are seen in early stage disease (stages IA and IB) and increased life expectancy is seen in advanced stage disease. The salubrious effect of these interventions is graphically seen in the fall in the mortality rate for cervical cancer compared with that of ovarian carcinoma, for which no treatable precursor lesion can be easily identified (Fig. 42.1).

Of the means by which the "control" of CIN/cervical cancer has occurred, the annual Pap smear is most important. The recognition of the 1 to 10% of Pap smears that are abnormal and their appropriate evaluation and treatment before progression to cancer make one of the great success stories of modern medicine. In the years to come, it is hoped that similar progress will be made in further identification of the causes of CIN/cervical cancer and development of a preventive treatment.

In this chapter, we review the natural history, evaluation, and treatment of CIN and cervical cancer, with special attention to the precursor lesion CIN and its early recognition, a responsibility of all physicians who see women for primary care.

Within the clinical context, certain *epidemiologic factors* relating to cervical neoplasia must be kept in mind (Table 42.1). It should be remembered that these factors represent epidemiologic characteristics and, in any given patient, individual factors may not apply. Of the factors listed, special emphasis should be placed on those factors relating to early sexual intercourse with multiple partners; the role of cigarette smoking; male factors, including the "high-risk" consort; immunologically deprived patients, such as those who are receiving immunosuppressive therapy; and of particular note, human papilloma virus.

CERVICAL INTRAEPITHELIAL NEOPLASIA

Pathology: The Squamocolumnar Junction

An understanding of the pathophysiology of CIN and its association with the *squamocolumnar junction* and *transformation zone* of the cervix is necessary to understand the rationale behind cervical Pap smear screening, diagnostic colposcopy, and the treatment of CIN. As the uterus and cervix grow during puberty and adolescence, the original squamocolumnar junction (SCJ) "rolls out," or everts, from its position just inside the cervical os to a position on the enlarged cervical surface. In this process, original columnar endocervical tissue is also rolled to the cervical surface. This fleshy, reddened tissue area is often misnamed erosion (as it looks like a pathologic, or eroded, tissue), although it is actually normal endocervical tissue in a new location. This area is exposed to vaginal

423

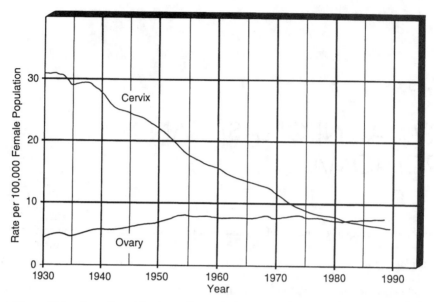

Figure 42.1. Age-adjusted death rate for cervical cancer in the United States, 1930–1987.

Table 42.1.
Potential Factors in Cervical Neoplasia

Epidemiologic characteristics	Other Factors
Early intercourse	Immune status
Multiple sex partners	Oral contraceptives
Early childbearing	Cigarette smoking
Male factors:	Intrauterine DES
"high-risk" consort	exposure
Socioeconomic status,	
race	Viral relations
Venereal infection	Papilloma virus

secretions and irritants and to a changing hormonal milieu, and the process of squamous metaplasia begins as a new squamocolumnar junction is formed farther inward from the old one.

The area between the old and new squamocolumnar junctions, where squamous metaplasia occurs, is called the transformation zone. In the menopausal years, the uterus and cervix again decrease in size, and the new SCJ comes to lie upward into the endocervical canal, often out of direct visual contact (Fig. 42.2).

In certain patients, *carcinogen exposure* may cause an abnormal maturation process at the transformation zone and begin the process of intraepithelial neoplasia. *Approximately 95% of squamous intraepithelial neoplasia occurs within the transformation zone.* Although the carcinogenicity of most suspected

carcinogens remains unproven, certain agents are known to be associated with the development of dysplasia (abnormal growth, in this case CIN). These include *cigarette smoke* (secreted through the endocervical glandular mucus), undefined factors transmitted through intercourse at a young age when the transformation zone is immature, and the human papilloma virus (HPV). Although it is unclear if HPV is a direct cervical carcinogen, *it is clear that HPV of certain types (16, 18, 31, 33, 35, 39, 45, 51, 52, 56, or 58) is closely associated with the development of dysplasia.* It is speculated that HPV may serve as a cofactor in the abnormal maturation and mitotic process of the epithelial cells. A distinct rise in the incidence of intraepithelial neoplasia in association with cytologic confirmation of HPV is well known.

Large-scale studies that have specifically searched for HPV in the genital tract squamous epithelium have revealed the high prevalence of the virus. *As many as 50 to 60% of young college-age women who have been screened with this technique have been shown to have HPV in the absence of specific cytologic changes or gross condyloma.* This suggests that other factors besides the presence of the papilloma virus are important for the genesis of intraepithelial neoplasia.

Currently, the role of DNA detection by the use of relatively simple office kits is of unproven value when used as part of the cytologic screening

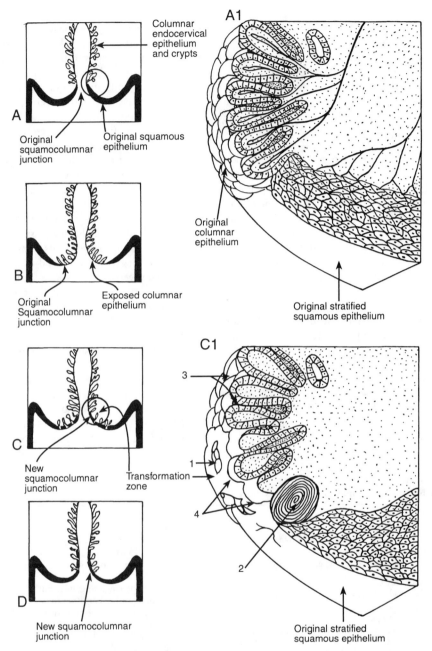

Figure 42.2. Squamocolumnar junction and transformation zone. **A,** Before puberty and adolescence, the original SCJ is at or just above the external os, with the original squamous epithelium being outside and the original columnar endocervical epithelium, inside. **A1,** Three-dimensional representation of the original SCJ. **B,** As the cervix matures and grows, the original SCJ rolls outward, followed by endocervical columnar epithelium, which is now exposed to the vagina and its contents. **C,** As the endocervical tissue is exposed and comes under the influence of mature hormone levels, the process of squamous metaplasia occurs, with a new SCJ forming inward from the old one. The area in between is the transformation zone, the site of this squamous metaplasia. **C1,** Three-dimensional representation of mature SCJ, showing islets of columnar epithelium (*1*), nabothian cyst (*2*), gland openings (*3*), and metaplastic epithelium (*4*). **D,** In menopause, the process reverses, and the new SCJ rolls inward to lie at or above the cervical os, often out of direct visual observation.

process. Limited reports suggest that in selected patients, particularly those at high risk for infection, DNA typing may be of some benefit in identifying the so-called high-risk viruses, particularly types 16, 18, and 31. Routine DNA typing of genital squamous epithelium is not recommended at this time.

Screening: The Pap Smear

During the early 1940s, George Papanicolaou developed a method to examine single-cell morphology based on an exfoliative cell specimen scraped from the cervix at the time of routine pelvic examination. The accuracy of this cytologic assessment by *Pap smear* depends on a number of factors, including the degree of cervical inflammation and concomitant infection, which may obscure early dysplastic changes; adequacy of the specimen obtained; and expeditious fixation of the specimen on the glass slide to avoid air-drying cytologic artifacts. Currently, the most accurate samples are obtained by using both the cervical spatula and the endocervical brush.

At the present time, the American College of Obstetricians and Gynecologists (ACOG) recommends obtaining the *first Pap smear at the time a woman becomes sexually active or by the age of 18 and yearly thereafter.* Reasons cited for these recommendations include the ease with which the Pap

smear is obtained, the improvement in the morbidity and mortality from CIN and cervical cancer associated with Pap smear screening, and the health promotion benefits of the examination. However, the indications and frequency for obtaining a Pap smear have been questioned by other professional groups. They suggest that low-risk patients (defined as women who have had three consecutive normal Pap smears, who have become sexually active after the age of 25, and who have had only one sexual partner) may have intervals of Pap smear screening of up to 3 years. Those who advocate this delayed interval as more appropriately cost-effective cite the observation that cervical intraepithelial neoplasia is generally a slowly progressing process in its transformation to more severe degrees of CIN and to frank cervical cancer. However, in most office settings the performance of the Pap smear at the time of an annual examination remains the accepted standard of care.

Pap smear classification is confusing because different classification systems are in current use. The most common systems are the *class system* (class I to V); the cervical intraepithelial neoplasia system, or *CIN system*, which provides a description of the degree of abnormality (CIN I to CIN III); and a more recently advocated convention, which describes squamous intraepithelial le-

---

Table 42.2.
The 1991 Bethesda System: Categories of Reported Information

Adequacy of the specimen	Intrauterine devices
Satisfactory for evaluation	Other
Satisfactory for evaluation but limited by (specify reason)	Epithelial cell abnormalities
	Squamous cells
Unsatisfactory for evaluation (specify reason)	Atypical squamous cells of undetermined significance
Descriptive diagnoses	Low-grade squamous intraepithelial lesion, encompassing HPV, mild dysplasia/CIN I
Benign cellular changes	High-grade squamous intraepithelial lesion, encompassing moderate and severe dysplasia, carcinoma in situ/CIN II and CIN III
Infection	
Trichomonas vaginalis	Squamous cell carcinoma
Fungal organisms morphologically consistent with *Candida* sp.	Glandular cells
	Endometrial cells, cytologically benign, in a postmenopausal woman
Predominance of coccobacilli consistent with shift in vaginal flora	Atypical glandular cells of undetermined significance
Bacterial morphologically consistent with *Actinomyces* sp.	Endocervical adenocarcinoma
Cellular changes associated with herpes simplex virus	Endometrial carcinoma
	Extrauterine adenocarcinoma
Reactive changes	Adenocarcinoma, not otherwise specified
Reactive cellular changes associated with:	Other malignant neoplasms (specify)
Inflammation (includes typical repair)	
Atrophy with inflammation ("atrophic vaginitis")	
Radiation	

Table 42.3.
Comparisons of Pap Smear Descriptive Conventions

Descriptive Convention						
Class system	Class I (normal)	Class II inflammation	Class III — Mild dysplasia	Class III — Moderate dysplasia	Class IV severe dysplasia CIS[a]	Class V suggestive of cancer or CIS[a]
CIN system	Normal	Inflammatory	CIN I *or*	CIN II	CIN III	Suggestive of cancer
Bethesda system	Within normal limits	Inflammatory a. Without atypia b. With atypia or cellular changes associated with HPV	Low grade SIL	High grade SIL	High grade SIL	Squamous cell cancer

Histology — Basal cells — Basement membrane — WBCs[a] — Invasive cervical cancer

[a]CIS, carcinoma in situ; WBCs, white blood cells.

sions, the *SIL system.* This most recent convention is also called the Bethesda system and was designed to provide an evaluation of the adequacy of the Pap smear preparation and a description of the cells found rather than just a classification without further identification of the abnormality. Within this system, lesions are described as "low-grade SIL" (LGSIL) and "high-grade SIL" (HGSIL). In addition, when cellular architecture suggests the involvement of human papilloma virus, this description is added to either the low-grade or the high-grade SIL description. Table 42.2 lists the information that can be obtained and the order in which it is reported in the Bethesda system. Currently, the class and CIN systems are still widely used, although many advocate conversion to the Bethesda system, which is being adopted by more and more cytological laboratories. Table 42.3 compares and contrasts the three systems.

Because of the evolution to a more standard reporting mechanism using the Bethesda system, there is concern about this transitional time in the application of these descriptive changes. This is coupled with the fact that not all laboratories are willing to accept the new classification system. As a result, many investigators are concerned that the new classification system "overreads" nonneoplastic epithelial cell abnormalities and thus obligates the clinician to unindicated and expensive follow-up, including unnecessary colposcopy and conization of the cervix.

The basis for these classification systems is the likelihood of the progression of precursor lesions to more advanced degrees of cervical intraepithelial neoplasia and eventually to carcinoma. Generally, more severe intraepithelial lesions progress more quickly, whereas less severe intraepithelial lesions may take as long as 7 to 8 years to progress to carcinoma. The term *dysplasia* is used to describe these intraepithelial cellular abnormalities, including an altered nuclear:cytoplasmic ratio, an increased staining of chromatin material, and other cellular characteristics that suggest a less orderly maturation process. For example, considering all cases of mild dysplasia (CIN I, classes II and III, or low-grade SIL), approximately 65% of these lesions will spontaneously regress, whereas approximately 20% will remain the same, leaving 15% to progress to worsening disease.

Because there is no way to predict which of these lesions is destined to progress and which is not, the predominant school of thought in the United States has been that *further investigation is warranted for even mildly abnormal Pap smears.* This philosophy of management also includes the idea that further investigation is indicated to identify women with disease that is more severe than indi-

Table 42.4.
Management Options for Abnormal Cervical Cytology (Bethesda System)

Bethesda Classification	Management
Atypical squamous cells of undetermined significance (ASCUS)[a]	There are several options, depending on the clinical circumstances and whether the diagnosis of ASCUS was accompanied by further qualification 1. Repeat Pap smear every 4–6 months for 2 years until there are three consecutive negative smears; if a second ASCUS is obtained, colposcopy should be considered 2. If the Pap report of ASCUS is qualified by severe inflammation, any specific infection should be treated and the Pap repeated in 2–3 months 3. ASCUS in a postmenopausal patient should be followed by a course of vaginal estrogen and a repeat Pap smear; if the Pap is still abnormal, colposcopy should be considered 4. If the Pap report of ASCUS is qualified by a statement favoring a neoplastic process, the Pap should be managed as LGSIL 5. If the patient is at special high risk for dysplasia, colposcopy should be considered
Low-grade squamous intraepithelial lesion (LGSIL)	Most LGSIL lesions will revert spontaneously without therapy. Some patients, however, will develop a precancerous lesion, so that several management options exist 1. Repeat Pap smear every 4–6 months for 2 year until there are three consecutive negative smears; if a second abnormality is obtained, colposcopy should be considered 2. Colposcopy with endocervical curettage and directed biopsies as indicated
High-grade squamous intraepithelial lesion (HGSIL)	Colposcopy with endocervical curettage and directed biopsies as indicated
Atypical glandular cells of undetermined significance	The Pap smears subsume a group of situations from exuberant benign reactive changes to adenocarcinoma in situ; each case must be individualized by clinical situation and risk factors; Options include the following 1. Repeat Pap, using endocervical brush 2. Endometrial biopsy 3. Cone biopsy

[a] No more than 5% of Pap smears should be reported as ASCUS. A greater frequency may indicate overuse of the classification. ASCUS does not correspond to the previous terms *inflammatory atypia* and *Class II*.

cated by their screening Pap smear. *Specifically, this investigation involves histologic diagnosis of the nature and grade of dysplasia/carcinoma that is suggested by the screening cytologic evaluation obtained at Pap smear.* This is accomplished by means of colposcopy and directed biopsy or cone biopsy of the cervix.

Recently, it has been pointed out that most mild lesions (LGSIL) regress spontaneously and do not proceed to more severe lesions. Based on this, some suggest that colposcopy and direct biopsy are excessive for these lesions and, instead, that inexpensive repetitive Pap smears will, over time, separate the two groups, identifying those who truly need the more expensive evaluation (Table 42.4). It should be remembered that these are treatment *guidelines only* rather than therapeu-

tic rules. Risks and benefits of both approaches should be assessed to plan diagnosis and treatment on an individual basis.

Histologic Evaluation of the Abnormal Pap Smear

A colposcope is a sophisticated binocular stereomicroscope with variable magnification (usually ×1 to 14) and a variable intensity light source with green filters, which aid in the identification of blood vessels. With *colposcopy*, small, often subtle areas of dysplastic change on the cervix can be evaluated and appropriate sites for biopsy chosen. Colposcopic criteria such as white epithelium, abnormal vascular patterns, and punctate lesions help identify such areas. To facilitate the examination, the cervix is washed with a dilute 3 to 4% acetic acid solution, which also acts as an epithelial desiccant, enhancing visualization of dysplastic lesions, which usually appear with relatively discrete borders at or near the squamocolumnar junction. *Visualization of the entire squamocolumnar junction is required for a satisfactory colposcopic examination,* since approximately 95% of the CIN/cervical cancer will arise in the transformation zone. If the squamocolumnar junction is not visualized in its entirety or if the margins of abnormal areas are not seen in their entirety, the colposcopic assessment is termed *unsatisfactory* and other evaluation is needed. This is the *first reason for cervical conization: unsatisfactory colposcopy.* Conization is described in the section on surgical excision.

The number of colposcopically directed biopsies obtained will vary, depending on the number of abnormal areas found and the severity of the involvement based on colposcopically defined criteria. After sampling the colposcopically identified lesions, an *endocervical curettage* (ECC), using a small curette, is performed. This simple sampling procedure may be performed without cervical dilation. This endocervical sample is obtained so that potential disease farther inside the cervical canal, which is not visualized by the colposcope, may be detected. The cervical biopsies and endocervical curettage are then submitted separately for pathologic assessment. Endocervical curettage will be positive for dysplasia in 5 to 10% of women with a dysplastic Pap smear. Because of the absence of tissue orientation from endocervical curettings, the degree of dysplasia determined from them is difficult to assess. This is *the second reason for cervical conization: positive endocervical curettage.*

In approximately 10% of colposcopies with directed biopsies and endocervical curettage, there will be a discrepancy between the screening Pap smear and the histologic data from biopsy and ECC, e.g., if the Pap smear is read as severely dysplastic (CIN III or high-grade SIL) and the directed biopsies only show mild dysplasia (CIN I or low-grade SIL). Directed biopsy of the cervix should vary no more than one grade with the reference Pap smear. When a "two-step" discrepancy occurs, further tissue diagnosis by cervical conization is necessary so that the most severe abnormality can be explained histologically. By obtaining the cone-shaped biopsy of the entire squamocolumnar junction and identified lesions as well as a portion of the endocervical canal, the pathologist can determine the most severe lesions by histologic, hence diagnostic, criteria. Often, the cone biopsy may prove to be therapeutic as well as diagnostic, since the entire lesion is removed. This is *the third indication for cervical conization: a two-step discrepancy between Pap smear and biopsy results.*

Cervical conization, or cone biopsy of the cervix, is a minor surgical procedure performed under general or regional anesthesia. Usually performed with scalpel and scissors (*cold knife conization, CKC*), conization is now also performed with a laser or with a heated wire loop, the *LLETZ (large loop excision of the transformation zone)* or *LEEP (loop electrosurgical excision procedure).* As seen in Figure 42.3, a cone-shaped specimen is removed from the cervix, which encompasses the SCJ, all identified lesions on the exocervix, and a portion of the endocervical canal, the extent of which depends on whether the ECC was positive or negative. This more extensive specimen allows the pathologist to fully ascertain the extent and severity of disease so that appropriate therapy may be selected.

If the margins of disease cannot be established, the patient will then require either further conization therapy or close follow-up, depending on the severity of the lesions encountered and the wishes of the patient for future childbearing. The risks of the procedure include infection, blood loss, and anesthesia. For women who may want children in

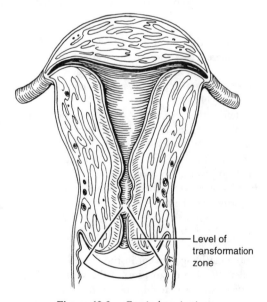

Level of transformation zone

Figure 42.3. Cervical conization.

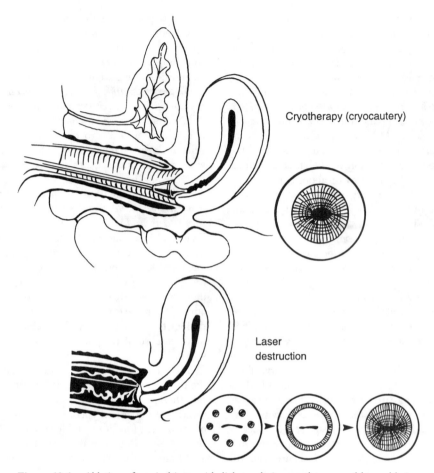

Cryotherapy (cryocautery)

Laser
destruction

Figure 42.4. Ablation of cervical intraepithelial neoplasia: cryotherapy and laser ablation.

the future, there are the additional risks of cervical incompetence, if the internal cervical os is compromised, and reduced cervical capacity to facilitate sperm transport, because of loss of mucus-secreting glands.

Before the advent of colposcopic evaluation of abnormal Pap smears, most patients with abnormal screening Pap smears were destined to undergo cervical conization, necessitating an anesthetic and brief hospitalization. Colposcopy in the clinic setting has eliminated the need for conization in the majority of patients.

Treatment

The underlying concept in the treatment of CIN is that excision or ablation of the superficial precursor lesion will avoid progression to carcinoma. Because these lesions are superficial and usually

confined to the visible and easily accessible SCJ, simple office techniques that require minimal or no anesthesia and that have little risk usually suffice. Controversy exists about the appropriateness of specific therapies for lesions of different severity and extent; ongoing research is designed to determine optimal therapies for each situation.

Cryocautery is a popular outpatient method used to treat low-grade CIN. The procedure involves covering the SCJ and all identified lesions with a "mushroom-tipped" stainless-steel probe, which is then supercooled with circulating liquid nitrogen or carbon dioxide. The size and shape of the probe depends on the size and shape of the cervix. The most commonly employed freezing technique involves a 3-min freeze followed by a 5-min thaw, with a repeat 3-min freeze (Fig. 42.4). The thaw period between the two freezing episodes allows the damaged tissue from the first freeze to become edematous and swell with intracellular fluid. With the second freeze, the edematous cellular architecture is refrozen and extends the damaged area slightly deeper into the tissue. Healing after cryotherapy may take up to 4 or 5 weeks, since the damaged tissue slowly sloughs and is replaced by new cervical epithelium. This process is associated with profuse watery discharge often mixed with necrotic cellular debris. It can be assumed that the entire healing process has been completed within 2 months, and usually, the next follow-up Pap smear is done 12 weeks following the freezing to ascertain the effectiveness of the procedure. The cure rates for low-grade cervical intraepithelial neoplasia using this technique approach 90%.

More recently, colposcopically directed *laser therapy* has been employed to ablate lesions involving cervical intraepithelial neoplasia. Because of the precision imparted by the colposcopic direction of the fine laser beam as well as the precise control of depth of ablation available by varying the laser beam's power and width, many physicians prefer laser ablation to "less precise" techniques. Each lesion may be addressed separately and ablated. In addition, ablation of the entire SCJ is often performed (see Fig. 42.4). Although the technology is more sophisticated than cryocautery, long-term cure rates with this technique are similar to that for cryocautery. An advantage of laser therapy is that it can be used for high-grade intraepithelial lesions, because the depth of ablation can be adjusted to accommodate the extent of the lesion.

On occasion, low-grade epithelial lesions involving only focal areas of the squamocolumnar junction are treated by *excisional biopsy* performed at the time of colposcopy. There are no data comparing the outcomes of this therapy to limited lesion ablation by either laser or cryocautery.

The most commonly employed technique of surgical excision is cervical conization. Cervical conization can be done for diagnostic purposes. If an entire lesion is removed (i.e., the lesion margins are clear), the procedure may also be therapeutic. This is especially valuable for women who wish future pregnancy. An alternative to conization is excision of the cone by hot wire loop, the LLETZ procedure, performed in the office setting. Long-term follow-up data of this treatment modality are not yet available, although preliminary findings are promising.

Advocates of this technique cite less marginal tissue destruction, making pathologic assessment

more reliable; less postoperative bleeding; better visualization of the regenerated squamocolumnar junction; and ease of performance with attendant decreased costs.

Follow-Up to Treatment

Patients who have been treated for cervical intraepithelial neoplasia need to be followed more frequently than patients presenting for annual health examinations. The patient is usually advised to return for a follow-up examination and Pap smear in approximately 3 months. At this time, the healing process has been completed, and the generation of new cells from the squamocolumnar junction should be free of inflammation and reparative changes that were caused by the treatment. If a follow-up Pap smear is done too soon after ablative or excisional treatment, it may be misinterpreted because of the abnormal-appearing cellular architecture resulting from the healing process. The patient usually receives repeat Pap smear assessment at 3-month intervals for 1 year and then at 6-month intervals for the 2nd year. If Pap smears remain normal, patients may resume having annual Pap smear assessments beginning the 3rd year. However, these patients should be counseled that they are at greater risk for recurrent abnormalities of the Pap smear and should be encouraged to avail themselves of annual health care checkups to include the Pap smear.

CERVICAL CARCINOMA

Until approximately 10 years ago, cervical cancer was the most common gynecologic malignancy, with a ratio of 2:1 over endometrial carcinoma. Now the cervical carcinoma:endometrial carcinoma ratio has almost reversed; endometrial carcinoma rates are twice that for invasive cervical carcinoma. Approximately 16,000 new cases of invasive cervical carcinoma are diagnosed annually.

The average age at diagnosis for invasive cervical cancer is approximately 50, although the disease may occur in the very young as well as the very old patient. In studies following patients with advanced cervical intraepithelial neoplasia, this precursor lesion precedes invasive carcinoma by approximately 10 years. In some patients, however, this time of progression may be considerably less; for still other patients, cervical cancer may not be preceded by CIN at all.

The *etiology* of cervical cancer is unknown. There is ample evidence that advanced *cervical in-*

traepithelial neoplasia arising in the squamous epithelium of the cervical transformation zone will often progress to invasive squamous cell cervical carcinoma. Similarly, the *human papilloma virus* has been implicated as an etiologic cofactor in the development of cervical carcinoma. Studies involving genetic probes have identified papilloma virus DNA fragments within areas of invasive cervical carcinoma. Other etiologic associations are also similar to those for CIN, including *factors related to the male ejaculate, the immature transformation zone, the number of different sexual partners, and cigarette smoking. Immunocompromised patients* (e.g., transplant patients or patients with HIV infection) are a special group who seem more susceptible to this disease.

About 85% of cervical cancer is of the squamous cell variety. Approximately 15% of cervical cancers are adenocarcinomas, arising from the endocervical glands.

Three rare types of cervical cancer are also encountered: *clear cell carcinoma* associated with diethylstilbestrol (DES) exposure in utero, *sarcoma*, and *lymphoma*. In general, the evaluation and treatment of squamous cell and adenocarcinoma

of the cervix are similar. The discussions that follow reflect this similarity and apply to these two most common cervical carcinomas.

Survival rates for cervical carcinoma reflect the extent of disease at the time of diagnosis. Stage I has more than 91% 5-year survival, whereas 5-year survival for stages IIA, IIIA, and IV are 83, 45, and 14%, respectively.

Clinical Evaluation

There is *no classic historical presentation* for cervical cancer. Two symptoms are often associated with cervical carcinoma, although both have other more common causes: *postcoital bleeding and abnormal uterine bleeding*. Other symptoms are determined by the organs or organ systems involved as the cancer spreads, and hence by the pattern of spread: direct invasion to contiguous structures and by lymphatics to distant sites of metastasis.

Visible lesions on the cervix should be biopsied. Lesions that should be considered for immediate biopsy include all new exophytic, friable, or bleeding lesions. These are readily differentiated from more common, normal variations of cervical anatomy such as nabothian cysts or condylomata. Pap

Table 42.5.
Clinical Stages of Carcinoma of the Cervix Uteri[a]

Stage	Characteristics
I	Carcinoma is strictly confined to cervix (extension to corpus should be disregarded)
IA	Preclinical carcinoma
IA1	Minimal microscopically evident stromal invasion
IA2	Microscopic lesions no more than 5 mm depth measured from base of epithelium surface or glandular from which it originates; horizontal spread not to exceed 7 mm
IB	All other cases of stage I: occult cancer should be marked "occ"
II	Carcinoma extends beyond cervix but has not extended to pelvic wall; involves vagina but not as far as lower third
IIA	No obvious parametrial involvement
IIB	Obvious parametrial involvement
III	Carcinoma has extended to pelvic wall; on rectal examination there is no cancer-free space between tumor and pelvic wall; tumor involves lower third of vagina; all cases with hydronephrosis or nonfunctioning kidney should be included, unless they are known to have another cause
IIIA	No extension to pelvic wall, but involvement of lower third of vagina
IIIB	Extension to pelvic wall, hydronephrosis, or nonfunctioning kidney caused by tumor
IV	Carcinoma has extended beyond true pelvis or has clinically involved mucosa of bladder or rectum
IVA	Spread of growth to adjacent pelvic organs
IVB	Spread to distant organs

[a] FIGO, revised 1985.

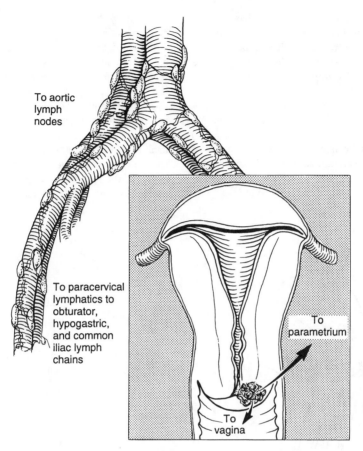

To aortic lymph nodes

To paracervical lymphatics to obturator, hypogastric, and common iliac lymph chains

To parametrium

To vagina

Figure 42.5. Spread patterns of cervical carcinoma.

smears are sometimes negative in this situation because exfoliative cells from frank cancer may be so distorted as to be uninterpretable. When a visible lesion is present, colposcopic assessment need not be done unless the results of the direct biopsy do not confirm cancer.

The *clinical staging of cervical carcinoma is the process by which the severity and extent of disease are assessed so that appropriate therapy may be undertaken*. Staging is based on the International Federation of Gynecology and Obstetrics (FIGO) Staging Classification of 1985 (Table 42.5). This is a convention based both on the histologic assessment of the tumor sample and on physical examination and laboratory study to ascertain the extent of disease. It is useful because of the very predictable manner in which *cervical carcinoma spreads by direct invasion and by lymphatic metastasis*.

Cervical carcinoma spreads through the cervical and paracervical lymphatics, through the parametria, and into the regional lymph nodes. Cervical carcinoma also spreads by direct extension proximal into the endocervical canal or distally into the vagina. In patients with primary lymphatic spread, the ascent of disease from the regional lymph glands proceeds to the deep pelvic nodes, including the external and internal iliac node chain, the common iliac node chain, and periaortic node chain (Fig. 42.5). Accordingly, advanced stages include a description of tumor beyond the cervix, into the vagina or parametria (stage II); directly to the lateral pelvic wall or the lower third of the vagina (stage III); or widespread disease, including but not limited to the bladder or rectum (stage IV).

Other studies that may be used in staging include intravenous pyelography and cystoscopy, proctosigmoidoscopy or barium enema, blood chemistries with emphasis on liver and renal function, and computed tomography studies on a selective basis. Computed tomography has been of special value in evaluating the extent of lymphatic involvement, given the difficulty in performing and interpreting bipedal lymphangiography, the other procedure used in some institutions for this evaluation.

Management

Once there has been histologic confirmation of invasive cervical carcinoma, it is imperative to refer the patient to a gynecologic oncologist for appropriate surgical and/or radiation therapy.

The mainstays of treatment for invasive cervical carcinoma include *radical surgical therapy and/or pelvic irradiation.* In general, surgical therapy is indicated for most patients with stage I disease and selected patients with stage II disease, because of the limited yet predictable extent of spread in these early stages. *Radical surgical therapy* includes radical hysterectomy aimed at removing all of the central disease, i.e., disease not only in the cervix itself but in all the adjacent paracervical, parametrial, and vaginal tissue. In addition, surgical eradication of the local and regional lymph nodes is an important part of radical surgical therapy (pelvic

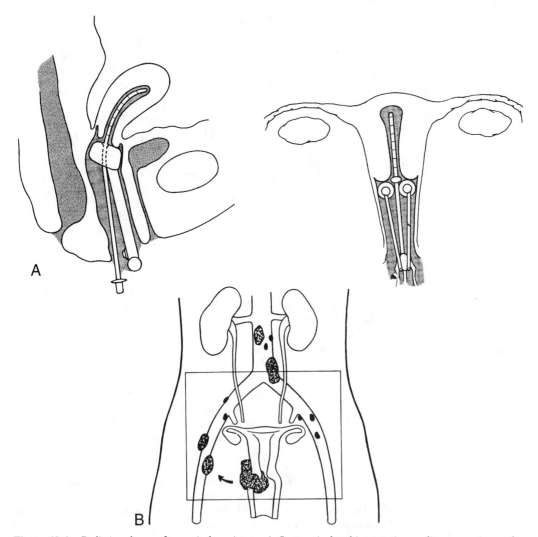

Figure 42.6. Radiation therapy for cervical carcinoma. **A,** Intravaginal and intrauterine applicators are inserted to irradiate the cervix, vagina, and uterus. **B,** External beam radiation is used along the paths of lymphatic spread of the tumor.

Table 42.6.
5-Year Survival for Treated Cervical Carcinoma

FIGO Stage	5-Year Survival (Percent)
0	100
IA	99
IB	85–90
IIA	73–80
IIB	68
IIIA	45
IIIB	36
IVA	15
IVB	2

lymphadenectomy). The presence or absence of tumor in the lymph nodes sampled defines, in part, the extent of disease and the need for further therapy, either radiation therapy or perhaps chemotherapy. It should be emphasized that simple hysterectomy with removal of the cervix is inadequate treatment for invasive cervical carcinoma. In young women who are treated surgically, ovarian preservation is usually advisable to provide the patient with the long-term benefits from endogenous estrogen secretion. Ovarian retention presents no additional risk to the patient, since cervical carcinoma neither spreads through the adnexal structures nor is estrogen dependent.

Radiation therapy is reserved for patients with stage IB or IIA disease who are poor surgical candidates and for all patients with more advanced disease. The basis for radiation therapy in more advanced disease is the likelihood for more extensive regional nodal involvement. Even with stage III disease extending to the lateral pelvic wall, approximately one-third of patients will be cured with primary radiation therapy. Both high-dose external beam therapy and intracavitary irradiation are used for most patients. Intrauterine and intravaginal applicators containing radioactive materials are placed to direct treatment of the uterus, cervix, and vagina as needed, and external beam radiation is applied primarily along the paths of lymphatic extension of cervical carcinoma (Fig. 42.6).

Fortunately, the adjacent nongynecologic structures, such as the bladder and distal colon,

tolerate these treatments fairly well, without significant untoward effects. Radiation therapy doses are calculated by individual patient needs to maximize radiation to the tumor sites and potential spread areas, while minimizing the amount of radiation to adjacent uninvolved tissues. *Complications of radiation therapy* include radiation cystitis and proctitis, which are usually relatively easy to manage when appropriate radiation doses have been calculated. Other more unusual complications include intestinal fistula, small bowel obstruction, or difficult to manage hemorrhagic proctitis or cystitis. It should be remembered that the tissue damage and fibrosis incurred by radiation therapy progresses over many years, and that these effects may complicate long-term management.

Most authorities believe that radical surgical excision and pelvic lymphadenectomy offer distinct advantages over radiation therapy for earlier stage disease. These include the potential for preservation of ovarian function in young women, preservation of sexual function, and avoidance of long-term radiation effects. On the other hand, certain operative complications such as hemorrhage, damage to local nerves supplying the bladder, and urinary vaginal fistula may develop from radical pelvic surgery. It is important for the risks and benefits of each form of therapy to be explained to the patient, and treatment should be performed based on individual patient selection.

Follow-up of patients with cervical carcinoma is best done by gynecologic oncologists who will use established protocols. Most oncology centers will follow patients in a specialized clinic for at least 5 years. When there is recurrence, 90% will reoccur within this time period. The 5-year survival for various stages of cervical carcinoma are shown in Table 42.6.

Treatment for recurrent disease is associated with poor cure rates. Most chemotherapeutic protocols have only limited usefulness and are reserved for palliative efforts. Likewise, specific "spot" radiation to areas of recurrence also provides only limited benefit. Occasional patients with central recurrence—i.e., recurrence of disease in the upper vagina or the residual cervix and uterus in radiation patients—may benefit from ultraradical surgery with partial or total pelvic exenteration. These candidates are few, but when properly selected, may benefit from this aggressive therapy.

CASE STUDIES

Case 42A

A 24-year-old college student, G1 P0010, presents for her annual pelvic examination and Pap smear and renewal of her oral contraceptive. History and physical examination are unremarkable. Her Pap smear is subsequently reported as HGSIL.

Questions Case 42A

The most appropriate next step in this patient's management is

A. Repeat Pap smear in 1 year
B. Repeat Pap smear now
C. Colposcopy with ECC and directed biopsy
D. Excisional biopsy
E. Cervical conization

Answer: C

HGSIL on screening examination requires histologic diagnosis so that appropriate treatment can be selected. Repeat Pap smear is another screening test and is thus inappropriate. Conization for diagnostic purposes is needed only if colposcopy and biopsy prove inadequate.

The colposcopy was satisfactory with areas of whitened epithelium. Subsequently, the ECC done at colposcopy was reported as negative as were the two biopsies that were taken. The most appropriate next step in this patient's management is

A. Repeat Pap smear in 1 year
B. Repeat Pap smear now
C. Colposcopy with ECC and directed biopsy
D. Excisional biopsy
E. Cervical conization

Answer: E

There is a two-step discrepancy between the screening Pap smear (high-grade SIL) and diagnostic biopsy results ("normal"), i.e., the source of the original abnormal Pap smear has yet to be found. This must be resolved before appropriate therapy can be suggested. Conization is appropriate and may, in addition, be curative.

A conization is performed and subsequently reported as three foci of moderate to severe dysplasia without extension beyond the surgical limits. The most appropriate next step in this patient's management is

A. Repeat Pap smear in 3 months
B. Repeat Pap smear now

C. Repeat colposcopy with ECC and directed biopsy
D. Excisional biopsy at four quadrants
E. Repeat cervical conization

Answer: A

The antecedent colposcopy was satisfactory, the conization has uninvolved surgical margins and is reported as CIN II–III, so that the conization has also been therapeutic. Follow-up with Pap smears every 3 months for at least 1 year is indicated, with further evaluation if new cytological abnormalities are discovered.

Case 42B

A 46-year-old mother of four presents with a complaint of postcoital spotting. Her last Pap smear was 2 years ago and was normal. On physical examination, a 1 × 0.5 cm friable mass is found on the anterior lip of her cervix. The remainder of her physical examination is normal.

Questions Case 42B

The most appropriate next step in this patient's management is

A. No further management indicated
B. Pap smear
C. Colposcopy with ECC and directed biopsy
D. Biopsy
E. Cervical conization

Answer: B, D

Both a Pap smear and immediate biopsy are indicated. If cervical carcinoma is discovered, staging and appropriate therapy may be begun immediately. The Pap smear may be unreliable in frank carcinoma and should not be relied on solely in the presence of a grossly visible lesion.

The Pap smear is reported as squamous cell carcinoma. The biopsy is reported as squamous cell carcinoma extending to the margins of the specimen. The most appropriate next step in this patient's management is

A. Radical hysterectomy
B. Radiation therapy
C. Colposcopy with ECC and directed biopsy
D. Repeat excisional biopsy to go past previous biopsy margins
E. Cervical conization

Answer: A or B

Invasive cervical carcinoma has been diagnosed and now requires treatment. Radical hysterectomy or radiation therapy may be indicated, depending on the patient's staging evaluation.

Case 42C

A 24-year-old G0 presents for annual physical examination and renewal of oral contraceptives, which she has used without difficulty since age 15. She has no history of sexually transmitted diseases and reports sexual relations with three partners during her life.

The patient's physical examination is normal and routine screening tests are performed with renewal of her oral contraceptive. The Pap smear is reported as satisfactory, LGSIL without inflammation.

Question Case 42C

The most appropriate next step in this patient's management is

A. No further management indicated
B. Pap smear in 3 to 4 months
C. Colposcopy with ECC and directed biopsy
D. Excisional biopsy
E. Cervical conization

Answer: B or C

Follow-up is required, but there is controversy whether the likelihood that LGSIL will progress warrants repeat Pap smears in 3 months or whether colposcopy is indicated at this time. Either management is correct. More aggressive and/or less focused biopsy for diagnostic purposes is inappropriate.

chapter 43

UTERINE LEIOMYOMA AND NEOPLASIA

Uterine enlargement as a result of leiomyoma (fibroids, myomas) is *common* in clinical practice. It is estimated that up to *30% of American women have these benign tumors,* although the majority do not present with significant symptoms and do not require hysterectomy. Despite this, leiomyomata are the most common indication for hysterectomy, accounting for approximately 30% of all such cases.

Traditionally, leiomyomata account for a large number of more conservative operations including myomectomy, uterine curettage, and operative hysteroscopy. Histologically, these benign tumors represent *localized proliferation of smooth muscle cells surrounded by a pseudocapsule of compressed muscle fibers.* When these tumors are symptomatic, the most *frequent clinical manifestations* include

1. *Pain,* including secondary dysmenorrhea;
2. *Bleeding,* most commonly menorrhagia (increased amount and duration of flow);
3. *Pressure symptoms,* related to the size and number of tumors filling the pelvic cavity; pressure against bladder, bowel, and pelvic floor.

Leiomyoma also represents an important clinical entity since, as *pelvic masses,* there may be a necessity to investigate them as if they were a malignancy. They are considered *hormonally responsive* tumors because the growth potential of these tumors is related to estrogen production, often with rapid growth occurring in the late reproductive or perimenopausal years. Menopause generally brings about cessation of tumor growth and even atrophy.

In 0.1 to 1% of cases, *malignancy* as *leiomyosarcoma* may develop. These are not thought to represent "degeneration" of a fibroid but, rather, a new neoplasm. Malignancy is more typical in older patients, especially postmenopausal patients who present with rapidly enlarging uterine masses and postmenopausal bleeding, unusual vaginal discharge, and pelvic pain. An enlarging uterine mass in a postmenopausal patient should be evaluated with considerably more concern for malignancy than one in a younger woman. Other cell types may be involved in this form of malignancy. These *heterologous* mixed tumors contain other sarcomatous tissue elements not necessarily found only in the uterus.

There are three quite rare variants of apparently benign uterine myomas. All are generally thought to be benign and somewhat estrogen dependent. *Intravenous leiomyomatosis* is described as invasion of the pelvic veins and even vena cava with histologically mature and benign smooth muscle tumor. *Benign metastasizing leiomyoma* has been reported in cardiac, lymphatic, and pulmonary nodules, presumed to be the result of either intravenous or lymphatic embolization. *Leiomyomatosis peritonealis disseminata* involves implants on peritoneal surfaces identical to uterine myomas.

LEIOMYOMAS

Symptoms

The symptoms associated with uterine fibroids frequently lead women to seek medical advice. Although smooth muscle tumors may occur anywhere in the body in women, they most commonly occur within the uterus or as an appendage to the uterus (Fig. 43.1). Gross and histologic changes may occur in uterine fibroids, and historically, these changes have been termed forms of "degeneration." The most common types of change include *red degeneration,* hemorrhagic changes associated with rapid growth; *hyaline degeneration,* hyalinization of the smooth muscle elements, occurring commonly after menopause; *calcification* and calcific replacement of inactive smooth muscle elements, occurring after menopause.

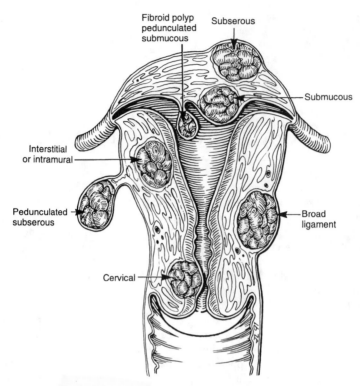

Figure 43.1.   Common types of uterine fibroids.

Bleeding is the most common presenting symptom in uterine fibroids. Although the kind of abnormal bleeding may vary, the most common presentation includes the development of progressively heavier menstrual flow that lasts longer than the normal duration (*menorrhagia*) and is defined as menstrual blood loss of >80 mL. This bleeding may result from significant distortion of the endometrial cavity by the underlying tumor. This contributes to three generally accepted but unproven *mechanisms for increased bleeding:*

1. Alteration of normal myometrial contractile function in the small artery and arteriolar blood supply underlying the endometrium;
2. Inability of the overlying endometrium to respond to the normal estrogen/progesterone menstrual phases, which contribute to efficient sloughing of the endometrium;
3. Pressure necrosis of the overlying endometrial bed, which exposes vascular surfaces that bleed in excess of that normally found with endometrial sloughing.

   Characteristically, the best example of a type of leiomyoma contributing to this bleeding pattern is

the so-called submucous leiomyoma. In this variant, the majority of the distortion created by the smooth muscle tumor projects toward the endometrial cavity rather than toward the serosal surface of the uterus. Enlarging intramural fibroids likewise may contribute to excessive bleeding if they become large enough to significantly distort the endometrial cavity.

Blood loss from this type of menstrual bleeding may be heavy enough to contribute to chronic iron-deficiency anemia and, rarely, to profound acute blood loss. The occurrence of isolated submucous (subendometrial) leiomyomata is unusual. Commonly, these are found in association with other types of leiomyomata (see Fig. 43.1).

Another common presenting complaint from uterine leiomyomata is that of a *progressive increase in "pelvic pressure."* This may be a sense of progressive pelvic fullness, "something pressing down," and/or the sensation of a pelvic mass. Most commonly, this is caused by slowly enlarging intramural or subserous myomas, which on occasion, may attain a massive size (Fig. 43.2). This type of leiomyoma is the most easily palpated on bimanual or abdominal examination and

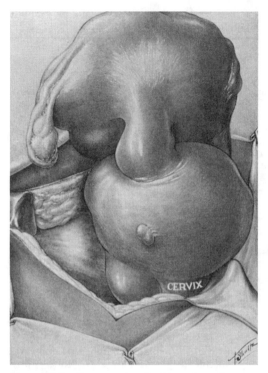

Figure 43.2. Large uterine fibroids at time of abdominal hysterectomy.

contributes to a characteristic "lumpy-bumpy," or cobblestone, sensation when multiple myomas are present. Occasionally, these large myomas present to the physician as a large asymptomatic pelvic or even abdominopelvic mass. Such very large leiomyomas may cause an uncommon but significant clinical problem: pressure on the ureters as they traverse the pelvic brim leading to *hydroureter and on occasion hydronephrosis.*

Another spectrum of presentation includes patients who develop progressively worsening *pelvic pain.* For many patients, this pain is manifest by the onset of secondary dysmenorrhea. Other pain symptoms, although rare, may be the result of rapid enlargement of a leiomyoma, resulting in areas of tissue necrosis or areas of subnecrotic vascular ischemia, which contribute to alteration in myometrial response to prostaglandins similar to the mechanism described for primary dysmenorrhea. Occasionally, torsion of a pedunculated myoma can occur, resulting in acute pain. Dull, intermittent low midline cramping pain is the clinical presentation when a submucous (subendometrial) myoma becomes pedunculated

and progressively prolapses through the internal os of the cervix.

Diagnosis

The *diagnosis* of these tumors is usually made by clinical examination, including abdominal and bimanual palpation, or imaging studies. In addition, irregularities of the uterine cavity can be detected at the time of endometrial curettage. Often the diagnosis is made incidentally by pathologic assessment of a uterine specimen removed for other indications.

When appreciated clinically by *abdominopelvic examination,* uterine leiomyomata have characteristic qualities. These include the presence of a large midline mobile pelvic mass with an irregular contour; the mass usually has a characteristic "hard feel" or solid quality. The degree of enlargement is usually stated in terms (weeks size) that are used to estimate equivalent gestational size. This is often appreciated as separate from adnexal disease, although on *occasion a subserosal pedunculated myoma may be difficult to distinguish from a solid adnexal mass.*

Of the available *imaging studies, pelvic ultrasound* is the most commonly used for confirmation of uterine myomas. The ultrasonographer can demonstrate areas of acoustic shadow hypoechogenicity amid otherwise normal myometrial patterns and can see a distorted endometrial stripe. Although solid leiomyomata share these characteristics, occasionally cystic components may also be seen as hypoechogenic areas and are consistent in appearance with myomas undergoing degeneration. Adnexal structures, including the ovaries, are usually identifiable separate from these masses. This is reassuring information, i.e., the pathology is uterine in nature and not adnexal, which has an associated higher risk of malignancy. Other studies that may be used include *computerized axial tomography and magnetic resonance imaging,* neither of which is cost-effective in diagnosing uterine myomas. They are expensive, time-consuming tests that usually give no more information than can be obtained with clinical examination alone or clinical examination plus ultrasonography.

Endometrial cavity tissue sampling, through either office biopsy or dilation and curettage, usually does not provide additional information toward making the diagnosis of leiomyomata uteri. Office sampling is unreliable to confirm

Table 43.1.
Criteria for Myomectomy[a]

Indication
  Leiomyomata in infertility patients, as a probable factor in failure to conceive or in recurrent pregnancy loss

Confirmation of indication
  In the presence of failure to conceive or recurrent pregnancy loss:

  1. Presence of leiomyomata of sufficient size or specific location to be a probable factor
  2. No more likely explanation exists for the failure to conceive or recurrent pregnancy loss

Actions before procedure
  1. Evaluate other causes of male and female infertility or recurrent pregnancy loss
  2. Evaluate the endometrial cavity and fallopian tubes, e.g., hysterosalpingogram
  3. Document discussion that complexity of disease process may require hysterectomy

Modified from the American College of Obstetricians and Gynecologists. Quality assessment and improvement in obstetrics and gynecology. Washington, DC: 1994.

this diagnosis, since most of the sampling devices are not large enough to obtain the leiomyomatous elements and only scratch the surface of the endometrial cavity. However, an indirect appreciation for uterine enlargement may be gained by uterine sounding, which is part of this procedure. If there is irregular uterine bleeding and the patient's clinical presentation or age makes endometrial carcinoma a significant probability, endometrial sampling is useful to evaluate for this possibility.

Dilation and curettage may provide relevant information, because larger tissue specimens, including small submucous (subendometrial) myomas, may be obtained. In addition, exploration by the sharp curette will often confirm the distortion of the uterine cavity suggestive of impingement by intramural myomas. For the patient with pedunculated intracavitary myomas, curettage may be not only diagnostic but also therapeutic, as removal of the pedunculated intracavitary myomas results in relief from the patient's bleeding and pain symptoms.

Hysteroscopy may also be used to evaluate the enlarged uterus by directly visualizing the endometrial cavity. The increased size of the cavity can be documented and submucous fibroids can be visualized and removed. Although the efficacy of hysteroscopic removal (resection) of submucous myomas has been documented, long-term followup suggests that up to 20% of patients will require additional treatment when reexamined 10 years later.

Treatment of Uterine Fibroids

The majority of patients with uterine myomas do not require surgical treatment. For example, if patients

present with menstrual aberrations, the endometrial cavity may be sampled to rule out endometrial hyperplasia or cancer. This is of particular importance for patients in the late reproductive or perimenopausal years. If the patient's bleeding is not heavy enough to cause significant alteration in hygiene or lifestyle and is not contributing to iron-deficiency anemia, reassurance and observation may be all that are necessary. Assessment of further uterine growth may be done by repeat pelvic examinations and assisted by serial pelvic ultrasound measurements. Rarely, uterine fibroids impinge on the ureter, causing hydroureter and hydronephrosis. This is more likely the case when the fibroid grows laterally from the uterus between the leaves of the broad ligament.

An attempt may be made to minimize uterine bleeding by using intermittent progestin supplementation, if patients are anovulatory, and/or prostaglandin synthetase inhibitors, which decrease the amount of secondary dysmenorrhea and in some cases the amount of menstrual flow. If there is significant endometrial cavity distortion by intramural or submucous myomas, hormonal supplementation will be of minimal benefit, since the excessive bleeding is usually related to profound anatomic and vascular distortion. This conservative approach can potentially be utilized until the time of the menopause.

Of the surgical options available, *myomectomy* is occasionally warranted in younger patients whose fertility is compromised by the presence of myomas, creating significant intracavitary distortion. However, there are potential complications of myomectomy, including excessive intraoperative blood loss and risk of postoperative hemorrhage, which are slightly greater than the complications associ-

Table 43.2.
Criteria for Hysterectomy for Leiomyomata[a]

Indication
  Leiomyomata

Confirmation of indication
  Presence of 1, 2, or 3:
    1. Asymptomatic leiomyomata of such size that they are palpable abdominally and are a concern to the patient
    2. Excessive uterine bleeding evidenced by either of the following:
      a. Profuse bleeding with flooding or clots or repetitive periods lasting >8 days
      b. Anemia caused by acute or chronic blood loss
    3. Pelvic discomfort caused by myomata (a, b, or c):
      a. Acute and severe
      b. Chronic lower abdominal or low back pressure
      c. Bladder pressure with urinary frequency not caused by urinary tract infection

Actions before procedure
  1. Confirm the absence of cervical malignancy
  2. Eliminate anovulation and other causes of abnormal bleeding
  3. When abnormal bleeding is present, confirm the absence of endometrial malignancy
  4. Assess surgical risk from anemia and need for treatment
  5. Consider patient's medical and psychologic risks concerning hysterectomy

Contraindications
  1. Desire to maintain fertility, in which case myomectomy should be considered
  2. Asymptomatic leiomyomata of size <12 weeks gestation determined by physical examination or ultrasound examination

Modified from the American College of Obstetricians and Gynecologists. Quality assessment and improvement in obstetrics and gynecology. Washington, DC: 1994.

ated with hysterectomy. Recently published criteria for myomectomy have been published to help guide the clinician's decision making (Table 43.1).

Although *hysterectomy* is commonly performed for uterine myomas, it should be considered as definitive treatment only in symptomatic women who have completed childbearing. *Indications* should be specific and well documented (Table 43.2).

Because uterine leiomyomata are "estrogen-dependent" benign neoplasms, newer treatments that include *pharmacologic inhibition of estrogen secretion have been used as temporizing measures*. This is particularly applicable in the perimenopausal years when women are more likely anovulatory with relatively more endogenous estrogen. Pharmacologic removal of the ovarian estrogen source can be achieved by suppression of the hypothalamic-pituitary-ovarian axis through the use of gonadotropin-releasing hormone agonists (GnRH analogs). This treatment is commonly used for 3 to 6 months before planned hysterectomy, but it can also be used as a temporizing medical therapy until natural menopause occurs. GnRH agonists not only can result in a reduction in uterine size, often by as much as 40 to 60%, but can also lead to a technically easier surgery with markedly diminished blood loss.

In patients with an adequate endogenous estrogen source, this treatment will not permanently reduce the size of uterine myomas, as withdrawal of the medication predictably results in regrowth of the myomas. Although less successful, other pharmacologic agents such as danazol have also been used as medical treatment for myomas by reducing endogenous production of ovarian estrogen.

The ultimate decision to perform a hysterectomy or not should include an assessment of the patient's future reproductive plans as well as careful assessment of clinical factors, including the amount and timing of bleeding, the degree of enlargement of the tumors, and the associated disability rendered to the individual patient. The presence of uterine myomas alone does not necessarily warrant hysterectomy.

Although leiomyoma are equivocally associated with infertility, patients with leiomyoma do become pregnant. *Pregnancy with leiomyoma* is usually unremarkable, with a normal antepartum course, labor, and delivery. Myomas may grow or become symptomatic, sometimes associated with *red or carneous degeneration*. Bedrest and strong analgesics are usually sufficient as treatment, although on occasion myomectomy may be needed. The risk of abortion or preterm labor is relatively high, so that prophylactic β-adrenergic tocolytics are sometimes used. *Vaginal birth after myomectomy* is controversial and must be decided on a case-by-case basis. Rarely, myomas are located below the fetus, in the lower uterine segment or cervix, causing a soft tissue dystocia, leading to cesarean birth.

LEIOMYOSARCOMA

Uterine sarcomas represent an *unusual gynecologic malignancy* accounting for approximately *3% of cancers involving the body of the uterus*. Progressive uterine enlargement occurring in the postmenopausal years should not be assumed to be the result of simple uterine leiomyomata, as appreciable endogenous ovarian estrogen secretion is absent, thereby minimizing this as a potential cause for progressive uterine enlargement. In addition, postmenopausal women on low-dose hormone-replacement therapy are not at risk for stimulation of uterine enlargement, since the doses of estrogen given are low and unlikely to stimulate regrowth of preexisting uterine fibroids. In this situation, uterine sarcoma (leiomyosarcoma) should be considered. Other symptoms of uterine sarcoma include postmenopausal bleeding, unusual pelvic pain coupled with uterine enlargement, and an increase in unusual vaginal discharge. As with endometrial sampling in patients with myomas, this procedure in the postmenopausal patient may not provide the sufficient histologic information to diagnose sarcoma. This leaves surgical removal as the method of most reliable diagnosis. Accordingly, hysterectomy is usually indicated in patients with documented, and especially progressive, uterine enlargement.

The *virulence of uterine sarcoma* is directly related to the number of mitotic figures and cellular proliferation as defined histologically. In addition, these tumors are more likely to spread hematogenously than endometrial adenocarcinoma. When uterine sarcoma is suspected, patients should undergo typical tumor survey to include assessment for distant metastatic disease. At the time of hysterectomy, it is necessary to thoroughly explore the abdomen and sample commonly affected node chains, including the iliac and periaortic areas. The staging for uterine sarcoma is surgical and identical to that for endometrial adenocarcinoma.

The overall rate of survival for patients with uterine sarcoma is considerably worse than that for those with endometrial adenocarcinoma. Only 50% of patients survive 5 years. Adjunctive radiation therapy and chemotherapy provide little additional benefit as primary adjuvant therapy or as therapy for recurrent disease. Unlike the adenocarcinoma endometrial counterparts, these tumors are not responsive to hormonal treatment with high-dose progestins.

CASE STUDIES

Case 43A

A 47-year-old G3 P3 woman presents with an 8-month history of progressively longer and heavier menstruation. Her last two cycles have included clotted blood flow for the first 5 days of each menstrual period with another 5 days of relatively normal menstrual flow. Before 8 months ago, her menstruation included 6 days of "average flow." She has no other problems except that in the last few months she has felt tired.

Physical examination reveals a woman of normal height and weight with a resting pulse of 76. Her blood pressure is normal. General physical examination is unremarkable with the exception of a suprapubic "fullness." On pelvic examination, there is old menstrual blood in the vault. The cervix is smooth and on bimanual examination the uterus is consistent with approximately 14-week gestational size with multiple surface irregularities. Finger stick hematocrit done by the office nurse is 27%.

Questions Case 43A

The most likely diagnosis is

A. Endometrial hyperplasia
B. Uterine fibroids
C. Endometrial carcinoma
D. Gestational trophoblastic disease
E. Leiomyosarcoma of the uterus

Answer: B

This patient typifies the history and physical findings of a perimenopausal woman with probable fibroid tumors of the uterus. Significant aspects of her history include progressive menorrhagia with associated anemia as detected in your office. Physical examination is consistent with uterine fibroids as the most likely diagnosis.

What studies are appropriate to adequately evaluate this patient?

A. Pelvic ultrasound
B. Pap smear
C. Endometrial biopsy
D. Complete blood count (CBC) and reticulocyte count (retic. ct.)

E. Iron/total iron-binding capacity (Fe/TIBC) and fo-late/B_{12}
F. CT scan of pelvis

Answer: A, B, C, D

Ultrasound is primarily indicated to evaluate the ad-nexae for ovarian pathology and to evaluate the ureters for hydroureter secondary to obstruction by the pelvic mass. A Pap smear and endometrial biopsy are requi-site to evaluate for malignancy. A blood count and retic-ulocyte count will be consistent with an iron-deficiency anemia or will point to additional diagnoses. Fe/TIBC and folate/B_{12} are acceptable tests but add little to the management in most instances. A CT scan is not needed in these circumstances.

The Pap smear is satisfactory, the endomerial biopsy shows disordered normal endometrium, the pelvic ultra-sound is consistent with a large fibroid uterus with no adnexal abnormalities. The possibility of hormonal sup-pression should be discussed. Finally, a risk/benefit dis-cussion regarding the possibility of hysterectomy should be undertaken, particularly in light of her age and sever-ity of symptoms.

Case 43B

A 64-year-old woman is referred to you by another phy-sician requesting a second opinion. This patient had an uneventful menopause at the age of 54 and has not been on hormone-replacement therapy. In the last 3 months she has had intermittent vaginal bleeding, and on physical examination the referring physician de-tected a uterus that he thought was consistent with ap-proximately 12-week gestational size and somewhat ir-regular. A previous examination done by him 1.5 years ago was entirely normal. Endometrial sampling done by him last week revealed atrophic endometrium. The uter-ine cavity sounded to 11 cm at that time. Your physical examination confirms his findings.

Question Case 43B

Definitive treatment for this patient should include

A. Long-term progestin hormonal suppression
B. Gonadotropin-releasing hormone agonists
C. Dilation and curettage
D. Total abdominal hysterectomy and bilateral sal-pingo-oophorectomy
E. Vaginal hysterectomy

Answer: D

This patient illustrates features highly suggestive of uter-ine sarcoma. She is postmenopausal and has little po-tential for endogenous stimulation of preexisting fib-roids. Knowledge of a normal examination 1.5 years earlier with current findings of a markedly enlarged uterus in this age group should alert the clinician to the possibility of uterine leiomyosarcoma. Although imag-ing studies might be useful and endometrial sampling is mandatory, definitive treatment for this patient is an abdominal hysterectomy with bilateral salpingo-oophorectomy.

chapter 44

ENDOMETRIAL HYPERPLASIA AND CANCER

Endometrial carcinoma is the most common genital tract malignancy, accounting for approximately 35,000 new cases annually. It is considered the best example of an "estrogen-dependent" neoplasm. Fortunately, patients with this disease usually present early in the disease course with some form of abnormal uterine bleeding, particularly postmenopausal bleeding. Accordingly, the *detection of this disease by endometrial sampling is highly accurate and should be used liberally in patients at risk.* Risk factors for the development of endometrial carcinoma include clinical conditions associated with an estrogen-rich environment. With early diagnosis and surgical treatment, survival rates can be excellent.

Endometrial carcinoma may represent the end point of precursor lesions, including atypical hyperplasias and/or intraepithelial neoplasia of the endometrial lining. This chapter includes a discussion of the spectrum of abnormal changes found in the endometrium, ranging from simple hyperplasia to invasive adenocarcinoma of the endometrium.

The *underlying pathophysiologic process* in development of endometrial hyperplasia and endometrial cancer is overgrowth of the endometrium in response to an estrogen-dominant hormonal milieu. Sources of estrogen may be glandular (ovarian) or extraglandular (peripheral conversion or exogenous source) (Table 44.1). As explained below, endometrial hyperplasia may range from a simple hyperplastic response through an atypical hyperplastic response to an overt carcinomatous change. Endometrial hyperplasia is more common in perimenopausal women who do not ovulate regularly and postmenopausal women. Postmenopausal women not only are subject to residual estrogen stimulation from the ovary but also produce estrogen by conversion of androgenic pre-cursors in peripheral fat stores (androstenedione to estrone, the principal source of endogenous estrogen in postmenopausal women). Obese women are, therefore, at higher risk for endometrial hyperplasia and carcinoma.

Approximately three-quarters of patients with endometrial carcinoma are diagnosed in their postmenopausal years. Of the remaining cases of endometrial cancer, most occur at the time of anovulation during the perimenopausal years (from their mid-40s through their early 50s), whereas a small number occur in younger patients who have been chronically anovulatory.

ENDOMETRIAL HYPERPLASIA

The relationship between estrogen production and endometrial growth (proliferation) is clear. Endometrial proliferation represents a normal part of the menstrual cycle and occurs during the follicular or estrogen-dominant phase of the cycle. With continued estrogen stimulation through either endogenous mechanisms or by exogenous administration, simple endometrial proliferation will become endometrial hyperplasia (Fig. 44.1). *Endometrial hyperplasia is the "abnormal proliferation of both glandular and stromal elements showing altered histologic architecture."* True endometrial proliferation is a simple overabundance of normal endometrium, whereas endometrial hyperplasia involves histologic features with cellular architectural abnormalities. When proliferation becomes hyperplasia is not clear, although studies showing sequential change suggest it requires 6 months or longer of "unopposed estrogen" stimulation.

Histologic *variations of endometrial hyperplasia include cystic glandular hyperplasia, adenomatous hyperplasia, and atypical adenomatous hyperplasia.* Unlike cervical carcinoma precursors, there is no uni-

Table 44.1.
Estrogen Sources

Endogenous
  Glandular
    Estradiol (ovary)
    Estrone (ovary)
  Peripheral
    Estrone (fat, conversion of androstenedione)
  Tumor
    Granulosa cell of ovary (an uncommon tumor and
      source)

Exogenous
  Medications
    Conjugated estrogen (mostly estrone)
    Lyophilized estradiol
    Cutaneous patches
    Vaginal creams

form agreement that each of these lesions will progress to endometrial cancer if left untreated. In addition, these histologic variants can occur in only small foci of an otherwise normal endometrium, revealing that these changes may not necessarily involve the entire endometrial cavity at the same time. Therefore, the microscopic picture as judged by a pathologist may not represent the complete anatomic picture.

There are two different terminologies used to describe endometrial hyperplasia. The parameters used by both include amount of endometrium, density of glands, structural abnormalities of glands, and cytologic features of glandular epithelium. *Traditional terminology uses descriptive terms: cystic hyperplasia, adenomatous hyperplasia, and atypical adenomatous hyperplasia,* with degrees of architectural or cytologic atypia. The most recent terminology

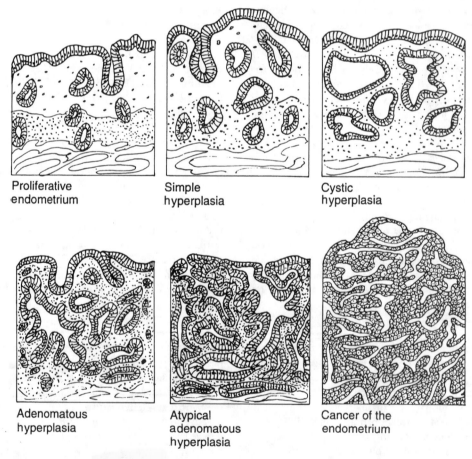

Figure 44.1. Endometrial histology: hyperplasia to carcinoma.

Table 44.2.
Classifications of Endometrial Hyperplasias

Traditional Histologic	ISGYP
Cystic hyperplasia	Simple hyperplasia
Adenomatous hyperplasia	Complex hyperplasia (adenomatous hyperplasia without cytologic atypia)

Atypical adenomatous hyperplasia
  Architectural atypia
    (mild, moderate, severe)
  Cytologic atypia
    (mild, moderate, severe)
	Atypical hyperplasia (adenomatous hyperplasia with cytologic atypia)

Table 44.3.
Patients at Risk for Unopposed Estrogen Exposure

Patients using exogenous estrogen alone
Patients with history of chronic anovulation
Obese postmenopausal women
Patients with "late" menopause (>55 years old)

adopted by the International Society of Gynecologic Pathologists (ISGYP) presents the endometrial hyperplasias in a slightly different way to better describe their premalignant potential: *simple hyperplasia, complex hyperplasia without cytologic atypia, and atypical hyperplasia*, which includes adenomatous hyperplasia with cytologic atypia. The classifications are compared in Table 44.2.

Risk factors for endometrial hyperplasia are the same as for endometrial carcinoma, i.e., any features contributing to an increased estrogen environment. The sources of estrogen are listed in Table 44.1. Table 44.3 identifies those patients at increased risk for unopposed estrogen stimulation.

Cystic Endometrial Hyperplasia (Simple Hyperplasia)

Cystic endometrial hyperplasia is the *least significant form* of endometrial hyperplasia. It is not commonly associated with progression to or the occurrence of endometrial carcinoma, although it is considered a modest risk factor as a precursor lesion. In this variety of hyperplasia, both glandular elements and stromal cell elements proliferate excessively. Histologically, glands that are simple tubules demonstrate marked variation in size, from small to enlarged cystically dilated glands (the hallmark of this hyperplasia). Cystic glandular hyperplasia should not be confused with a normal postmenopausal variant — cystic involution of the endometrium — which is histologically not a hyperplastic condition.

Adenomatous Hyperplasia (Complex Hyperplasia)

Endometrial adenomatous hyperplasia represents an *abnormal proliferation of primarily glandular elements without concomitant proliferation of stromal elements.* This increased gland:stroma ratio gives the endometrium a "crowded" picture, frequently with glands appearing almost back to back. As the severity of the hyperplasia increases, the glands become more crowded and more structurally bizarre. It is thought that adenomatous hyperplasia represents a true intraepithelial neoplastic process and is occasionally found coexisting with areas of endometrial adenocarcinoma; however, it may also be found microscopically in small areas within normal proliferative endometrium.

Atypical Adenomatous Hyperplasia (Atypical Hyperplasia with Cytologic Atypia)

Adenomatous hyperplasia, which *contains significant numbers of glandular elements that exhibit cytologic atypia and disordered maturation,* is considered particularly important as a precursor lesion to endometrial carcinoma. This so-called *carcinoma in situ of the endometrium* has at least a 20 to 30% risk for malignant transformation.

Diagnosis and Management

The diagnosis of endometrial hyperplasia can be made by taking a sample of the endometrium for histologic evaluation. This is most easily accomplished by any of a number of different atraumatic aspiration devices available for office use (e.g., Pipelle, Vabra). The routine *Pap smear is not reliable* in diagnosing endometrial hyperplasia or cancer; however, this diagnosis must be considered when atypical endometrial cells are found on the Pap smear (atypical glandular cells of undetermined significance, AGUS) and an appropriate evaluation undertaken. The most common *indication for endometrial sampling is abnormal bleeding*, with liberal consideration given to obtaining a specimen *in patients over the age of 35 who present with abnormal uterine bleeding.* After ruling out pregnancy by simple urine pregnancy testing, patients can be adequately sampled with relatively little discomfort. Further management is usually dictated by the results of the biopsy specimen. Dilation and curettage (D&C) can also be used for diagnostic sampling of the endometrium, although it is usually reserved for patients in whom outpatient sampling is technically difficult or in cases where outpatient sampling has been nondiagnostic.

Sometimes the office endometrial biopsy will be reported as "insufficient tissue for diagnosis." In a postmenopausal woman not on estrogen replacement, these data may be sufficient, as it is compatible with the suspected atrophic condition of the endometrium. In other cases, the clinical suspicion of a possible hyperplastic endometrial process may be high enough to warrant D&C to more fully sample the endometrial cavity. Although office endometrial biopsy is considered a sufficient technique for endometrial sampling, clinical judgment as to its interpretation must be applied in each situation.

Another approach is hysteroscopic evaluation of the endometrium with directed biopsies of suspicious areas. This technique also allows direct diagnosis of polyps, myomas, and structure abnormalities. Although somewhat more expensive and inconvenient for the patient, it offers some theoretical advantages over a blind biopsy, especially because traditional endometrial biopsy techniques sample only a small part of the surface area of the endometrial cavity.

If *simple hyperplasia, cystic hyperplasia, or adenomatous hyperplasia* of the simple variety has been diagnosed by tissue sample, medical treatment is usually offered. In most cases, *medical treatment* involves the administration of a form of synthetic progesterone (progestin) in doses that will inhibit and eventually reverse the hyperplastic response evoked by estrogen stimulation. Probably the most common regimen is Provera (medroxyprogesterone acetate), 10 mg per day for 10 days each month. Progestin therapy works to alter the enzymatic pathways, which eventually convert endogenous estradiol to weaker estrogens, as well as to decrease the number of estrogen receptors in the endometrial glandular cells. Progestins have a net effect of decreasing endometrial glandular proliferation and, when administered for sufficient period of time or in high enough doses, will actually render the endometrium atrophic. In addition, with progestin withdrawal, the endometrium is sloughed, analogous to corpus luteum progesterone withdrawal in a normal menstrual cycle (the so-called chemical D&C).

Atypical adenomatous hyperplasia is usually treated surgically by hysterectomy, since it is this variant that is much more likely to become endometrial carcinoma. This treatment decision is usually fairly clear, because the majority of patients with this disorder will be in their late reproductive or perimenopausal years. In selected patients (e.g., younger women who may wish to become pregnant), longer term *progestin management* after thorough endometrial curettage may be employed to avoid a hysterectomy. Typical regimens might include depomedroxyprogesterone acetate (Depo-Provera), 1000 mg/week i.m. for 4 weeks, followed by 5 months of monthly therapy with 400 mg/month, or megestrol acetate (Megace), 80 mg per day for 6 to 12 weeks. Patients who are treated medically for atypical adenomatous hyperplasia should also be followed with periodic endometrial sampling (3 months after therapy and then once to twice per year) so that treatment response can be gauged.

ENDOMETRIAL POLYPS

Most endometrial polyps represent focal accentuated benign hyperplastic processes. Their histologic architecture is characteristic and may commonly be found in association with other types of endometrial hyperplasia or even carcinoma. Polyps occur most frequently in perimenopausal or immediately postmenopausal women, when the ovary is characterized by unopposed estrogen production because of chronic anovulation. The most common presenting symptom is abnormal bleeding. Often small polyps may be incidentally found as part of endometrial aspiration or curettage done for evaluation of the bleeding problem. Rarely, a large polyp may begin to protrude through the cervical canal, and the patient will present not only with bleeding irregularities but also with low dull midline pain as the cervix is slowly dilated and effaced. The appearance of these on speculum examination is quite striking. In these cases, surgical removal is necessary to reduce the amount of bleeding and to prevent infection from the exposed endometrial surface. *Less than 5% of polyps show malignant change,* and when they do, they may represent any endometrial histologic variant. Polyps in postmenopausal women are more likely to be associated with endometrial carcinoma than are those found in reproductive age women.

ENDOMETRIAL CARCINOMA

Although the *relationship between endometrial hyperplasias and estrogen* is clear (Table 44.4), the mechanism behind the ultimate change from hyperplastic variations to endometrial carcinoma is less clear. Certainly, estrogen is implicated because of its association with the antecedent hyperplasia, but the actual stimulus to malignant degeneration is unknown. It remains standard teaching to consider endometrial carcinoma as an "estrogen-dependent neoplasm."

Endometrial carcinoma is typically a disease of the postmenopausal woman. Approximately 75% of patients with endometrial carcinoma are postmenopausal, while 15 to 20% are perimenopausal and only 5 to 10% are menstrual. Between 15 and 25% of postmenopausal women with bleeding have uterine malignancy.

Most primary endometrial carcinomas are adenocarcinomas and are described according to their histologic and glandular architecture. Since squamous epithelium appears to co-exist with the glandular elements in an adenocarcinoma, descriptive terms that include the squamous element may be used, depending on the amount of squamous tissue present in the histologic specimen. In cases where the squamous element makes up >10% of the histologic picture, and it appears benign, the term *adenoacanthoma* is used. Uncommonly, the squamous element may appear malignant on histologic assessment, and this is referred to as *adenosquamous carcinoma*. Other descriptions such as clear cell carcinoma and papillary serous adenocarcinoma may be applied, depending on the histologic architecture. Knowledge of these unusual subtypes is less important than an overall appreciation of the fact that all of these carcinomas are considered under the general category of adenocarcinoma of the endometrium.

The diagnosis of endometrial cancer is most frequently made by endometrial sampling after a patient presents with abnormal uterine bleeding. Special consideration should be given to the patient who presents with postmenopausal bleeding, i.e., bleeding that occurs after 6 months of amenorrhea in a patient who has been diagnosed as menopausal. In this group of patients, it is mandatory to assess the endometrium histologically, since the chance of having an endometrial carcinoma is approximately 15%. Other gynecologic assessments should also be made, including careful physical and pelvic examination as well as a screening Pap smear.

Because of the current International Federation of Gynecology and Obstetrics (FIGO) staging of endometrial carcinoma (Table 44.5), which is surgical rather than clinical, differential sampling of the endocervical canal and endometrial cavity before therapy is less important now than with previous staging criteria. Fractional curettage should, however, be kept in mind for patients who are not surgical candidates because of other risk factors, e.g., patients whose primary treatment is radiotherapy.

Route of Spread

Knowledge of the route of spread of endometrial cancer guides the surgeon toward thorough surgical assessment of potentially involved tissues and serves as the basis for the FIGO staging system. Endometrial carcinoma usually spreads throughout the endometrial cavity first and then begins to invade the myometrium, endocervical canal, and eventually, lymphatics. Hematogenous spread occurs with endometrial carcinoma more readily than in cervical cancer or ovarian cancer. Invasion of adnexal structures may occur via lymphatics or direct implantation through the fallopian tubes. Once there is extrauterine spread to the peritoneal

Table 44.4.
Factors Affecting the Risk of Endometrial Carcinoma

Increases the Risk	Diminishes the Risk
Unopposed estrogen stimulation	Ovulation
Unopposed menopausal estrogen-replacement therapy (4–8 ×)	Progestin therapy
Menopause after 52 years (2.4 ×)	Combination oral contraceptives
Obesity (3 ×: 21–50 lb; 10 ×: >50 lb)	Menopause before 49 years
Nulliparity (2–3 ×)	Normal weight
Diabetes (2.8 ×)	Multiparity
Feminizing ovarian tumors (granulosa theca cell tumors of the ovary)	
Chronic anovulation; polycystic ovarian syndrome[a]	

[a] Less than 5% of endometrial carcinoma is in women <40 years old; yet of these, approximately 20% have chronic anovulation, polycystic ovarian syndrome.

G-1 Highly Differentiated Adenocarcinoma
with Partially Solid Areas
G-2 Moderately "
G-3 Mostly Solid or Undifferentiated

Table 44.5.
FIGO Surgical Staging of Endometrial Carcinoma (1988)

Stage	Description
IA G123	Tumor limited to endometrium
IB G123	Invasion to less than one-half of the myometrium
IC G123	Invasion to more than one-half of the myometrium
IIA G123	Endocervical glandular involvement only
IIB G123	Cervical stromal invasion
IIIA G123	Tumor invading serosa, adnexa, or both and/or positive peritoneal cytology
IIIB G123	Vaginal metastases
IIIC G123	Metastases to pelvic and/or periaortic lymph nodes
IVA G123	Tumor invades bladder, bowel mucosa, or both
IVB	Distant metastases, including intraabdominal and/or inguinal lymph node

Rules related to staging

1. Because corpus cancer is now surgically staged, procedures previously used for differentiation of stages are no longer applicable, e.g., the findings of D&C to differentiate between stage I and stage II. It is appreciated that there may be a small number of patients with corpus cancer who are treated primarily with radiation therapy. If that is the case, the clinical staging adopted by FIGO in 1971 would still apply, but use of that staging system would be noted.

2. Ideally, the width of the myometrium is measured along with the width of tumor invasion.

cavity, cancer cells have access to the entire abdominal pelvic cavity and may spread in a fashion similar to ovarian cancer.

Unusual histologic subtypes, including *papillary serous adenocarcinoma and clear cell adenocarcinoma* of the endometrium, tend to be more aggressive in abdominopelvic spread than the more common adenocarcinoma of the endometrium. Microscopic spread may also be present despite the absence of gross abdominal pelvic lesions. Accordingly, cytologic assessment of peritoneal washings is important at the outset of surgical treatment for endometrial carcinoma. The current FIGO guidelines for the staging of endometrial carcinoma emphasizes the need for thorough surgical assessment of the abdominopelvic cavity, including sampling of both periaortic and pelvic lymph nodes when depths of invasion are more than one-third of the myometrial thickness and in cases where there are obvious peritoneal foci of tumor.

Prognostic Factors

The single most important prognostic factor for endometrial carcinoma is histologic grade. Histologically, poorly differentiated or undifferentiated tumors are associated with a considerably poorer progno-sis because of the likelihood of extrauterine spread through adjacent lymphatics and peritoneal fluid. This is true even of relatively limited lesions. Therefore, this finding is important in the initial surgical management of the patient and is of significance in deciding on adjunctive therapy via radiation or chemotherapy.

The grading system of the *FIGO adopted in 1988 lists three grades of endometrial carcinoma:* G1 is highly differentiated adenomatous carcinoma, G2 is moderately differentiated adenomatous carcinoma with partly solid areas, and G3 is predominately solid or entire undifferentiated carcinoma. The majority of patients with endometrial carcinoma have G1 or G2 lesions by this classification, with 15 to 20% having undifferentiated or poorly differentiated G3 lesions.

Depth of myometrial invasion is the second most important prognostic factor. When the tumor has invaded greater than one-third of the thickness of the myometrium, the prognosis is markedly worsened. Worsening grade of tumor closely parallels depth of myometrial invasion and lymph node metastasis. Other factors that have prognostic value include the original tumor volume both within the uterus and defined by extrauterine spread, lymphatic involvement, and hematogenous spread.

Survival rates vary widely, depending on the grade of tumor and depth of penetration into the myometrium. A patient with a G1 tumor that does not invade the myometrium has a 95% 5-year survival rate, whereas a patient with a poorly differentiated (G3) tumor with deep myometrial invasion may have a 5-year survival rate of only 20%.

Treatment

As a surgically staged disease, *primary surgical treatment is the cornerstone of management.* After opening the abdomen, peritoneal washings are obtained. The abdominopelvic cavity is manually and visually explored, and then a *total abdominal hysterectomy with bilateral salpingo-oophorectomy* is performed. The decision to include pelvic and/or periaortic nodes is determined by the depth of myometrial invasion as judged by the attending pathologist. *Vaginal hysterectomy* has been used successfully in the treatment of stage I disease in selected patients and may be especially useful in patients for whom the stress of abdominal surgery may be problematic. There is a 5 to 10% incidence of *vaginal apex recurrence* after simple hysterectomy for endometrial carcinoma, probably because of paravaginal lymphatic involvement in most cases. This incidence of apex recurrence is reduced by one-half with the use of preoperative radiation, although the 5-year survival rates for those receiving preoperative radiation and those who do not are not different.

Many gynecologic oncologists advise routine *sampling of the common iliac nodes* regardless of depth of penetration or histologic grade, citing as their reason, the inherent inaccuracies of gross myometrial inspection and frozen section assessment of the histologic grade and depth of penetration. In addition, they cite the incidence of pelvic nodal metastasis as between 2 and 10% for all stage I lesions, G1–3.

Adjunctive therapy after hysterectomy, which may include external beam radiation, has been shown to significantly reduce the risk of pelvic and vaginal recurrence. *Postoperative radiation* therapy may be especially valuable in patients with deeply invasive cancers, those with cervical involvement, and those with poorly differentiated tumors. *Preoperative radiation* may be useful to those patients with obvious endocervical involvement and/or may be important in reducing a bulky endometrial tumor.

The first line of *treatment for recurrent disease* is hormonal and includes various *progestin preparations* given in high doses (Depo-Provera, 400 mg/week for at least 12 weeks; if there is a positive response, progestin at a lower dosage is recommended for life). Approximately one-third of these patients will have a short-term (<5 years) response, and approximately 15% will have a long-term response (>5 years). A major advantage of high-dose progestin therapy is its minimal complication rate. *Chemotherapy* with drugs, including Adriamycin (doxorubicin) and cisplatin, produces occasional favorable short-term results, but long-term remissions with these therapies are rare.

The use of *estrogen-replacement therapy* in patients previously treated for endometrial carcinoma is controversial. Recent data suggest that for well-differentiated, minimally invasive endometrial carcinoma that has not recurred within 5 years, estrogen with progestin-replacement therapy may be safe. However, cautious assessment of long-term risk versus benefits of hormone-replacement therapy should be accorded each patient.

CASE STUDIES

Case 44A

A 62-year-old woman whose last normal menstrual period was 7 years ago presents with a 2-month history of intermittent vaginal bleeding. She has had two children (ages 39 and 40) and is in generally good health and currently taking no medications. Physical examination reveals a patient of average height and weight and normal blood pressure. Pelvic examination shows some atrophy of the vaginal mucosa with a small and smooth cervix without evidence of blood. Bimanual examination demonstrates a small, firm, anteflexed uterus of normal size with an unremarkable adnexal examination. Rectovaginal examination is negative and the stool is guaiac negative.

Questions Case 44A

Having performed a Pap smear, including samples of both the exocervix and cervical canal, your next diagnostic assessment should be to:

A. Await results of Pap smear before further assessment
B. Obtain vaginal maturation index for estrogen production
C. Obtain pelvic ultrasound
D. Perform endometrial biopsy
E. Schedule for dilation and curettage

Answer: D

This case illustrates a high-risk history for endometrial carcinoma: new onset postmenopausal bleeding. Despite having normal physical and pelvic examinations, this patient has approximately a 15% risk of endometrial carcinoma. The Pap smear is unreliable in detecting this neoplasm, and it is mandatory to obtain endometrial sampling. The preferable technique for this is by office biopsy. Dilation and curettage is reserved for patients in whom the clinician encounters technical difficulty or there is an inadequate office sample.

The Pap smear is satisfactory and negative. The Pipelle endometrial biopsy is reported as insufficient tissue for pathologic diagnosis. Your management should now entail

A. Progestin therapy: medroxyprogesterone 10 mg p.o. q.d. for 10 days
B. Estrogen therapy: premarin 0.625 mg p.o. q.d. and medroxyprogesterone 2.5 mg p.o. q.d.
C. Schedule for dilation and curettage
D. Pelvic ultrasound
E. Repeat Pipelle endometrial biopsy

Answer: B

This postmenopausal women is estrogen deficient, and her bleeding is from the scant endometrium left. A lack of tissue is expected; no further sampling is required at this time. Progestin therapy will not help and, indeed, may worsen the bleeding. Hormone-replacement therapy should stop the bleeding and benefit the patient in other ways, including beneficial effects on her risk of cardiovascular disease and osteoporosis.

Case 44B

A 27-year-old patient comes in with a 3-year history of progressively infrequent menstrual periods. Her menarche was age 17, she has never had "monthly periods" but has always had six or seven periods per year. In the last 3 years she has had only two or three menstrual periods per year. She has also been unable to become pregnant. Her last bleeding episode was 2 months ago. Physical examination reveals a woman 5 feet 4 inches tall weighing 210 pounds with a normal pelvic examination. After a negative pregnancy test, an endometrial biopsy performed as part of her infertility assessment reveals adenomatous hyperplasia.

Question Case 44B

The most efficacious treatment for this patient would be

A. Pharmacologic ovulation induction
B. Intermittent short-term progestin therapy
C. Oral contraceptives
D. Dilation and curettage
E. Artificial insemination

Answer: A

This patient has chronic anovulation with resultant hyperplasia of the endometrium. Because she is also infertile, the optimal treatment of ovulation induction may help enable her to become pregnant, also reversing the hyperplasia by the production of progesterone. Other therapy such as intermittent progestin use and/or oral contraceptive use may treat the endometrial hyperplasia problem but would not address the infertility concern. Adenomatous hyperplasia without atypia carries a low risk for malignancy. Therefore, aggressive surgical treatment such as D&C is not warranted. Likewise, dilation and curettage is no better a diagnostic tool than office sampling. Artificial insemination is of no value in a chronically anovulatory patient. For completeness, other etiology for oligomenorrhea in the patient should also be assessed, e.g., pituitary or thyroid dysfunction.

Case 44C

A 32-year-old G3 P3003 who had a postpartum tubal ligation with her last pregnancy presents with irregular vaginal bleeding for 6 months. She has had a recent significant weight gain, now weighing 245 pounds. Her pelvic examination reveals a normal cervix, normal-size midposition uterus, no adnexal masses, and a negative rectovaginal examination with negative guaiac. A Pap smear and cultures were performed. Because of her history of irregular bleeding, a Pipelle endometrial biopsy is also performed.

The Pap smear is reported as satisfactory and negative. The endometrial biopsy is reported as adenomatous hyperplasia with marked atypia.

Question Case 44C

You should now recommend

A. Dilation and curettage
B. Hysteroscopy
C. Progestin therapy
D. Hormone-replacement therapy
E. Hysterectomy

Answer: E

Adenomatous hyperplasia with marked atypia is also called "endometrial carcinoma in situ," as it carries a high risk of becoming endometrial carcinoma. Because this patient has completed her childbearing, hysterectomy, with adjuvant therapy as indicated by the pathology specimen results, is the best management. If this patient had wanted more children or wished to avoid hysterectomy if possible, progestin therapy could be attempted, but with close monitoring of her endometrium to document efficacious results.

chapter 45

OVARIAN AND ADNEXAL DISEASE

The area between the lateral pelvic wall and the cornu of the uterus medially is referred to as the *adnexal space or adnexae*. This area includes the ovaries, fallopian tubes, the upper portion of the broad ligament and mesosalpinx, and remnants of the embryonic müllerian duct. Within the adnexal space, the organs most commonly affected by disease processes are the ovaries and fallopian tubes.

This chapter describes the physiologic variations of the ovary and fallopian tubes that can mimic disease as well as the benign and malignant ovarian and fallopian tube neoplasms. It also illustrates how nongynecologic structures in the region, such as the bowel and bladder, may produce symptoms that can be confused with "gynecologic" adnexal disease. Pelvic infection, ectopic pregnancy, and endometriosis are discussed in separate chapters.

ADNEXAL SPACE AND ASSOCIATED NONGYNECOLOGIC DISEASE

In addition to the reproductive organs, parts of the urinary and gastrointestinal tracts are located in the adnexal space. The most common urologic disorders are upper and lower *urinary tract infection*, and the less common, *renal and ureteral calculi*. Even rarer are anatomic abnormalities such as a *ptotic kidney*, which may present as a solid pelvic mass. An isolated pelvic kidney may likewise present as an asymptomatic solid cul-de-sac mass. Right adnexal signs and symptoms are associated with acute *appendicitis*, which should be considered in the differential diagnosis of acute right lower quadrant pain. Less commonly, symptoms in the right adnexa may be related to intrinsic *inflammatory bowel disease* involving the ileocecal junction. Left-sided bowel disease involving the rectosigmoid is seen more often in older patients, as in acute or chronic diverticular disease. Because of the age of these patients and the proximity of the

left ovary to the sigmoid, *sigmoid diverticular disease* is included in the differential diagnosis of a left-sided adnexal mass. Finally, left-sided pelvic pain or a mass may be related to *rectosigmoid carcinoma*.

THE OVARIES

Pelvic examination is central in evaluation of the ovary. Symptoms that may arise from physiologic and pathologic processes of the ovary must be correlated with physical examination findings. Also, since some ovarian conditions are asymptomatic, incidental physical examination findings may be the only information available when an evaluation begins. Interpretation of examination findings requires knowledge of the physical characteristics of the ovary during the stages of the life cycle.

In the *premenarchal age group*, the *ovary should not be palpable*. If it is, a pathologic condition is presumed and further evaluation is necessary.

In the *reproductive age group*, the normal *ovary is palpable about half of the time*. Important considerations include ovarian size, shape, consistency (firm or cystic), and mobility. In reproductive age women taking oral contraceptives, the ovaries are palpable less frequently and are smaller and more symmetrical than in women who are not using contraceptives.

In the *postmenopausal* patient, the ovaries are functionally quiescent except for some androgen production. These ovaries are no longer responsive to gonadotropin secretion, and therefore, their surface follicular activity diminishes over time, disappearing in most women within 3 years of the onset of natural menopause. Women who are close to the natural menopause are more likely to have residual functional cysts. In general, palpable ovarian enlargement in a postmenopausal patient should be assessed more critically than in a younger woman, because the incidence of ovarian malignant neoplasm is increased in this group.

455

One-quarter of all ovarian tumors in postmenopausal women are malignant, while in reproductive age women only about 10% of ovarian tumors are malignant. Indeed, this risk was considered so great in the past that the presence of any ovarian enlargement in a postmenopausal woman was an indication for surgical investigation, the so-called palpable postmenopausal ovary (PPO) syndrome. With the advent of more sensitive pelvic imaging techniques to assist in diagnosis, routine removal of minimally enlarged postmenopausal ovaries is no longer recommended. If the patient is within 3 years of natural menopause, and transvaginal ultrasonography confirms the presence of a simple, unilocular cyst of less than 5 cm in diameter, the management may be serial pelvic and transvaginal ultrasound examinations. Masses that are larger or appear complex on ultrasonography are best managed surgically.

Functional Ovarian Cysts

Functional ovarian cysts are not neoplasms but rather anatomic variations, arising as a result of normal ovarian function. They may present as an asymptomatic adnexal mass or become symptomatic, requiring evaluation and possibly treatment.

When an ovarian follicle fails to rupture during follicular maturation, ovulation does not occur and a *follicular cyst* may develop. This, by definition, will involve a lengthening of the follicular phase of the cycle with resultant secondary amenorrhea. Follicular cysts are lined by normal granulosa cells and the fluid contained within them is rich in estrogen.

A follicular cyst becomes clinically significant if it is large enough to cause pain or if it persists beyond one menstrual interval. For poorly understood reasons, the granulosa cells lining the follicular cyst persist through the time when ovulation should have occurred and continue to enlarge through the second half of the cycle. A cyst may enlarge beyond 5 cm and continue to fill with estrogen-rich follicular fluid from the thickened granulosa cell layer. Symptoms associated with a follicular cyst may include mild to moderate unilateral lower abdominal pain and alteration of the menstrual interval. The latter may be the result of both failed subsequent ovulation and bleeding stimulated by the large amount of estradiol produced within the follicle. This estrogen-rich environment along with the lack of ovulation overstimulates the endometrium and causes irregular bleeding. Pelvic examination findings may include unilateral tenderness with a palpable mobile, cystic adnexal mass.

Given a patient with these findings, the physician must decide whether further diagnostic assessment and treatment are necessary. Pelvic ultrasonography is occasionally warranted in reproductive age patients who have cysts larger than 5 cm in diameter. Ultrasound characteristics include a unilocular simple cyst without evidence of blood or soft tissue elements and without evidence of external excrescences. For most patients, however, ultrasound confirmation is not required. Instead, the patient may be reassured and followed with a repeat pelvic examination in about 6 to 8 weeks.

Most follicular cysts will spontaneously resolve during this time. Alternatively, an estrogen- and progesterone-containing oral contraceptive may be given to suppress gonadotropin stimulation of the cyst. Although this practice has not been shown to "shrink" the existing follicle cyst, it may suppress the development of a new cyst and permit resolution of the existing problem. If the cyst persists despite expectant management, the presence of another type of cyst or neoplasm should be suspected, and further evaluated by imaging studies and/or surgery. The role of transvaginal sonography with directed needle aspiration of such cysts is controversial but being investigated in prospective studies.

On occasion, *rupture of a follicular cyst* may cause acute pelvic pain. Because release of follicular fluid into the peritoneum produces only transient symptoms, surgical intervention is rarely necessary.

A *corpus luteum cyst* is the other common type of functional ovarian cyst. It is related to the postovulatory, i.e., luteal-dominant phase of the menstrual cycle. Two variations of corpus luteum cysts are encountered. The first is a slightly enlarged corpus luteum, which may continue to produce progesterone for longer than the usual 14 days. Menstruation is delayed from a few days to several weeks, although it usually occurs within 2 weeks of the missed period. Persistent corpus luteum cysts are often associated with dull lower quadrant pain. This pain and a missed menstrual period are the most common complaints associated with persistent corpus luteum cysts. Pelvic examination usually discloses an enlarged, tender, cystic or solid adnexal mass. Because of the triad of missed menstrual period, unilateral lower quadrant pain, and adnexal enlargement, ectopic pregnancy is often considered in the differential diagnosis. A negative pregnancy test eliminates this possibility, whereas a positive pregnancy test mandates further evaluation as to the location of the pregnancy. Patients with recurrent persistent corpus luteum cysts may benefit from cyclic oral contraceptive therapy.

The second common type of corpus luteum cyst is the rapidly enlarging luteal-phase cyst into which there is spontaneous hemorrhage. Sometimes called the *corpus hemorrhagicum*, this hemorrhagic cyst may rupture late in the luteal phase, resulting in the following clinical picture: a patient not using oral contraceptives, with regular periods, who presents with acute pain late in the luteal phase. Some patients present with evidence of hemoperitoneum as well as hypovolemia and require surgical resection of the bleeding cyst. In others, the acute pain and blood loss are self-limited. These patients may be managed with mild analgesics and reassurance.

Benign Ovarian Neoplasms

Although most ovarian enlargements in the reproductive age group are functional cysts, about 25% will prove to be nonfunctional ovarian neoplasms. In the reproductive age group, 90% of these neoplasms are benign, whereas the risk of malignancy rises to approximately 25% when postmenopausal patients are also included. Thus ovarian masses in older patients and in reproductive patients where there is no response to oral contraceptives are of special concern. Unfortunately, unless the mass is particularly large or becomes symptomatic, these masses may remain undetected for some time. Many ovarian neoplasms are first discovered at the time of routine pelvic examination.

Ovarian neoplasms are usually categorized by the cell type of origin: (a) epithelial cell tumors, the largest class of ovarian neoplasm; (b) *germ cell tumors,* which include the most common ovarian neoplasm in reproductive age women, the benign cystic teratoma or dermoid; and (c) *stromal cell tumors.* The classification of ovarian tumors by cell line of origin is presented in Table 45.1.

Benign Epithelial Cell Neoplasms

The exact cell source for the development of epithelial cell tumors of the ovary is unclear; however, the cells are characteristic of typical glandular epithelial cells. They contain microscopic glandular and

Table 45.1.
Histogenic Classification of All Ovarian Neoplasms

From celomic epithelium (epithelial)	From germ cell
Serous	Dysgerminoma
Mucinous	Teratoma
Endometrioid	Endodermal sinus
Brenner	(yolk sac)
	Choriocarcinoma
From gonadal stroma	Miscellaneous cell line
Granulosa theca	sources
Sertoli-Leydig	Lymphoma
(arrhenoblastoma)	Sarcoma
Lipid cell fibroma	Metastatic
	Colorectal
	Breast
	Endometrial

secretory apparatus, they secrete into a luminal surface, and they are separated from underlying stroma by a basement membrane. Evidence exists to suggest that these cells are derived from mesothelial cells lining the peritoneal cavity. Since the müllerian duct-derived tissue becomes the female genital tract by differentiation of the mesothelium from the gonadal ridge, it is hypothesized that these tissues are also capable of differentiating into glandular tissue. Accordingly, the more common epithelial tumors of the ovary are grouped into serous, mucinous, and endometrial neoplasms as shown in Table 45.2.

The most common epithelial cell neoplasm is the *serous cystadenoma.* A total of 70% of serous tumors are benign; approximately 10% will have intraepithelial cellular characteristics, which suggest that they are of low malignant potential; and the remaining 20% are frankly malignant by both histologic criteria and by clinical behavior. Benign tumors usually present clinically as cystic adnexal masses, which may be bilateral about 15% of the time. Typically, they are larger than functional ovarian cysts and may cause perceptible increasing abdominal girth. These tumors may occur in any age group, although they are more common in the perimenopausal and postmenopausal patient. On ultrasonography, these cysts tend to appear multilocular, especially if they are large. The *treatment of serous tumors* is surgical because of the relatively high rate of malignancy. In the younger patient with smaller tumors, an attempt can be made to perform an ovarian cystectomy to try to minimize the amount of ovarian tissue removed. For large unilateral serous tumors in young patients, unilateral oophorectomy with preservation of the contra-

Table 45.2.
Histologic Classification of the Common Epithelial Tumors of the Ovary

Serous tumors
  Serous cystadenomas
  Serous cystadenomas with proliferating activity of the
    epithelial cells and nuclear abnormalities but with
    no infiltrative destructive growth (low potential
    malignancy)
  Serous cystadenocarcinoma

Mucinous tumors
  Mucinous cystadenomas
  Mucinous cystadenomas with proliferating activity of
    the epithelial cells and nuclear abnormalities but
    with no infiltrative destructive growth (low
    potential malignancy)
  Mucinous cystadenocarcinoma

Endometrioid tumors (similar to adenocarcinomas in
  the endometrium)
  Endometrioid benign cysts
  Endometrioid tumors with proliferating activity of
    the epithelial cells and nuclear abnormalities but
    with no infiltrative destructive growth (low
    potential malignancy)
  Adenocarcinoma

Brenner tumor

Unclassified carcinoma

---

lateral ovary is indicated to maintain fertility. In patients past the reproductive age, bilateral oophorectomy along with hysterectomy may be indicated, not only because of the chance of future malignancy but also because of the increased risk of a similar occurrence in the contralateral ovary.

Mucinous tumors are also of epithelial (mesothelial) cell origin. The *mucinous cystadenoma* is the second most common epithelial cell tumor of the ovary. The malignancy rate of 15% is lower than that for serous tumor, as is the 5% rate of bilaterality. These cystic tumors can become very large, sometimes filling the entire pelvis and extending into the abdominal cavity. In fact, when enormous cystic adnexal masses are found, mucinous cystadenomas should be suggested. Ultrasound assessment shows multilocular septation. Surgery is the treatment of choice.

A third type of benign epithelial neoplasm is the *endometrioid tumor*. The majority of benign endometrioid tumors take the form of endometriomas, which are cysts lined by well-differentiated endometrial-like glandular tissue. There is further discussion of this neoplasm in "Malignant Ovarian Neoplasms," below.

The *Brenner cell tumor* is an uncommon benign epithelial cell tumor of the ovary. This tumor is usually described as a solid ovarian tumor because of the large amount of stroma and fibrotic tissue that surrounds the epithelial cells. It is more common in older women and occasionally occurs in association with mucinous tumors of the ovary. When discovered as an isolated tumor of the ovary, it is relatively small compared with the large size attained often by the serous and especially by the mucinous cystadenomas, It is rarely malignant.

Benign Germ Cell Neoplasms

Germ cell tumors are derived from the primary germ cells. The tumors arise in the ovary and may contain relatively differentiated structures such as hair or bone. The most common tumor found in women of all ages is the *benign cystic teratoma*, also called a *dermoid cyst or dermoid*. Dermoids may contain differentiated tissue from all three embryonic germ layers (ectoderm, mesoderm, and endoderm). The most common elements found are of ectodermal origin, primarily squamous cell tissue such as skin appendages (sweat, sebaceous glands) with associated hair follicles and sebum. It is because of this predominance of dermoid derivatives that the term *dermoid* is used. Other constituents of dermoids include central nervous system tissue, cartilage, bone, teeth, and intestinal glandular elements, most of which are found in well-differentiated form. One unusual variant is the *struma ovarii*, in which functioning thyroid tissue is found.

A dermoid cyst is frequently encountered as an asymptomatic unilateral cystic adnexal mass, which is mobile, nontender, and often felt anterior to the broad ligament, i.e., just under the abdominal examining fingers rather than deep in the pelvis. The diagnosis can be confirmed by ultrasound, because of the peculiar pattern of echogenicity from inside the cyst caused by its contents.

Treatment of benign cystic teratomas is necessarily surgical, even though the rate of malignancy is less than 1%. Surgical removal is required because of the possibility of ovarian torsion and rupture, resulting in intense chemical peritonitis and a potential surgical emergency. Between 10 and 20% of these cysts are bilateral, underscoring the need for examination of the contralateral ovary at the time of surgery.

Benign Stromal Cell Neoplasms

Stromal cell tumors of the ovary are usually considered solid tumors and are derived from specialized sex cord stroma of the developing gonad. These tumors may develop along primarily female cell type into *granulosa theca cell tumors* or into primarily male gonadal type of tissue, which are described as *Sertoli-Leydig cell tumors*. Both of these tumors are referred to as functioning tumors because of their hormone production. *Granulosa theca cell tumors primarily produce estrogenic components* and may be manifest in patients through feminizing characteristics, and *Sertoli-Leydig cell tumors produce androgenic components*, which may contribute to hirsutism or virilizing symptoms. These neoplasms occur with approximately equal frequency in all age groups, including pediatric patients. When the granulosa cell tumor occurs in the pediatric age group, it may contribute to signs and symptoms of precocious puberty, including precocious thelarche and vaginal bleeding. Vaginal bleeding may also occur when this tumor develops in the postmenopausal years. Both the granulosa cell tumor and the Sertoli-Leydig cell tumor have malignant potential as discussed below.

The *ovarian fibroma* occurs in approximately 10% of patients with ovarian neoplasms, but is unlike the other stromal cell tumors in that it does not secrete sex steroids. It is usually a small solid tumor with a smooth surface and occasionally will be clinically misleading because of the presence of ascites. The combination of benign ovarian fibroma coupled with ascites and right unilateral hydrothorax has historically been referred to as *Meigs syndrome.*

In summary, the following points regarding benign ovarian neoplasms can be made: (*a*) they are more common than malignant tumors of the ovary in all age groups, (*b*) the chance for malignant transformation increases with increasing age, (*c*) they warrant surgical treatment because of their potential for malignancy, (*d*) preoperative assessment may be assisted by the use of pelvic imaging techniques such as ultrasound, and (*e*) surgical treatment may be conservative for benign tumors, especially if future reproduction is desired.

Malignant Ovarian Neoplasms

Ovarian cancer is the *fifth most common of all cancers in women* in the United States and the *third most common gynecologic malignancy*, having a frequency of approximately one-fourth that of endometrial carcinoma. Yet the *mortality rate of this disease is the highest of all the gynecologic malignancies*, primarily because early detection of the disease before widespread dissemination is difficult. Ovarian neoplasms are rarely symptomatic in early stages of disease, becoming symptomatic only after extensive metastasis. As yet, there is no effective screening test for ovarian cancer similar to the Pap smear for cervical cancer, so that approximately two-thirds of the patients with ovarian cancer have advanced disease at the time of diagnosis. It is estimated that there will be approximately 22,000 new cases of ovarian cancer in 1995, and that 60% of these patients will die within 5 years. The most important demographic observation regarding ovarian cancer is that it *presents most commonly in the fifth and sixth decade of life*. There is a higher incidence of ovarian cancer in western European countries and in the United States, with a five to seven times greater incidence than age-matched populations in the Far East. Whites are 50% more likely to develop ovarian cancer than blacks living in the United States.

A woman's risk of developing ovarian cancer during her lifetime is approximately 1%. The risk increases with age until approximately 70 years, at which time it declines modestly. The certain epidemiologic factors associated with developing ovarian cancer include low parity, decreased fertility, and delayed childbearing. In small groups of patients, there appears to be a familial predisposition to the development of ovarian cancer (*cancer family syndrome*) with an autosomal dominant genetic transmission pattern. Some investigators have suggested a possible carcinogenic source introduced into the lower genital tract by way of the vagina that eventually reaches the ovary. Inert agents such as asbestos and talc can be found in the peritoneal mesothelial cells, although the role of these and other potentially carcinogenic agents is unclear. An association with viral exposure, in particular with prior infection with mumps virus, has been suggested.

Long-term suppression of ovulation may protect against the development of ovarian cancer, at least for epithelial cell tumors. It has been suggested that so-called incessant ovulation may predispose to neoplastic transformation of the epithelial cell surfaces of the ovary. Oral contraceptives that cause anovulation appear to be modestly protective against the occurrence of ovarian cancer. No evidence exists to implicate the use of postmenopausal hormone-replacement therapy in the development of ovarian cancer.

Pathogenesis and Diagnosis

Malignant ovarian epithelial cell tumors spread primarily by direct extension within the peritoneal cavity because of direct cell sloughing from the ovarian surface. This process explains the observation that there is often widespread peritoneal dissemination of these cancers at the time of diagnosis, even with relatively small primary ovarian lesions. Although epithelial cell ovarian cancers also spread by lymphatic and blood-borne routes, it is the direct extension into the virtually unlimited space of the peritoneal cavity that contributes to their late clinical presentation.

The early diagnosis of ovarian cancer is also made difficult by the *lack of effective screening tests*. Approximately 60% of patients have advanced disease at the time of diagnosis. Refined imaging techniques (especially transvaginal ultrasonography) and serum tumor markers — such as the monoclonal antibody OC125, which recognizes the antigen Ca125 (which is present in serous ovarian tumors but not in mucinous or nonepithelial ovarian tumors) — offer promise for the future. Much work remains, however, before these or similar tests are considered accurate or cost-effective. Currently, serum tumor markers have been shown to be useful in the follow-up of previously treated epithelial cell neoplasms of the ovary but not for detection. Until these techniques are shown to be efficacious, detection is limited by the physician's index of suspicion and skill in the assessment of women who present with persistent but vague abdominopelvic symptoms or findings. The clinician is cautioned against the application of seemingly exacting technology while abandoning the exercise of sound clinical judgment. Further study of imaging techniques and serum tumor markers is ongoing in hopes of enabling earlier diagnosis of these tumors.

Histologic Classification

Malignant ovarian neoplasms are usually categorized by the cell type of origin similar to their benign counterparts: (*a*) *malignant epithelial cell tumors,* which are the most common type; (*b*) *malignant germ cell tumors;* and (*c*) *malignant stromal cell tumors* (see Table 45.1). Most malignant ovarian tumors have histologically similar but benign counterparts. The relationship between a benign ovarian neoplasm and its malignant counterpart

is clinically important. If the benign counterpart is found in a patient, removal of both ovaries is strongly considered, because of the possibility of future malignant transformation in the remaining ovary. The decision as to removal of one or both ovaries, however, must be individualized based on age, type of tumor, and future risks. For example, it has been shown that approximately 10% of seemingly benign epithelial cell tumors may contain histologic evidence of intraepithelial neoplasia, commonly referred to as borderline malignancies, or "tumors of low malignant potential."

Staging

The staging of ovarian carcinoma is based on extent of spread of tumor and histologic evaluation of the tumor. The International Federation of Gynecology and Obstetrics (FIGO) classification of ovarian cancer is presented in Table 45.3.

Epithelial Cell Ovarian Carcinoma

About 90% of all ovarian malignancies are of the epithelial cell type. These are thought to represent abnormalities in the differentiation of the pleuripotential mesothelial cells (which were derived embryologically from the gonadal ridge) that occupy parts of the visceral peritoneum. The ovary contains these cells as part of an ovarian capsule just overlying the actual stroma of the ovary. When these mesothelial cell elements are situated over developing follicles, they go through metaplastic transformation whenever ovulation occurs. Repeated ovulation is, therefore, associated with the histologic change in these cells derived from celomic epithelium.

Malignant epithelial serous tumors (serous cystadenocarcinoma) are the most common malignant epithelial cell tumors. About 50% of these cancers are thought to be derived from their benign precursors (serous cystadenoma), and as many as 30% of these tumors are bilateral at the time of clinical presentation. They are typically multiloculated and often have external excrescences on an otherwise smooth capsular surface.

Another epithelial cell variant, which contains cells reminiscent of endocervical glandular mucous secreting cells, is the *malignant mucinous epithelial tumor (the mucinous cystadenocarcinoma).* These tumors have a lower rate of bilaterality (10 to 15%) and can be among the largest of ovarian tumors, often measuring >20 cm. They may be associated with widespread peritoneal extension

Table 45.3.
FIGO Staging for Primary Carcinoma of the Ovary

Stage	Description
I	Growth limited to the ovaries
Ia	Growth limited to one ovary; no ascites containing malignant cells; no tumor on the external surface; capsule intact
Ib	Growth limited to both ovaries; no ascites containing malignant cells; no tumor on the external surface; capsule intact
Ic	Tumor either stage Ia or Ib but with tumor on the surface of one or both ovaries; or with capsule ruptured, or with ascites present containing malignant cells, or with positive peritoneal washings
II	Growth involving one or both ovaries with pelvic extension
IIa	Extension and/or metastases to the uterus and/or tubes
IIb	Extension to other pelvic tissues
IIc	Tumor either stage IIa or IIb but with tumor on the surface of one or both ovaries; or with capsule(s) ruptured, or with ascites present containing malignant cells, or with positive peritoneal washings
III	Tumor involving one or both ovaries with peritoneal implants outside the pelvic and/or positive retroperitoneal or inguinal nodes; superficial liver metastasis equals stage III; tumor is limited to the true pelvis, but histologically proven malignant extension is to small bowel or omentum
IIIa	Tumor grossly limited to the true pelvis with negative nodes but with histologically confirmed microscopic seeding of abdominal peritoneal surfaces
IIIb	Tumor of one or both ovaries with histologically confirmed implants of abdominal peritoneal surfaces; none exceeding 2 cm in diameter; nodes negative.
IIIc	Abdominal implants >2 cm in diameter and/or positive retroperitoneal or inguinal nodes
IV	Growth involving one or both ovaries with distant metastasis; if pleural effusion is present, there must be positive cytologic test results to deem a case stage IV; parenchymal liver metastasis equals stage IV

with thick mucinous ascites, termed *pseudomyxomatous peritonei*.

Endometrioid Tumors

Endometrioid epithelial cell tumors are the second most common type of epithelial cell malignancy of the ovary, constituting about 20% of all ovarian cancers. These tumors contain histologic features similar to endometrial carcinoma. Endometrioid tumors may arise in association with a primary endometrial carcinoma, making it difficult to determine whether they are primary to the ovary or metastatic from the endometrium. Only about 10% of these tumors are found in association with endometriosis and even fewer are known to have progressed from benign endometriotic precursors.

Of the remaining epithelial cell carcinomas of the ovary, *clear cell carcinomas* are thought to arise from mesonephric elements and Brenner tumors are thought to arise uncommonly (less than 5%) from their benign counterpart. Interestingly, Brenner tumors occur approximately 10% of the time in the same ovary that contains mucinous cystadenoma; the reason for this is unclear.

Germ Cell Tumors

Germ cell tumors constitute less than 5% *of all ovarian malignancies*. However, they are the *most common ovarian cancers in women under the age of 20*, making up 60% of the malignant tumors discovered in this age group. Germ cell tumors may be functional, producing human chorionic gonadotropin (hCG) or α-fetoprotein (AFP), both of which can be used as tumor markers. The most common germ cell malignancies are *dysgerminoma* and *immature teratoma*. Other tumors are recognized as *mixed germ cell tumors, endodermal sinus tumors, and embryonal tumors*. There has been remarkable progress in treatment of this group of tumors in the last 10 years. Improved chemotherapeutic and radiation protocols have resulted in greatly improved 5-year survival rates.

Dysgerminomas are unilateral in about 90% of patients. They are the *most common type of germ cell tumor seen in patients with gonadal dysgenesis*. These tumors often arise in benign counterparts called the gonadoblastoma. The tumors are particularly *radiosensitive*, rendering adjunctive therapy efficacious.

Because of the young age of patients with dysgerminomas, removal of only the involved ovary with preservation of the uterus and contralateral tube and ovary may be considered if the tumor is less than approximately 10 cm and if there is no evidence of extraovarian spread. Unlike the epithelial cell tumors, these malignancies are more likely to spread via lymphatic channels, and therefore, the pelvic and periaortic lymph nodes must be assessed carefully at the time of surgery. If disease has spread outside the ovaries, conventional hysterectomy and bilateral salpingo-oophorectomy are necessary, usually followed by postoperative radiation to the abdomen and pelvis. Chemotherapy is usually reserved for primary treatment failures. The prognosis of these tumors is generally excellent. The overall 5-year survival rate for patients with dysgerminoma is 90 to 95% when the disease is limited to one ovary that is <10 cm in size.

Immature teratomas are the malignant counterpart of benign cystic teratomas (dermoids). These are the *second most common germ cell cancer* and are *most often found in women under the age of 25.* They are usually unilateral, although on occasion a benign counterpart may be found in the contralateral ovary. Because these tumors are rapidly growing, they may produce painful symptomatology relatively early, because of hemorrhage and necrosis during the rapid growth process. As a result, the diagnosis is made when the disease is limited to one ovary in two-thirds of these young women. As with dysgerminoma, if an immature teratoma is limited to one ovary, unilateral oophorectomy is sufficient. Dramatic progress has been made in the treatment of these tumors in the past 15 years, with 5-year survival being >80% for patients with well-differentiated tumors.

Rare Germ Cell Tumors

Endodermal sinus tumors and embryonal cell carcinomas are uncommon malignant ovarian tumors for which there has been a remarkable improvement in cure rate. Before about 10 years ago, these tumors were almost uniformly fatal. New chemotherapeutic protocols have resulted in an overall 5-year survival of >60%. These tumors typically occur in childhood and adolescence, with the primary treatment being surgical resection of the involved ovary followed by combination chemotherapy. The endodermal sinus tumor produces α-fetoprotein, whereas the embryonal cell carcinoma produces both α-fetoprotein and β-hCG.

Gonadal Stromal Cell Tumors

The gonadal stromal cell tumors make up an unusual group of tumors, which is characterized by hormone production, hence these tumors are called *functioning tumors.* The hormonal output from these tumors is usually in the form of female or male sex steroids or, on occasion, adrenal steroid hormones.

The *granulosa cell tumor* is the *most common in this group.* These tumors occur in all ages, although in older patients they are more likely to be benign. Granulosa cell tumors may *secrete large amounts of estrogen, which in 15 to 20% of older women may cause endometrial hyperplasia or endometrial carcinoma.* Thus endometrial sampling is especially important when ovarian tumors such as the granulosa tumor are estrogen producing. Measurement of estrogen levels as a reflection of tumor dissemination has not been found useful, nor has follow-up of estrogen production been suggested as a useful tumor marker. The survival of patients with this neoplasm is contingent on factors similar to those for other tumors, in particular, whether or not the tumor has ruptured at the time of surgical exploration.

Surgical treatment should include extirpation of the uterus and both ovaries in postmenopausal women as well as in women of reproductive age who no longer wish to remain fertile. In a young woman with the lesions limited to one ovary with an intact capsule, unilateral oophorectomy with careful surgical staging may be adequate. This tumor may demonstrate recurrences up to 10 years later. This is especially true with large tumors, which have a 20 to 30% chance of late recurrence.

Sertoli-Leydig cell tumors (arrhenoblastoma) are the rare testosterone-secreting counterparts to granulosa cell tumors. They usually occur in older patients and should be suspected in the differential diagnosis of perimenopausal or postmenopausal patients with hirsutism or virilization and an adnexal mass. Treatment of these tumors is similar to that for other ovarian malignancies in this age group and is based on extirpation of uterus and ovaries.

Other stromal cell tumors include *fibromas* and *thecomas*, which very rarely demonstrate malignant counterparts, the *fibrosarcoma and malignant thecoma.*

Other Ovarian Malignancies

Very rarely, the ovary may be the site of initial manifestation of *lymphoma.* These are usually found in association with lymphoma elsewhere,

Table 45.4.
Surgical Staging for Primary Tubal Carcinoma

Stage	Description
I	
IA	Disease confined to one tube with no ascites
IB	Disease confined to both tubes with no ascites
IC	Disease confined to one or both tubes but ascites present with malignant cells in the fluid
II	
IIA	Extension to the uterus or ovaries of both
IIB	Extension to the uterus or ovaries and to other intraperitoneal organs or tissues beyond the true pelvis
III	Extension to the uterus or ovaries and to other intraperitoneal organs and tissues beyond the true pelvis
IV	Metastases present in organs or tissues outside the peritoneal cavity

although there have been case reports of primary ovarian lymphoma. Once the diagnosis has been made, management is similar to that for lymphoma of other origin.

Malignant mesodermal sarcomas are another rare type of ovarian tumor, which usually show aggressive behavior and are diagnosed at late stages. The survival rate is poor and clinical experience with these tumors is limited.

Cancer Metastatic to the Ovary

Classically, the term *Krukenberg tumor* describes an ovarian tumor that is metastatic from other sites such as the gastrointestinal tract (80% from stomach, remainder from colon), breast, and endometrium. Most of these tumors are characterized as infiltrative, mucinous carcinoma of predominately signet-ring cell type and as bilateral and associated with widespread metastatic disease. On occasion, these tumors are associated with abnormal uterine bleeding or virilization, leading to the supposition that some may produce estrogens or androgens. Cancers metastatic to the ovary account for 5 to 10% of ovarian malignancies. In 10% of patients with cancer metastatic to the ovary, an extraovarian primary site cannot be demonstrated. In this regard, it is important to consider ovarian preservation versus "prophylactic" oophorectomy at the time of hysterectomy in patients who have a strong family history (first-degree relatives) of epithelial ovarian cancer, primary gastrointestinal tract cancer, or breast cancer. In

patients previously treated for cancer or gastrointestinal cancer, consideration should be given to the incidental removal of the ovaries at the time of hysterectomy, because these patients have a high predilection for development of ovarian cancer. The prognosis for most patients with carcinoma metastatic to the ovary is dismal, with 5 to 10% 5-year survival rates being quoted.

FALLOPIAN TUBES

Normal fallopian tubes cannot be palpated and are generally not considered in the differential diagnosis of adnexal disease *in the asymptomatic patient*. There are common problems involving the fallopian tubes, including ectopic pregnancy, salpingitis/hydrosalpinx/tuboovarian abscess, and endometriosis (which can present as masses or be symptomatic). These conditions are discussed in other chapters.

Benign Disease of the Fallopian Tube and Mesosalpinx

Paraovarian cysts develop in the mesosalpinx from vestigal wolffian structures, tubal epithelium, and peritoneum inclusions. These are differentiated from *paratubal cysts*, which are found near the fimbriated end of the fallopian tube and are common, called *hydatids of Morgagni*. Both are usually small and symptomatic, although rarely they can reach large proportions.

Carcinoma of the Fallopian Tube

Primary fallopian tube carcinoma is usually an adenocarcinoma, although other cell types, including adenosquamous carcinoma and sarcoma, are rarely reported. About two-thirds of patients with this rare gynecologic malignancy (<1% of gynecologic malignancies) are postmenopausal. Grossly, these tumors are often rather large, resembling a hydrosalpinx, with a normal contralateral tube in 95% of cases. Microscopically, most are typical papillary serous cystadenocarcinomas of the ovary. The symptoms of this tumor are so slight that the tumor is often advanced before recognition of a problem. The most common complaint associated with fallopian tube carcinoma is postmenopausal bleeding followed by abnormal vaginal discharge. If such a discharge is profuse and serosanguineous, it is termed *hydrotubae profluens*, sometimes considered diagnostic of this tumor. Staging is surgical, *similar to that for ovarian carcinoma* (Table 45.4); progression is similar to ovarian carcinoma, with intraperitoneal metastases and ascites. Treatment is total abdominal hysterectomy with bilateral removal of the adnexae; careful exploration of the diaphragm, liver, paracolic gutters, omentum, and bowel; and biopsy of the omentum and retroperitoneal nodes. The overall 5-year survival rate is 35 to 45%, with stage I having the best rate, approaching 70%. There are too few data to ascertain whether adjunctive therapy is useful, and this management must be made on a case-by-case basis.

Carcinoma metastatic to the fallopian tube is far more common than primary fallopian tube carcinoma, including uterine and ovarian tumors. A few cases of *other very rare tumors of the fallopian tube are reported*, including malignant mixed müllerian tumors, primary choriocarcinoma, fibroma, and adenomatoid tumors.

GENERAL PRINCIPLES IN THE SURGICAL MANAGEMENT OF OVARIAN AND FALLOPIAN TUBE MALIGNANCY

Primary surgical therapy is indicated in the majority of ovarian malignancies, regardless of stage. This surgery is based on the principle of *cytoreductive surgery, or "tumor debulking."* The rationale for cytoreductive surgery is that adjunctive radiotherapy and chemotherapy are more effective when all tumor masses are reduced to <1 cm in size (see Chapter 40). Because direct peritoneal seeding is the primary method of intraperitoneal spread, multiple adjacent structures commonly contain tumor, resulting in cytoreductive procedures that are often quite extensive. Each procedure includes the following.

1. Peritoneal cytology is obtained; this is used to assess microscopic spread of tumor. Samples are taken immediately after entering the abdomen before extensive surgery has been undertaken. Gross ascites is aspirated and submitted for cytologic analysis. If there is no gross ascites, saline irrigation is used to "wash" the peritoneal cavity in an attempt to find microscopic disease. The wash is then submitted for cytologic assessment.
2. To visually and by palpation determine the extent of disease, thorough inspection and palpation are done, including the uterus, fallopian tubes and ovaries, surfaces of the pelvis, right and left pericolic gutters, omentum, upper abdominal viscera including the surface of the liver and spleen, and undersurface of the diaphragm.
3. Partial omentectomy is usually performed, with or without evidence of tumor involvement.
4. Sampling of the pelvic and periaortic lymph nodes is done in earlier stage disease of stromal cell and germ cell tumors, which have a higher likelihood of lymphatic spread. In the absence of gross disease, biopsies are obtained from the pelvic peritoneum and peritoneum of the right and left upper and lower pericolic gutters.

Based on the histologic evaluation of all samples, a rational program of adjunctive radiotherapy or chemotherapy may be undertaken.

Follow-up currently consists of clinical history and examination; various imaging studies, such as ultrasound and/or CT; and in epithelial cell tumors, the use of serum tumor markers such as Ca125. One other area of special consideration for ovarian cancer patients is the *second-look laparotomy.* This procedure is reserved for patients who have no clinically evident disease after the completion of primary surgical therapy and a standard course of adjunctive chemotherapy. If the patient has been rendered clear of gross disease at the time of surgery and if she has undergone a course of standard chemotherapy for presumed microscopic residual disease, it is often difficult to know whether residual disease remains. Therefore, many ovarian cancer treatment protocols include second-look laparotomy to ascertain if residual disease remains.

CASE STUDIES

Case 45A

A 23-year-old G1 P1001 describes a new, crampy pain in her right pelvis over the last 3 days. Her last menstrual period (LMP) was 3 weeks ago and was normal. She uses a diaphragm for contraception and her urine pregnancy test is negative. On pelvic examination a 3 × 4 cm tender cystic mass is found in the right adnexa. The remainder of her examination is normal.

Questions Case 45A

The best management at this time would be to schedule

A. A return visit in 1 week
B. A return visit to the office in 2 months
C. A return visit to the office in 1 year
D. A diagnostic laparoscopy
E. An exploratory laparotomy

Answer: B

Although the differential diagnosis includes various tumors and benign gynecologic pathology, the most likely diagnosis is a "functional" ovarian cyst, i.e., a follicular or corpus luteum cyst. A return visit is necessary, as a functional cyst will resolve, whereas other pathology will not; 2 months is a reasonable time, but 1 year is too long. Surgical intervention is far too aggressive a measure at this time. Transvaginal or transabdominal ultrasound will provide additional information as to size and consistency of the mass and should be ordered on a case-by-case basis.

Which medications are appropriate for this patient at this time?

A. Oral contraceptives
B. Oral progesterone
C. Oral estrogen
D. Gonadotropin-releasing hormone (GnRH) agonist
E. Oral doxycycline

Answer: A

Gonadotropin suppression with oral contraceptives can be used in a patient with a functional ovarian cyst, although this is not a "required" management. It would be particularly appropriate if the patient were to express a desire to switch to oral contraceptives for birth control purposes also. Indeed, no medication, i.e., watchful expectation, would also be an acceptable management. Progesterone and estrogen would not aid in cyst resolution. No evidence of infection was given, hence antibiotic therapy is not indicated. GnRH agonist would eliminate gonadotropin stimulation of the ovary but would be overtreating this clinical situation.

The mass persists after 2 months of oral contraceptive therapy; in fact, it is now 2 cm larger. Ultrasound examination confirms a cystic mass. Ca125 is within normal ranges, as are all other laboratory evaluations. At exploratory laparotomy, a cystic mass is found without any other pelvic abnormalities. An ovarian cystectomy is performed. The final pathology report is serous cysadenoma.

What options should be presented to the patient at this time?

A. Total abdominal hysterectomy and bilateral salpingo-oophorectomy
B. Unilateral salpingo-oophorectomy
C. Radiation therapy
D. Chemotherapy
E. Observation

Answer: E

This benign ovarian neoplasm requires no specific follow-up, although yearly examinations are important in this young women who has had a benign ovarian neoplasm.

Case 45B

A 53-year-old woman notices increased facial and body hair and a deepening tone of voice. On physical examination, the patient has considerable coarse facial hair and a 3 × 4 cm, firm left adnexal mass.

Questions Case 45B

The serum concentration of which of the following hormones would most likely be elevated?

A. hCG
B. Progesterone
C. Estradiol
D. Testosterone

Answer: D

The history and physical examination are most consistent with a Sertoli-Leydig cell tumor, the rare testosterone-secreting counterpart to the granulosa cell tumor.

The best management at this time would be to schedule

A. A transvaginal pelvic ultrasound examination
B. A return visit to the office in 2 months
C. A return visit to the office in 1 year
D. A diagnostic laparoscopy
E. An exploratory laparotomy

Answer: E

Exploratory laparotomy and total abdominal hysterectomy with bilateral salpingo-oophorectomy are indicated. Temporizing with a probable ovarian malignancy in a postmenopausal patient is not appropriate. Ultrasound evaluation might offer more information about the characteristics of the adnexal mass but would not alter the surgical management.

Case 45C

A 17-year-old G0 complains of a painful full sensation in her right lower quadrant. She has had regular menstrual periods since age 14 and uses a low-dose oral contraceptive. She has no history of sexually transmitted diseases, admits to one sexual partner, and has had serial negative cultures as part of her annual examinations. She had a normal pelvic examination with satisfactory, negative Pap smear 9 months before her visit with this complaint. On physical examination you find a nervous young lady weighing 105 pounds with a normal general physical examination and pelvic examination except for a 5 × 5 cm firm mobile mass in the right adnexae. Her urine pregnancy test is negative.

Questions Case 45C

Your immediate evaluation should include

A. Repeat Pap smear
B. Endometrial biopsy
C. Pelvic ultrasound
D. Carcinoembryonic antigen (CEA)
E. β-hCG

Answer: C

Repeat Pap smear and endometrial biopsy are not consistent with this complaint and finding. Hormonal markers are likewise of little value. The mass feels solid, and ultrasound will help establish its internal structure.

The ultrasound confirms a 5 × 5 cm right adnexal mass that is described as composed of mixed cystic and solid components, some of which are calcified. There is no evidence of ascites, and the left adnexae appears unremarkable. Your management suggestion should now be

A. Observation, as there is no evidence of ascites, hence malignancy

B. Observation, as malignancy is uncommon in this age group and the risks of intervention are not warranted
C. Observation with serial ultrasound examinations, as adnexal masses are common in young women and resolve spontaneously in most cases
D. Diagnostic laparoscopy
E. Exploratory laparotomy or operative laparoscopy

Answer: E

This is a new and symptomatic mass, solid in nature, so that benign follicular tumor is unlikely. Further observation is not appropriate, as an adnexal accident may occur (torsion, etc.), and the tumor may be malignant, however unlikely. Diagnostic laparoscopy is not indicated, as removal of the mass is required. Either exploratory laparotomy or operative laparoscopy may be used to remove the mass, depending on the operator's skills and training.

At exploratory laparotomy, a unilateral cystic mass is discovered. When opened at the operating table, it contained mature structures such as hair and teeth. Subsequently, the pathology report was benign cystic teratoma.

chapter 46

GESTATIONAL TROPHOBLASTIC DISEASE

Gestational trophoblastic neoplasia (GTN), which represents a *rare variation of pregnancy*, is limited in most instances to a benign disease called *molar pregnancy*. This disorder includes neoplasms that are derived almost entirely from abnormal placental (trophoblastic) proliferation. Molar pregnancy may in turn be divided into *complete mole* (no fetus) and *incomplete mole* (fetus plus molar degeneration). Fewer than 10% of patients with GTN will develop persistent or malignant disease. Fortunately, persistent or malignant GTN is very responsive to effective chemotherapy.

Key clinical features of gestational trophoblastic neoplasia include its consistent clinical presentation, reliable means of diagnosis with pathognomonic ultrasound findings, presence of specific tumor marker (quantitative serum hCG), availability of effective surgical treatment, sensitivity to chemotherapy when GTN is persistent or malignant, and reliable long-term follow-up through assessment of quantitative hCG levels.

The disease has a number of *characteristic features*, including (*a*) the potential for malignant transformation, (*b*) clinical presentation as a pregnancy, (*c*) profound hormonal changes found in association with the abnormal proliferation of trophoblastic tissue, (*d*) genetic makeup, and (*e*) and high sensitivity to chemotherapeutic agents.

The *etiology* of this disorder is unknown. It has been observed that the incidence varies among different national and ethnic groups with the highest occurring among Oriental women living in Asia (up to 1 in 200 pregnancies) and the lowest incidence occurring in Caucasian women of western European and U.S. origins (approximately 1 in 2000 pregnancies). The recurrence rate is approximately 2%. It is more common in very young women and in women at the end of their reproductive years. It is also associated with dietary deficiencies, such as folic acid. The classification of gestational trophoblastic disease is described in Table 46.1. Since persistent gestational trophoblastic neoplasia may follow simple molar pregnancy, an appreciation of the latter's clinical presentation, histology, clinical risk factors, and long-term follow-up are necessary to thoroughly treat the patient with this unusual tumor.

HYDATIDIFORM MOLE (MOLAR PREGNANCY)

A complete hydatidiform mole includes abnormal proliferation of the syncytiotrophoblast and replacement of normal placental trophoblastic tissue by *hydropic placental villi*. Complete moles do not include the formation of a fetus, and fetal membranes are characteristically absent. *Partial moles* are characterized by focal trophoblastic proliferation and degeneration of the placenta and are associated with a chromosomally abnormal fetus. In this form of molar pregnancy, trophoblastic proliferation is largely from the cytotrophoblast (Fig. 46.1).

The *genetic constitutions* of these two types of molar pregnancy are different (Table 46.2). Complete moles are entirely of paternal origin as a result of the fertilization of a blighted ovum by a haploid sperm, which then reduplicates. Accordingly, the karyotype of a complete mole is 46,XX. The fetus of a partial mole is usually a triploidy, the most common being 69,XXY. The triploidy is comprised of one haploid set of maternal chromosomes and two haploid sets of paternal chromosomes, which arise from dispermic fertilization. Of the two varieties, the complete mole is more common (approximately 90% of molar pregnancies). Although the potential for malignant transformation is greater in complete moles, partial moles may also undergo this change, and therefore, both varieties should be followed in a similar fashion to minimize the chance for malignant sequelae.

Table 46.1.
Classification of Gestational Trophoblastic Disease

Molar pregnancy
  Complete mole
  Partial mole

Persistent gestational trophoblastic neoplasia
  Histologically benign
  Persistent histologically benign
  Persistent histologically malignant

Clinical Presentation

Clinically, patients with molar pregnancy of either variety may present with findings consistent with pregnancy but also with uterine size/dates discrepancy, exaggerated subjective symptoms of pregnancy, and bleeding suggestive of spontaneous abortion. Of these symptoms, *bleeding* is the most characteristic and occurs in most patients early in the second trimester of pregnancy. The bleeding is usually painless. The patient also may experience the passage of tissue, as fragments of the edematous trophoblast are passed through the dilated cervical os. Most patients have already been *diagnosed as pregnant*, having had a positive pregnancy test. There is a *uterine dates/size discrepancy* in two-thirds of patients. The uterus may be either too large or too small for gestational age, usually larger than expected. This discrepancy, coupled with late first or early second trimester bleeding, usually leads the clinician to perform ultrasound imaging of the uterus, which confirms the diagnosis of molar pregnancy by its characteristic "snowstorm" appearance (Fig. 46.2).

Molar pregnancies may present with *other signs and symptoms*, including visual disturbances, severe nausea and vomiting, marked pregnancy-induced hypertension (preeclampsia), proteinuria, and rarely, clinical hyperthyroidism. Some patients experience tachycardia and shortness of breath, arising from intense hemodynamic changes associated with acute hypertensive changes. In these patients, hyperreflexia may also be found. Physical examination reveals not only the dates/size discrepancy of the uterine fundus and absent fetal heart tones but also changes associated with developing preeclampsia. Occasionally, bimanual pelvic examination may reveal large *adnexal masses* (theca lutein cysts), which represent marked enlargement of the ovaries as a result of high levels of hCG stimulation.

The clinical presentation of partial molar pregnancy is similar to that for complete mole, although typically

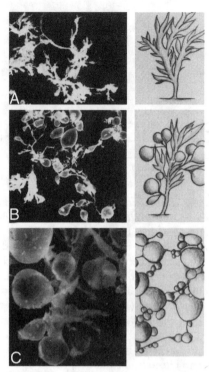

Figure 46.1. Villi gross morphology. **A,** Normal chorionic villi. **B,** Partial mole with normal villi admixed with swollen ones (case of triploidy, 69,XX4). **C,** Complete mole with swollen, vesicular villi.

the patient presents at a more advanced gestational age (after the 20th week of pregnancy). Vaginal bleeding is less common than with complete moles. Uterine growth that is less than that expected for the gestational age, especially if coupled with rapidly developing hypertension, may be the first clinical indication. Because of the growth/dates discrepancy, ultrasonography is obtained, which reveals molar degeneration of the placenta and frequently a grossly abnormal fetus.

Laboratory Assessment

The laboratory assessment of molar pregnancy is critical for both treatment and follow-up. After the molar pregnancy has been confirmed by imaging studies, laboratory documentation is necessary to ascertain the *level of hCG*. These levels are extremely high in molar pregnancy and not only *help classify risk category but also serve as a sensitive tumor marker in the follow-up* of these patients. Other valuable studies include a baseline chest x-ray to

Table 46.2.
Complete and Incomplete Hydatidiform Moles

Characteristic	Complete	Incomplete
Synonyms	True; classic	Partial
Villi	All edematous	Some normal
Capillaries	Few, no fetal RBCs	Some; fetal RBCs
Embryo	None	Abnormal fetus
hCG titer	High	Moderately elevated to high
Karyotype	Mostly 46,XX	Triploid
Malignant potential	15–20%	Slight

check for metastatic disease, assessment of hemoglobin and hematocrit, and selected other tests, depending on clincal evidence of preeclampsia and/or hyperthyroidism. Before treatment, blood should be obtained for blood type and Rh and screened for antibodies in case blood replacement is necessary. This is particularly important for patients who undergo uterine evacuation, as there is the potential for extensive blood loss during the procedure. Similar laboratory studies should be obtained whether the patient has partial or complete mole.

Treatment

In most cases of *molar pregnancy*, the definitive treatment is prompt *removal of the intrauterine contents*. Uterine evacuation is done most expeditiously by dilation of the cervix followed by *suction curettage*. After suction curettage with an atraumatic plastic cannula, *gentle sharp curettage* may be performed to provide small amounts of myometrial tissue for separate pathologic assessment. This is used to ascertain whether there has been myometrial invasion. The evacuation of larger moles is sometimes associated with uterine atony and excessive blood loss, so that appropriate preparations should be made for oxytocic administration and blood transfusion if they are needed.

In cases of *partial mole*, a similar procedure may be carried out, with the additional need for larger grasping instruments to remove the abnormal fetus. With cases involving enlargement of the uterus beyond 24 weeks gestational size, an alternative to suction evacuation is induction of labor with prostaglandin vaginal suppositories. In general, *the larger the uterus, the greater the risk of pulmonary complications* associated with trophoblastic

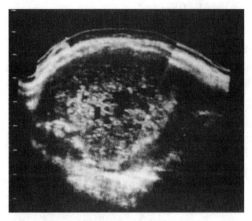

Figure 46.2. "Snowstorm" appearance of complete mole on ultrasound examination.

emboli, fluid overload, and anemia. This is particularly true in patients with extreme degrees of associated pregnancy-induced hypertension (preeclampsia), since patients may experience concomitant hemoconcentration and alteration in vascular hemodynamics. In these patients, uterine evacuation by prostaglandin stimulation may be safer.

Occasional patients in the older reproductive age group may be best served by hysterectomy, which ensures removal of the entire primary neoplasm. This is especially true in patients with "high-risk" disease, as described in Table 46.3. This treatment should be reserved for patients who have no interest in further childbearing and/or have other indications for hysterectomy.

The *bilaterally enlarged multicystic ovaries (theca lutein cysts)*, arising from massive follicular stimulation by large amounts of systemic hCG, do not represent malignant changes. This enlargement invariably regresses after the molar pregnancy has been evacuated and, therefore, does not require surgical removal. Understanding the physiology of these cysts is especially important in the patient undergoing abdominal hysterectomy as the primary treatment.

Postevacuation Management

Because of the predisposition for recurrent non-malignant or malignant disease, patients should

Table 46.3.
Conditions That Define High Risk Gestational Trophoblastic Disease

Uterus >16 week size

Theca-lutein cysts

Marked trophoblastic proliferation and/or anaplasia

Hyperthyroidism

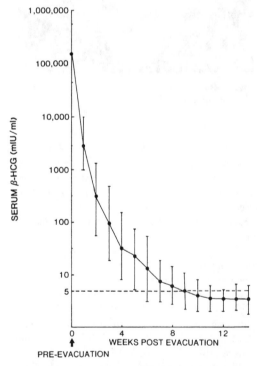

Figure 46.3. Normal regression curve and smoothed 95% confidence limits of serum β-hCG following evaluation of a hydatidiform mole. Time 0 is time of evacuation.

be followed closely for at least 1 year. The *removed molar tissue* should be examined carefully to identify hyperplastic and/or anaplastic proliferation. The small tissue sample provided by the sharp curettage specimen pivotal in determining myometrial invasion. RhoGAM should be given as indicated in a normal pregnancy.

Follow-up consists primarily of *periodic physical examination,* including pelvic examination and the *assessment of quantitative hCG levels,* according to the schedule outlined in Table 46.4. Quantitative serum β-hCG values fall after evacuation in a characteristic manner (Fig. 46.3), with plateauing being an indication of persistent disease and the need for further treatment. Following this guideline, assures the physician that recurrent disease is not developing; that an intercurrent pregnancy (within 1 year) is not causing an increase in hCG levels, and that for future pregnancy another molar pregnancy is ruled out early, since the recurrence rate for these patients is approximately five times the initial rate (1 in 400 in the United States). Effective contraception is recommended in the 1st year of follow-up.

METASTATIC/MALIGNANT GESTATIONAL TROPHOBLASTIC NEOPLASIA

Recurrent benign gestational trophoblastic neoplasia and/or malignant transformation of this disease (choriocarcinoma) occurs in less than 10% of patients with antecedent molar pregnancy. Early identification and treatment of recurrence is critically important. Failure of quantitative hCG levels to regress following initial therapy suggests that

Table 46.4.
Posttreatment Follow-up for Molar Pregnancy

General physical and pelvic examination and baseline chest x-ray at 2 weeks

Serum quantitative hCG level every 2 weeks until normal (0-5 mIU)

Serum quantitative hCG monthly for 1 year after obtaining first normal level

Assurance of contraception for 1 year (oral contraceptives preferred unless contraindicated)

Early ultrasound examination and quantitative hCG level for future pregnancy further treatment is needed. Common sites of persistent or metastatic disease include the uterus, adjacent pelvic structures, the lungs, and the brain. Treatment of persistent gestational trophoblastic disease may involve the use of a number of potentially effective chemotherapeutic agents. What should be remembered is that gestational trophoblastic neoplasia, even in its malignant form, is highly sensitive to chemotherapy and is considered a "prototype" for tumors that are sensitive to these agents. The indications for chemotherapy for persistent or malignant trophoblastic disease are presented in Table 46.5.

Generally, nonmetastatic persistent gestational trophoblastic neoplasia is completely treated by single-agent chemotherapy. The prognosis for malignant GTN is more complex, divided into good and poor prognosis categories (Table 46.6). The World Health Organization (WHO) has developed a prognostic scoring system for gestational trophoblastic neoplasia, which takes into account a number of epidemiologic and laboratory findings (Table 46.7). Chemotherapeutic agents used include both single-agent treatment with methotrexate and actinomycin as well as combination chemotherapy ("triple therapy"), which includes methotrexate, actinomycin, and chlorambucil (MAC) (Table 46.8).

Other chemotherapeutic agents are being tested and may be effective as well. Where chemotherapy is indicated, the treatment protocol depends on whether patients fall into the "good" or "poor" prognosis metastatic group. Adjunctive radiation therapy is usually recommended for patients with brain or liver metastases, although the data in support of this therapy are scant.

CASE STUDIES

Case 46A

A 38-year-old woman presents for prenatal care. Her last normal menstrual period was approximately 10 weeks ago. For the past 5 or 6 days, she has experienced light vaginal spotting, and she has been bothered by rather intense "morning sickness" for the past 4 weeks. She has been able to tolerate fluids and a few small meals, but generally does not have a normal appetite.

Physical examination reveals a blood pressure of 150/100, urine shows 3+ protein, the uterine fundus is approximately 16 weeks size, and there is an absence of fetal heart tones. Pelvic examination shows the cervix to be fingertip dilated with a small amount of blood at the os. Bimanual examination confirms an enlarged uterus consistent with approximately 16 week size, and there is a suggestion of bilateral adnexal masses.

Question Case 46C

Which of the following should be done immediately?

A. Obtain quantitative serum hCG
B. Obtain pelvic ultrasound
C. Begin 24-hr urine collection for total protein
D. Obtain fetal heart rate reading with fetal monitor
E. Initiate hypertension workup

Answer: A, B

This problem typifies a number of features of molar pregnancy, including uterine dates/size discrepancy,

Table 46.5.
Indications for Chemotherapy for Trophoblastic Disease

Histologic diagnosis of choriocarcinoma

Evidence of metastatic disease

Indications based on quantitative serum β-hCG levels
  Plateaued or rising titer after evacuation
  Titer that has not returned to normal after 12 weeks postevacuation

Reelevated level after a normal level has been obtained, exclusive of a new pregnancy

Table 46.6.
Clinical Classification of Malignant GTN

Nonmetastatic GTD (not defined in terms of good versus poor prognosis)

Metastatic GTD
  Good prognosis: absence of high-risk factors
    Pretreatment hCG level <40,000 mIU/mL serum β-hCG
    <4-months' duration of disease
    No evidence of brain or liver metastasis
    No significant prior chemotherapy
    No antecedent term pregnancy

  Poor prognosis: any single high-risk factor
    Pretreatment hCG level >40,000 mIU/mL serum β-hCG
    >4-months' duration of disease
    Brain and/or liver metastases
    Failed prior chemotherapy
    Antecedent term pregnancy

Table 46.7.

WHO Prognostic Scoring System for Gestational Trophoblastic Disease[a]

Prognostic Factor	0	1	2	3
Age	<39	>39		
Antecedent pregnancy	HM[b]	Abortion; ectopic	Term	
Interval (months)[c]	<4	4–6	7–12	>12
hCG level (IU/liter)	<10^3	10^3–10^4	10^4–10^5	>10^5
ABO blood groups (female × male)		O × A	B	
		A × O	AB	
Largest tumor (cm)	<3	3–5	>5	
Site of metastasis		Spleen, kidney	GI[b] tract, liver	Brain
Number of metastases		1–3	4–8	>8
Prior chemotherapy			Single drug	Multiple drugs

[a] Low risk, 4; intermediate risk, ≤5–7; high risk, ≥8.

[b] HM, hydatidiform mole; GI, gastrointestinal.

[c] Time between antecedent pregnancy and start of chemotherapy.

Table 46.8.

Chemotherapy for Gestational Trophoblastic Disease

Single agent
  Methotrexate (15–25 mg i.m. or I.V. daily for 5 days)
  Actinomycin D (0.015 mg/kg or 0.5 mg I.V. daily for 5 days)
  Treatment courses are repeated as often as toxicity will allow

Triple therapy
  Methotrexate (15–25 mg I.V. daily for 5 days)
  Actinomycin D (0.5 mg I.V. daily for 5 days)
  Clorambucil (10 mg orally daily for 5 days)
  or
  Cytoxan (150–250 mg I.V. daily for 5 days)

Leucovorin "rescue"
  Methotrexate (1.0 mg/kg I.M.) followed in 12–24 hr by citrovorum factor (0.01 mg/kg I.M.); the
    methotrexate is given every other day for four doses or until toxicity develops

acute pregnancy-induced hypertension (preeclampsia), absence of fetal development, and bilateral theca-lutein cysts. The diagnosis can be most readily made by obtaining an ultrasound. This should be done first to confirm the diagnosis, after which treatment will include treatment of the preeclampsia to prevent seizures and plans for expeditious uterine evacuation. A quantitative serum β-hCG is drawn as a baseline value against which postevacuation β-hCG evacuations may be compared.

Case 46B

A 22-year-old woman returns for her fourth postoperative follow-up examination since undergoing a suction curettage for an incomplete mole (trophoblastic degeneration of the triploidy fetus) 5 weeks ago. The initial quantitative hCG titer drawn at the time of her diagnosis was 40,000 mIU. The serum titer drawn 2 weeks ago was 1,500 mIU. The serum titer obtained yesterday shows a quantitative hCG level of 4,500 mIU.

Question Case 46B

The most appropriate therapy at this point should be

A. A simple hysterectomy

B. Hysterectomy and bilateral salpingo-oophorectomy

C. Radiation therapy

D. Dilation and curettage

E. Chemotherapy

Answer: D, then E

This case is typical of a patient with persistent trophoblastic disease, as illustrated by rapidly falling serum β-hCG titers followed by resurgence a few weeks later. Given her young age and low-risk category, single-agent chemotherapy is most appropriate to treat this problem. Before beginning chemotherapy, she should have another dilation and curettage to obtain enough tissue to characterize the type of persistent trophoblast. It should be remembered, however, that dilation and curettage may not always reveal the presence of persistent trophoblast, since it can be present outside the uterine cavity and/or in metastatic sites.

chapter 47

ETHICS IN OBSTETRICS AND GYNECOLOGY

Ethics in obstetrics and gynecology has some unique characteristics that are illustrated by the following cases.

First Case: A Jehovah's Witness patient, hemorrhaging from a placenta previa needs a cesarean section. Do we give blood against the patient's expressed wishes (a form of battery), even to save her life? Do we allow her to die while we deliver her child safely but motherless?

Second Case: A pregnant woman who uses cocaine. Should the mother-to-be who uses cocaine be held accountable for the condition (including death) of her unborn child?

Third Case: A markedly neurotic child-abusing mother with several children who refuses contraception. Should we require Norplant implants or Depo-Provera injections for this woman?

Fourth Case: A 33-year-old woman dying of cervical cancer who has been given a high dose of morphine to try to abate her increasing and prolonged pain but whose respirations have dropped to 3/min. Should we give her a narcotic antagonist or let her die sooner with a side effect of the medication for her intractable pain?

The ethical quandaries demonstrated in these four cases present a challenge to clarify the way we think about ethical problems in medicine that is relevant to whatever area of medicine is eventually chosen as a specialty.

There is a substantial literature that presents methods of thinking about ethical issues, which is quite helpful. By using this literature, you will not solely depend on your personal reaction to a problem or on your intuition. Indeed, the use of ethical principles allows us to make better medical choices by standing back and reflecting on these problems rather than either by not dealing with them or by reacting randomly based on emotions, personal bias, or social pressures.

How can you identify the basic ethical dilemmas of a confusing case? What sort of systematic approach is helpful? The answers to these questions are illustrated by detailed analysis of the first case.

A 24-year-old G2 P1001 Jehovah's Witness with a complete placenta previa is transferred from the antepartum care unit to labor and delivery with the onset of bleeding (2 cups of bright red blood in 10 min). Her husband, also a Jehovah's Witness, and her mother who is not a member of that group accompany her. She rapidly loses 1 liter of blood, and evidence of fetal distress is found on the electronic fetal monitor. She reaffirms her absolute refusal of blood or blood products, even though an emergency cesarean section is proposed for her own and her fetus's survival. Her blood pressure is dropping despite rapid hydration. She becomes unconscious. The anesthesiologist says the patient will probably die with the insults of anesthesia and surgery without blood transfusion. The patient's mother demands that you give her daughter blood. The husband refuses. The fetal heart tracing demonstrates severe fetal distress consistent with profound fetal damage or death, and you begin the cesarean section and deliver a healthy 7-lb girl with Apgar scores of 2 and then 8 with resuscitation. The patient survives the surgery, but in recovery her blood pressure drops to 50/0 postoperatively, and she remains unconscious and on a ventilator with a central venous pressure of 0. The patient's mother screams, "You are killing her! She is my only child!" Her husband firmly reminds you of the religious beliefs he and his wife share and warns you that his attorney is available if needed. What is the right thing to do?

The first step is to try to separate this emotional case into ethically separate concerns. An analytical scheme from the book *Clinical Ethics* is useful for this purpose (Table 47.1). Separating a case into four areas of concern allows us to fit each particular problem in a family of ethical issues that are associated with particular principles central to medical ethics. This process of systematic analysis and reflection is basic to medical ethics.

Considering this first case, we would ask, "What was the *medical indication* for the cesarean section?" Clearly, both child and mother would die without surgery. Continuing acute hemorrhage from placenta previa has no potential therapy other than surgical delivery and removal of the placenta. Support of the cardiovascular system with blood products is medically indicated. Yet this patient has clearly stated her *preference:* she will not accept blood products, both while no acute problem is present or after. She believes that blood is directly opposed to God's will and that receiving blood, even against her wishes, will permanently and negatively affect her spiritual self. She does not feel life under such circumstances (i.e., after receiving blood) to be acceptable.

From her caregiver's viewpoint, blood transfusion is more likely to produce a better quality of life, i.e., survival without neurologic or major organ sequelae. Without blood products, her survival is questionable, and even with survival, her risk for prolonged ICU stay, cardiac failure, renal failure, and hematologic sequelae are much greater.

Considering *contextual issues,* we wonder how this newborn child will do *without her mother.* In addition, what is the validity of the cost of care in an ICU for the sequelae resulting from the patient's choice when other patients need the ICU bed? What about the grandmother's concerns? Is the husband coercing the patient to not accept blood? Is he coercing the physician with comments about his attorney or is that his right to protect his wife? What would the law say if we gave the patient blood without permission?

The first case is complex, but it is clear that the patient's choice to refuse blood products is an underlying issue. Does this patient's autonomous refusal constitute a real choice, and if so, should we accept it? While the law has much to say about the rights of individuals to choose or refuse care, the choice here to not give blood is based on the great respect caregivers must have for the right of patients to determine their care that medical ethics has supported. There is much literature regarding autonomy and refusal of blood products that can be accessed to illuminate these choices.

In more general terms, the medical indications for a proposed management always need to be as clear and as "scientific" as possible. Is the benefit of what is proposed clearly greater than the harm that might be caused or is the benefit at a level that makes the harm acceptable? Consider the fourth case: the 33-year-old dying slowly of cervical cancer. She is at risk from the pain medication needed to alleviate her suffering. Is the relief of pain so great a benefit that the decreased respiratory rate and potential respiratory arrest are acceptable? Consider the third case: the mother

Table 47.1.

Areas of Concern and Associated Ethical Principles in Clinical Medical Ethics: A Functional Scheme for Clinical Ethical Decision Making

Ethical concern:	MEDICAL INDICATION What is the best treatment? What are the alternatives?	Ethical concern:	PATIENT PREFERENCES What does the patient want?
Ethical principle:	BENEFICENCE The duty to promote the good of the patient	Ethical principle:	AUTONOMY Respect for the patient's right to self-determination
Ethical concern:	QUALITY OF LIFE What impact will the proposed treatment or lack of it have on the patient's life?	Ethical principle:	SOCIOECONOMIC ISSUES What does the patient want? What are the needs of society?
Ethical principle:	NONMALEFICENCE The duty not to inflict harm or injury	Ethical principle:	JUSTICE The patient should be given what is "due."

who refuses contraception yet abuses her children. Is Norplant medically indicated for the child-abusing patient? Does she have a medical contra-indication to its use? Remember that before proceeding with a proposed treatment, the benefit to the patient must be clear. If the benefit is unclear but the treatment ongoing, the issues are still more complex.

Consider a variation in the case of the patient with cervical cancer. She is also not able to eat because of the pain and the family requests total parenteral nutrition (TPN). It will make them "feel better about things." Many would consider that TPN was medically futile and question the ethics of its continued use. The group of cases related to *medical indications* involve such concerns as benefit (or *beneficence*) and the related concept of futility.

The cases that can be categorized under *patient preferences* revolve around the principle of *autonomy*, the respect we hold for the patient's right to choose care. It is important to note that the physician-patient relationship emphasizes a relationship between *the* physician and *the* patient. Even in obstetrics, where the consequences of patient choices on another potential life can be significant, the primacy of the physician-patient (versus physician-fetus) relationship is paramount. What the patient wants and her capacity to make those choices are in question here. Consider the second case: Does the drug-using mother have the capacity to make decisions about her unborn child? By reason of the effect of the drugs, has she lost the capacity for acceptable decision making? Is society bound by her decision making? What about the rights of the unborn child? Consider the fourth case: Is the dying patient whose mentation is potentially clouded by impending death and the medications used for pain relief capable of decisions about her care?

Quality of life issues are always important. The absence of pain in a terminal cancer patient may significantly improve the quality of her living, even if the length of time is shortened. Some patients may consider the diminution of quality of life with potential permanent neurologic damage or loss of time with children arising as a result of blood loss (as in the first case) so significant that they will accept blood despite their religious beliefs. So the harms of treatment or no treatment viewed in the context of a particular patient's life are what must be considered. In a sense, this deals with *nonmaleficence:* the duty to not harm patients

while treating them. Harm clearly must also be framed in the patient's framework. In the fourth case, prolonged life may not be valued if significant pain or an elongated hospital stay is the quality of life that must be accepted. That becomes unacceptable "harm" to that patient. Yet, as in the first case, the quality of life after blood transfusion may be acceptable for the added time to be spent with her children and the diminished risk of major organ damage. The benefits of proposed therapy must be framed in the outcome of that therapy for good or ill.

Finally, all the *contextual and socioeconomic issues* that surround a particular case should be considered. It is here that the concerns of the children and mother and father and other relatives and concerns about legal issues and issues of cost are addressed. Threats to sue, angry families, and "dumping" of patients without health insurance or money to pay for health care, for examples, can so overwhelm the health care team that the real ethical issues of a case (e.g., the capacity to choose or futility) are not considered. Socioeconomic issues, while important in making final choices about care, generally should not override clear medical indications or clear patient preferences. When socioeconomic considerations are deeply divided from what is medically indicated or what a patient prefers, they cause problems. For example, imagine this in the fourth case: the 33-year-old mother cannot die at home near her children because of medical cost regulations; in the first case, the sequelae of refused blood products and prolonged ICU stay deny a bed to a patient with complications of leukemia therapy so that this care has to be delivered in another institution away from trusted physicians. These outcomes appear unfair or unjust and illustrate cases dealing with the ethical principle of *justice* and how to determine allocation of resources.

What are the unique ethical problems of obstetrics and gynecology? Clearly, maternal and fetal conflicts and how we define procreation and family are uniquely poignant in obstetrics and gynecology. The primary concern of physicians is the best care of their patients. This has been true since Hippocrates admonished us "to do away with the suffering of the sick." Special-interest groups have variously defined the "rights" of the fetus so that, at times, the primacy of duty to the patient (mother) seems in question. Yet there never has been a time in the development of medical ethics or in the opinions expressed by the American College of

Obstetricians and Gynecologists that the fetus is considered to take precedence over the mother in considerations of medical care or the therapeutic alliance of physician and patient. This is valuable to keep in mind when considering these problems.

Abortion would be the first example of these considerations, where the controversy can be so emotional and damaging that an ethical discussion cannot occur. Consistent with our primary duty to the patient, those circumstances where survival of the mother would be seriously compromised by the maintenance of pregnancy are the least controversial. Clearly, preservation of the patient/mother's life and loss of the fetus would be supported by many viewers. As the "case" gets further away from this clearer situation, the discussion becomes more complex. To understand these controversies, it is valuable to explore what elements we use to define life as "human" before we define loss of a fetus as loss of a human life. What are elements of humanness and when are they achieved in pregnancy? Is ability to survive independent of the mother significant? Is the potential to achieve those elements defining *human* pertinent? These are important issues to explore before considering, for example, a case such as elective abortion at 12 weeks or selective pregnancy reduction.

Defining these issues also helps in consideration of the "rights" of pregnant women to engage in behavior or activities that put the fetus at some risk, such as use of cocaine, alcohol, smoking, or refusal of cesarean section for fetal indication. At what level of human development or potential, if at all, does concern for fetal outcomes override the patient/mother's autonomous choices? In what sort of case might we reasonably override expressed patient wishes to preserve fetal life? For example, how does drug use interact with capacity to choose? Consider the second case: Is the drug-using mother's decision to continue to use drugs during pregnancy acceptable? What are the consequences of incarcerating such mothers as a solution? Is an acutely intoxicated mother's decision to refuse cesarean section for fetal indications acceptable?

Looking at the many changes in reproductive endocrinology, the idea of a clearest case, sometimes called a paradigm case, may help sort out the ethical discussions. What, for example, is the clearest set of relationships between parents and children? Biologically, the relationship between mother donating the egg and a father donating the sperm in vivo without augmentation is the para-

digm case. The relationship of this family unit, with the parental responsibilities for financial support, history, culture, and education has been the traditional paradigm for family in our culture. How these elements change with a group of cases will vary. Adoption by mother/father pair, adoption by single parent, adoption by two mothers or two fathers, in vitro combination of egg from mother and father, in vitro combination of unrelated sperm with the maternal egg, and the varieties of gestational pattern with surrogacy and egg and sperm donation are all variations on the original theme. How far from our paradigm family is acceptable? Why? What do we do with the "extra" fertilized or harvested eggs from in vitro fertilization? How is this different or the same as the issue of humanness or potential for humanness that we raised when discussing abortion?

SUMMARY

In obstetrics-gynecology, as in all medicine, there is potential to utilize the skills and concepts of medical ethics. To do so requires methods of systematic reflection to delineate the ethical problems and to analyze these problems further. The analytical framework shown earlier in this chapter helps identify ethical issues, placing them in specific areas, associating them with some principles and families of cases. Further analysis comparing a case to a paradigm case, may be helpful. Finally, obtaining recent papers on the issues from MED-ETHX in Medline or the medical library will bring together various authors' views on the ethical issues surrounding a given clinical situation.

CASE STUDIES

There are no clear answers in medical ethics, only questions to which we should apply a logical scheme for analysis to make best decisions possible. Consider the following situations. Apply the decision matrix presented in this chapter to decide how *you* would analyze each.

Case 47A

Your patient is a 28-year-old G3 P3003 whose ethnic background and religious views place high value on a male offspring. She has had three girls. She is now 12 weeks pregnant and requests you test for gender and abort a female pregnancy. She notes she must have a son for her husband and can barely afford a fourth child in any event.

Questions Case 47A

Do you do the test? Do you abort the pregnancy if it is female? If you do and she returns with another pregnancy, do you continue the process to its logical conclusion: a male fetus or a complication so that further pregnancy is not possible? What if the husband insists? What if the mother is unsure? What if her attorney reminds you that it is her body, not yours, and her decision? What if your attorney reminds you that the public relations outcome of this case stinks either way you choose?

Case 47B

A 26-year-old G7 P6006 arrives at an estimated 37 to 41 weeks gestation in labor. She has had no prenatal care. She is an abuser of drugs and alcohol and is high on cocaine she ingested just before entering the hospi-tal. When placed on an electronic fetal monitor with external probes, decelerations are noted but the patient will not permit adjustment of the tocodynamometer to allow characterization of the decelerations, nor will she permit rupture of membranes for placement of a scalp electrode.

Questions Case 47B

What do you do? A cesarean section because you cannot evaluate the fetus effectively and it may be in distress? Wait and see if the patient will calm down and allow appropriate fetal assessment? Is the patient competent to make decisions having just taken cocaine? Does the fetus have a right to a "good birth"? If you let the patient labor and deliver vaginally and the baby is brain damaged, are you liable? If you do a cesarean section and the baby is okay but the mother has a serious complication, are you liable?

STUDY QUESTIONS

INSTRUCTIONS FOR STUDY QUESTIONS

The study questions are designed to help you test how well you learned the content of each chapter. To maximize the usefulness of the questions, you should

1. Read the chapter through completely at least once;
2. Answer all of the study questions (do not check your answer after each question);
3. Reread the parts of the chapter related to the questions you answered incorrectly.

The correct answer to each question is contained in the chapter. Questions do not necessarily follow the order that information is presented in the chapter.

The questions are in several formats: multiple choice, true-false, and matching. For true-false and matching questions, more than one option may be correct. Read the questions carefully and follow the instructions for the different item formats.

Chapter 1 Final Questions (61 questions)

1.1   The last menstrual period (LMP) is dated from

    a. The first day of the last normal period
    b. The last day of the last normal period
    c. The first day of the last bleeding episode
    d. The last day of the last bleeding episode

1.2   Postmenopausal bleeding is defined as

    a. Bleeding beginning 6 months after cessation of menses
    b. Irregular bleeding continuing for 6 months after cessation of regular menses
    c. Bleeding beginning 12 months after cessation of menses
    d. Irregular bleeding continuing for 12 months after cessation of regular menses

1.3   Any passage of clots during menstruation is abnormal.

    a. True
    b. False

1.4–1.8   Instructions: Match the abbreviation in the obstetric history with its appropriate definition.

    G _____ P _____ _____ _____ _____

1.4   G refers to _____

1.5   The first number after P refers to _____

1.6   The second number after P refers to _____

1.7   The third number after P refers to _____

1.8   The fourth number after P refers to _____

    a. Number of living children
    b. Number of pregnancies
    c. Number of term pregnancies
    d. Number of preterm pregnancies
    e. Number of abortions

1.9   Inquiry concerning adult and child history of sexual abuse and assault should be routinely included in the sexual history.

    a. True
    b. False

1.10   Tanner's classification with respect to the breast concerns changes in

    a. The breast before and after lactation
    b. The breast associated with malignancy
    c. The breast associated with maturation
    d. Breast configuration associated with galactorrhea

1.11   Breast examination is done in the

    a. Supine position
    b. Sitting position
    c. Both
    d. Neither

1.12   Peau d'orange change in the breast is associated with

    a. Edema of the lymphatics
    b. Jaundice
    c. Too vigorous breast-feeding
    d. Galactorrhea

1.13   Which kind of speculum is usually more suitable for examination of the nulliparous patient?

    a. Graves speculum
    b. Pederson speculum
    c. Mogans speculum
    d. Ling speculum

1.14   The use of vaginal lubricant should be minimized when performing the speculum examination because lubricant interferes with

    a. Cervical cytology
    b. Cervical cultures
    c. Wet prep evaluation
    d. Visualization of the cervix

Answers (1.1-1.14)

1.1 a	1.5 c	1.9 a	1.12 a
1.2 a	1.6 d	1.10 c	1.13 b
1.3 b	1.7 e	1.11 c	1.14 a, b, c
1.4 b	1.8 a		

1.15 Which uterine configuration is most difficult to assess for size, shape, configuration, and mobility?

a. Anteverted
b. Anteverted, anteflexed
c. Midposition
d. Retroverted
e. Retroverted, retroflexed

1.16 Pap smears should be fixed no more than _____ second(s) after preparation?

a. 1
b. 10
c. 20
d. 30

1.17 The rectovaginal examination is necessary only when there are symptoms of pelvic relaxation, fecal incontinence, or bleeding from the rectum.

a. True
b. False

1.18–1.22 Instructions: Match the condition with the appropriate screening examination recommendation.

1.18 Thyroid disease, TSH _____

1.19 Cervical dysplasia, Pap _____

1.20 Cholesterol/lipid, profile _____

1.21 Breast cancer, mammography _____

1.22 Bowel cancer, sigmoidoscopy _____

a. Every 5 years from age 19; every 3–4 years after age 65
b. Every other year from age 40, yearly after age 50
c. Every 3–5 years after age 65
d. Annual from puberty or onset sexual activity
e. Every 3–5 years after age 40

1.23–1.26 Instructions: Match the diseases with the appropriate recommendations for immunization.

1.23 Tetanus-diphtheria _____

1.24 Influenza vaccine _____

1.25 Pneumococcal vaccine _____

1.26 Hepatitis B vaccine _____

a. Every 10 years from age 19 to age 64 when at risk
b. Once when 14–16 years old
c. For at risk groups
d. Every 10 years from age 19 to age 64 when at risk; yearly after age 65

1.27 Obstetrician-gynecologists provide primary as well as speciality care for over _____ of women in the United States.

a. 1/4
b. 1/2
c. 3/4

1.28–1.31 Instructions: From the list below, select the leading cause(s) of morbidity for women in each of the following age categories.

1.28 12–18 years of age _____

1.29 19–39 years of age _____

1.30 40–64 years of age _____

1.31 Greater than 65 years of age _____

a. HEENT conditions
b. Upper respiratory infections (URI)
c. Infection (viral, parasites, bacterial)
d. Sexual abuse
e. Accidental injury
f. Digestive tract conditions
g. Acute urinary conditions
h. Osteoperosis/arthritis
i. Hypertension
j. Orthopaedic conditions
k. Heart disease
l. Hearing and vision impairment
m. Urinary incontinence

1.32–1.35 Instructions: From the list of conditions/situations below, select the leading cause(s) of death for women in the following age categories.

1.32 12–18 years of age _____

1.33 19–39 years of age _____

1.34 40–64 years of age _____

1.35 Greater than 65 years of age _____

a. Motor vehicle accidents
b. Homicide
c. Suicide
d. Leukemia
e. Cardiovascular disease
f. Coronary artery disease
g. AIDS
h. Breast cancer
i. Uterine cancer
j. Lung cancer
k. Cerebrovascular accident
l. Colorectal cancer
m. Obstructive lung disease
n. Ovarian cancer
o. Pneumonia/influenza
p. Accidents

Answers (1.15-1.35)

1.15 e	1.21 b	1.26 c	1.31 a, b, e, h, i, k, l, m
1.16 b	1.22 e	1.27 b	1.32 a, b, d
1.17 b	1.23 b	1.28 a, b, c, d, e, f, g	1.33 a, b, e, f, g, h, i, m
1.18 c	1.24 a	1.29 a, b, c, e, g	1.34 e, f, h, j, k, l, m, n
1.19 d	1.25 d	1.30 a, b, h, i, j, k, l	1.35 e, f, h, j, k, l, m, o, p
1.20 a			

1.36–1.42   Instructions: Match the risk factor or condition with the appropriate screening test or intervention recommendation.

1.36   Cervical dysplasia _____

1.37   Skin cancer _____

1.38   Anemia _____

1.39   Hypercholesteremia, coronary artery disease _____

1.40   Breast cancer _____

1.41   Colorectal cancer _____

1.42   Thyroid disease _____

  a.   Sickle cell preparation
  b.   Cholesterol/lipid profile
  c.   Yearly physician examination
  d.   Self-examination
  e.   Screening mammography
  f.   Hemogram
  g.   Physical examination of suspicious lesions
  h.   Fecal occult blood test
  i.   TSH
  j.   Sigmoidoscopy
  k.   Pap smear

1.43   Which of the following is *not* a task for the physician at the time of the initial patient evaluation?

  a.   Establishing and developing a professional relationship of mutual trust and respect with the patient
  b.   Gathering historical information
  c.   Gathering physical information
  d.   Making a differential diagnosis
  e.   Making a definitive diagnosis
  f.   Identifying issues involving health maintenance and disease prevention

1.44   Surnames should generally be used in the professional physician-patient relationship.

  a.   True
  b.   False

1.45   When a patient is obviously becoming uncomfortable with a topic during a history taking session, the best response of the physician is to

  a.   Ignore the discomfort and proceed with questioning
  b.   Discontinue discussion of the topic to avoid further patient discomfort and damage to the patient-physician relationship
  c.   Address the patient's discomfort in a positive and supportive manner

1.46   The chief complaint should always be recorded in the medical record as a direct quote to avoid altering or obscuring the patient's intent.

  a.   True
  b.   False

1.47   Inquiry about pelvic pain that interferes with daily activities or requires more analgesia than provided by plain aspirin or acetaminophen should include questions about

  a.   Duration and quality of pain
  b.   Relationship of pain in time to menses
  c.   Radiation of pain to areas outside of the pelvis
  d.   Association of pain with body position

1.48   Inquiry about menses should include all *except*

  a.   Estimation of menstrual flow in milliliters
  b.   Number of pads or tampons during heavy part of menstrual flow
  c.   Whether pads or tampons are soaked at the time of removal
  d.   Presence and size of clots
  e.   Intermenstrual bleeding

1.49   In the gynecologic history, differentiation of vaginitis and pelvic inflammatory disease is often possible by inquiring about the route of medical therapy employed, that is, topical therapy or oral or parenteral therapy.

  a.   True
  b.   False

1.50   Which of the following should be included in the history of a patient with infertility?

  a.   Previous fertility
  b.   Previous diseases in the patient
  c.   Previous disease in the patient's partner
  d.   Sexual practices
  e.   Duration of time that pregnancy has been attempted

1.51   The most cost-effective and reliable means of early detection of breast cancer is

  a.   A yearly mammogram alone
  b.   A yearly physician examination alone
  c.   A breast examination, combined with appropriately scheduled mammography.

1.52   Palpation and inspection of the breast should be done simultaneously to expedite the examination.

  a.   True
  b.   False

1.53   In which of the following ways does elevating the head of the examining table about 30° facilitate the pelvic examination?

  a.   It allows the patient to comfortably read materials provided to distract her from the examination
  b.   It relaxes the abdominal wall muscle groups making examination easier
  c.   It allows observation of the patient's responses
  d.   It allows eye contact between the physician and the patient

---

Answers (1.36-1.53)

1.36 k	1.41 h, j	1.46 b	1.50 all
1.37 g	1.42 i	1.47 all	1.51 c
1.38 a, f	1.43 e	1.48 a	1.52 b
1.39 b	1.44 a	1.49 a	1.53 b, c, d
1.40 c, d, e	1.45 c		

1.54 Unless there is a history of STDs, gloving both hands for the routine pelvic examination is unnecessary.

a. True
b. False

1.55 Dissymmetry on inspection of the external genitalia

a. Is usually normal and needs no follow up
b. May be caused by disease and should be evaluated
c. Should only be followed-up if there is accompanying pain or pressure sensation

1.56–1.57 Instructions: Match the type of speculum with the primary indications for its use.

1.56 Graves speculum _____

1.57 Pederson speculum _____

a. Parous menstrual woman
b. Multiparous woman
c. Prepubertal girl
d. Menopausal woman not on hormone replacement

1.58 Lubricants should be used liberally to facilitate speculum insertion during the routine pelvic examination, whether or not a Pap smear will be performed or cytologic specimens obtained.

a. True
b. False

1.59 Which of the following statements about the bimanual examination is *incorrect*?

a. The dominant hand should be used vaginally and the nondominant hand abdominally
b. Pressure with the abdominal hand should be applied with the flat and not the tips of the fingers
c. The uterus should be evaluated for size, shape, consistency, configuration, and mobility
d. An anterior cervix is usually associated with a antiverted uterus
e. Sharp flexion of the uterus may alter the expected relationships between the cervix and uterus

1.60 Normal ovaries are palpable in the menstrual-aged woman about _____ of the time.

a. 30%
b. 40%
c. 50%
d. 60%
e. 70%

1.61 The differential diagnosis is

a. Based on one or more of the historical, physical, or laboratory findings
b. An exhaustive list meant to include all possibilities
c. Used as an alternative list if the presumptive diagnosis is in error
d. Used so that laboratory testing can address all possible conditions

---

Answers (1.54-1.61)

1.54 b	1.56 a	1.58 b	1.60 c
1.55 b	1.57 b, c, d	1.59 a	1.61 a, c

Chapter 2 Final Questions (17 questions)

2.1 Chorionic villus sampling is generally associated with what percent risk of fetal loss?

    a. 0.5%
    b. 1.5%
    c. 2.5%
    d. 3.5%

2.2 Obstetric forceps are used to _____ the expulsive forces of the second stage of labor.

    a. Augment
    b. Supplant
    c. Overcome
    d. Replace

2.3 Which type of forceps delivery is not practiced because of its unacceptable risk to mother and fetus?

    a. Outlet forceps
    b. Low forceps
    c. Low forceps rotation
    d. Midforceps rotation
    e. High forceps

2.4 Which type of uterine incision at the time of cesarean section is generally accepted to require cesarean section with subsequent pregnancies?

    a. Low transverse
    b. Low vertical
    c. Classical

2.5 The limitations of ultrasonography make it impossible to use to evaluate fetal anatomy.

    a. True
    b. False

2.6 Ultrasonography should routinely be used to confirm pelvic examination findings.

    a. True
    b. False

2.7 The primary indication for circumcision of the male infant is

    a. Reduction and prevalence of penile carcinoma
    b. Penile hygiene
    c. Social-religious considerations

2.8 A profuse watery vaginal discharge is most commonly associated with which therapy for cervical dysplasia?

    a. Colposcopy
    b. Cryotherapy
    c. Laser therapy
    d. Conization

2.9 *Total abdominal hysterectomy* refers to the removal of the

    a. Uterus
    b. Ovaries
    c. Fallopian tubes
    d. Bladder

2.10–2.12 Instructions: Match the surgical procedure involvng the uterus with its correct definition.

2.10 Removal of uterus and contiguous structures _____

2.11 Removal of uterine corpus _____

2.12 Removal of uterus _____

    a. Total hysterectomy
    b. Subtotal hysterectomy
    c. Radical hysterectomy

2.13 Which of the following are indications for cervical conization?

    a. Two-step discrepancy between Pap smear and colposcopically directed biopsy
    b. Colposcopy where the squamocolumnar junction cannot be visualized
    c. Therapy of cervical dysplasia

2.14 Cervical conization is associated with a high incidence of cervical stenosis and incompetence.

    a. True
    b. False

2.15–2.16 Instructions: Match the procedure with the appropriate description(s)

2.15 Abdominal hysterectomy _____

2.16 Vaginal hysterectomy _____

    a. Used when substantial pathology is expected
    b. Requires longer operating time
    c. Appropriate for repair of cystocele or rectocele
    d. Associated with shorter recovery period
    e. Appropriate when additional abdominal procedures are contemplated

2.17 Hysteroscopy can be used for which of the following?

    a. Staging of cancer
    b. Polypectomy
    c. Endometrial ablation
    d. Evaluation of bleeding

Answers (2.1-2.17)

2.1 a	2.6 b	2.10 c	2.14 b
2.2 a	2.7 c	2.11 b	2.15 a, b, e
2.3 e	2.8 b	2.12 a	2.16 c, d
2.4 c	2.9 a	2.13 all	2.17 all
2.5 b			

Chapter 3 Final Questions (65 questions)

3.1 The genital system develops from embryonic

    a. Ectoderm
    b. Mesoderm
    c. Endoderm

3.2 The urogenital ridges give rise to elements of the

    a. Cardiovascular system
    b. Reproductive system
    c. Urinary system
    d. Skeletal system

3.3 In the ovary, it is the _____ that comes to contain the developing follicles.

    a. Cortex
    b. Medulla

3.4 The first indication of the sex of the embryo is the

    a. Entry of primordial germ cells
    b. Formation of the tunica albuginea
    c. Formation of primordial follicles
    d. Degeneration of the genital ducts

3.5 The primordial germ cells can be identified during the 4th week of development in the

    a. Yolk sac
    b. Gonadal ridge
    c. Urogenital sinus
    d. Cortical cords

3.6 In the female, the _____ persist to form the major parts of the reproductive tract.

    a. Paramesonephric (müllerian) ducts
    b. Mesonephric (wolffian) ducts

3.7 The formation of the uterus and fallopian tubes _____ dependent on the presence of ovaries.

    a. Is
    b. Is not

3.8 Absence of the ovary is usually a single event without other associated abnormalities.

    a. True
    b. False

3.9–3.10 Instructions: Match the developmental abnormality of the uterus with the underlying cause.

3.9 Absence of uterus _____

3.10 Double uterus (uterus didelphys) _____

    a. Inferior parts of the paramesonephric ducts do not fuse
    b. Paramesonephric ducts degenerate

3.11–3.12 Instructions: Match the developmental abnormality of the vagina with the underlying cause.

3.11 Absence of the vagina _____

3.12 Vaginal atresia _____

    a. Vaginal plate does not canalize
    b. Vaginal plate does not develop

3.13 The urogenital sinus gives rise to which of the following?

    a. Urethra
    b. Hymen
    c. Epithelium of the urinary bladder
    d. Rectum

3.14 The external genitalia _____ pass through an indifferent (undifferentiated) stage.

    a. Do
    b. Do not

3.15 The labia minora develop from the

    a. Genital tubercle
    b. Urogenital folds
    c. Labioscrotal swellings
    d. Urogenital sinus

3.16 The labia majora develop from the

    a. Genital tubercle
    b. Urogenital folds
    c. Labioscrotal swellings
    d. Urogenital sinus

3.17 The clitoris develops from the

    a. Genital tubercle
    b. Urigenital folds
    c. Labioscrotal swellings
    d. Urogenital sinus

Answers (3.1–3.17)

3.1 b	3.6 a	3.10 a	3.14 a
3.2 b, c	3.7 b	3.11 b	3.15 b
3.3 a	3.8 b	3.12 a	3.16 c
3.4 b	3.9 b	3.13 a, b, c	3.17 a
3.5 a			

3.18 The embryological origin of the fallopian tube is from the

a. Wolffian (mesonephric) ducts
b. Metanephric ducts
c. Müllerian (paramesonephric) ducts
d. Urogenital sinus

3.19 The embryologic origin of the vagina is from the

a. Urogenital sinus and müllerian ducts
b. Müllerian ducts and wolffian ducts
c. Mesonephric ducts and metanephric ducts
d. Urogenital sinus and wolffian ducts

3.20 The frenulum is the embryologic homologue of the penis

a. True
b. False

3.21 The innominate bones are composed of the

a. Ilium
b. Tibia
c. Ischium
d. Pubis
e. Sacrum

3.22 The false pelvis and true pelvis are separated by the

a. Acetabulum
b. Sacrospinous ligament
c. Linea terminalis
d. Obturator membrane
e. Obturator foramen

3.23 The dimensions of the _____ must be adequate to permit passage of the fetus during labor.

a. True pelvis
b. False pelvis

3.24 The _____ separates the false pelvis from the true pelvis.

a. Plane of the pelvic inlet
b. Plane of the greatest diameter
c. Plane of the least diameter
d. Plane of the pelvic outlet

3.25 Arrest of fetal descent occurs most commonly at the

a. Plane of the pelvic inlet
b. Plane of the greatest diameter
c. Plane of the least diameter
d. Plane of the pelvic outlet

3.26–3.29 Instructions: Match the pelvic plane diameter with the appropriate average value in centimeters.

3.26 Obstetric conjugate _____

3.27 Transverse diameter of inlet _____

3.28 Bispinous diameter of midplane _____

3.29 Transverse diameter of greatest diameter _____

a. 10.0–11.0
b. 10.5
c. 12.5
d. 13.5

3.30 Based on the Caldwell and Moloy classification, the most common pelvic type is the

a. Gynecoid
b. Android
c. Anthropoid
d. Platypelloid

3.31–3.32 Instructions: Match the part of the vulva with the structures that it contains.

3.31 Labia majora _____

3.32 Labia minora _____

a. Sebaceous glands
b. Sweat glands
c. Hair follicles

3.33–3.37 Instructions: Match the structure with the type of epithelium that lines it.

3.33 Bartholin's duct _____

3.34 Skene's duct _____

3.35 Urethra _____

3.36 Vagina _____

3.37 Endocervical canal _____

a. Squamous
b. Columnar
c. Transitional

3.38 The anterior wall of the vagina is _____ the posterior wall.

a. Longer than
b. The same length as
c. Shorter than

Answers (3.18-3.38)

3.18 c	3.24 a	3.29 c	3.34 c
3.19 a	3.25 c	3.30 a	3.35 c
3.20 b	3.26 a	3.31 a, b, c	3.36 a
3.21 a, c, d	3.27 d	3.32 a, b	3.37 b
3.22 c	3.28 b	3.33 c	3.38 c
3.23 a			

3.39A   The part of the uterus where the fallopian tubes enter is called the

    a. Fundus
    b. Cornu
    c. Mesosalpinx
    d. Cardinal ligament
    e. Lower uterine segment

3.39B   The two main anatomical divisions of the uterus are the

    a. Corpus and fundus
    b. Cornu and fundus
    c. Corpus and cervix
    d. Cervix and isthmus

3.40   The blood supply of the uterus comes from the

    a. Ovarian artery
    b. Uterine artery
    c. Vaginal artery

3.41   The uterine veins enter the

    a. Common iliac veins
    b. Internal iliac veins
    c. Inferior vena cava
    d. Femoral veins
    e. External iliac veins

3.42   The portion of the fallopian tube that borders on the ovary is the

    a. Isthmus
    b. Ampulla
    c. Infundibulum

3.43   The uterus is supported by the

    a. Uterosacral ligaments
    b. Cardinal ligaments
    c. Round ligaments
    d. Broad ligaments
    e. Ovarian ligaments

3.44   Before puberty, the ratio of the length of the body of the uterus to the length of the cervix is approximately

    a. 1:1
    b. 2:1
    c. 3:1
    d. 4:1

3.45   Which of the following statements about the uterine artery is *incorrect*?

    a. It is a branch of the hypogastric artery
    b. It anastomoses with the ovarian vessels
    c. It anastomoses with the vaginal vessels
    d. It penetrates the uterus at a level of the internal cervical os after passing under the ureter

3.46   The portion of the broad ligament between the ovaries and the fallopian tube is called the

    a. Round ligament
    b. Ligament of Jacobs
    c. Cardinal ligament
    d. Mesosalpinx

3.47   The uterosacral ligaments

    a. Arise from the lateral wall of the uterus
    b. Attach to the sacrum at S3–4
    c. Prevent prolapse of the uterus into the vagina
    d. Cause tension of the cervix ventrally

3.48   Which of the following statements about the ovary is *correct*?

    a. The ovary is attached to the broad ligament by the mesovarium
    b. The ovary is attached to the uterus by the ovarian ligament
    c. The ovary is attached to the side of the pelvis by the infundibulopelvic ligament
    d. The ovary is attached to the fallopian tube by the ovarian ligament

3.49   Hilus cells are found in the

    a. Ovarian cortex
    b. Ovarian medulla
    c. Mesoovarium
    d. Graafian follicle

3.50   The streak ovary is associated with

    a. Klinefelter's syndrome
    b. Asherman's syndrome
    c. Osteogenesis imperfecta
    d. Embryonic gonadal death

3.51   The blood supply to the fallopian tubes is solely from the ovarian arteries.

    a. True
    b. False

3.52   As compared to the reproductive years, the size of the ovary of a menopausal woman is

    a. Increased
    b. Unchanged
    c. Decreased

3.53   The diploid number of chromosomes in humans is

    a. 23
    b. 32
    c. 46
    d. 84
    e. 92

Answers (3.39-3.53)

3.39A	b	3.42	c	3.46	d	3.50	d
3.39B	c	3.43	a, b, c, d	3.47	c	3.51	b
3.40	a, b	3.44	a	3.48	a, b, c	3.52	c
3.41	b	3.45	d	3.49	b	3.53	c

3.54 Which of the following statements about human chromosomes is *incorrect*?

a. Genes are located along the length of a chromosome in a linear fashion
b. Genes are lengths of DNA that encode a specific peptide sequence
c. Chromosomes are composed of DNA associated with histones
d. Human chromosomes are formed in 23 heterologous pairs
e. The normal human chromosome complement is 44 autosomes and two sex chromosomes

3.55 Which of the following should not be part of genetic counseling?

a. Obtaining information from patients
b. Reviewing appropriate diagnostic modalities
c. Assessing risk in future pregnancies
d. Guiding the patient to the most appropriate management option
e. Providing empathetic support for a patient's decision

3.56 Which of the following chromosome abnormalities is the most common among live borns?

a. Trisomy 21
b. Trisomy 18
c. Trisomy 13
d. Turner syndrome (monosomy X)
e. Cri-du-chat (del 5p) syndrome

3.57 Test results are available soonest from which of the following procedures?

a. Amniocentesis
b. Chorionic villus sampling
c. Fetal skin sampling
d. Parental blood chromosome analysis

3.58 Chorionic villus sampling can be used for the detection of

a. Neural tube defects
b. Fetal omphalocele
c. Trisomy 18
d. Achondroplasia
e. Marfan syndrome

3.59 The most common chromosomal abnormality reliably diagnosed by amniocentesis is

a. Trisomy 13
b. 21/22 translocation
c. 13–15/21 translocation
d. Trisomy 18
e. Trisomy 21

3.60 Which of the following statements about the cri-du-chat syndrome is *incorrect*?

a. It is caused by deletion of part of the short arm of chromosome 5
b. The infants are macrosomic
c. Individuals with the syndrome have low-set ears and a moonlike face
d. It is not associated with older than average parents
e. Females are affected more often than males

3.61 In autosomal dominant inheritance

a. The inheritance is usually independent of sex
b. Both sexes are equally affected
c. The inheritance is a result of a pair of mutant genes situated on an autosome
d. One-half of the children of an affected person are affected
e. One-half of the siblings of an affected person are affected

3.62 If there is complete failure of testicular formation following the formation of an XY zygote

a. The individual will develop as a female with uterus, tubes, vagina, and vulva
b. The individual will develop as a male with undescended testes and hypospadias
c. The external genitalia will be normal
d. The external genitalia will be ambiguous and there is an absence of vagina, uterus, and tubes
e. The individual will become a transsexual

3.63 Which of the following is a Mendelian dominant hereditary bleeding disorder that affects both sexes?

a. Hemophilia
b. Christmas disease
c. Von Willebrand's disease
d. Down syndrome

3.64 Alpha-fetoprotein is normal in amniotic fluid in which of the following?

a. Spina bifida
b. Anencephaly
c. Esophageal atresia
d. Rh isoimmunization
e. Postmaturity

3.65 In which of the following may an afflicted individual live to at least 10 years of age?

a. Trisomy 21
b. Trisomy 18
c. Trisomy 16
d. Trisomy 13
e. Turner syndrome

Answers (3.54-3.65)

3.54 d	3.57 b	3.60 b	3.63 c
3.55 d	3.58 c	3.61 a, b, d, e	3.64 e
3.56 a	3.59 e	3.62 a	3.65 a, e

Chapter 4 Final Questions (79 questions)

4.1   The neonatal mortality rate is

a. Synonymous with the stillbirth rate
b. The number of neonatal deaths per 1000 births
c. The number of neonatal deaths per 1000 live births
d. The number of neonatal deaths per 1000 population
e. The number of neonatal deaths in the first 7 days of life

4.2   The maternal mortality rate is

a. The number of deaths in pregnant women per 1,000 population
b. The number of deaths in pregnant women
c. The number of deaths in pregnant women per 100,000 live births

4.3   Which of the following may be indications of ovulation?

a. Midcycle abdominal pain (Mittelschmerz)
b. An upward shift in basal body temperature
c. A prolactin surge at midcycle
d. A change in cervical mucus
e. Increased plasma levels of progesterone

4.4   In a normal singleton pregnancy, maternal blood volume

a. Increases by 10–15%
b. Increases by 45%
c. Decreases by 10–15%
d. Decreases by 45%

4.5   Which of the following is *not* characteristic of a normal pregnancy?

a. Cardiac volume increases by 10%
b. The electrocardiogram shows deviation to the left
c. Arterial blood pressure and vascular resistance increase
d. The resting pulse rate increases by about 10–15 bpm
e. The heart is displaced upward and to the left

4.6   Which of the following is the cause of the leukocytosis of pregnancy?

a. A response to infection
b. An increase in adrenocortical activity
c. An increased stimulation of lymphocyte production
d. An unknown cause

4.7–4.9   Instructions: Match the molecule with the mechanism(s) by which it crosses the placenta.

4.7   Oxygen _____

4.8   Glucose _____

4.9   Amino acids _____

a. Simple diffusion
b. Facilitated diffusion
c. Active transport
d. Pinocytosis

4.10–4.15   Instructions: Match the gastrointestinal tract activity with the change that is expected in pregnancy.

4.10   Appetite _____

4.11   Gastric motility _____

4.12   Intestinal transit time _____

4.13   Bile composition _____

4.14   Liver enzyme levels _____

4.15   Gastric reflux _____

a. Increases
b. Decreases
c. Remains the same

4.16   "Morning sickness" typically begins during which weeks of pregnancy?

a. 1–3
b. 4–8
c. 10–12
d. 14–18

4.17   Morning sickness in the first trimester is typically associated with nutritional deprivation.

a. True
b. False

4.18   Treatment of morning sickness includes

a. Reassurance
b. Frequent small meals
c. Three large meals with antacids
d. Inclusion of bland foods

4.19   Hyperemesis gravidarum is a transient nausea of pregnancy associated with no adverse effects to mother and infant.

a. True
b. False

Answers (4.1-4.19)

4.1 c	4.6 d	4.11 b	4.16 b
4.2 c	4.7 a	4.12 a	4.17 b
4.3 a, b, d, e	4.8 b	4.13 c	4.18 a, b, d
4.4 b	4.9 c	4.14 a	4.19 b
4.5 c	4.10 a	4.15 a	

4.20   Ptyalism is caused by

   a. Excess production of saliva
   b. Excess production of gastric acid
   c. Inability of the patient to swallow normal amounts of saliva
   d. Allergic reactions to various foods during pregnancy

4.21   Decreased gastrointestinal motility during pregnancy is related to increased levels of

   a. Progesterone
   b. Human chorionic gonadotropin
   c. Estrogen
   d. Androstenedione
   e. Thyrotropin-releasing factor

4.22   Epulis is a pregnancy-related vascular swelling of the

   a. Gums
   b. Nares
   c. Epiglottis
   d. Nailbeds
   e. Larynx

4.23   Pica can include craving for which of the following?

   a. Ice
   b. Fatty foods
   c. Laundry starch
   d. Clay

4.24–4.33   Instructions: For each pulmonary function, indicate whether it is increased, unchanged, or decreased in pregnancy.

4.24   Oxygen requirement _____

4.25   Arterial pH _____

4.26   Carbon dioxide pressure _____

4.27   Oxygen pressure _____

4.28   Tidal volume _____

4.29   Expiratory reserve volume _____

4.30   Inspiratory capacity _____

4.31   Vital capacity _____

4.32   Residual volume _____

4.33   Minute volume _____

   a. Increased
   b. Unchanged
   c. Decreased

4.34   The increased nasal stuffiness and perception of increased nasal secretions during pregnancy are associated with

   a. Mucosal hyperemia
   b. Increased immuoglobulin production
   c. Increased interluminal production of mast cell toxins

4.35   The acid base status in pregnancy is characterized by

   a. Mild respiratory alkalosis
   b. Mild metabolic alkalosis
   c. Mild respiratory acidosis
   d. Mild respiratory metabolic acidosis

4.36   The tidal volume increases by _____ percent during pregnancy.

   a. 10–20
   b. 30–40
   c. 50–60
   d. 70–80

4.37   Blood flow to which of the following organs is increased during pregnancy?

   a. Uterus
   b. Kidney
   c. Breast
   d. Skin
   e. Brain

4.38   Inferior vena cava syndrome is caused by

   a. Baroreceptor changes in cardiac function associated with changes in position
   b. Transient release of epinephrine associated with uterine displacement caused by fetal movement
   c. Transient cardiac arrhythmias secondary to positional changes in the mother
   d. Spasm of the inferior vena cava secondary to fetal movement
   e. Compression of the inferior vena cava by the gravid uterine corpus

4.39   The peripheral vascular resistance decreases during pregnancy because of increasing levels of

   a. Estrogen
   b. Progesterone
   c. Androstenedione
   d. Estrone

4.40   Which of the following normal physical findings arise from the fact that the cardiovascular system is in a hyperdynamic state during pregnancy?

   a. Increased second heart sound split with inspiration
   b. Distended neck veins
   c. Low grade systolic ejection murmurs
   d. Diastolic murmurs

4.41   On chest X-ray the heart appears to demonstrate cardiomegaly during pregnancy because it is displaced

   a. Upward and to the left
   b. Upward and to the right
   c. Downward and to the left
   d. Downward and to the right

Answers (4.20-4.41)

4.20 c	4.26 c	4.32 c	4.37 a, b, c, d
4.21 a	4.27 a	4.33 a	4.38 e
4.22 a	4.28 a	4.34 a	4.39 b
4.23 a, c, d	4.29 c	4.35 a	4.40 a, c
4.24 a	4.30 a	4.36 b	4.41 a
4.25 b	4.31 a		

4.42 Plasma volume begins to increase at the 6th week of pregnancy and reaches it maximum at approximately

   a. 20–24 weeks
   b. 25–29 weeks
   c. 30–34 weeks
   d. 35–39 weeks
   e. Term

4.43–4.52 Instructions: For each hematologic parameter listed below, indicate whether it is increased, decreased, or remains the same during pregnancy.

4.43 Plasma volume _____

4.44 Hemoglobin concentration _____

4.45 Hematocrit _____

4.46 Total erythrocyte volume _____

4.47 Mean cell volume _____

4.48 Erythrocyte sedimentation rate (ESR) _____

4.49 Serum iron _____

4.50 Total iron binding capacity _____

4.51 Serum transferrin _____

4.52 Serum ferritin _____

   a. Increased
   b. Decreased
   c. Remains the same

4.53 During pregnancy, the risk for thromboembolism

   a. Increases
   b. Decreases
   c. Remains the same

4.54 Because iron is passively transported to the fetus, maternal iron concentrations are critical to maintain fetal iron concentrations.

   a. True
   b. False

4.55 Bleeding time and clotting time are increased during a normal pregnancy.

   a. True
   b. False

4.56–4.62 Instructions: Identify whether the renal parameters listed below are increased, unchanged, or decreased during pregnancy.

4.56 Renal plasma flow _____

4.57 Glomerular filtration rate _____

4.58 Urinary output _____

4.59 Renin _____

4.60 Angiotensin I and II _____

4.61 Renin substrate _____

4.62 24 hr protein excretion _____

   a. Increased
   b. Unchanged
   c. Decreased

4.63 Typically, the ureteral dilation associated with the relaxing effect of progesterone in pregnancy is greater on the right side than on the left.

   a. True
   b. False

4.64 The decreased bladder tone in pregnancy caused by progesterone is associated with which of the following?

   a. Increased residual volume
   b. Dilated collecting systems
   c. Urinary stasis
   d. Increased incidence of pyelonephritis in patients with asymptomatic bacteria

4.65 In normal pregnancy, serum levels of creatinine, uric acid, and blood urea nitrogen

   a. Increase
   b. Decrease
   c. Remain the same

4.66 In virtually all pregnant patients, glucose excretion

   a. Increases
   b. Decreases
   c. Remains the same

Answers (4.42-4.66)

4.42 c	4.49 b	4.55 b	4.61 a
4.43 a	4.50 a	4.56 a	4.62 b
4.44 b	4.51 a	4.57 a	4.63 a
4.45 b	4.52 b	4.58 b	4.64 all
4.46 a	4.53 a	4.59 a	4.65 b
4.47 a	4.54 b	4.60 a	4.66 a
4.48 a			

4.67   Striae gravidarum, which appear on the abdominal, breast, and thigh skin of pregnant patients, are caused by excessive weight gain.

a.   True
b.   False

4.68   Because the rate of bone turnover increases during pregnancy, there typically is a loss of bone density.

a.   True
b.   False

4.69   Blurred vision during pregnancy is caused by swelling of the lens.

a.   True
b.   False

4.70   What percent of total cardiac output is channeled to the uterus at term?

a.   5%
b.   10%
c.   15%
d.   20%
e.   25%

4.71   Pregnancy is characterized by

a.   Hyperglycemia
b.   Hypoglycemia
c.   Hyperinsulinemia
d.   Hypoinsulinemia
e.   Hypertriglyceridemia
f.   Hypotriglyceridemia

4.72–4.77   Instructions: For each of the following pituitary hormones, indicate whether it is increased, unchanged, or decreased during pregnancy.

4.72   Prolactin _____

4.73   Follicle-stimulating hormone (FSH) _____

4.74   Luteinizing hormone (LH) _____

4.75   Adrenocorticotropic (ACTH) _____

4.76   Thyroid-stimulating hormone (TSH) _____

4.77   Oxytocin _____

a.   Increased
b.   Unchanged
c.   Decreased

4.78   During pregnancy, cortisol, androstenedione, deoxycorticosterone, and aldosterone produced by the adrenal gland, are

a.   Increased
b.   Unchanged
c.   Decreased

4.79   Approximately what percent of the umbilical blood supply goes through the ductus venosus?

a.   25%
b.   50%
c.   75%
d.   100%

Answers (4.67–4.79)

4.67 b	4.71 a, c, e	4.74 c	4.77 b
4.68 b	4.72 a	4.75 a	4.78 a
4.69 a	4.73 c	4.76 b	4.79 b
4.70 b			

Chapter 5 Final Questions (38 questions)

5.1 A positive pregnancy test may be associated with

   a. Spontaneous abortion
   b. Intrauterine pregnancy
   c. Ectopic pregnancy
   d. Trophoblastic disease

5.2 Congestion and a bluish color of the vagina is called

   a. Chadwick's sign
   b. Hegar's sign
   c. Newman's sign
   d. Herbert's sign
   e. Bate's sign

5.3 A softening of the cervix on physical examination is referred to as

   a. Chadwick's sign
   b. Hegar's sign
   c. Newman's sign
   d. Smith's sign
   e. Barzansky's sign

5.4 Fetal heart tones in a viable and normal pregnancy may routinely be heard by simple auscultation at or beyond how many weeks gestational age?

   a. 12–14
   b. 15–17
   c. 18–20
   d. 21–23

5.5 Commonly used electronic Doppler devices will detect fetal heart tones at approximately how many weeks of gestation?

   a. 8
   b. 10
   c. 12
   d. 14
   e. 16

5.6 Routinely used urine pregnancy tests become positive approximately how many weeks following the 1st day of the last normal menstrual period?

   a. 3
   b. 4
   c. 5
   d. 6
   e. 8

5.7 A serum progesterone level of greater than 25 ng/mL is usually consistent with

   a. Incomplete abortion
   b. Nonviable intrauterine pregnancy
   c. Ectopic pregnancy
   d. Viable intrauterine pregnancy

5.8 Intrauterine pregnancy is generally detectable by transvaginal ultrasonography when the β-hCG concentration is greater than

   a. 500–1000 mIU/mL
   b. 1500–2500 mIU/mL
   c. 3000–4000 mIU/mL
   d. 5000–6000 mIU/mL

5.9–5.13 Instructions: Match the laboratory test with its use in antenatal testing.

5.9 Complete blood count _____

5.10 Urinalysis and urine culture _____

5.11 Blood groups/Rh _____

5.12 Antibody screen _____

5.13 Glucose screen _____

   a. To screen for glucose intolerance
   b. To screen for anemia
   c. To determine hematologic status
   d. To evaluate for UTI and renal function
   e. To detect antifetal antibodies
   f. To determine risk of isoimmunization

5.14 In approximately what percentage of pregnant women are rubella titer positive?

   a. 55%
   b. 65%
   c. 75%
   d. 85%
   e. 95%

5.15 Specific screening for treponema is required following a positive

   a. Sickle cell test
   b. Rubella titer
   c. Hepatitis B surface antigen
   d. RPR
   e. Maternal serum α-fetoprotein

5.16 Maternal serum α-fetoprotein testing is best done at

   a. 7–10 weeks
   b. 11–14 weeks
   c. 15–18 weeks
   d. 19–22 weeks

5.17 "Normal" pregnancy lasts 40 ± _____ weeks calculated from the 1st day of the last normal menstrual period.

   a. 1
   b. 2
   c. 3
   d. 4

Answers (5.1-5.17)

5.1 all	5.6 b	5.10 d	5.14 d
5.2 a	5.7 d	5.11 f	5.15 d
5.3 b	5.8 b	5.12 e	5.16 c
5.4 c	5.9 b, c	5.13 a	5.17 b
5.5 c			

5.18   The fertilization age or conception age is how many weeks less than the menstrual or gestational age?

   a. 1
   b. 2
   c. 3
   d. 4

5.19   In a normal singleton pregnancy, from approximately 16 to 18 weeks gestation until approximately 36 weeks gestation the fundal height in centimeters is roughly equal to

   a. One-half the number of weeks gestational age
   b. The number of weeks gestational age
   c. Twice the number of weeks gestational age
   d. Four times the number of weeks gestational age

5.20   During antepartum care, a trace of glucosuria should be evaluated by glucose tolerance testing.

   a. True
   b. False

5.21   The generally prescribed recommendation for weight gain during pregnancy is

   a. 15–20 lb
   b. 25–30 lb
   c. 40–45 lb
   d. 50–55 lb

5.22   After "lightening" has occurred, the fundal height has generally

   a. Increased
   b. Stayed the same
   c. Decreased

5.23–5.25   Instructions: Match the fetal presentation with the estimated incidence of its occurrence.

5.23   Cephalic presentation _____

5.24   Breech presentation _____

5.25   Shoulder presentation _____

   a. 95%
   b. 1%
   c. 3.5%
   d. 15%

5.26   In regards to Ultrasonography, earlier in pregnancy there is more deviation in normal values of gestational age and the information obtained is less accurate than later in pregnancy.

   a. True
   b. False

5.27   Quantification of fetal activity is a common test that allows assessment of fetal well-being.

   a. True
   b. False

5.28   The normal fetal heart rate at term is

   a. 50–75 bpm
   b. 80–100 bpm
   c. 120–160 bpm
   d. 175–190 bpm

5.29   A reactive NST is characterized when the fetal heart rate increases by _____ beats per minute over a period of 15 sec following fetal movement, two such accelerations occurring in a 20-min span.

   a. 5
   b. 15
   c. 25
   d. 50

5.30   A nonreactive NST should be repeated in 3–4 days.

   a. True
   b. False

5.31   In an abnormal contraction stress test, you would expect the fetal heart rate to _____ in response to a uterine contraction.

   a. Increase
   b. Remain the same
   c. Decrease

5.32   The number of contractions in a 10-min window that must occur for a CST to be measurable are

   a. 1
   b. 2
   c. 3
   d. 4
   e. 5

5.33   Tests of fetal well-being have a high incidence of false-positive results.

   a. True
   b. False

5.34   A biophysical profile where there is one or more episodes of fetal breathing in 30 min, three or more discrete movements in 30 min, opening/closing of the fetal hand, a nonreactive NST, and no pockets of amniotic fluid greater than 1 cm would have a total score of

   a. 2
   b. 4
   c. 6
   d. 8

Answers (5.18-5.34)

5.18 b	5.23 a	5.27 a	5.31 c
5.19 b	5.24 c	5.28 c	5.32 c
5.20 b	5.25 b	5.29 b	5.33 a
5.21 b	5.26 b	5.30 b	5.34 c
5.22 c			

5.35 Exclusive of the fetal heart rate reactivity, which of the following elements of the biophysical profile is generally considered most important?

a. Fetal breathing
b. Gross body movement
c. Fetal tone
d. Qualitative amniotic fluid volume

5.36 Tests of fetal lung maturity are generally utilized when delivery of a fetus less than _____ weeks gestational age is contemplated.

a. 30
b. 32
c. 34
d. 36
e. 38

5.37 Phospholipid production generally increases at approximately _____ weeks gestational age so that the PG test is positive.

a. 27–29
b. 30–31
c. 32–33
d. 34–35
e. 36–37

5.38 What percent of correctly performed positive tests of fetal lung maturity are associated with a subsequent development of respiratory distress syndrome?

a. 0
b. 2
c. 4
d. 6
e. 8

Answers (5.35-5.38)

5.35 d   5.36 d   5.37 c   5.38 b

Chapter 6 Final Questions (160 questions)

6.1 Anemia in pregnancy is generally defined as a hemo-globin less than

    a. 6 g/dL
    b. 8 g/dL
    c. 10 g/dL
    d. 12 g/dL

6.2 The most frequent type of anemia in pregnancy is

    a. Iron-deficiency anemia
    b. Folate-deficiency anemia
    c. Sickle-cell anemia
    d. Vitamin B_{12}-deficiency anemia
    e. Thalassemia anemia

6.3 During pregnancy, the serum iron usually is

    a. Increased
    b. Unchanged
    c. Decreased

6.4 During pregnancy, the total iron-binding capacity is

    a. Increased
    b. Unchanged
    c. Decreased

6.5 Which of the following statements concerning iron deficiency anemia in pregnancy is *correct*?

    a. One pregnancy can cause anemia in the next pregnancy
    b. Adequate treatment is 100 mg ferrous gluconate daily
    c. With absent iron stores, a patient with iron-deficiency anemia can be treated with 60 mg of elemental iron daily
    d. A daily supplement of 30 mg of elemental iron is sufficient to meet the total requirements during pregnancy

6.6 Women with sickle-cell trait (HbAS disease) have in-creased

    a. Incidence of spontaneous abortion
    b. Perinatal mortality
    c. Incidence of urinary tract infections
    d. Incidence of preterm births
    e. Incidence of low-birth-weight babies

6.7 Which of the following is *not* characteristic of von Willebrand's disease?

    a. Decreased factor VII
    b. Decreased factor VIII
    c. Family history of the disease
    d. Prolonged bleeding time
    e. Prolonged partial thromboplastin time

6.8 When iron therapy is initiated during a normal preg-nancy, there is routinely a significant increase in the hematocrit within 2–4 weeks.

    a. True
    b. False

6.9 Anemia associated with folate deficiency can be asso-ciated with

    a. Multiple gestation
    b. Patients with a high alcohol intake
    c. Patients taking Dilantin
    d. Patients eating the normal adult intake of folate

6.10 Vitamin B_{12} deficiency is associated with which of the following diseases?

    a. Chronic malabsorption syndrome
    b. Pancreatic disease
    c. Crohn's disease
    d. Ulcerative colitis

6.11 A mixed iron and folate deficiency is characterized by

    a. Normocytic and normochromic anemia
    b. Microcytic and normochromic anemia
    c. Microcytic and megaloblastic anemia
    d. Normocytic and megaloblastic anemia

6.12 Which of the following hereditary hemolytic anemias are rare causes of anemia in pregnancy?

    a. Hereditary spherocytosis
    b. Autosomal dominant defect of the erythrocyte membrane
    c. Glucose-6-phosphate dehydrogenase deficiency
    d. Pyruvate kinase deficiency

6.13 Which of the following anemias presents as micro-cytic and hypochromic but with a normal serum iron and total iron-binding capacity?

    a. Iron-deficiency anemia
    b. Thalassemia trait
    c. Sickle-cell anemia
    d. Sickle-cell trait

6.14 Which of the following is most reliable in making the diagnosis of iron deficiency during pregnancy?

    a. Red cell morphology
    b. Serum iron values
    c. Fe/TIBC
    d. MCV
    e. MCHC

6.15 Which of the following hemoglobinopathies can lead to significant adverse effects during pregnancy?

    a. Sickle-cell trait
    b. Sickle-cell disease
    c. Sickle-cell–β-thalassemia
    d. Sickle-cell–hemoglobin C

Answers (6.1-6.15)

6.1 c	6.5 a, d	6.9 all	6.13 b
6.2 a	6.6 c	6.10 all	6.14 c
6.3 c	6.7 b, e	6.11 a	6.15 b, c, d
6.4 a	6.8 b	6.12 all	

6.16 Patients are defined as having sickle-cell trait (HbSA disease) when the quantitative hemoglobin electrophoresis shows _____ hemoglobin HgS.

a. 40%
b. 60%
c. 80%
d. 100%

6.17 Prophylactic red cell transfusion should be utilized for

a. All patients with hemoglobinopathies
b. Only patients with complications such as congestive heart failure

6.18–6.20 Instructions: Match the hemoglobinopathy with its incidence in pregnancy.

6.18 Sickle-cell trait (HbSA disease) _____

6.19 Sickle-cell disease (HbSS disease) _____

6.20 Sickle-cell–β-thalassemia _____

a. 1 in 12
b. 1 in 500
c. 1 in 1700

6.21 The pH of urine in pregnancy is _____ as compared to the nonpregnant state.

a. Increased
b. The same
c. Decreased

6.22 Pregnant patients with asymptomatic bacteriuria _____ routinely treated.

a. Are
b. Are not

6.23 What percent of patients with asymptomatic bacteriuria during pregnancy will develop symptomatic urinary tract infection?

a. 25
b. 50
c. 75
d. 100

6.24 Approximately _____ of patients with symptomatic pyelonephritis in pregnancy will demonstrate increased uterine activity and/or preterm labor.

a. 20%
b. 40%
c. 60%
d. 80%
e. 100%

6.25 If a pregnant patient with pyelonephritis does not improve on appropriate intravenous antibiotic therapy within 48–72 hrs, consideration should be given to

a. The possibility of urinary tract obstruction
b. Reevaluation of the antibiotic used for treatment
c. The use of single-shot intravenous pyelogram or ultrasonography
d. The possibility of another source of infection

6.26 The most common organism cultured from the urine of pregnant patients with urinary tract symptoms is

a. *Pseudomonas*
b. *E. Coli*
c. *Proteus*
d. *N. gonorrhoeae*

6.27 Because of the relative urinary stasis in pregnancy, urinary calculi are a particularly dangerous complication, usually requiring surgical correction.

a. True
b. False

6.28 The glomerular filtration rate increases by nearly _____ in pregnancy.

a. 25%
b. 50%
c. 75%
d. 100%

6.29 Preconception counseling for patients with preexisting renal disease should include the recommendation that pregnancy be avoided unless the blood creatinine level is _____ mg % or less.

a. 1
b. 2
c. 3
d. 4
e. 5

6.30 Pregnancy following renal transplantation has a generally _____ prognosis.

a. Favorable
b. Unfavorable

6.31 What factor in association with preexisting renal disease results in a particularly poor prognosis for baby and mother?

a. Retinopathy
b. Hypertension
c. Atrophic skin changes
d. Obesity
e. Anemia

Answers (6.16–6.31)

6.16 a	6.20 c	6.24 a	6.28 b
6.17 b	6.21 a	6.25 all	6.29 b
6.18 a	6.22 a	6.26 b	6.30 a
6.19 b	6.23 a	6.27 b	6.31 b

6.32 Of pregnant patients with bronchial asthma, approximately what percent will have one or more severe attacks during pregnancy?

a. 15
b. 30
c. 45
d. 60
e. 75

6.33 Which of the following interventions are appropriate in the pregnant patient with an acute exacerbation of asthma?

a. Oxygen therapy
b. Electronic fetal monitoring
c. β-adrenergic receptor stimulants
d. Theophylline

6.34 The risk of uterine growth retardation associated with chronic asthma is _____ if glucocorticoid therapy is required.

a. Increased
b. Unchanged
c. Decreased

6.35 Pregnant patients who smoke have an increased risk of

a. Spontaneous abortion
b. Ectopic pregnancy
c. Preterm labor and delivery
d. Abruptio placentae
e. Intrauterine growth retardation

6.36 Congenital tuberculosis is _____ complication of maternal infection.

a. A common
b. An uncommon

6.37 The incidence and severity of the common cold (URI) are _____ in pregnancy.

a. Increased
b. Unchanged
c. Decreased

6.38 Patients with the following cardiac diseases are best advised not to become pregnant.

a. Primary pulmonary hypertension
b. Uncorrected tetralogy of Fallot
c. Eisenmenger syndrome
d. Patent ductus arteriosus

6.39 In normal patients, cardiac output in pregnancy increases about

a. 20%
b. 40%
c. 60%
d. 80%
e. 100%

6.40–6.43 Instructions: Match the New York Heart Association functional classification of heart disease with the appropriate description.

6.40 Class I _____

6.41 Class II _____

6.42 Class III _____

6.43 Class IV _____

a. No symptoms of cardiac decompensation at rest, marked limitation of physical activity
b. No cardiac decompensation or limitation of physical activity
c. No symptoms of cardiac decompensation at rest, minor limitations of physical activity
d. Symptoms of cardiac decompensation at rest, increased discomfort with any physical activity

6.44 The fetuses of patients with functionally significant cardiac disease are at increased risk for

a. Low birth weight
b. Sepsis
c. Premature birth
d. Congenital heart defects

6.45 The majority of obstetric patients with severe cardiac disease who die do so during the

a. Antepartum period
b. Intrapartum period
c. Postpartum period

6.46 Most pregnant patients with mitral valve prolapse experience severe left atrial and ventricular enlargement and dysfunction.

a. True
b. False

6.47 Pregnant patients with rheumatic heart disease and severe associated valvular lesions have an increased incidence of _____ during pregnancy.

a. Thromboembolic disease
b. Subacute bacterial endocarditis
c. Cardiac failure
d. Pulmonary edema

Answers (6.32-6.47)

6.32 a	6.36 b	6.40 b	6.44 a, c
6.33 all	6.37 a	6.41 c	6.45 c
6.34 a	6.38 a, b, c	6.42 a	6.46 b
6.35 all	6.39 b	6.43 d	6.47 all

6.48   Which of the following is characteristic of patients at increased risk for peripartum cardiomyopathy?

    a.   African-American heritage
    b.   History of preeclampsia
    c.   Under 25 years of age
    d.   First pregnancy

6.49   Counseling about the benefits of sterilization is warranted for patients with peripartum cardiomyopathy.

    a.   True
    b.   False

6.50   Patients with Marfan's syndrome in pregnancy may expect

    a.   A 25–50% maternal mortality
    b.   A 50% chance of inheritance of the disease by offspring
    c.   Both A and B
    d.   Neither A nor B

6.51–6.53   Instructions: Match the American Diabetic Association (ADA) classification with the appropriate description.

6.51   Type I diabetes _____

6.52   Type II diabetes _____

6.53   Gestational diabetes _____

    a.   Adult-onset glucose intolerance
    b.   Glucose intolerance diagnosed in childhood
    c.   Glucose intolerance identified during pregnancy

6.54   In pregnancy, human placental lactogen has which of the following effects?

    a.   Increased levels of free fatty acids
    b.   Increased gluconeogenesis
    c.   Decreased glucose uptake
    d.   Increased lipolysis

6.55–6.62   Instructions: Match the White classification of diabetes with the appropriate description.

6.55   A _____

6.56   B _____

6.57   C _____

6.58   D _____

6.59   E _____

6.60   F _____

6.61   R _____

6.62   T _____

    a.   Onset between ages 10 and 13, duration 10–19 years, no vascular disease
    b.   Pelvic arteriosclerosis by x-ray
    c.   Onset under age 10, duration greater than 20 years, some vascular disease
    d.   Onset after 20 years, duration less than 10 years, no vascular disease
    e.   Transplantation
    f.   Proliferative retinopathy
    g.   Vascular nephritis
    h.   Gestational diabetes, onset in pregnancy

6.63   The normal glucosuria of pregnancy is commonly about _____ mg per day.

    a.   10
    b.   100
    c.   300
    d.   500
    e.   700

6.64   Infants of diabetic mothers are at an increased risk for which of the following congenital anomalies?

    a.   Cardiac deformities
    b.   Craniofacial deformities
    c.   Limb deformities
    d.   Situs inversus

6.65   Infants born to mothers with insulin-dependent diabetes are at higher risk for

    a.   Neonatal hyperbilirubinemia
    b.   Neonatal hypoglycemia
    c.   Hypocalcemia
    d.   Polycythemia

6.66   A complication of pregnancy in diabetic patients is

    a.   Oligohydramnios
    b.   Polyhydramnios

Answers (6.48–6.66)

6.48 a, b	6.53 c	6.58 c	6.63 c
6.49 a	6.54 a, c, d	6.59 b	6.64 a, c
6.50 c	6.55 h	6.60 g	6.65 all
6.51 b	6.56 d	6.61 f	6.66 b
6.52 a	6.57 a	6.62 e	

6.67 Which of the following are known risk factors for gestational diabetes?

    a. History of giving birth to an infant weighing more than 4000 g
    b. History of repeated spontaneous abortion
    c. History of unexplained stillbirth
    d. Obesity
    e. Family history of diabetes

6.68 Beginning at about 30–32 weeks gestation in pregnant diabetics, which of the following measures of fetal well-being are commonly applied?

    a. Daily fetal kick counts
    b. Serial nonstress testing
    c. Serial biophysical profile testing
    d. Serial ultrasonography

6.69 Most pregnant diabetics are maintained on a daily calorie intake of approximately

    a. 1600–1700
    b. 2300–2400
    c. 2800–2900
    d. 3300–3400

6.70 Serial sonography for insulin-dependent diabetics is important in the latter part of pregnancy because of the risk of

    a. Macrosomia and polyhydramnios
    b. Intrauterine growth retardation and polyhydramnios
    c. Macrosomia and oligohydramnios
    d. Intrauterine growth retardation and oligohydramnios

6.71 For a diabetic patient taking a mixed regimen of NPH and regular insulin in the morning and evening, the fasting glucose reflects the

    a. Regular insulin given in the morning
    b. NPH insulin given in the morning
    c. NPH insulin given the previous evening
    d. Regular insulin given in the evening

6.72 In the well-controlled diabetic with no complications, induction of labor at _____ weeks is often undertaken based on the risks of continued pregnancy.

    a. 40–42
    b. 38–40
    c. 36–38
    d. 34–36
    e. 32–34

6.73 What percent of gestational diabetics return to a normal glucose status postpartum?

    a. over 95
    b. 85–95
    c. 75–85
    d. 65–75
    e. 55–65

6.74 The currently recognized upper normal limit for the 1-hr Glucola test is _____ mg %.

    a. 120
    b. 140
    c. 160
    d. 180
    e. 200

6.75 The patient is considered to have gestational diabetes when _____ of the four test results of the 3-hr. glucose-tolerance test (Glucola) are abnormal.

    a. 1
    b. 2
    c. 3
    d. 4

6.76 Of the patients screened by the 1-hr Glucola test between 24 and 28 weeks gestation, approximately 15% will be found to have an abnormal glucose value. Of these, approximately _____ will be found to have gestational diabetes using a 3-hr glucose-tolerance test.

    a. 5%
    b. 15%
    c. 30%
    d. 45%
    e. 60%

6.77 "Ideal" control for a pregnant diabetic would be maintaining fasting plasma glucose measurements in the range of

    a. 60–70 mg %
    b 90–100 mg %
    c. 100–110 mg %
    d. 110–120 mg %

6.78 To avoid toxoplasma infection, pregnant women should be advised to

    a. Eat only well cooked meat
    b. Avoid exposure to cats
    c. Avoid exposure to cat feces
    d. Avoid vegetables that have not been well washed

Answers (6.67–6.78)

6.67 all	6.70 a	6.73 a	6.76 b
6.68 all	6.71 c	6.74 b	6.77 b
6.69 b	6.72 b	6.75 b	6.78 a, b, c

6.79 The clinical triad of fetal toxoplasmosis gondii infection is

   a. Uveitis, hemoglobinuria, and hydrothecosis
   b. Atrial septal defect, mandibular overgrowth, and chorioretinitis
   c. Hepatomegaly, convulsions, and icterus
   d. Chorioretinitis, hydrocephalus, and cerebral calcifications
   e. Anencephaly, pneumonia, and thrush

6.80 All cats, whether they hunt and eat their prey or consume only prepared foods, are considered reservoirs of toxoplasmosis and should be avoided by women while they are pregnant.

   a. True
   b. False

6.81 In toxoplasmosis, infection in the first trimester causes _____ fetal disease than infection in the third trimester.

   a. More severe
   b. As severe
   c. Less severe

6.82 Causes of polyhydramnios include

   a. Diabetes
   b. Intestinal atresia
   c. Anencephaly
   d. Toxoplasmosis

6.83 Which of the following statements about the newborn of a myasthenic patient is *correct*?

   a. The infant is never affected
   b. The infant may develop a transient type of the disease
   c. The infant will develop the disease

6.84 Relapses in the myasthenic patient are treated most commonly by

   a. Ergotrate
   b. Neostigmine
   c. Pyridostigmine
   d. Progesterone

6.85 Which of the following statements about Hodgkin's disease and pregnancy is *correct*?

   a. Pregnancy is quite unusual
   b. Pregnancy exacerbates the disease
   c. Pregnancy prevents effective treatment
   d. The infant is not adversely influenced
   e. The rate of spontaneous abortions is high

6.86 Microcephaly, chorioretinitis, deafness, and mental retardation are the characteristic results of which intrauterine infection?

   a. Cytomegalovirus
   b. Coxsackie B
   c. Mumps
   d. Rubeola
   e. Rubella

6.87 Which of the following antibiotics, when given to a mother during pregnancy, may produce enamel defects and yellowing of the teeth of the fetus?

   a. Cephaloridine
   b. Colistimethate sodium
   c. Penicillin
   d. Tetracycline
   e. Chloramphenicol

6.88 T_4 and T_3 serum concentrations are lowered during pregnancy because of

   a. Estrogen-induced alterations of thyroid gland production
   b. Progesterone-induced alterations of thyroid gland production
   c. Estrogen-induced increases in thyroxin-binding globulin
   d. Progesterone-induced increases in thyroxin-binding globulin

6.89 Which of the following is the preferred treatment for hyperthyroidism in pregnancy because of its relatively lower placental transfer to the fetus?

   a. Propylthiouracil (PTU)
   b. Methimazole (Tapazole)

6.90 Which of the following statements concerning hypothyroidism in pregnancy is *incorrect*?

   a. The fetus of a myxedematous mother will be a cretin or develop mental retardation unless treated as a neonate
   b. Myxedema does not affect fertility or libido
   c. The pituitary-thyroid axis of the fetus develops independently
   d. Hypothyroidism is encountered infrequently in pregnancy because it usually occurs after the reproductive age
   e. Prompt treatment of myxedema in pregnancy will allow normal outcome

6.91 What neonatal complication occurs in over 50% of babies born of mothers who suffer from hyperparathyroidism?

   a. Hyperbilirubinemia
   b. Alopecia
   c. Hiatal hernia
   d. Neonatal tetany
   e. Low birth weight

Answers (6.79-6.91)

6.79 d	6.83 b	6.86 a	6.89 a
6.80 b	6.84 b, c	6.87 d	6.90 b
6.81 a	6.85 d	6.88 c	6.91 d
6.82 a, b, c			

6.92 Approximately what percent of pregnant women have asymptomatic cervical colonization of B-hemolytic streptococci?

a. 10
b. 30
c. 50
d. 70
e. 90

6.93 While awaiting B-hemolytic streptococci cultures, it is generally recommended to proceed with prophylactic treatment with penicillin or ampicillin because of the risk to the neonate of transcervical colonization.

a. True
b. False

6.94 *Treponema pallidum* can cross the placenta of the fetus only after approximately the 20th week of gestation.

a. True
b. False

6.95 Hutchinson's teeth, mulberry molars, saddle nose, and saber shins are characteristic of congenital

a. Rubella
b. Syphilis
c. Toxoplasmosis
d. Bacterial vaginosis

6.96 *Treponema pallidum* reaches the fetus by

a. Direct contact through the chorion
b. Transplacental circulation
c. The amniotic fluid
d. Lymphatics

6.97 Which of the following are associated with congenital syphillis?

a. Cutaneous lesions
b. Osteochondritis of the long bones
c. Pseudoparalysis
d. Hepatosplenomegaly

6.98 If the VDRL titer is greater than 1:8, a treponemal-specific test is not needed to confirm the diagnosis of syphilis in pregnancy.

a. True
b. False

6.99 What increase in the serologic titer for syphilis indicates either inadequate treatment or reinfection and is an indication for further therapy?

a. 2-fold
b. 4-fold
c. 6-fold
d. 8-fold
e. 10-fold

6.100 Prophylactic treatment of the newborn of a woman with *Neisseria gonorrhoeae* infection with which of the following is successful in preventing neonatal gonococcal ophthalmia?

a. Penicillin
b. Silver nitrate
c. Tetracycline
d. Ampicillin

6.101 Bacterial vaginosis in the antepartum period has been associated with an increased incidence of

a. Postpartum metritis
b. Premature rupture of membranes
c. Amniotic fluid infection
d. Preterm labor

6.102 Approximately what percent of women with bacterial vaginosis in pregnancy are asymptomatic?

a. 10
b. 25
c. 50
d. 75
e. 100

6.103 Delivery of an infant through a birth canal with primary herpes infection is associated with a neonatal infection rate of

a. 10%
b. 20%
c. 30%
d. 40%
e. 50%

6.104 Routine culturing for herpes simplex virus should be performed near term to ascertain whether vaginal delivery is safe.

a. True
b. False

6.105 Active cytomegalovirus infection in the lower genital tract _____ an indication for cesarean delivery.

a. Is
b. Is not

6.106 Intrapartum acyclovir treatment is effective in reducing the risk of neonatal infection with cytomegalovirus.

a. True
b. False

6.107 What percent of reproductive age women lack immunity to the rubella virus?

a. 5
b. 15
c. 25
d. 35
e. 45

Answers (6.92-6.107)

6.92 b	6.96 b	6.100 b, c	6.104 b
6.93 a	6.97 all	6.101 all	6.105 b
6.94 b	6.98 b	6.102 c	6.106 b
6.95 b	6.99 b	6.103 e	6.107 b

6.108 The risk of congenital rubella syndrome is _____ if a woman develops an infection in the first trimester as compared to the third trimester.

 a. Increased
 b. Unchanged
 c. Reduced

6.109 Which of the following is *not* a neonatal abnormality associated with congenital rubella infection?

 a. Cataracts and/or retinopathy
 b. Patent ductus arteriosus or pulmonary artery hyperplasia
 c. Musculoskeletal anomalies, including phocomelia
 d. Deafness or impaired hearing
 e. Hepatosplenomegaly

6.110 A pregnant woman exposed to rubella should immediately be vaccinated.

 a. True
 b. False

6.111 The most classic eye finding in fetal congenital rubella is

 a. Retinopathy
 b. Cataracts
 c. Glaucoma
 d. Microphthalmia
 e. Myopia

6.112 Because the rubella vaccine utilizes a live attenuated rubella virus, administration of the vaccine to a woman who is breast-feeding is contraindicated.

 a. True
 b. False

6.113 It is believed that about _____ of pediatric HIV infection is secondary to vertical transmission from mother to fetus.

 a. 20%
 b. 40%
 c. 60%
 d. 80%
 e. 100%

6.114 Antepartum, intrapartum, and postpartum administration of zidovudine has been associated with a decreased risk of transmission of HIV infection from mother to infant.

 a. True
 b. False

6.115 The sensitivity and specificity of the combined use ELISA and Western blot tests for HIV infection is

 a. 59%
 b 69%
 c. 79%
 d. 89%
 e. 99%

6.116 The management of labor for a HIV-infected woman should include

 a. Avoiding the use of fetal scalp electrodes
 b. Avoiding fetal scalp blood sampling
 c. Intrapartum administration of zidovudine as part of an intrapartum-antepartum-postpartum regime
 d. Cesarian section to avoid infection

6.117 The risk of deep-vein thrombosis during pregnancy is _____ in the immediate postpartum period.

 a. Higher than
 b. The same as
 c. Lower than

6.118 The goal of intravenous heparin anticoagulation for deep thrombophlebitis in pregnancy is to maintain a partial thromboplastin time (PTT) prolonged _____ over the baseline value for 7–10 days.

 a. 0.5–1-fold
 b. 1.5–2-fold
 c. 2.5–3-fold
 d. 3.5–4-fold

6.119 Coumadin and heparin are equally recommended for the treatment of deep venous thrombosis during pregnancy.

 a. True
 b. False

6.120 Recurrent pulmonary embolization from pelvic thrombophlebitis is best treated with

 a. Anticoagulation
 b. Ligation of femoral veins
 c. Ligation of inferior vena cava
 d. Paravertebral block of sympathetic chain

6.121 When considering the diagnosis of pulmonary embolism in pregnancy, PaO_2 of _____ mm Hg or below is suggestive, indicating the need for further evaluation.

 a. 70
 b. 75
 c. 80
 d. 85
 e. 90

Answers (6.108-6.121)

6.108 a	6.112 b	6.116 a, b, c	6.119 b
6.109 c	6.113 d	6.117 c	6.120 c
6.110 b	6.114 a	6.118 b	6.121 c
6.111 b	6.115 e		

6.122   Which of the following neurologic disorders is *not* expressly associated with pregnancy?

a.   Peripheral nerve compressions syndrome
b.   Eclampsia
c.   Chorea gravidarum
d.   Bell's palsy

6.123   Pregnancy is associated with an increase in epileptic seizures in about three-quarters of affected women.

a.   True
b.   False

6.124   Patients with epilepsy appear to have a _____ increased risk of bearing children with congenital anomalies.

a.   2-fold
b.   4-fold
c.   6-fold
d.   8-fold

6.125   During an epileptic seizure, the immediate risk(s) to the fetus include

a.   Uteroplacental insufficiency
b.   Abruptio placentae
c.   Placenta previa
d.   Vasa previa

6.126   Because of concerns about teratogenesis, which is the most commonly used anticonvulsant drug during pregnancy?

a.   Phenytoin
b.   Dilantin
c.   Carbamazepine
d.   Phenobarbital

6.127   The risk of cerebral vascular accident in pregnancy is _____ from that of the nonpregnant state.

a.   Increased
b.   Unchanged
c.   Decreased

6.128   Anticholinesterases such as neostigmine or pyridostigmine are commonly used in the treatment of what neurologic disease in pregnancy?

a.   Cerebral vascular accident
b.   Multiple sclerosis
c.   Epilepsy
d.   Myasthenia gravis

6.129   Infants of multiple sclerosis victims have _____ lifetime risk of developing the disease as compared with the general population.

a.   An increased
b.   An unchanged
c.   A decreased

6.130–6.134   Instructions: Match the alterations in gastrointestinal functioning during pregnancy with the appropriate clinical manifestation(s).

6.130   Reduced resting lower esophageal sphincter pressure and altered esophageal motility _____

6.131   Decreased gastric emptying and increased residual volume _____

6.132   Altered propulsive motility and increased transit time _____

6.133   Increased activity and efficiency of brush borders _____

6.134   Reduced contractility and increased water and sodium absorption _____

a.   Stasis and bacterial overgrowth, pseudo-obstruction, and sequestration of bile salts
b.   Gastroesophageal reflux, heartburn, and erosive esophagitis
c.   Increased risk of anesthesia-associated aspiration and a decreased incidence of duodenal ulcer
d.   Increased absorption of some nutrients
e.   Constipation and pseudo-obstruction

6.135   Approximately 25% of women with first trimester nausea and vomiting will develop the more severe hyperemesis gravidarum.

a.   True
b.   False

6.136   Peptic ulcer disease most usually is _____ during pregnancy

a.   Exacerbated
b.   Unchanged
c.   Improved

6.137   The treatment of pancreatitis in pregnancy includes

a.   Nasogastric suction
b.   Intravenous fluid therapy to correct electrolyte imbalance
c.   Insulin therapy for hyperglycemia
d.   Calcium gluconate therapy for hypocalcemia

6.138   The maternal morbidity and mortality associated with appendicitis in pregnancy is _____ as compared to the nonpregnant state.

a.   Increased
b.   Unchanged
c.   Decreased

Answers (6.122–6.138)

6.122 d	6.127 a	6.131 c	6.135 b
6.123 b	6.128 d	6.132 a	6.136 b
6.124 b	6.129 a	6.133 d	6.137 all
6.125 a, b	6.130 b	6.134 e	6.138 a
6.126 c			

6.139 The most common perinatal complication associated with appendicitis in pregnancy is

   a. Premature rupture of membranes
   b. Premature labor
   c. Placenta previa
   d. Abruptio placentae

6.140 The morbidity of regional enteritis in pregnancy is primarily related to

   a. Abdominal abscesses
   b. Intestinal obstruction
   c. Toxic megacolon
   d. Colonic perforation
   e. Colonic stricture

6.141 Routine dental care during pregnancy should be avoided because the risk of local anesthetics, either with or without epinephrine, is great to the fetus.

   a. True
   b. False

6.142–6.146 Instructions: Match the type of hepatitis with the appropriate description(s).

6.142 Hepatitis A _____

6.143 Hepatitis B _____

6.144 Hepatitis C _____

6.145 Hepatitis D _____

6.146 Hepatitis E _____

   a. Often associated with fulminant hepatitis
   b. Represents 50% of cases of hepatitis in pregnancy
   c. Spread by water, food, or fecal contamination
   d. Spread primarily by blood or blood product transfusion
   e. Associated with unexpectedly high maternal mortality

6.147 The clinical course of hepatitis B infection is significantly exacerbated by pregnancy.

   a. True
   b. False

6.148 If a mother is identified as a carrier of hepatitis B or develops hepatitis B during pregnancy, the neonate should receive

   a. Active immunization for hepatitis (hepatitis B vaccine)
   b. Passive immunization with hepatitis B antibody immunoglobulin (HBIG)

6.149 Cholestasis of pregnancy is often recurrent in subsequent pregnancies

   a. True
   b. False

6.150 Patients with cholestasis of pregnancy present with which of the following?

   a. Pruritis
   b. Fatigue
   c. Jaundice
   d. Fever

6.151 Because of the high maternal morbidity and mortality associated with acute fatty liver of pregnancy, delivery as soon as feasible is recommended.

   a. True
   b. False

6.152 The most important obstetric consideration involving blunt abdominal trauma to the abdomen is

   a. Uterine perforation
   b. Abruptio placentae
   c. Premature rupture of the membranes
   d. Uterine rupture

6.153 Excluding genetic causes, alcohol use during pregnancy is the most common cause of mental retardation.

   a. True
   b. False

6.154 Fetal alcohol syndrome is associated with

   a. Mental retardation
   b. Prenatal and postnatal growth retardation
   c. Cardiovascular and central nervous system anomalies
   d. Craniofacial anomalies

6.155 Segmental intestinal atresia, limb-reduction defects, disruptive brain anomalies, congenital heart defects, and prune-belly syndrome are associated with the ingestion of

   a. Marijuana
   b. Cocaine
   c. Alcohol
   d. Caffeine

Answers (6.139-6.155)

6.139 b	6.144 d	6.148 a, b	6.152 b
6.140 a, b	6.145 a	6.149 a	6.153 a
6.141 b	6.146 e	6.150 a, b, c	6.154 all
6.142 c	6.147 b	6.151 a	6.155 b
6.143 b			

6.156 Thrombocytopenia-associated spontaneous bleed-
       ing during pregnancy usually occurs with platelet
       concentration of less then

       a. 100,000/mm³
       b. 80,000/mm³
       c. 60,000/mm³
       d. 40,000/mm³
       e. 20,000/mm³

6.157 The initial treatment of immune thrombocytopenic
       purpura in pregnancy is

       a. Administration of γ-globulin
       b. Splenectomy
       c. Administration of corticosteroids
       d. Transfusion of platelets

6.158 Patients with lupus anticoagulant have a rate of re-
       productive wastage in excess of

       a. 30%
       b. 50%
       c. 70%
       d. 90%

6.159 While it is uncertain whether vaginal delivery
       through a cancerous cervix worsens the prognosis
       for the cancer, abdominal delivery is generally rec-
       ommended.

       a. True
       b. False

6.160 Stage for stage, the prognosis for cervical cancer in a
       pregnant patient is _____ for a nonpregnant pa-
       tient.

       a. Worse than
       b. The same as
       c. Better than

Answers (6.156–6.160)

6.156 e   6.158 d   6.159 a   6.160 b
6.157 c

Chapter 7 Final Questions (27 questions)

7.1   Amniotic fluid

  a. Protects against infection of the fetus
  b. Protects against fetal trauma
  c. Protects the fetus from umbilical cord compression
  d. Allows for fetal respiration

7.2   Premature rupture of the membranes (PROM) is defined as rupture of the chorioamniotic membrane

  a. Prior to the onset of labor
  b. At the onset of labor
  c. During the active phase of labor
  d. Prior to complete effacement

7.3   Premature rupture of the membranes occurs in what percent of all pregnancies?

  a. Less than 2
  b. 2–5
  c. 10–15
  d. 20–25

7.4   The presence of sexually transmitted diseases is associated with increased incidence of premature rupture of membranes.

  a. True
  b. False

7.5–7.6   Instructions: Match the anomalous result from the Nitrazine test with the situations likely to cause it.

7.5   False-negative Nitrazine test

7.6   False-positive Nitrazine test

  a. Basic urine
  b. Presence of cervical mucus
  c. Blood contamination
  d. Previous premature rupture of the membranes with little residual fluid
  e. Some antiseptic solutions
  f. Vaginitis (especially *Trichomonas*)
  g. Presence of semen
  h. Minimal amniotic fluid leakage

7.7   The most common situation that can be confused at term with premature rupture of membranes is

  a. Bloody show
  b. Passage of cervical mucus
  c. Intermittent urinary leakage
  d. Yeast vaginitis

7.8   The Nitrazine test is used to assess for premature rupture of membranes based on the fact that amniotic fluid is

  a. Acid
  b. Alkaline
  c. Of higher specific gravity than water
  d. Of lower specific gravity than water

7.9   In order to decide upon the appropriate management for a patient with premature rupture of membranes, assessment of the cervical Bishop score by digital examination is required.

  a. True
  b. False

7.10   The presence of bacteria on Gram stain of amniotic fluid obtained by amniocentesis after premature rupture of membranes is a better predictor of intrauterine infection than the presence of white cells.

  a. True
  b. False

7.11   Which of the following factors should be considered in developing a management plan for a patient with premature rupture of the membranes?

  a. The gestatational age at the time of rupture
  b. The presence of uterine contractions
  c. The amount of amnotic fluid around the fetus
  d. Maternal age

7.12   The use of betamethasone to enhance pulmonary maturity is contraindicated in the presence of premature rupture of membranes because of the risk of intrauterine infection.

  a. True
  b. False

7.13   Prior to _____ weeks of gestational age, premature rupture of the membranes presents the risks of pulmonary hypoplasia and amniotic band syndrome.

  a. 25
  b. 27
  c. 29
  d. 31

7.14   The expectant management of premature rupture of membranes in a fetus that is significantly preterm usually includes which of the following?

  a. Daily WBC counts for the first few days
  b. Frequent ultrasound assessment for amniotic fluid volume
  c. Serial cervical digital examinations to detect the onset of labor
  d. Daily fetal movement monitoring
  e. Intermittent electronic monitoring

Answers (7.1-7.14)

7.1 all	7.5 d, h	7.9 b	7.12 b
7.2 a	7.6 a, b, c, e, f, g	7.10 a	7.13 a
7.3 c	7.7 c	7.11 a, b, c	7.14 a, b, d, e
7.4 a	7.8 b		

7.15 After the initial leakage of amniotic fluid, the fetal membranes will seal over in more than half of cases, allowing the patient to leave the hospital.

    a. True
    b. False

7.16 Premature rupture of membranes refers to rupture of membranes

    a. Before 40 weeks gestation
    b. Before delivery
    c. Before the onset of labor
    d. Before viability

7.17 The diagnosis of rupture of membranes may be based on all of the following *except*

    a. Nitrazine test
    b. Patient history
    c. White blood cell count
    d. Ultrasound findings

7.18 Mechanisms of amniotic fluid production are thought to include which of the following?

    a. Fetal urine production
    b. Fetal bowel movements
    c. Fetal pulmonary effluent
    d. Passage of fluid across the fetal membranes
    e. Passage of fluid across the fetal skin

7.19 Complete fetal respiratory system development is dependent in part on adequate amniotic fluid volume.

    a. True
    b. False

7.20 Premature rupture of membranes occurs in approximately _____ of all pregnancies.

    a. 5–10%
    b. 10–15%
    c. 15–20%
    d. 20–25%
    e. 25–30%

7.21 About _____ of gravidas with premature rupture of membranes will have a preterm birth.

    a. 1%
    b. 5%
    c. 10%
    d. 15%
    e. 20%

7.22 The incidence of chorioamnionitis increases with increasing gestational age in the presence of premature rupture of the membranes.

    a. True
    b. False

7.23 Which of the following statements about premature rupture of the membranes and intrauterine infections is *incorrect*?

    a. Intact membranes with normal amniotic fluid volume fully protect the fetus from infection
    b. Subclinical intraamniotic infection may play a role in premature rupture of the membranes
    c. Metabolites from intrauterine infection may weaken the amniotic membranes
    d. Metabolites from intrauterine infection may initiate uterine contractions through stimulation of prostaglandin synthesis

7.24 Which of the following statements about premature rupture of the membranes and chorioamnionitis are correct?

    a. Purulent discharge often preceeds fever and uterine tenderness by several hours
    b. Gravidas in this situation often enter into tulmultous, spontaneous labor
    c. Fever greater than 100.5° is common
    d. This situation is often associated with fetal tachycardia
    e. Treatment consists of antibiotic therapy and prompt delivery

7.25 After premature rupture of membranes, the static intrauterine pressure caused by the resting tone of the uterus usually forces most of the amniotic fluid from the uterine cavity.

    a. True
    b. False

7.26 The differential diagnosis of premature rupture of the membranes includes

    a. Urinary incontinence
    b. Increased vaginal secretions in pregnancy
    c. Vaginal discharge associated with vaginitis
    d. Vesicovaginal fistula

7.27 Which of the following is *not* a component of the physical examination of the gravida with premature rupture of membranes?

    a. Speculum examination and confirmation of rupture of membranes with Nitrazine and/or fern testing
    b. Speculum examination and culturing for *N. gonorrhoeae*, β-hemolytic streptococcus, and chlamydia
    c. Testing of pooled fluid for phosphatidylglycerol if the fetal age warrants
    d. Digital examination of the cervix to ascerain if there is associated preterm labor

Answers (7.15–7.27)

7.15 b	7.19 a	7.22 b	7.25 b
7.16 c	7.20 b	7.23 a	7.26 all
7.17 b	7.21 b	7.24 b, c, d, e	7.27 d
7.18 a, c, d, e			

Chapter 8 Final Questions (30 questions)

8.1 Which of the following is a predisposing factor to respiratory distress syndrome?

    a. Short gestation
    b. Cesarean section
    c. Perinatal asphyxia
    d. Maternal diabetes

8.2 The 10% of babies born prematurely in the United States account for what percent of all perinatal morbidity and mortality?

    a. 10
    b. 30
    c. 50
    d. 70
    e. 90

8.3 An infant born at 30 weeks of gestation and weighing 2600 g would be defined as

    a. Low birth weight
    b. Preterm
    c. Both low birth weight and preterm
    d. Neither low birth weight nor preterm

8.4 Premature birth is associated with which of the following perinatal complications?

    a. Respiratory distress syndrome
    b. Intraventricular hemorrhage
    c. Skeletal abnormalities
    d. Sepsis
    e. Seizures

8.5 Which of the following factors has *not* been associated with preterm labor?

    a. Maternal infections
    b. Maternal age
    c. Uterine distortion
    d. Placental abnormalities
    e. Substance abuse

8.6 Which of the following indicators often precede preterm labor?

    a. Increased uterine irritability
    b. Increased frequency of contractions
    c. Rapid weight gain
    d. Pelvic pressure

8.7 Which of the following are recognized signs and symptoms associated with preterm labor?

    a. Low dull backache
    b. Pelvic pressure
    c. Abdominal cramps
    d. Change in vaginal discharge

8.8 Which of the following should be included in the evaluation of suspected preterm labor?

    a. Status of the cervix
    b. CAT scan for gestational age
    c. Electronic fetal monitor for frequency of contractions
    d. Abdominal palpation for strength of contractions

8.9 Which of the following laboratory studies are useful in the evaluation of a patient at risk for preterm labor?

    a. Urinalysis and urine culture
    b. Culture for β-streptococcus
    c. Culture of *N. gonorrhoeae*
    d. Wet preparation for bacterial vaginosis

8.10–8.13 Instructions: Match the tocolytic agent with its proposed mode of action.

8.10 Magnesium sulfate _____

8.11 β-adrenergic agents (ritodrine or terbutaline) _____

8.12 Prostaglandin-synthetase inhibitors (indomethacin) _____

8.13 Calcium-channel blockers (nifedipine) _____

    a. Increases cyclic AMP in cell, which decreases free calcium
    b. Competes with calcium for entry into cells
    c. Prevents calcium entry into muscle cells
    d. Decreases prostaglandin production

8.14–8.17 Instructions: Match the tocolytic agent with possible complications.

8.14 Magnesium sulfate _____

8.15 β-adrenergic agents (ritodrine or terbutaline) _____

8.16 Prostaglandin-synthetase inhibitors (indomethacin) _____

8.17 Calcium-channel blockers (nifedipine) _____

    a. Maternal hypotension, tachycardia, anxiety, chest tightening, and ECG changes
    b. Premature constriction of ductus arteriosus, especially after 34 weeks gestation
    c. Maternal flushing and headache, respiratory depression at high doses
    d. Possible decrease in uteroplacental blood flow with fetal hypoxia and hypercarbia

---

Answers (8.1–8.17)

8.1 all	8.6 a, b, d	8.10 b	8.14 c
8.2 c	8.7 all	8.11 a	8.15 a
8.3 b	8.8 a, c, d	8.12 d	8.16 b
8.4 a, b, d, e	8.9 all	8.13 c	8.17 d
8.5 b			

8.18 It is customary to stop tocolytic therapy at

    a. 30 weeks
    b. 32 weeks
    c. 34 weeks
    d. 36 weeks
    e. 38 weeks

8.19 Which of the following is not a contraindication to tocolysis?

    a. Mature fetus
    b. Anomalous fetus
    c. Intrauterine infection
    d. Maternal age greater than 35 years
    e. Presence of advanced labor

8.20 The efficacy of tocolytic agents is difficult to establish, in part because of difficulty in separating true preterm labor from premature uterine activity.

    a. True
    b. False

8.21 In regard to preterm labor: Overall, the tocolytic agent generally considered to have the highest degree of safety is

    a. Terbutaline
    b. Indomethacin
    c. Magnesium sulfate
    d. Nifedipine

8.22 In patients with preterm labor prior to 32 weeks gestation, corticosteroids are often given to

    a. Decrease uterine activity
    b. Stabilize vascular membranes
    c. Enhance fetal lung maturity
    d. Prevent infection

8.23 Preterm birth resulting from preterm labor is the most common cause of perinatal morbidity and mortality.

    a. True
    b. False

8.24 Most cases of preterm labor are defined as idiopathic, that is, no specific etiology can be found.

    a. True
    b. False

8.25 Surgically correctable causes of preterm birth include

    a. Incompetent cervix
    b. Uterine leiomyomas
    c. Septate uterus
    d. Vaginal stenosis

8.26 Maternal smoking is strongly associated with

    a. Intrauterine growth retardation
    b. Preterm labor
    c. A and B
    d. Neither A nor B

8.27–8.29 Instructions: Match the category of factors associated with preterm labor with the appropriate specific examples.

8.27 Excessive uterine enlargement _____

8.28 Uterine distortion _____

8.29 Placental abnormalities _____

    a. Multiple gestation
    b. Septate uterus
    c. Leiomyomas
    d. Placenta previa
    e. Abruptio placentae
    f. Hydramnios

8.30 A routine pelvic examination is often performed at 24–28 weeks to discover asymptomatic dilation and effacement of the cervix which is associated with an increased likelihood of preterm labor.

    a. True
    b. False

Answers (8.18–8.30)

8.18 d	8.22 c	8.25 a, b, c	8.28 b, c
8.19 d	8.23 a	8.26 c	8.29 d, e
8.20 a	8.24 a	8.27 a, c, f	8.30 a
8.21 c			

Chapter 9 Final Questions (39 questions)

9.1 Approximately what percent of women will experience bleeding during the second and third trimesters of pregnancy?

 a. 5
 b. 10
 c. 15
 d. 20
 e. 25

9.2 Bleeding in the second half of pregnancy can come from which of the following sources?

 a. Varicose veins
 b. Vaginal tears or lacerations
 c. Cervical carcinoma
 d. Cervicitis

9.3 An 18-year-old primigravida at term, not in labor, has sudden onset of severe continuous lower abdominal pain with a rapid pulse, low blood pressure, fetal bradycardia, and a tender abdomen. Which of the following is the most likely diagnosis?

 a. Abruptio placentae
 b. Placenta previa
 c. Uterine rupture
 d. Amniotic fluid embolus
 e. Supine hypotensive syndrome

9.4 A primigravida at term has profuse vaginal bleeding. Fetal heart tones are normal. The cervix is 2–3 cm dilated with an edge of placenta palpable. Which of the following is the most appropriate treatment?

 a. Voorhees' bag
 b. Braxton-Hicks version
 c. Cesarean delivery
 d. Rupture of the fetal membranes to stimulate delivery
 e. Replace blood loss and await vaginal delivery

9.5 Which of the following is *not* associated with massive placental abruption?

 a. Painless vaginal bleeding
 b. Uterine rigidity
 c. Uterine pain
 d. Maternal cardiovascular collapse
 e. Absent fetal heart sounds

9.6 Vasa previa diagnosed in early labor is best treated with

 a. Voorhees' bag
 b. Forceps delivery
 c. Spontaneous delivery
 d. Cesarean section
 e. Willet clamp

9.7–9.10 Instructions: Match the type of placenta previa with the appropriate description.

9.7 Complete or total placenta previa _____

9.8 Partial placenta previa _____

9.9 Marginal placenta previa _____

9.10 Low-lying placenta _____

 a. The margin of the placenta extends across part but not all of the internal os
 b. The entire cervical os is covered by the placenta
 c. The placenta is located near but not directly adjacent to the internal os
 d. The edge of the placenta lies adjacent to the internal os

9.11 Which of the following factors is *not* associated with placenta previa?

 a. Increasing maternal age
 b. Increasing parity
 c. Previous cesarean section
 d. Presence of a twin pregnancy
 e. Maternal hypertension

9.12 Placenta previa occurs, on average, in 1 in _____ pregnancies.

 a. 100
 b. 250
 c. 500
 d. 1000
 e. 1500

9.13 The incidence of placenta previa in nulliparas is _____ in multiparas.

 a. Less than
 b. The same as
 c. Greater than

9.14 The position of the placenta in relation to the internal cervical os remains constant throughout pregnancy.

 a. True
 b. False

9.15 In placenta previa, the first bleeding episode occurs most commonly at what gestational age?

 a. 23–24 weeks
 b. 25–26 weeks
 c. 27–28 weeks
 d. 29–30 weeks
 e. 31–32 weeks

Answers (9.1-9.15)

9.1	a	9.5	a	9.9	d	9.13	a
9.2	b, c, d	9.6	d	9.10	c	9.14	b
9.3	a	9.7	b	9.11	e	9.15	d
9.4	c	9.8	a	9.12	b		

9.16 Placenta previa is coincident with abruptio placentae in approximately what percent of cases?

a. less than 5
b. 10
c. 20
d. 40

9.17 Transvaginal ultrasonography is especially useful in the diagnosis of what type of placenta previa?

a. Anterior
b. Lateral
c. Posterior
d. All types of placenta previa

9.18 The initial management of a patient with placenta previa and a bleeding episode always includes which of the following?

a. Hospitalization
b. Immediate cesarean section
c. Immediate pitocin induction of labor
d. Blood transfusion

9.19 Which of the following are criteria for outpatient care of a patient with known placenta previa?

a. Highly motivated patient
b. Evidence of understanding of and compliance with instructions
c. Immediate access to the hospital
d. Primigravid patient only

9.20 The current perinatal mortality rate associated with placenta previa is

a. Less than 10%
b. 15%
c. 20%
d. 30%
e. 40%

9.21 Vaginal delivery with known placenta previa may be indicated if

a. The fetus is dead
b. There are major fetal malformations, leading to likely fetal demise
c. The pregnancy is clearly previable
d. The placental location and stage of labor are such that it is anticipated that vaginal delivery can be accomplished with a relatively small blood loss.

9.22 The incidence of congenital anomalies in cases of placenta previa is _____ the average for all pregnancies.

a. The same as
b. Twice
c. Three times
d. Four times

9.23 In placenta previa accreta, the trophoblast tissue invade the

a. Cervix
b. Lower uterine segment
c. Upper uterine segment
d. Mesosalpinx

9.24 Which of the following are common to both placenta previa and abruptio placentae?

a. Vaginal bleeding
b. Abdominal discomfort
c. Painful uterine contractions
d. Presence of a normal fetal heart rate

9.25 Placental abruption is defined as

a. Abnormal position of the placenta
b. Abnormal separation of the normally implanted placenta
c. Abnormal morphology of the placenta

9.26 Placental abruption is associated with

a. Maternal hypertension
b. Polyhydramnios
c. Maternal trauma
d. Maternal cocaine use

9.27 In abruptio placentae, the amount of vaginal bleeding is always proportional to the degree of placental abruption.

a. True
b. False

9.28 Couvelaire uterus is associated with

a. Placenta previa
b. Abruptio placentae
c. Both
d. Neither

9.29 The degree of fetal compromise is typically greatest in

a. Placenta previa
b. Placental abruption

9.30 The diagnosis of placental abruption is made primarily by

a. Clinical presentation and evaluation
b. Ultrasound
c. Amniocentesis
d. Laboratory evaluation

Answers (9.16-9.30)

9.16 b	9.20 a	9.24 a	9.28 b
9.17 d	9.21 all	9.25 b	9.29 b
9.18 a	9.22 b	9.26 all	9.30 a
9.19 a, b, c	9.23 b, c	9.27 b	

9.31–9.34 Instructions: Match the blood component with the appropriate factors.

9.31   Packed red blood cells _____

9.32   Fresh frozen plasma _____

9.33   Cryoprecipitate _____

9.34   Fresh whole blood _____

a. Fibrinogen, factors VIII XIII
b. RBCs only
c. All procoagulants, no platelets
d. RBCs and all procoagulants

9.35   Which of the following is *not* part of the classic "clinical presentation" of abruptio placentae?

a. Vaginal bleeding
b. Tender uterus
c. Frequent painful uterine contractions
d. Normal fetal heart rate

9.36   In vasa previa, the umbilical cord inserts into the

a. Central mass of the placenta
b. Membranes of the placenta
c. Internal os

9.37   The Kleihauer-Betke test may be used effectively in the evaluation of

a. Abruptio placentae
b. Vasa previa
c. Placenta accreta

9.38   The appropriate treatment for a ruptured vasa previa is

a. Augmentation of labor to expedite delivery
b. Tocolysis to decrease blood loss
c. Cesarean section to effect delivery as rapidly as possible
d. Paraumbilical artery transfusion to stabilize the infant in utero

9.39   In the absence of massive blood loss, coagulation defects are _____ in placenta previa than in abruptio placentae.

a. More common
b. As common
c. Less common

Answers (9.31–9.39)

9.31 b	9.34 d	9.36 b	9.38 c
9.32 c	9.35 d	9.37 b	9.39 c
9.33 a			

Chapter 10 Final Questions (46 questions)

10.1–10.2 Instructions: Match the blood pressure levels associated with a diagnosis of hypertension in pregnancy.

10.1   Systolic blood pressure _____

10.2   Diastolic blood pressure _____

    a. 80 mm Hg
    b. 90 mm Hg
    c. 100 mm Hg
    d. 120 mm Hg
    e. 140 mm Hg
    f. 160 mm Hg

10.3   Hypertension in pregnancy is defined as a rise in the diastolic blood pressure of at least (A) _____ mm Hg or in the systolic blood pressure of at least (B) _____ mm Hg.

1	5
2	10
3	15
4	20
5	25
6	30

10.4   The blood pressure is lowest if measured with the patient

    a. Lying in the lateral position
    b. Standing
    c. Sitting
    d. Lying in the prone position

10.5   During the course of pregnancy, blood pressure typically _____ in the middle trimester

    a. Increases slightly
    b. Decreases slightly
    c. Fluctuates irregularly

10.6   Pregnancy-induced hypertension develops in what percentage of pregnancies that proceed beyond the first trimester?

    a. less than 5
    b. 5–10
    c. 11–15
    d. 16–20
    e. 21–25

10.7   In multiple gestation, the incidence of pregnancy induced hypertension is _____ in a singleton pregnancy.

    a. Lower than
    b. The same as
    c. Higher than

10.8   Which of the following are characteristic of preeclampsia?

    a. Hypertension
    b. Proteinuria
    c. Edema
    d. Tonic-clonic seizures

10.9   What is the most likely diagnosis of a patient who presents with hypertension in the 12th week of pregnancy?

    a. Preeclampsia
    b. Eclampsia
    c. Chronic hypertension

10.10   Approximately what percent of women with chronic hypertension develop superimposed preeclampsia or eclampsia?

    a. 25
    b. 50
    c. 75
    d. 100

10.11   The intrauterine growth retardation often associated with hypertensive disease in pregnancy is most likely related to

    a. Chronic uteroplacental insufficiency
    b. Congenital anomalies of the fetus
    c. Anomalies of placental structure
    d. Associated placental abruption

10.12   In the patient with preeclampsia, visual disturbances such as scotomata and persistent severe headache are usually considered to arise from

    a. Infarct
    b. Vasospasm
    c. Partial embolic occlusion

10.13   The right upper quadrant pain seen in preeclampsia arises from

    a. Hepatic infarction
    b. Hepatic capsule distension
    c. Hepatic rupture

10.14   In a patient with preeclampsia, a _____ hematocrit may signify a worsening disease process.

    a. Increasing
    b. Decreasing

Answers (10.1–10.14)

10.1 e	10.5 b	10.9 c	10.12 b
10.2 b	10.6 b	10.10 a	10.13 b
10.3 (a) 3; (b) 6	10.7 c	10.11 a	10.14 a
10.4 a	10.8 a, b, c		

10.15 Which of the following is not included in the definition of severe preeclampsia?

   a. Oliguria (500 mL or less in 24 hr) and a rising plasma creatinine level
   b. Severe thrombocytopenia or overt intravascular hemolysis
   c. The development of convulsions in the absence of neurologic disease
   d. Proteinuria of 5 g or more in 24 hr
   e. A persistent blood pressure of 160 mm Hg or more systolic, or 110 mm Hg or more diastolic

10.16 In general, antihypertensive therapy is indicated in preeclampsia when the diastolic blood pressure is repeatedly above

   a. 90 mm Hg
   b. 100 mm Hg
   c. 110 mm Hg
   d. 120 mm Hg
   e. 130 mm Hg

10.17 The general goal of antihypertensive therapy in pregnancy is to rapidly return the patient to normal blood pressure levels for her age group.

   a. True
   b. False

10.18 Which of the following should be part of the management of a patient with mild preeclampsia who is being cared for at home?

   a. Bedrest
   b. Recording of daily fetal movement
   c. Daily dosing with magnesium sulfate
   d. Daily weighing

10.19 Which of the following is not indicative of worsening preeclampsia?

   a. Increasing hematocrit
   b. Increased renal function
   c. Thrombocytopenia
   d. Rapid patient weight gain

10.20 Intravenous magnesium sulfate is used to prevent convulsions and treat blood pressure elevation in preeclampsia.

   a. True
   b. False

10.21 Muscular paralysis and respiratory difficulty are noted at what serum concentration of magnesium sulfate?

   a. 4–7 mg/dL
   b. 8–12 mg/dL
   c. 15–17 mg/dL
   d. greater than 30 mg/dL

10.22 Magnesium sulfate toxicity is treated with the slow intravenous administration of

   a. Insulin
   b. Calcium gluconate
   c. Potassium hydroxide
   d. Magnesium gluconate

10.23–10.29 Instructions: Match the antihypertensive medication with its mechanism of action.

10.23 Thiazide _____

10.24 Methyldopa _____

10.25 Hydralazine _____

10.26 Propranolol _____

10.27 Labetalol _____

10.28 Nifedipine _____

10.29 Prazosin _____

   a. Calcium-channel blocker
   b. β-adrenergic blockade
   c. α and β-adrenergic blockade
   d. Direct vasodilator and cardiac effects
   e. Decreased plasma volume and cardiac output
   f. False neurotransmission, CNS effect
   g. Direct peripheral vasodilation

10.30 Magnesium sulfate given intravenously in a large single dose for eclampsia may be associated with all of the following except

   a. Transient loss of beat-to-beat variation
   b. Bone deposition of magnesium
   c. Hypermagnesemia in the fetus
   d. Reduction in glomerular filtration rate
   e. Diminished patellar reflex

10.31 In the postpartum period, reversal of the vasospastic process associated with preeclampsia is manifest by

   a. Decreased deep tendon reflexes
   b. Rapid fall in blood pressure
   c. Brisk diuresis
   d. Continued weight gain

10.32 If a preeclampsia patient does not seize during her pregnancy or within the first 24 hr after delivery, there is virtually no risk of her developing eclampsia.

   a. True
   b. False

Answers (10.15-10.32)

10.15 c	10.20 b	10.25 g	10.29 d
10.16 c	10.21 c	10.26 b	10.30 d
10.17 b	10.22 b	10.27 c	10.31 c
10.18 a, b, d	10.23 e	10.28 a	10.32 b
10.19 b	10.24 f		

10.33 In a patient with hypertension, midepigastric pain in the last trimester is suggestive of

    a. Ruptured splenic aneurysm
    b. Impending eclampsia
    c. Crohn's disease
    d. Hepatic hemorrhage
    e. Abruptio placentae

10.34 Which of the following are elements of the HELLP syndrome?

    a. Seizures
    b. Hemolysis
    c. Hepatic dysfunction
    d. Low platelets

10.35 Platelet transfusion for the HELLP syndrome is usually indicated on the platelet count falls below

    a. 10,000/mm^3
    b. 20,000/mm^3
    c. 30,000/mm^3
    d. 40,000/mm^3
    e. 50,000/mm^3

10.36 If fetal bradycardia is noted during an eclampsia seizure, immediate delivery by cesarean section is mandatory to salvage the fetus.

    a. True
    b. False

10.37 In patients with hypertension in pregnancy, each rise of 5 mm Hg of mean arterial pressure is associated with a progressive rise in perinatal mortality.

    a. True
    b. False

10.38 Preeclampsia occurs in about what percent of deliveries?

    a. 3
    b. 7
    c. 10
    d. 14

10.39 Placental size is usually _____ in patients with chronic hypertension/preeclampsia.

    a. Increased
    b. Normal
    c. Decreased

10.40 Patients with chronic hypertension/preeclampsia generally demonstrate all of the following *except*

    a. Fetal macrosomia
    b. Intrauterine growth retardation
    c. Oligohydramnios
    d. Dysmaturity

10.41 Compared to normotensive patients, patients with chronic hypertension/preeclampsia are _____ to develop intrapartum uteroplacental insufficiency.

    a. Less likely
    b. Equally likely
    c. More likely

10.42–10.46 Instructions: Match the pathology associated with hypertension in pregnancy with the most appropriate laboratory evaluations.

10.42 Vasoconstriction and decreased intravascular volume _____

10.43 Coagulopathy _____

10.44 Hepatocellular dysfunction _____

10.45 Renal dysfunction _____

10.46 Effects of the fetus _____

    a. NST/OCT/biophysical profile
    b. Amniotic fluid volume evaluation
    c. Fetal weight and growth evaluation
    d. 24-hr urine for creatinine clearance
    e. Coagulation profile
    f. Complete blood count
    g. Platelet count
    h. Liver function studies
    i. Fibrin split products
    j. Total urinary protein for 24 hr

Answers (10.33-10.46)

10.33 b	10.37 a	10.41 c	10.44 e, h
10.34 b, c, d	10.38 b	10.42 f	10.45 d, j
10.35 b	10.39 c	10.43 e, f, g, i	10.46 a, b, c
10.36 b	10.40 a		

Chapter 11 Final Questions (33 questions)

11.1 When the father is homozygous Rh+ and the mother is Rh–, what is the probability that the fetus will be Rh+?

 a. 25%
 b. 50%
 c. 75%
 d. 100%

11.2 Which of the following statements about isoimmunization is incorrect?

 a. It involves the development of fetal antibodies in response to maternal red blood cells
 b. The antibodies involved in isoimmunization cross the placental barrier
 c. The ability of the fetus to produce red blood cells can counter the isoimmunization process, to a greater or lesser extent
 d. The father must be Rh+ and the mother Rh– for Rh isoimmunization to occur.

11.3 The major class of antibody responsible for Rh isoimmunization is

 a. IgG
 b. IgM
 c. IgE

11.4 Complications for the fetus arising from an Rh+ fATHon tus and an Rh– mother will usually first appear in which pregnancy?

 a. First
 b. Second
 c. Third
 d. Fourth

11.5 The bilirubin produced in Rh isoimmunization that collects in the fetal system is responsible for a significant part of the morbidity of the disease.

 a. True
 b. False

11.6 Pregnancies with severely affected Rh-immunized fetuses may be complicated by

 a. Polyhydramnios
 b. Fetal hydrops
 c. Fetal cardiac failure
 d. Fetal anemia

11.7 Hydrops fetalis involves

 a. Severe fluid retention due to renal failure in the fetus
 b. Irreversible carbohydrate metabolic failure
 c. Decreased fetal aldosterone secretion
 d. The inability of the fetal hematopoietic tissue to compensate for anemia resulting from red cell destruction

11.8 Which of the following is not an element in hydrops fetalis?

 a. Fetal ascites
 b. Low output cardiac failure
 c. Anemia
 d. Decreased oncotic pressure in the fetal intravascular space

11.9–11.13 Instructions: Match the event with the risk of sensitization.

11.9 Mismatched blood transfusion _____

11.10 Spontaneous abortion _____

11.11 Ectopic pregnancy _____

11.12 Full-term delivery _____

11.13 Induced abortion _____

 a. less than 1%
 b. 1–2%
 c. 3–4%
 d. 5–6%
 e. 15%
 f. 25%
 g. 50%
 h. 90%

11.14 In fetal Rh isoimmunization, the degree of fetal hypoproteinemia is _____ fetal hepatic red cell production.

 a. Positively correlated with
 b. Negatively correlated with
 c. Unrelated to

11.15 Once Rh isoimmunization has occurred, the severity of disease always increases with each subsequent pregnancy.

 a. True
 b. False

Answers (11.1-11.15)

11.1 d	11.5 b	11.9 h	11.13 d
11.2 a	11.6 all	11.10 c	11.14 a
11.3 a	11.7 d	11.11 a	11.15 b
11.4 b	11.8 b	11.12 e	

11.16 Antibody development will occur in about what percent of cases of an Rh– mother and an Rh+ fetus?

    a. 5
    b. 15
    c. 25
    d. 35
    e. 45
    f. 75

11.17 The Liley curve reflects the status of the sensitized fetus based on the measurement of _____ in the amniotic fluid.

    a. Whole red blood cells
    b. Hemoglobin
    c. Rh-D antigen
    d. Bilirubin
    e. Albumin

11.18 In the second sensitized pregnancy where the mother is Rh– and the fetus is Rh+, antibody titers are _____ to the fetal condition.

    a. Directly related
    b. Unrelated

11.19 The major factor allowing fetal erythrocytes to enter the maternal circulation is

    a. Labor and delivery
    b. Normal placental circulation
    c. Spontaneous abortion
    d. Premature rupture of the membranes
    e. Low level placental abruption

11.20 Isoimmunization during pregnancy is caused exclusively by the Rh system.

    a. True
    b. False

11.21 Rh immune globulin is effective against which antigen of the Rh system?

    a. A
    b. B
    c. D
    d. Rh

11.22 RhoGAM should be administered to an Rh– patient during pregnancy at which of the following times?

    a. At 28 weeks gestation
    b. Within 3 days of delivery of a Rh+ infant
    c. At the time of amniocentesis
    d. After an ectopic pregnancy
    e. After a spontaneous abortion

11.23 The administration of Rho-D immune gobulin (Rho GAM) in the first 72 hr postpartum decreases the risk of subsequent sensitization from approximately 15% in the untreated state to 0%.

    a. True
    b. False

11.24 Human Rho-D immune globulin (RhoGAM)

    a. Prevents the transfer of incompatible fetal cells to the mother
    b. Attaches to the fetal Rh+ cells in the maternal circulation and obscures the antigen sites
    c. Prevents antibody production in the maternal hematopoietic system

11.25 The administration of a 300-mg dose of RhoGAM to Rh– patients at 28 weeks gestation is found to reduce the risk of sensitization to about

    a. 0.1%
    b. 0.2%
    c. 0.3%
    d. 0.4%
    e. 0.5%

11.26 The standard 300-mg dose of Rh immune globin will effectively neutralize how many milliliters of fetal red blood cells?

    a. 5
    b. 10
    c. 15
    d. 20
    e. 25

11.27 Non-Rh(D) non-ABO hemolytic disease is frequently associated with blood transfusions.

    a. True
    b. False

11.28 ABO hemolytic disease is _____ associated with fetal kernicterus than Rh hemolytic disease.

    a. Less often
    b. As often
    c. More often

11.29 Direct fetal transfusion into the umbilical cord under ultrasound guidance carries with it a risk of fetal death of up to

    a. 1%
    b. 3%
    c. 5%
    d. 7%
    e. 15%

Answers (11.16-11.29)

11.16 b	11.20 b	11.24 b	11.27 a
11.17 d	11.21 c	11.25 b	11.28 a
11.18 b	11.22 all	11.26 c	11.29 b
11.19 a	11.23 b		

11.30 The amount of fetal red cells required to elicit an antibody response is estimated at about

    a. 0.001 mL
    b. 0.01 mL
    c. 0.1 mL
    d. 1.0 mL
    e. 10.0 mL

11.31 Which of the following statements about the Kleihauer-Betke test is *not* correct?

    a. It is used to detect fetomaternal hemorrhage
    b. A negative test result is an indication to administer Rh immunglobulin
    c. It identifies fetal cells in the maternal circulation
    d. The ratio of fetal:maternal cells are assessed microscopically

11.32 The relative proportion of patients with ABO hemolytic disease and non-Rh(D) non-ABO hemolytic disease, as compared to patients with Rh isoimmunization, has

    a. Increased
    b. Remained the same
    c. Decreased

11.33 Which of the following statements about ABO hemolytic disease is not correct?

    a. It results in milder fetal kernicterus than Rh hemolytic disease
    b. It is rarely associated with hydrops fetalis
    c. The disease severity is probably related to the relatively smaller number of A and B antigenic sites on fetal red blood cells
    d. It usually occurs in the second trimester

Answers (11.30-11.33)

11.30 b   11.31 b   11.32 a   11.33 d

Chapter 12 Final Questions (29 questions)

12.1–12.4   Instructions: Match the clinical situation with the appropriate incidence in the general population.

12.1   Monozygotic twins _____

12.2   Dizygotic twins _____

12.3   Twinning with ovulation induction _____

12.4   Twinning with in vitro fertilization _____

   a.   1 of 3 pregnancies
   b.   1 of 12 pregnancies
   c.   1 of 90 pregnancies
   d.   1 of 250 pregnancies
   e.   1 of 500 pregnancies

12.5–12.8   Instructions: Match the time of division of the conceptus (twinning) with the corresponding organization of fetal membranes.

12.5   Twinning within 3 days of fertilization _____

12.6   Twinning between 4 and 8 days of fertilization _____

12.7   Twinning between 9 and 12 days of fertilization _____

12.8   Twinning 12 days or more after fertilization _____

   a.   Conjoined twins
   b.   Monoamniotic/monochorionic
   c.   Diamniotic/dichorionic
   d.   Diamniotic/monochorionic

12.9   Which of the following is *not* more commonly associated with multiple pregnancy?

   a.   Megaloblastic anemia
   b.   Fetal macrosomia
   c.   Vasa previa
   d.   Congenital anomalies
   e.   Polyhydramnios

12.10   Multifetal pregnancy is associated with an increased incidence of which of the following?

   a.   Perinatal morbidity
   b.   Fetomaternal hemorrhage
   c.   Intrauterine growth retardation
   d.   Umbilical cord prolapse
   e.   Postpartum hemorrhage

12.11   In monozygotic twins, oligohydramnios and anemia of one twin and hydramnios with polycythemia of the other twin are due to

   a.   Congenital anomalies of the fetuses
   b.   Vascular anastomoses between the fetuses
   c.   Umbilical cord compression
   d.   Maternal diabetes

12.12–12.13   Instructions: Match the type of twinning with its apprpriate mechanism.

12.12   Dizygotic twins _____

12.13   Monozygotic twins _____

   a.   Two separate ova fertilized by two separate sperm
   b.   Division of the fertilized ovum at various times after conception

12.14   The incidence of triplets is approximately

   a.   1:1000
   b.   1:4000
   c.   1:8000
   d.   1:10,000

12.15   A familial factor is present in twinning that follows the

   a.   Maternal lineage
   b.   Paternal lineage
   c.   Both maternal and paternal lineages

12.16–12.19   Instructions: Match the number of fetuses with the average time at delivery.

12.16   Singleton pregnancy _____

12.17   Twin pregnancy _____

12.18   Triplet pregnancy _____

12.19   Quadruplet pregnancy _____

   a.   25 weeks
   b.   29 weeks
   c.   33 weeks
   d.   37 weeks
   e.   40 weeks

12.20   A twin pregnancy where one twin is characterized by impaired growth, anemia, and hypovolemia and the other twin by hypervolemia, hypertension, polycythemia, and congestive heart failure is suffering from

   a.   Conjoined twin syndrome
   b.   Twin-twin transfusion syndrome
   c.   Single umbilical artery syndrome

12.21   Multifetal pregnancy is associated with an increased risk of

   a.   Maternal diabetes
   b.   Preeclampsia
   c.   Rh isoimminization
   d.   Preterm labor and delivery

Answers (12.1-12.21)

12.1 d	12.7 b	12.12 a	12.17 d
12.2 c	12.8 a	12.13 b	12.18 c
12.3 b	12.9 b	12.14 c	12.19 b
12.4 a	12.10 a, c, d, e	12.15 a	12.20 b
12.5 c	12.11 b	12.16 e	12.21 b, d
12.6 d			

12.22 Which of the following should be included in the differential diagnosis when uterine size is excessively large compared to the calculated gestational age?

   a. Twins
   b. Polyhydramnios
   c. Uterine fibroids
   d. Hydatidiform mole

12.23 Diagnosis of multiple gestation is usually made by

   a. Ultrasound
   b. Leopolds maneuvers
   c. Pelvic examination
   d. Fundal height measurement

12.24 When should women carrying multifetal pregnancies begin to limit their activities to avoid premature labor?

   a. 18–20 weeks
   b. 21–23 weeks
   c. 24–26 weeks
   d. 27–29 weeks

12.25 The chief antenatal assessment to evaluate the progress of twin pregnancy is periodic

   a. Fundal height measurements
   b. Ultrasonography
   c. Pelvic examination
   d. Urinary estriols

12.26 Discordant growth in twins is generally defined as a _____ difference in weight beween the larger and smaller fetus.

   a. 10%
   b. 20%
   c. 30%
   d. 40%
   e. 50%

12.27 Which of the following obstetric maneuvers would be accomplished with the membranes ruptured?

   a. External cephalic version
   b. Internal cephalic version

12.28 Antenatal concerns in twin pregnancies include

   a. Adequate nutrition
   b. Pregnancy-induced hypertension
   c. Post-term morbidity
   d. Inadequate fetal growth

12.29 Intrapartum management of twin pregnancies at term is usually determined by

   a. Gestational age
   b. Presentation of the twins
   c. Local custom
   d. Size of the twins

Answers (12.22-12.29)

12.22 all	12.24 c	12.26 b	12.28 a, b, d
12.23 a	12.25 b	12.27 b	12.29 b

Chapter 13 Final Questions (30 questions)

13.1 The fetus or infant whose weight is at or below the _____ percentile of the normal population is defined as having intrauterine growth retardation (IUGR).

   a. 5th
   b. 10th
   c. 15th
   d. 20th

13.2 Low birth weight is synonomous with intrauterine growth retardation.

   a. True
   b. False

13.3 Intrauterine growth retardation is based on weight for a

   a. Given parity
   b. Specific gestational age
   c. Specific population

13.4 A fetus with IUGR is at higher risk for which of the following?

   a. Neonatal death
   b. Meconium aspiration
   c. Hyperglycemia
   d. Hyperthermia
   e. Asphyxia during labor

13.5–13.6 Instructions: Match the time of onset of intrauterine growth retardation with the appropriate description(s).

13.5 Early onset IUGR _____

13.6 Delayed onset IUGR _____

   a. Irreversible reduction in organ size
   b. Reversible decrease in cell size
   c. Associated with genetic/immunologic factors
   d. Associated with uteroplacental insufficiency

13.7 Which of the following are causes of intrauterine growth retardation?

   a. Recent onset maternal diabetes
   b. Smoking
   c. Hypertension
   d. Fetal rubella
   e. Maternal obesity
   f. Multiple pregnancy

13.8 This most common factor associated with intrauterine growth retardation is

   a. Hypertensive disease
   b. Rubella infection
   c. Alcohol use
   d. Drug use
   e. Smoking

13.9 Congenital anomalies account for what percent of all cases of IUGR?

   a. 5%
   b. 15%
   c. 25%
   d. 35%
   e. 45%

13.10–13.11 Instructions: Match the type of IUGR with the appropriate description(s).

13.10 Asymmetric IUGR _____

13.11 Symmetrical IUGR _____

   a. Unequal decrease in the size of structures
   b. Equal decrease in the size of structures
   c. Associated with congenital anomalies or early intrauterine infection
   d. Associated with severe nutritional deficiencies or hypertension

13.12 Morbidity with symmetrical IUGR is _____ with asymmetrical IUGR.

   a. Greater than
   b. The same as
   c. Less than

13.13 Diminished organ size and function is primarily associated with

   a. Early onset intrauterine growth retardation
   b. Delayed onset intrauterine growth retardation

13.14 Restoration of normal size with adquate nutrition is primarily associated with

   a. Early onset intrauterine growth retardation
   b. Delayed onset intrauterine growth retardation

13.15 Fundal height measurements should advance in centimeter increments in close parallel with gestational age between approximately 15 and 36 weeks gestation.

   a. True
   b. False

13.16 An efficient screening procedure for intrauterine growth retardation is

   a. Clinical estimations of fetal weight
   b. Serial fundal height measurements
   c. Maternal weight gain

Answers (13.1-13.16)

13.1	b	13.5	a, c	13.9	b	13.13	a
13.2	b	13.6	b, d	13.10	a, d	13.14	b
13.3	b	13.7	b, c, d, f	13.11	b, c	13.15	a
13.4	a, b, e	13.8	a	13.12	a	13.16	b

13.17 In patients with suspected intrauterine growth retardation and uncertain dates, ultrasonographic measurement of the _____ may be especially useful in establishing gestational age.

a. Biparietal diameter
b. Intraorbital diameter
c. Cerebrum
d. Cerebellum
e. Femur length

13.18 The addition of oligohydramnios to intrauterine growth retardation leads to _____ than intrauterine growth retardation alone

a. A worse outcome
b. An unchanged outcome
c. An improved outcome

13.19–13.21 Instructions: Match the technique for direct studies of the fetus with the appropriate use(s).

13.19 Amniocentesis _____

13.20 Percutaneous umbilical blood sampling _____

13.21 Chorionic villus sampling _____

a. Chromosomal analysis
b. Viral culture
c. Evaluation of free floating fibroblasts
d. Immunoglobulin studies
e. Oxygenation and acid-base studies

13.22 Bedrest is often recommended for patients with intrauterine growth retardation in order to

a. Regulate fetal heart rate
b. Increase uteroplacental blood flow
c. Increase maternal nutritional intake
d. Decrease maternal catecholamine release

13.23 Which of the following may be used to evaluate fetal well-being in cases of intrauterine growth retardation?

a. Fetal "kick-counts"
b. Nonstress test
c. Biophysical profile
d. Doppler ultrasound of blood flow through the umbilical cord

13.24 Amnioinfusion may be useful in the treatment of fetal heart rate decelerations in a patient with intrauterine growth retardation and associated oligohydraminos.

a. True
b. False

13.25 Fetal macrosomia is defined as weight greater than _____ g.

a. 3000
b. 4000
c. 5000

13.26 An fetus is defined as having macrosomia if it is above the _____ percentile in weight for gestational age.

a. 70th
b. 80th
c. 90th

13.27 Which of the following can be consequences of fetal macrosomia?

a. Prolonged second stage of labor
b. Hypothermia
c. Shoulder dystocia
d. Intrapartum fetal injury

13.28 Which of the following should be included in the differential diagnosis of a larger than expected uterine size?

a. Large but normal fetus
b. Polyhydramnios
c. Uterine leiomyomata
d. Other gynecologic tumor
e. Multiple pregnancy

13.29 Recommended weight gain in pregnancy is about _____ lb.

a. 20–30
b. 25–35
c. 30–40
d. 35–45
e. 40–50

13.30 The mechanism involved in the development of macrosomic infants in diabetics is thought to be

a. Transfer of glucose from mother to fetus
b. Transfer of insulin from fetus to mother
c. Transfer of growth hormone from mother to fetus
d. Transfer of insulin from mother to fetus

Answers (13.17-13.30)

13.17 d	13.21 a	13.25 b	13.28 all
13.18 a	13.22 b	13.26 c	13.29 b
13.19 a, c	13.23 all	13.27 a, c, d	13.30 a
13.20 a, b, d, e	13.24 a		

Chapter 14 Final Questions (26 questions)

14.1   A normal pregnancy is defined to last from 38 to _____ weeks.

    a. 40
    b. 41
    c. 42
    d. 43
    e. 44

14.2   A patient who has not delivered by the end of the _____ week from the 1st day of the last menstrual period is postterm.

    a. 41st
    b. 42nd
    c. 43rd
    d. 44th

14.3   Postterm pregnancy occurs in what percent of pregnancies?

    a. 8–10
    b. 11–13
    c. 14–16
    d. 17–19
    e. 20–22

14.4   Approximately what percent of patients having one postterm pregnancy will have a prolonged pregnancy with their next gestation?

    a. 0
    b. 25
    c. 50
    d. 75
    e. 100

14.5–14.8   Instructions: Match the "cause" of postterm pregnancy with the appropriate description(s).

14.5   Inaccurate or unknown dates _____

14.6   Anencephaly _____

14.7   Placental sulfatase deficiency _____

14.8   Extrauterine pregnancy _____

    a. Altered estrogen production
    b. Labor impossible due to fetal position
    c. X-linked disease
    d. Most common cause
    e. High association with late or no prenatal care

14.9   Which of the following statements about the dysmaturity (postmaturity) syndrome is *correct*?

    a. Occurs in about one-fifth of true postterm pregnancies
    b. Associated with growth retardation
    c. Integumentary changes (scaling epidermis, meconium staining) are seen
    d. Increased amounts of subcutaneous fat are common

14.10   In macrosomia associated with postterm pregnancy, there is the possibility of

    a. Hyperglycemia
    b. Hyperbilirubinemia
    c. Shoulder dystocia
    d. Fetopelvic disproportion

14.11   Postterm pregnancy may be associated with

    a. Increased incidence of fetal compromise
    b. Placental dysfunction
    c. Meconium aspiration
    d. Oligohydramnios

14.12   Amniotic fluid reaches its maximum volume at about

    a. 34 weeks
    b. 36 weeks
    c. 38 weeks
    d. 40 weeks
    e. 42 weeks

14.13–14.14   Instructions: Match the birth injury with its best description.

14.13   Erb or Duchenne palsy _____

14.14   Klumpke paralysis _____

    a. Injury to the upper roots of the brachial plexus
    b. Injury limited to the lower nerves of the brachial plexus

14.15   The passage of meconium and subsequently meconium aspiration syndrome is primarily associated with postterm pregnancy, being a relatively rare event in term pregnancies.

    a. True
    b. False

Answers (14.1-14.15)

14.1	c	14.5	d, e	14.9	a, b, c	14.13	a
14.2	b	14.6	a	14.10	b, c, d	14.14	b
14.3	a	14.7	a, c	14.11	all	14.15	b
14.4	c	14.8	b	14.12	b		

14.16 If upon rupture of membranes, meconium stained amniotic fluid is discovered in the intrapartum patient, the next management should be

 a. Immediate cesarean section
 b. Periumbilical blood gas measurement
 c. Amnioinfusion
 d. Fetal scalp blood sampling
 e. Close electronic monitoring of fetal status

14.17 Amniocentesis is required for the evaluation of fetal lung maturity in postdate pregnancies, preparatory to possible delivery.

 a. True
 b. False

14.18 If a patient's "due date" is November 11, she is said to be postterm on

 a. November 18
 b. November 25
 c. November 12
 d. December 2

14.19 The fragile, small, newborn with postmaturity syndrome is especially susceptible to brachial plexus injury.

 a. True
 b. False

14.20 Brachial plexus injury is reported in about 1 in _____ term deliveries.

 a. 250
 b. 500
 c. 750
 d. 1000

14.21 Brachial plexus injury usually results in severe damage to the brachial plexus nerve roots and significant, permanent dysfunction of the deltoid and infraspinatus muscles.

 a. True
 b. False

14.22 Once a patient approaches _____ weeks gestation, the management options that should be considered are either to induce labor or to initiate (or continue) surveillance of fetal well-being.

 a. 38
 b. 39
 c. 40
 d. 41
 e. 42

14.23 Which of the following may be included in assessments of fetal well-being during postterm pregnancy?

 a. Daily fetal movement counts
 b. Biweekly nonstress testing
 c. Biweekly biophysical profile testing
 d. Weekly oxytocin challenge testing
 e. Assessment of amniotic fluid volume by ultrasound

14.24 Labor must be induced (or cesarean birth performed) by the end of the 42nd week of gestation.

 a. True
 b. False

14.25 Cesarean birth should be considered with the estimated fetal weight is at least _____ g or greater.

 a. 3500–4000
 b. 4000–4500
 c. 4500–5000
 d. 5000–5500

14.26 The intrapartum management of postterm pregnancy should include artificial rupture of the membranes when possible.

 a. True
 b. False

Answers (14.16-14.26)

14.16 e	14.19 b	14.22 d	14.25 c
14.17 b	14.20 b	14.23 all	14.26 a
14.18 b	14.21 b	14.24 b	

Chapter 15 Final Questions (74 questions)

15.1 Which is *not* considered necessary for the diagnosis of true labor?

 a. Rhythmic contractions
 b. Cervical dilatation
 c. Cervical effacement
 d. Bloody show

15.2 Which of the following is *not* characteristic of "Braxton-Hicks" contractions?

 a. Rhythmic contractions
 b. Cervical dilatation
 c. Lower abdominal discomfort
 d. Bloody show

15.3 Late in pregnancy the fetal head descends into the pelvis and the contour of the abdomen changes. This is referred to as

 a. False descent
 b. Lightening
 c. Braxton-Hicks labor
 d. Effacement

15.4 Frequent urination found in late pregnancy is due to

 a. Increased clearance of free water
 b. Fluid shifts from diminishing amniotic fluid volume
 c. Decreased pressure on the maternal diaphragm
 d. Compression of the bladder caused by descent of the fetal head

15.5 With lightening, a patient may notice

 a. Increased urinary frequency
 b. Ease of respiratory effort
 c. A flatter abdomen
 d. Decreased weight

15.6 Which of the following are indications that a patient in late pregnancy should come to the hospital for evaluation?

 a. Regular contractions 15–20 min apart
 b. Sudden gush of fluid
 c. Continuing gradual leakage of fluid
 d. Vaginal bleeding
 e. Decreased fetal movement

15.7–15.9 Instructions: Match the terms related to fetal location with the appropriate description(s).

15.7 Lie _____

15.8 Presentation _____

15.9 Position _____

 a. Relationship of the fetal presenting part to the right and left side of the maternal pelvis
 b. Relationship of the long axis of the fetus with the maternal long axis
 c. Portion of the fetus lowest in the birth canal

15.10 The most common fetal lie found during early labor is

 a. Oblique
 b. Transverse
 c. Vertex
 d. Longitudinal

15.11 The most common fetal presentation found during early labor is

 a. Oblique
 b. Transverse
 c. Vertex
 d. Longitudinal

15.12 Leopold's maneuvers are used to establish

 a. Cervical effacement
 b. Fetal lie
 c. Fetal presentation
 d. Fetal position

15.13 Vaginal examination of a patient in early labor finds the cervix to be approximately 1 cm in length and 1 cm dilated. The effacement is

 a. 10%
 b. 25%
 c. 50%
 d. 75%
 e. 100%

15.14 The turning of the fetal head toward the sacrum is termed

 a. Transverse lie
 b. Anterior asynclitism
 c. Left side position
 d. Occipital presentation

15.15 Vaginal examination of a patient in early labor finds the presenting part (vertex) to be at the level of the ischial spines. The station is reported as

 a. +2
 b. +1
 c. 0
 d. −1
 e. −2

15.16 At 0 station, the biparietal diameter of the fetal head _____ the pelvic inlet.

 a. Has not yet reached
 b. Is at
 c. Has passed below

15.17 Cervical effacement relates to

 a. How far the cervix is opened
 b. The degree of cervical thinning
 c. The relationship of the presenting part to the cervix
 d. The softness of the cervix

Answers (15.1-15.17)

15.1 d	15.6 b, c, d, e	15.10 d	15.14 b
15.2 b, d	15.7 b	15.11 c	15.15 c
15.3 b	15.8 c	15.12 b, c, d	15.16 c
15.4 d	15.9 a	15.13 c	15.17 b
15.5 a, b, c			

15.18 Engagement is
   a. When the widest diameter of the presenting part has passed through the pelvic inlet
   b. When the occiput has passed through the pelvic inlet
   c. Synonymous with fixation

15.19 In the nulliparous patient, effacement _____ precedes dilatation.
   a. Often
   b. Rarely

15.20 Engagement of the fetal head is common in multiparous patients at the onset of labor.
   a. True
   b. False

15.21–15.24 Instructions: Match the stage of labor with the appropriate description(s).

15.21 First stage _____

15.22 Second stage _____

15.23 Third stage _____

15.24 Fourth stage _____
   a. Complete dilation to delivery the infant
   b. Delivery of infant to the delivery of the placenta
   c. Onset of labor to full cervical dilation
   d. Period extending up to 2 hr after delivery of the placenta

15.25 The active phase of the first stage of labor is generally defined from _____ cm dilation to complete dilation.
   a. 1 to 2
   b. 2 to 3
   c. 3 to 4
   d. 4 to 5
   e. 5 to 6

15.26 In nulliparas, the average length of the stages of labor are _____ in multiparas.
   a. Shorter than
   b. The same length as
   c. Longer than

15.27 The vertex presentation occurs in about what percent of term labors?
   a. 65
   b. 75
   c. 85
   d. 95

15.28–15.31 Instructions: Match the movements of the fetus during labor with the appropriate description(s).

15.28 External rotation _____

15.29 Extension _____

15.30 Flexion _____

15.31 Descent _____
   a. Movement of the presenting part through the birth canal
   b. Allows the smaller diameter of the head to present to the maternal pelvis
   c. Occurs when the head reaches the introitus
   d. Occurs after the delivery of the head

15.32 In order to assess a woman's progress in labor, a bimanual pelvic examination should be performed at a minimum of every 60 min.
   a. True
   b. False

15.33 Which of the following should occur after spontaneous rupture of membranes?
   a. Examination of the fluid for blood
   b. Examination of the fluid for meconium
   c. Auscultation or measurement of the fetal heart rate
   d. Measurement of the pH of fluid

15.34 If electronic fetal monitoring is not used during labor, the fetal heart rate should be auscultated every _____ min during the active phase of labor.
   a. 5
   b. 10
   c. 15
   d. 20
   e. 25
   f. 30

15.35 During the second stage of labor in the absence of electronic fetal monitoring, fetal heart rate auscultation should be performed after
   a. Each uterine contraction
   b. Every other uterine contraction
   c. Every third uterine contraction
   d. Every contraction generating more than 15–20 mm Hg pressure

15.36 An external tocodynamometer provides information about
   a. Contraction frequency
   b. Contraction duration
   c. Contraction strength
   d. Baseline uterine pressure

Answers (15.18-15.36)

15.18 a	15.23 b	15.28 d	15.33 a, b, c
15.19 a	15.24 d	15.29 c	15.34 c
15.20 b	15.25 c	15.30 b	15.35 a
15.21 c	15.26 c	15.31 a	15.36 a, b
15.22 a	15.27 d	15.32 b	

15.37–15.38 Instructions: Match the stage of labor with the neuropathway with which pain transmission is most associated.

15.37 First stage _____

15.38 Second stage _____

  a. T-10, T-11, T-12, and L-1
  b. S-2, S-3, and S-4

15.39 The sensory nerves from the cervix pass through the

  a. Pudendal nerve
  b. Ilioinguinal nerve
  c. Iliohypogastric nerve
  d. Lumbar 4, 5
  e. Sacral 2, 3, 4

15.40–15.42 Instructions: Match the obstetric anesthetic technique with the use with which it is best associated.

15.40 Epidural anesthesia _____

15.41 Spinal anesthesia _____

15.42 Pudendal anesthesia or block _____

  a. Provides perineal anesthesia for vaginal delivery
  b. Anesthesia for the active phase of labor and delivery
  c. Short-term anesthesia for vaginal or abdominal delivery

15.43–15.46 Instructions: Match the type of anesthesia with the major associated maternal risk(s).

15.43 General anesthesia _____

15.44 Spinal anesthesia _____

15.45 Epidural anesthesia _____

15.46 Pudendal anesthesia _____

  a. Hypotension
  b. Loss of desire to push
  c. Maternal aspiration
  d. Headache

15.47 Maternal aspiration syndrome is a particularly high risk of general anesthesia in obstetric cases because of

  a. High alkaline content of the maternal gut during pregnancy
  b. Decreased GI function during labor
  c. Pica-like eating habits of women just prior to labor
  d. Side effect of most general anesthetics causing reflex spasm of the stomach

15.48 The major cause of maternal mortality from obstetrical anesthesia is

  a. Cardiac arrest
  b. Aspiration of vomitus
  c. Hemorrhage and shock
  d. Fatal reaction to local anesthetic
  e. Excessive concentration causing respiratory failure

15.49 The most common outcome of compression of the fetal head during labor is

  a. Mental retardation
  b. Epilepsy
  c. Cerebral palsy
  d. Cleft lip
  e. Molding

15.50 Caput succedaneum is caused by molding of the fetal head.

  a. True
  b. False

15.51 The most important point of reference in the use of forceps is

  a. Posterior sagittal diameter
  b. Greatest plane
  c. Station of biparietal diameter
  d. Pelvic contour

15.52–15.54 Instructions: Match the type of forceps delivery with the appropriate description(s).

15.52 Outlet forceps _____

15.53 Low forceps _____

15.54 Midforceps _____

  a. Head engaged, leading edge of skull above +2 station
  b. Fetal skull at perineal floor, scalp visible, AP, ROA to LOA (45°s)
  c. Leading edge of skull beyond +2 station

15.55 Forceps are used to replace the maternal forces expelling the fetus.

  a. True
  b. False

15.56 Forceps may be used to

  a. Rotate the fetal head
  b. Augment maternal voluntary pushing efforts
  c. Control delivery of the fetal head
  d. Rotate the fetus to a vertex presentation

Answers (15.37-15.56)

15.37 a	15.42 a	15.47 b	15.52 b
15.38 b	15.43 c	15.48 b	15.53 c
15.39 e	15.44 a, b, d	15.49 e	15.54 a
15.40 b	15.45 a	15.50 b	15.55 b
15.41 c	15.46 b	15.51 c	15.56 a, b, c

15.57   The usual postpartum blood loss at vaginal delivery is
  a. 100 cc
  b. 300 cc
  c. 500 cc
  d. 700 cc
  e. 900 cc

15.58   What percent of patients will undergo spontaneous labor and delivery between 37 and 42 weeks?
  a. 80
  b. 85
  c. 90
  d. 95
  e. 99+

15.59–15.60   Instructions: Match the type of contraction with the appropriate description(s).

15.59   Braxton-Hicks contractions _____

15.60   True labor contractions _____
  a. Associated with cervical effacement and dilatation
  b. Resolved with ambulation
  c. Radiation of discomfort to the low back
  d. Pain confined to the lower abdomen and groin

15.61–15.64   Instructions: Match the category of obstetric laceration with the appropriate description(s).

15.61   First degree _____

15.62   Second degree _____

15.63   Third degree _____

15.64   Fourth degree _____
  a. Involves underlying fascia or muscle but not rectal sphincter or rectal mucosa
  b. Extends through the rectal sphincter but not into the rectum
  c. Extends into the rectal mucosa
  d. Involves the vaginal mucosa and perineal skin

15.65   A midline episiotomy has _____ risk of extension than a mediolateral episiotomy.
  a. A greater
  b. The same
  c. Less risk

15.66   A mediolateral episiotomy is _____ to repair than a midline episiotomy.
  a. Easier
  b. The same difficulty
  b. Harder

15.67   During delivery of the fetal head, the likelihood of laceration or extension of episiotomy is decreased by performance of
  a. Spinelli's maneuver
  b. Leopold's maneuver
  c. Ritgen's maneuver
  d. Marceaus's maneuver

15.68   Which of the following are signs of placental separation?
  a. Uterus rising in abdomen to become globular in shape
  b. Decreased sensation of pressure
  c. Gush of blood
  d. "Lengthening" of the umbilical cord

15.69   It is customary to wait up to about _____ min for spontaneous extrusion of the placenta.
  a. 10
  b. 20
  c. 30
  d. 40
  e. 50

15.70   If there was minimal blood loss after placental delivery in a birth that was spontaneous without instrumentation or episiotomy, inspection of the birth canal is unnecessary.
  a. True
  b. False

15.71   If a patient already has had a cesarean section, the risk of uterine rupture in a subsequent labors requires a repeat cesarean section.
  a. True
  b. False

15.72   What is the Apgar score of an infant with a heart rate above 100, some flexion of extremities, a slow irregular respiratory effort, grimacing, and a body that is somewhat pinkish?
  a. 10
  b. 8
  c. 6
  d. 4
  e. 2

15.73   The 5-min Apgar score is used as the guideline to decide whether fetal resuscitation efforts should start.
  a. True
  b. False

15.74   Newborns with Apgar scores of 7–4 are considered mildly to moderately depressed.
  a. True
  b. False

Answers (15.57-15.74)

15.57 c	15.62 a	15.67 c	15.71 b
15.58 b	15.63 b	15.68 a, c, d	15.72 c
15.59 b, d	15.64 c	15.69 c	15.73 b
15.60 a, c	15.65 a	15.70 b	15.74 a
15.61 d	15.66 b		

Chapter 16 Final Questions (49 questions)

16.1   Which of the following statements about prolapse of the umbilical cord is *incorrect*?

a. It occurs in approximately 0.5% of patients
b. It occurs more frequently in patients of high parity
c. It most frequently occurs in breech presentation, twins, and polyhydramnios
d. It is associated with an increased perinatal mortality
e. Manual replacement of the cord is indicated when the presenting part is not engaged in the pelvis

16.2   Which of the following may be associated with uterine rupture?

a. Amniocentesis
b. Previous cesarean section
c. Myomectomy
d. Administration of oxytocin
e. Difficult forceps delivery

16.3   Cephalopelvic disproportion is similar to a(n)

a. Arrest disorder.
b. Protraction disorder.

16.4   Older gravidas have an increased incidence of

a. Uterine inertia
b. Malpresentation
c. Hypertension

16.5   The breech hydrocephalus is best managed by

a. Cesarean section
b. Destructive procedure
c. Decompression of the head transvaginally
d. Decompression of the head transabdominally

16.6   Abnormal labor, or dystocia, can result from

a. Anatomic anomalies of the fetus
b. Anatomic anomalies of the maternal bony pelvis
c. Anatomic anomalies of the uterus
d. Functional abnormalities of the uterus

16.7–16.9   Instructions: Match the abnormal pattern of labor with the appropriate description(s).

16.7   Prolonged latent phase _____

16.8   Protraction disorder _____

16.9   Arrest disorder _____

a. No progress from latent to active phase of labor
b. Secondary arrest of dilatation
c. Prolonged active phase of labor

16.10   If cervical dilation proceeds at less than 1.2 cm/hr (for a nulligravida), this would be classified as a

a. Prolonged latent phase
b. Protraction disorder
c. Arrest disorder

16.11   If there has been no descent of the presenting part for over 1 hr during the second stage of labor, this would be classified as a(n)

a. Prolonged latent phase
b. Protraction disorder
c. Arrest disorder

16.12–16.13   Instructions: Match the type of measurement of the strength of uterine contractions with the appropriate example(s).

16.12   Qualitative (subjective) measurement _____

16.13   Quantitative measurement _____

a. Manual palpation of maternal abdomen
b. Intrauterine pressure catheter
c. "Indentation" of uterus on palpation during contraction
d. Tocodynamometer

16.14   In order for a tocodynamometer to be used effectively, the membranes must be ruptured.

a. True
b. False

16.15   For labor pattern to be considered optimal, contractions must generate an intrauterine pressure of about _____ mm Hg at maximum pressure.

a. 10–20
b. 30–40
c. 50–60
d. 70–80

16.16   If the fetus has an estimated weight of at least _____ g, the incidence of shoulder dystocia and the need for cesarean section increase markedly.

a. 2500
b. 3500
c. 4500
d. 5500

Answers (16.1-16.16)

16.1 e	16.5 a	16.9 b	16.13 b
16.2 b, c, d, e	16.6 all	16.10 b	16.14 b
16.3 a	16.7 a	16.11 c	16.15 c
16.4 all	16.8 c	16.12 a, c, d	16.16 c

16.17–16.19   Instructions: Match the abnormal presentation/position with the appropriate description(s).

16.17   Brow presentation _____

16.18   Face presentation _____

16.19   Compound presentation _____
   a.   About 1 in 600–1000 deliveries
   b.   About 1 in 3000 deliveries
   c.   Usually requires cesarean section
   d.   Typically converts to either a vertex or face presentation
   e.   Usually resolves spontaneously as labor continues

16.20   Persistent occiput posterior position always requires rotation to the vertex, either by forceps or manual rotation.
   a.   True
   b.   False

16.21   Measurements of the bony pelvis by x-ray or clinical pelvimetry are _____ predictors of successful vaginal delivery.
   a.   Good
   b.   Poor

16.22   Causes of dystocia may include
   a.   Contracted bony maternal pelvis
   b.   Distended bladder or colon
   c.   Adnexal mass
   d.   Uterine leiomyomata

16.23–16.24   Instructions: Match the method used to stimulate uterine contractions with the appropriate example(s).

16.23   Induction of labor _____

16.24   Augmentation of labor _____
   a.   Intravenous oxytocin (Pitocin)
   b.   Prostaglandin gel
   c.   Laminaria

16.25   A prolonged active phase in a primigravid patient lasts longer than
   a.   10 hr
   b.   12 hr
   c.   14 hr
   d.   16 hr
   e.   18 hr

16.26   In multiparous patients, a prolonged active phase is defined as lasting more than
   a.   2 hr
   b.   4 hr
   c.   6 hr
   d.   8 hr
   e.   10 hr

16.27   Secondary arrest of dilatation occurs when cervical dilatation during the active phase of labor stops for at least
   a.   1 hr
   b.   2 hr
   c.   3 hr
   d.   4 hr

16.28   A history of a previous successful vaginal birth is an excellent predictor of similar success in subsequent pregnancies.
   a.   True
   b.   False

16.29   In a low-dose protocol for the administration of oxytocin, there is _____ to the maximum infusion rate.
   a.   A limit
   b.   No limit

16.30   Pelvic examination shows a dilation of 1–2 cm, 60% effacement, a cephalic part of –1 station, a soft cervix that is midposition. The Bishop score is
   a.   9
   b.   7
   c.   5
   d.   3

16.31–16.32   Instructions: Match the methods for "ripening" the cervix with the corresponding risk factor(s).

16.31   Intravaginal prostaglandin gel _____

16.32   Laminaria _____
   a.   Uterine hyperstimulation
   b.   Failure to dilate the cervix
   c.   Inadvertent rupture of the membranes
   d.   Cervical laceration
   e.   Infection
   f.   Uterine rupture

16.33   A Bishop score of _____ points or below is associated with a significant likelihood of failed induction.
   a.   2
   b.   4
   c.   6
   d.   8
   e.   10

Answers (16.17-16.33)

16.17 b, d	16.22 all	16.26 c	16.30 b
16.18 a, c	16.23 all	16.27 b	16.31 a, f
16.19 a, e	16.24 a	16.28 b	16.32 b, c, d, e
16.20 b	16.25 b	16.29 a	16.33 b
16.21 b			

16.34–16.35   Instructions: Match the contractions characteristic of the types of labor with the appropriate
description(s).

16.34   True labor _____

16.35   False labor _____

   a.   Intensity increases over time
   b.   No cervical dilation
   c.   Irregular intervals and duration
   d.   No relief from sedation
   e.   Regular intervals
   f.   Intensity unchanged
   g.   Lower abdominal discomfort
   h.   Both back and abdominal discomfort
   i.   Relief from sedation
   j.   Cervical dilation occurs

16.36   The prolonged latent phase in labor may be managed by

   a.   Rest
   b.   Augmentation with pitocin
   c.   Amniotomy

16.37   If the second stage of labor lasts longer than 2 hr,
cesarean section or, if possible, operative vaginal delivery is mandatory.

   a.   True
   b.   False

16.38   Which of the following are risks to the fetus from
prolonged labor?

   a.   Sepsis
   b.   Subdural hematoma
   c.   Cerebral damage
   d.   Hemorrhage

16.39   Meconium aspiration syndrome is associated with

   a.   Prolonged labor
   b.   Postdates pregnancy
   c.   Intrauterine growth retardation
   d.   Chronic maternal hypertension

16.40   If amnioinfusion is used when meconium-stained amniotic fluid is noticed, immediate intubation to examine the area below the vocal cords for meconium

   a.   Is usually unnecesary
   b.   Should be carried out as routine

16.41   Breech presentation occurs in about _____ of singleton term deliveries.

   a.   1%
   b.   3%
   c.   5%
   d.   7%
   e.   9%

16.42   Which of the following factors are associated with
breech presentation?

   a.   Multiple pregnancy
   b.   Oligohydramnios
   c.   Prematurity
   d.   Hydrocephaly
   e.   Previous breech
   f.   Uterine anomalies

16.42   Vaginal delivery of the term breech is generally
avoided when the fetus weighs below _____ g.

   a.   1000
   b.   1500
   c.   2000
   d.   2500
   e.   3000

16.43   Which of the following should be present in candidates for external cephalic version?

   a.   Normal fetus
   b.   Reassuring fetal heart tracing
   c.   Oligohydramnios
   d.   Presenting part in pelvis.
   e.   Well-established uterine contractions
   f.   No uterine surgical scars

16.44   Which of the following are risks of external cephalic
version?

   a.   Uterine rupture
   b.   Sepsis
   c.   Cord accident
   d.   Placental abruption
   e.   Premature rupture of the membranes

16.45   In breech presentation, the use of anti-D immune
globulin in D– women is unnecessary.

   a.   True
   b.   False

16.46–16.48   Instructions: Match the type of vaginal
breech delivery with the appropriate description(s).

16.46   Total breech extraction _____

16.47   Partial breech extraction _____

16.48   Spontaneous breech delivery _____

   a.   Spontaneous delivery to umbilicus with remainder of body extracted
   b.   Total body extracted
   c.   No traction or manipulation of the fetus

16.49   Cesarean section is required in the breech presentation in approximately _____ of term breeches because of hyperextension of the fetal head.

   a.   5%
   b.   10%
   c.   15%
   d.   20%
   e.   25%

Answers (16.34-16.49)

16.34 a, d, e, g, h, j	16.39 all	16.42 c	16.46 b
16.35 b, c, f, g, i	16.40 b	16.43 a, b, f	16.47 a
16.36 all	16.41 b	16.44 a, c, d	16.48 c
16.37 b	16.42 a, c, d, e, f	16.45 b	16.49 a
16.38 a, b, c			

Chapter 17 Final Questions (36 questions)

17.1 Nonreassuring fetal status during labor occurs in about what percent of pregnancies?

a. Less than 1
b. 5–10
c. 15–20
d. 25–30

17.2 Which of the following are included in the criteria for the diagnosis of fetal asphyxia?

a. Metabolic or mixed acidemia
b. Persistent Apgar scores of 3 or below
c. Evidence of neonatal neurologic sequelae
d. Heart rate acceleration

17.3 All neonates who have Apgar scores of 0–3 for longer than 5 min have experienced fetal asphyxia.

a. True
b. False

17.4–17.6 Instructions: Match the causes of nonreassuring fetus status with the appropriate example(s).

17.4 Uteroplacental insufficiency _____

17.5 Umbilical cord compression _____

17.6 Fetal conditions, anomalies _____

a. Umbilical cord accidents such as umbilical cord prolapse
b. Placental edema as seen in maternal diabetes or hydrops fetalis
c. Maternal or fetal sepsis
d. Fetal congenital anomalies
e. Intrauterine growth retardation
f. Prematurity
g. Oligohydramnios
h. Placental accidents such as abruptio placentae or placenta previa
i. Uterine hyperstimulation
j. Postdates pregnancy

17.7 If there is progressive and unrecognized fetal hypoxia associated with uteroplacental insufficiency, metabolic acidosis _____ respiratory acidosis.

a. Preceeds
b. Follows

17.8 If a fetus experiences progressive and sustained hypoxia, the mixed metabolic and respiratory acidosis that may ensue is especially associated with

a. Aerobic glycolysis
b. Anaerobic glycolysis
c. Aerobic gluconeogenesis
d. Anaerobic gluconeogenesis

17.9 Baseline fetal tachycardia is defined as a heart rate greater than _____ beats per minute for 10 or more min.

a. 150
b. 160
c. 170
d. 180
e. 190

17.10 The most common cause(s) of fetal tachycardia is

a. Fetal anemia
b. Maternal anemia
c. Maternal hypothermia
d. Maternal hyperthermia

17.11 Baseline fetal bradycardia is defined as a heart rate of less than _____ beats per minute for 10 or more min.

a. 90
b. 100
c. 110
d. 120
e. 130

17.12 Fetal heart rates in the bradycardia range between 110 and 119 are commonly associated with fetal compromise whether or not accompanied by other evidence of nonreassuring fetal status.

a. True
b. False

17.13 A sinusoidal fetal heart rate pattern is frequently associated with

a. Rh isoimmunization
b. Umbilical cord prolapse
c. Placental abruption
d. Preeclampsia
e. Fetal anemia

17.14 Fetal arrhythmias are seen in what percent of monitored labors?

a. Less than 1
b. 5
c. 10
d. 15

17.15 The presence of fetal heart rate variability is an indication of

a. Fetal compromise
b. Fetal well-being

Answers (17.1-17.15)

17.1 b	17.5 a, g	17.9 b	17.13 a, e
17.2 a, b, c	17.6 c, d, e, f, j	17.10 d	17.14 a
17.3 b	17.7 b	17.11 d	17.15 b
17.4 b, h, i, j	17.8 b	17.12 b	

17.16–17.17 Instructions: Match the type of fetal heart rate variability with the appropriate description(s).

17.16 Short-term variability _____

17.17 Long-term variability _____

  a. Variation in amplitude seen on a beat-to-beat basis
  b. Irregular, crude "wave-like" patterns
  c. Amplitude of 5–15 beats per minute
  d. Amplitude of 3–8 beats per minute
  e. Normally encountered after approximately 28 weeks gestation

17.18 Both long- and short-term fetal heart rate variability may be measured only with the use of a fetal scalp electrode.

  a. True
  b. False

17.19 Fetal sleep is associated with _____ fetal heart rate variability.

  a. Increased
  b. Unchanged
  c. Decreased

17.20–17.21 Instructions: Match the fetal heart rate pattern with corresponding cause(s).

17.20 Fetal tachycardia _____

17.21 Fetal bradycardia _____

  a. Maternal fever and infection
  b. Maternal treatment with beta blockers
  c. Fetal immaturity
  d. Fetal hypoxia
  e. Fetal anoxia
  f. Fetal congenital heart block
  g. Maternal thyrotoxicosis
  h. Fetal anemia
  i. Fetal infection
  j. Maternal treatment with sympathomimetic or parasympatholytic drugs, e.g., atropine

17.22–17.24 Instructions: Match the type of fetal heart rate deceleration with the appropriate description(s).

17.22 Early deceleration _____

17.23 Variable deceleration _____

17.24 Late deceleration _____

  a. Associated with umbilical cord compression
  b. Associated with pressure on the fetal head
  c. Associated with uteroplacental insufficiency

17.25 The presence of persistent late decelerations and decreased beat-to-beat variability should lead to which of the following?

  a. Direct measurement of fetal acid-base status
  b. Monitoring the frequency of fetal movement
  c. Measurement of maternal blood pressure
  d. Measurement of amniotic fluid volume

17.26 A normal fetal scalp blood gas pH is in the range of

  a. 6.80–6.95
  b. 7.00–7.15
  c. 7.25–7.40
  d. 7.50–7.65

17.27 The type of fetal acidosis (respiratory, mixed, metabolic) is _____ for management decisions.

  a. Irrelevant
  b. Important

17.28 Fetal heart rate accelerations are generally believed to be

  a. Indicative of fetal well-being
  b. A sign of fetal stress and compromise

17.29 Which of the following describes a late fetal heart rate deceleration?

  a. Deceleration starts after uterine contraction begins, nadir after peak of uterine contraction, resolves to baseline after uterine contraction is over
  b. Deceleration begins with uterine contraction, nadir at peak of uterine contraction, returns to baseline at end of uterine contraction
  c. Deceleration may start before or after the start of the uterine contraction

17.30 Which of the following physiologic mechanisms are associated with periodic fetal heart rate changes?

  a. Intrinsic fetal heart rate control
  b. Extrinsic fetal heart rate control
  c. Response to fetal myocardial calcium depletion
  d. Response to fetal myocardial hypoxia

17.31 Acceleration of the fetal heart rate after fetal scalp stimulation is usually considered a sign of relative fetal well-being.

  a. True
  b. False

17.32 Repetitive late fetal heart rate decelerations are considered particularly ominous with respect to fetal well-being if associated with

  a. Variable decelerations
  b. Early decelerations
  c. Increased FHR variability
  d. Decreased FHR variability

Answers (17.16-17.32)

17.16 a, d, e	17.21 b, e, f	17.25 a	17.29 a
17.17 b, c, e	17.22 b	17.26 c	17.30 a, d
17.18 b	17.23 a	17.27 b	17.31 a
17.19 c	17.24 c	17.28 a	17.32 d
17.20 a, c, d, g, h, i, j			

17.33 If a scalp pH is taken because of concern about fetal status and the pH is in the range of _____, it is generally advisable to repeat the scalp pH measurement within 15–30 min unless the fetal condition has improved.

   a. Below 7.20
   b. 7.20–7.24
   c. 7.25–7.29
   d. Above 7.30

17.34 In a face of evidence of intrauterine fetal compromise, the administration of which drug may be considered to relax uterine tone and slow contraction rate?

   a. Atropine
   b. Meperidine
   c. Terbutaline
   d. Succinylcholine
   e. Morphine

17.35 The single most reliable indicator of fetal status using electronic fetal monitoring is

   a. Variability
   b. Baseline
   c. Accelerations
   d. Periodic decelerations

17.36 Uteroplacental insufficiency should be suspected with

   a. Maternal hypertension
   b. Diabetes mellitus
   c. Toxemia

Answers (17.33-17.36)

17.33 b   17.34 c   17.35 a   17.36 all

Chapter 18 Final Questions (46 questions)

18.1   The puerperium is the _____-week period following birth during which the reproductive tract returns to its normal nonpregnant state.

    a. 4
    b. 6
    c. 8
    d. 10
    e. 12

18.2   Uterine involution is the result of a decrease in the

    a. Number of cells in the uterine myometrium
    b. Size of cells in the uterine myometrium

18.3   The uterus returns to its prepregnancy position in the true pelvis by about _____ weeks postpartum.

    a. 1
    b. 2
    c. 3
    d. 4
    e. 5

18.4   The uterus returns to its prepregnancy size by about _____ weeks postpartum.

    a. 2
    b. 3
    c. 4
    d. 5
    e. 6

18.5–18.6   Instructions: Match the type of lochia with the appropriate description(s).

18.5   Lochia rubra _____

18.6   Lochia serosa _____

    a. Consists of blood and necrotic decidual debris
    b. Consists of degenerated decidual material and leukocytes
    c. Appears by the end of the 1st postpartum week
    d. Appears during the 1st several postpartum days

18.7   The cervix is substantively returned to its prepregnancy shape by approximately 1 week after delivery.

    a. True
    b. False

18.8   In the breast-feeding woman, the vaginal mucosa reflects the _____ state.

    a. Hyperestrogenic
    b. Hypoestrogenic

18.9   The remnants of the hymen in the postpartum woman appear as fleshy tags at the introitus that are called

    a. The hymenal ring
    b. Myrtiform caruncles
    c. Inclusion bodies
    d. Hyperplastic nodes of Ling

18.10   The mean time to ovulation in the nonlactating postpartum woman is approximately

    a. 2 weeks
    b. 4 weeks
    c. 6 weeks
    d. 8 weeks
    e. 10 weeks

18.11   The diastasis recti noted postpartum usually

    a. Requires surgical correction
    b. Resolves in time without intervention

18.12   During the immediate postpartum period, there is a shift of fluid into the

    a. Intravascular space
    b. Extracellular space

18.13   The elevated pulse rate characteristic of pregnancy

    a. Decreases at the end of the third stage of labor
    b. Decreases approximately 1 hr after delivery
    c. Persists for about 3 weeks postpartum

18.14   During the first few days postpartum, the glomerular filtration rate remains _____ as compared to the nonpregnant state.

    a. Elevated
    b. Decreased

18.15   Transitory urinary retention in the postpartum period following vaginal delivery is primarily related to

    a. Sympathometic discharge
    b. Peripartum cystitis
    c. Periurethral edema
    d. Progesterone-associated loss of bladder contractility

18.16   A normal uterus weighs approximately _____ g immediately after delivery.

    a. 500
    b. 1000
    c. 1500
    d. 2000

Answers (18.1-18.16)

18.1 b	18.5 a, d	18.9 b	18.13 b
18.2 b	18.6 b, c	18.10 e	18.14 a
18.3 b	18.7 b	18.11 b	18.15 c
18.4 b	18.8 b	18.12 a	18.16 b

18.17 Postpartum uterine contractile pain is greater in breast-feeding women because of the increased release of _____ during suckling.

   a. Progesterone
   b. Prostaglandins
   c. Oxytocin
   d. Estrogen

18.18 Breast-feeding _____ a contraindication to immunization for rubella in the immediate postpartum period.

   a. Is
   b. Is not

18.19 The use of oral contraceptives is contraindicated in the breast-feeding patient.

   a. True
   b. False

18.20–18.22 Instructions: Match the type of postpartum breast complication with the appropriate description(s).

18.20 Breast engorgement _____

18.21 Postpartum mastitis _____

18.22 Plugged duct _____

   a. Unilateral location, localized swelling, intense localized pain, generally feels ill
   b. Unilateral location, localized swelling, localized pain, generally feels well
   c. Bilateral location, generalized swelling, generalized pain, generally feels well
   d. Associated with fever

18.23 Generally, _____ of the total dosages of any medication is seen in breast milk.

   a. 1%
   b. 4%
   c. 7%
   d. 10%
   e. 13%

18.24 Which of the following medications would contraindicate breast-feeding?

   a. Lithium carbonate
   b. Tetracycline
   c. Bromocriptine
   d. Methotrexate
   e. Dicloxacillin

18.25 Milk begins to be produced on about the _____ postpartum day.

   a. 1st
   b. 3rd
   c. 5th
   d. 7th
   e. 9th

18.26 "Postpartum blues" or mild postpartum depression occurs in over one-half of deliveries, typically beginning on postpartum day

   a. 1
   b. 3
   c. 7
   d. 10
   e. 21

18.27 Postpartum mental disease is expected to recur in subsequent pregnancies in approximately what percent of patients?

   a. 25
   b. 50
   c. 75
   d. 100

18.28 Patients with breast engorgement and plugged ducts generally are relatively free of systemic symptoms.

   a. True
   b. False

18.29 Immediate postpartum uterine hemostasis is maintained by

   a. Primary clotting of blood in the uterine artery
   b. Contraction of the uterine smooth muscle
   c. Scar formation within the uterine cavity

18.30 In women who breast-feed, the lochia seems to resolve _____ in women who do not breast-feed.

   a. More slowly than
   b. At the same rate as
   c. More rapidly than

18.31 By the end of the _____ postpartum week, the endometrium is reestablished in most patients.

   a. 1st
   b. 2nd
   c. 3rd
   d. 4th
   e. 5th

18.32 Fifty percent of women ovulate within _____ days postpartum.

   a. 30
   b. 60
   c. 90
   d. 120
   e. 150

18.33 Ovulation can occur as early as _____ weeks postpartum in a women who does not breast-feed.

   a. 2
   b. 4
   c. 6
   d. 8
   e. 10

Answers (18.17-18.33)

18.17 c	18.22 b	18.26 b	18.30 c
18.18 b	18.23 a	18.27 a	18.31 c
18.19 b	18.24 a, b, c, d	18.28 a	18.32 c
18.20 c	18.25 b	18.29 b	18.33 b
18.21 a, d			

18.34   The silvery stripes seen on the abdominal skin post-
        partum are called

        a. Diastasis recti
        b. Tunica albuginea
        c. Striae
        d. Myrtiform caruncles

18.35   Drugs that are excreted by the renal system may be
        given in their nonpregnancy doses immediately after
        delivery as the GFR returns to normal within a few
        hours of delivery.

        a. True
        b. False

18.36   In a normal patient immediately after delivery, loss
        of fluid through diuresis and loss of extravascular
        fluid is approximately

        a. 1 kg
        b. 3 kg
        c. 5 kg
        d. 7 kg
        e. 9 kg

18.37   Bromocriptine functions to suppress lactation
        through inhibition of

        a. Prolactin
        b. Estrogen
        c. Progesterone
        d. Prostaglandin
        e. Serotonin

18.38   Breast engorgement in non-breast-feeding women
        typically occurs _____ days postpartum.

        a. 1
        b. 3
        c. 5
        d. 7
        e. 9

18.39   Infection of episiotomy sites occurs in what percent
        of patients?

        a. 0.1
        b. 1
        c. 10
        d. 25

18.40   Which vitamin is not found in human breast milk?

        a. A
        b. D
        c. C
        d. K
        e. E

18.41   Suicidal ideation is associated with postpartum de-
        pression in approximately 1 in _____ pregnancies.

        a. 500
        b. 1000
        c. 1500
        d. 2000
        e. 2500

18.42   Which of the following statements about colostrum
        is *incorrect*?

        a. The IgA content of colostrum may offer pro-
            tection to the newborn infant against enteric
            infection
        b. The secretion of colostrum persists for at least 2
            weeks
        c. Antibodies are readily demonstrable in colos-
            trum
        d. Colostrum contains more protein and minerals
            than breast milk
        e. Colostrum contains less sugar and fat than
            breast milk

18.43   Which of the following is *not* involved in stimulating
        milk production and secretion?

        a. Thyroid-stimulating hormone
        b. Progesterone and estrogen
        c. Human placental lactogen
        d. Prolactin
        e. Cortisol and insulin

18.44   During the first 5 months of pregnancy, breast de-
        velopment occurs because of

        a. Increased fat deposition
        b. Increased cardiac output
        c. Slowed venous return from the breasts
        d. Capillary dilation
        e. Synergistic hormone action

18.45   Breast-feeding in the postpartum period

        a. Markedly diminishes blood loss
        b. Slightly diminishes blood loss
        c. Does not affect the amount of blood loss
        d. Slightly increases blood loss
        e. Markedly increases blood loss

18.46   Mastitis followed by breast abscess is most fre-
        quently due to

        a. Bacterial vaginosis
        b. Pneumococcus
        c. *Escherichia coli*
        d. *Streptococcus pyogenes*
        e. *Staphylococcus aureus*

Answers (18.34-18.46)

18.34 c	18.38 b	18.41 d	18.44 e
18.35 b	18.39 a	18.42 b	18.45 c
18.36 c	18.40 d	18.43 a	18.46 e
18.37 a			

Chapter 19 Final Questions (30 questions)

19.1   The traditional definition of postpartum hemor-
       rhage is blood loss in excess of

    a. 250 cc
    b. 500 cc
    c. 750 cc
    d. 1000 cc

19.2   The most common cause of postpartum hemor-
       rhage is

    a. Uterine laceration
    b. Uterine atony
    c. Cervical laceration
    d. Retained uterine tissue
    e. Vaginal laceration

19.3   Excessive bleeding from the placental implantation
       site postpartum is primarily prevented by

    a. Muscular contraction of the uterus
    b. Coagulation of the uterine vascular bed
    c. Mechanical obstruction of vessels

19.4–19.6 Instructions: Match the factors predisposing to
uterine atony with the appropriate example(s).

19.4   Excessive uterine enlargement _____

19.5   Characteristics of labor _____

19.6   Interference with uterine contractility _____

    a. Use of magnesium sulfate
    b. Prolonged labor
    c. Augmentation of labor
    d. Polyhydramnios
    e. Uterine leiomyoma
    f. Multiple gestation
    g. Precipitous delivery

19.7   It is standard practice to infuse Pitocin diluted in
       intravenous fluids (usually _____ units in 1 liter of
       fluid run at 125–165 cc/hr) starting soon after deliv-
       ery of the placenta.

    a. 10
    b. 20
    c. 30
    d. 40

19.8   Intravenous administration of undiluted oxytocin
       can lead to

    a. Hypotension
    b. Hypertension

19.9–9.10 Instructions: Match the type of uterine atony
with the appropriate management measure(s).

19.9   Initial uterine atony _____ .

19.10 Persistent uterine atony _____

    a. Rapid infusion of oxytocin
    b. Uterine massage
    c. Methergine (methylergonovine maleate)
    d. Prostaglandin
    e. Uterine artery ligation
    f. Hypogastric artery ligation
    g. Hysterectomy
    h. Selective arterial embolization

19.11 Prostaglandin $F_2\alpha$ should not be administered into
       the myometrium because of the risk of myometrial
       tissue necrosis.

    a. True
    b. False

19.12 Lacerations of the lower genital tract are _____
       uterine atony as a cause of postpartum hemorrhage.

    a. More common than
    b. As common as
    c. Less common than

19.13 Predisposing factors to lower genital tract laceration
       include

    a. Forceps delivery
    b. Breech delivery
    c. Delivery of a macrosomic infant
    d. Precipitous delivery
    e. Premature rupture of the membranes

19.14 Because of the highly vascular nature of the cervix in
       the immediate postpartum period, any laceration re-
       quires suture to affect hemostasis.

    a. True
    b. False

19.15 Hematomas in the vulva/lower vagina are _____ in
       the upper vagina.

    a. More common than
    b. As common as
    c. Less common than

Answers (19.1-19.15)

19.1 b	19.5 b, c, g	19.9 a, b, c, d	19.13 a, b, c, d
19.2 b	19.6 a, e	19.10 all	19.14 b
19.3 a	19.7 b	19.11 b	19.15 a
19.4 d, f	19.8 a	19.12 c	

19.16   Which of the following statements about vulvar hematomas is *incorrect*?

   a. They usually are associated with exquisite pain.
   b. They usually are associated with shock.
   c. If less than 5 cm and stable in size, they may be managed expectantly.
   d. If the size is increasing, surgical management usually is required.

19.17   All cervical lacerations require suture repair to avoid future cervical incompetence.

   a. True
   b. False

19.18   The site of postpartum hematoma associated with the greatest morbidity is the

   a. Vulva
   b. Lower vagina
   c. Upper vagina
   d. Cervix

19.19–19.21   Instructions: Match the type of placental penetration into the uterus with the appropriate description(s).

19.19   Placenta accreta _____

19.20   Placenta increta _____

19.21   Placenta percreta _____

   a. Penetration into the uterine muscle
   b. Penetration into the superficial lining of the uterus
   c. Penetration involving the full thickness of the muscular uterine wall

19.22   Which of the following are predisposing factors to retained placenta?

   a. Uterine leiomyomas
   b. Previous cesarean delivery
   c. Multiple gestation
   d. Prior uterine curettage
   e. Succenturiate lobe

19.23   The theory behind treatment of partial uterine inversion is to induce uterine

   a. Contraction
   b. Relaxation

19.24   Postpartum hemorrhage secondary to uterine atony is characterized by firming of the uterus upon massage, with later muscular relaxation after massage ceases.

   a. True
   b. False

19.25   Patients treated intrapartum and postpartum with intravenous magnesium sulfate are predisposed to

   a. Uterine atony
   b. Retained placenta
   c. Uterine inversion

19.26   The presence of retained placental tissue can be identified through

   a. External palpation of the abdomen
   b. Ultrasound examination of the uterus
   c. Measurement of progesterone levels

19.27–19.29   Instructions: Match the time period with the appropriate measure(s) to prevent, minimize or manage postpartum hemorrhage in at-risk patients.

19.27   Before delivery _____

19.26   During delivery _____

19.29   In recovery room _____

   a. Avoid excessive traction on umbilical cord
   b. Identify any predisposing factors
   c. Determine baseline hematocrit
   d. Closely observe patient for excessive bleeding
   e. Send blood specimen to blood bank for group and screen
   f. Inspect placenta for complete removal
   g. Perform digital exploration of uterus
   h. Establish well-functioning intravenous line with large-bore catheter
   i. Massage uterus
   j. Visualize cervix and vagina
   k. Frequently palpate uterus with massage
   l. Determine vital signs frequently
   m. Obtain baseline coagulation studies and platelet count if indicated

19.30   The most common cause of death in amniotic fluid embolism is

   a. Cardiorespiratory collapse
   b. Afibrigenemia
   c. Massive hemorrhage
   d. Acute renal failure
   e. Cerebral infarction

Answers (19.16-19.30)

19.16 b	19.20 a	19.24 a	19.26 a, f, g, i, j
19.17 b	19.21 c	19.25 a	19.29 d, k, l
19.18 c	19.22 a, b, d, e	19.26 b	19.30 a
19.19 b	19.23 b	19.27 b, c, e, h, m	

Chapter 20 Final Questions (41 questions)

20.1 The definition of febrile morbidity is a temperature of _____ or higher on any 2 of the first 10 days postpartum exclusive of the first 24 hr.

 a. 37.5° C
 b. 38° C
 c. 38.5° C
 d. 39° C

20.2 Which of the following factors directly predispose to postpartum infection?

 a. Maternal obesity
 b. Anemia
 c. Prolonged labor
 d. Postdates pregnancy
 e. Premature rupture of the membranes

20.3–20.6 Instructions: Match the postpartum day with the site(s) where infection is most likely to appear.

20.3 Day 1 _____
20.4 Day 2 _____
20.5 Day 3 _____
20.6 Day 4 _____

 a. Urinary tract (cystitis, pyelonephritis)
 b. Lungs (atelectasis pneumonia)
 c. Wound (superficial infection, necrotizing fascitis)
 d. Extremities (thrombophlebitis)

20.7 The postcesarean birth incision site infection rate can be reduced by about one-half with the administration of prophylactic antibiotics.

 a. True
 b. False

20.8 The most common infection following cesarean delivery is

 a. Metritis
 b. Pneumonia
 c. Pyelonephritis
 d. Pelvic abscess
 e. Wound infection

20.9 The etiology of postpartum pelvic infections is most commonly

 a. Gram-positive aerobes
 b. Gram-negative aerobes
 c. Gram-positive anaerobes
 d. Gram-negative anaerobes
 e. Polymicrobial

20.10–20.13 Instructions: Match the classification of organisms associated with postpartum metritis with specific examples of organisms from that category.

20.10 Gram-positive aerobes _____
20.11 Gram-negative aerobes _____
20.12 Gram-positive anaerobes _____
20.13 Gram-negative anaerobes _____

 a. Enterococcus
 b. Proteus
 c. Peptococcus
 d. Staphylococcus
 e. Streptococcus
 f. Escherichia coli
 g. Klebsiella
 h. Bacteroides
 i. Peptostreptococcus
 j. Clostridium

20.14 Metritis usually

 a. Is confined to the endometrial lining of the uterus
 b. Extends into the myometrium and parametrium

20.15 Which of the following statements about metritis is incorrect?

 a. Fever is a characteristic feature
 b. Uterine tenderness is a characteristic feature
 c. Diminished or absent bowel sounds may indicate an extensive infection
 d. Infection usually is associated with a leukocytosis in the range of 15,000–30,000 cells/μL.

20.16 Blood cultures in the postpartum febrile patient are required prior to initiating any antibiotic therapy.

 a. True
 b. False

20.17 Culturing the endometrial cavity prior to treatment for presumed metritis is impractical because of the contamination with vaginal flora as the sampling device traverses the vagina and cervical opening.

 a. True
 b. False

20.18 Initial antibiotic therapy for metritis may consist of

 a. A single agent
 b. A combination of drugs

Answers (20.1-20.18)

20.1 b
20.2 a, b, c, e
20.3 b
20.4 a
20.5 c
20.6 d
20.7 a
20.8 a
20.9 e
20.10 a, d, e
20.11 b, f, g
20.12 c, i, j
20.13 h
20.14 b
20.15 b
20.16 b
20.17 a
20.18 all

20.19 Intravenous antibiotic therapy for metritis is continued until the patient

    a. Is asymptomatic
    b. Has normal bowel function
    c. Is afebrile for at least 24 hours
    d. Has been treated for a total of at least 7 days

20.20 It is customary to provide additional antibiotic therapy in a patient being treated for postpartum metritis if there has been no response to the initial therapy within

    a. 12–24 hr
    b. 24–36 hr
    c. 36–48 hr
    d. 48–72 hr
    e. 72–96 hr

20.21 Multidrug regimes such as clindamycin and azetreonam are virtually always required for the complete therapy of postpartum metritis.

    a. True
    b. False

20.22 A postpartum pseudomass associated with febrile morbidity is most commonly due to postcesarean

    a. Phlegmon
    b. Pelvic abscess
    c. Hematoma
    d. Urinoma

20.23 Which of the following is *not* characteristic of a pelvic abscess as a complication of postpartum metritis?

    a. Persistent fever
    b. Paradoxical sense of well-being
    c. Delayed return to gastrointestinal function
    d. Localized pain or tenderness on abdominal examination
    e. Evidence of pelvic mass on imaging

20.24 Which of the following statements about management of a pelvic abscess complicating postpartum metritis is *incorrect*?

    a. Ultrasound, CT, and/or MRI are often useful in diagnosis
    b. Initial therapy should include broad spectrum antibiotics
    c. Initial therapy should include drainage of the abcess
    d. Rupture may be associated with shock and is a surgical emergency

20.25 After vaginal delivery, postpartum urinary tract infection is _____ after cesarean birth.

    a. Less common than
    b. As common as
    c. More common than

20.26 Dysuria _____ a useful sign of urinary tract infection in the puerperium.

    a. Is
    b. Is not

20.27 Antibiotic therapy for urinary tract infection should not begin until the results of urine culture are obtained.

    a. True
    b. False

20.28 Which of the following is useful in identifying the presence of postpartum urinary tract infection?

    a. Dysuria
    b. Frequency of urination
    c. Costovertebral tenderness

20.29 Which of the following statements about infection of the incision site following cesarean delivery is *correct*?

    a. The incision should be probed to determine the extent of infection
    b. Broad spectrum antibiotic therapy is often utilized
    c. Culture of the wound is not usually required
    d. Drainage of the wound is required

20.30 Episiotomy site infection is _____ infection of the incision site following cesarean delivery.

    a. More common than
    b. As common as
    c. Less common than

20.31 Which of the following statements about infection of the episiotomy site is *correct*?

    a. Episiotomy site infection is relatively common
    b. Infections usually are characterized by low-grade fever and localized swelling and tenderness
    c. The initial treatment of episiotomy site infection is removal of sutures, drainage, and sitz baths
    d. It is best to allow the wound to close by secondary intention due to the location of the wound near potential site of contamination such as the vagina and rectum.

Answers (20.19-20.31)

20.19 a, b, c	20.23 b	20.26 b	20.29 a, b, d
20.20 d	20.24 c	20.27 b	20.30 c
20.21 b	20.25 a	20.28 c	20.31 b, c
20.22 a			

20.32 Which of the following statements about necrotizing fascitis is *correct*?

   a. It is a rare postpartum infection
   b. It is especially virulent, involving the adjacent fascia, muscle, and subcutaneous tissue
   c. It is frequently fatal
   d. It requires surgical debridement in all cases

20.33 Postpartum mastitis is more common in

   a. Lactating women
   b. Nonlactating women

20.34 Mastitis most often occurs

   a. At the onset of nursing
   b. In the 1st week postpartum
   c. 1 month postpartum
   d. 6 months postpartum

20.35 Localized breast pain is generally the first symptom of postpartum mastitis.

   a. True
   b. False

20.36 Patients with postpartum mastitis _____ be advised to discontinue nursing until the infection resolves.

   a. Should
   b. Should not

20.37 Respiratory complications following delivery

   a. Characteristically present in the 1st postpartum day
   b. Are often associated with atelectasis
   c. May involve pneumonia, especially in patients with predelivery respiratory disease
   d. Are more common if general anesthesia was used

20.38 Septic pelvic thrombophlebitis

   a. Is a sequella of postpartum pelvic infection
   b. Is associated with venous stasis and bacterial colonization
   c. May be complicated by microembolization to the lungs and other organs by way of the inferior vena cava
   d. Usually presents as residual fever and tachycardia during treatment for metritis

20.39 The standard treatment for septic pelvic thrombophlebitis in the postpartum period is

   a. A switch from double- to triple-antibiotic therapy
   b. Placement of an inferior vena case sieve
   c. Empiric treatment with heparin
   d. Administration of fever-reducing drugs and rest

20.40 Septic pelvic thrombophlebitis usually resolves within 24–48 hr following initiation of intravenous heparin therapy.

   a. True
   b. False

20.41 The recommended duration of anticoagulation therapy for septic pelvic thrombophlebitis after the resolution of fever varies from 7 to 30 days.

   a. True
   b. False

Answers (20.32–20.41)

20.32 all	20.35 b	20.38 all	20.40 a
20.33 a	20.36 b	20.39 c	20.41 a
20.34 c	20.37 all		

Chapter 21 Final Questions (44 questions)

21.1 In which of the following breast tissues may pathologic changes occur?

   a. Connective tissue
   b. Fatty tissue
   c. Glandular structures

21.2 The breast has a _____ blood and lymphatic supply.

   a. Sparse
   b. Rich

21.3 As a malignancy in women, breast cancer ranks _____ in frequency.

   a. First
   b. Second
   c. Third
   d. Fourth
   e. Fifth

21.4 Collecting ducts arising from breast lobes terminate (drain) at the

   a. Areola
   b. Nipple
   c. Montgomery's ducts
   d. Chest wall lymphatics

21.5 The most common benign breast condition is

   a. Ductal estasia
   b. Fibroadenoma
   c. Fibrocystic change
   d. Intraductal papilloma
   e. Galactocele

21.6 The most common benign breast condition mistaken for cancer is

   a. Fat necrosis
   b. Fibrocystic change
   c. Ductal ectasia
   d. Intraductal papilloma

21.7 The most common presenting complaint of women with fibrocystic breast change is

   a. Solitary breast mass
   b. Localized breast tenderness
   c. Bilateral, cyclic pain
   d. Nipple discharge
   e. Multiple breast masses

21.8 The usual sequence of events in the development of fibrocystic breast change is

   a. Obstruction of ducts, cyst formation, fibrosis
   b. Fibrosis, ductal expansion, cyclic breast pain
   c. Ductal atrophy, fibrosis, cyst formation
   d. Proliferation of stroma, adenosis, cyst formation

21.9 A 34-year-old patient complains of cyclic breast tenderness and diffuse nodularity on monthly breast self-examination. Your examination finds multiple firm, mobile masses, predominantly in the upper outer quadrants of each breast. You aspirate one of these masses and obtain clear, straw-colored fluid. The best initial manangement of this condition is

   a. Suggesting mechanical support of the breast
   b. Danazol sodium therapy
   c. Progesterone-only oral contraceptives
   d. GnRH agonist therapy
   e. Excisional biopsy

21.10 Breast self-examination should be performed

   a. Following menstruation
   b. Twice monthly
   c. 3–5 days prior to menstruation
   d. Weekly

21.11 Approximately what percent of breast cancers are found by the patient herself?

   a. 10
   b. 30
   c. 50
   d. 70
   e. 90

21.12 Approximately 1 in _____ women will develop breast cancer during her lifetime.

   a. 5
   b. 7
   c. 9
   d. 11
   e. 13

21.13 Historical risk factors identify what percent of breast cancer patients?

   a. 10
   b. 25
   c. 40
   d. 55
   e. 70

Answers (21.1-21.13)

21.1 all	21.5 c	21.8 d	21.11 e
21.2 b	21.6 a	21.9 a	21.12 c
21.3 a	21.7 c	21.10 a	21.13 b
21.4 b			

21.14–21.18 Instructions: Match the risk factor for breast cancer with the appropriate relative risk.

21.14 First-degree relative (sister or mother) with breast cancer _____

21.15 Oral contraceptive use _____

21.16 Estrogen-replacement therapy _____

21.17 Contralateral breast cancer _____

21.18 Atypical hyperplasia on breast biopsy _____

    a. No effect
    b. 1.2–3.0
    c. 4.0–6.0
    d. 5.0

21.19 What proportion of patients age 30 to 54 years of age with breast cancer are identified by specific risk factors?

    a. One-fifth
    b. Two-fifths
    c. Three-fifths
    d. Four-fifths

21.20 What percent of all breast cancer occurs after the age of 40?

    a. 95
    b. 85
    c. 75
    d. 65

21.21 Breast pain is a presenting symptom in approximately what percent of patients with breast cancer?

    a. 10
    b. 20
    c. 30
    d. 40
    e. 50

21.22 The average doubling time of breast cancer cells is

    a. 35 days
    b. 100 days
    c. 175 days
    d. 300 days
    e. 450 days

21.23 The most common form of breast cancer is

    a. Cystosarcoma phylloides
    b. Infiltrating intraductal carcinoma
    c. Noninfiltrating intraductal carcinoma
    d. Lobular carcinoma
    e. Paget's disease

21.24 Paget's disease accounts for approximately what percent of breast cancers?

    a. 1
    b. 3
    c. 5
    d. 7
    e. 9

21.25 Breast cancer may be detected by mammography _____ it is detectable by breast self-examination.

    a. Significantly before
    b. At about the same time as
    c. Significantly after

21.26 Approximately what percent of breast cancers present as a mass?

    a. 20
    b. 40
    c. 60
    d. 80
    e. 100

21.27 A 34-year-old patient with a family history of breast cancer undergoes a needle aspiration of a cystic breast mass. The fluid obtained is clear. Your next step in the management of this patient would be

    a. Send the fluid for cytology
    b. Obtain a mammogram
    c. Check the site for recurrence of the mass
    d. Perform a needle biopsy of the cyst wall

21.28 The advantage of mammography is that it can

    a. Identify suspicious lesions 2 or more years before they are palpable
    b. Assess the degree of spread of malignancy
    c. Differentiate between benign and malignant conditions
    d. Provide reassurance about suspicious masses

21.29 The accuracy of mammography in diagnosing breast cancer is approximately

    a. 65
    b. 75
    c. 85
    d. 95

21.30 The current use of mammography has been credited with reducing the mortality of breast cancer by

    a. 5
    b. 15
    c. 30
    d. 45
    e. 60

Answers (21.14-21.30)

21.14 b	21.19 a	21.23 b	21.27 c
21.15 a	21.20 b	21.24 a	21.28 a
21.16 a	21.21 a	21.25 a	21.29 c
21.17 d	21.22 b	21.26 d	21.30 c
21.18 c			

21.31 Current mammography techniques result in radiation exposure that approximates

    a. 0.5–1 rad
    b. 3–5 rad
    c. 8–10 rad
    d. 12–15 rad

21.32 A 23-year-old patient presents with a 2- to 3-cm firm, painless, freely movable mass in her left breast. She reports that the mass does not change during her menstrual cycle and has grown slowly over the past year. The mass was found by the patient during breast self-examination. The most likely diagnosis is

    a. Intraductal carcinoma
    b. Fibroadenoma
    c. Ductal estasia
    d. Fibrocystic change

21.33 Multiple fibroadenomas develop in approximately what percent of patients?

    a. less than 5
    b. 5–10
    c. 15–20
    d. 25–30
    e. 35–40

21.34 The recurrence rate of fibroadenomas of the breast is approximately

    a. 1–3%
    b. 5–8%
    c. 12–15%
    d. 18–20%
    e. 30–33%

21.35 A 42-year-old woman presents with a firm, non-tender mass in her right breast. You perform fine needle aspiration, which is reported as "negative for malignancy." The next step in the management of this patient should be

    a. Open biopsy
    b. Immediate mammography
    c. Repeat fine needle aspiration
    d. Mammography in 6 months
    e. Reassurance and mammography as per routine

21.36 The most common presenting complaint of patients with intraductal papillomas of the breast is

    a. Unilateral bloody nipple discharge
    b. Unilateral cyclic pain
    c. Subareolar palpable mass
    d. Bilateral milky discharge

21.37 Nipple discharge associated with burning, itching or nipple discomfort in older patients is suggestive of

    a. Intraductal papilloma
    b. Fibroadenoma
    c. Ductal ectasia
    d. Papillary carcinoma

21.38 Cytologic evaluation of nipple discharge is associated with a false-negative rate of approximately

    a. 3%
    b. 8%
    c. 12%
    d. 20%

21.39–21.44 Instructions: Match the TNM stage of breast cancer with the appropriate description(s).

21.39 T3 _____

21.40 T4 _____

21.41 N0 _____

21.42 N1 _____

21.43 N3 _____

21.44 M1 _____

    a. Distant metastases present
    b. Tumor greater than 5 cm
    c. Tumor of any size with direct extension to chest wall or skin
    d. No palpable ipsilateral axillary nodes
    e. Movable ipsilateral axillary nodes
    f. Ipsilateral supraclavicular or infraclavicular nodes considered to contain growth or edema of the arm

---

Answers (21.31-21.44)

21.31 a	21.35 a	21.39 b	21.42 e
21.32 b	21.36 a	21.40 c	21.43 f
21.33 c	21.37 c	21.41 d	21.44 a
21.34 d	21.38 d		

Chapter 22 Final Questions (72 questions)

22.1 In assessing the effectiveness of various contraceptive methods, the "method failure rate" reflects the rate of failure when the method is

   a. Used in actual practice
   b. Tested in the laboratory
   c. Used correctly 100% of the time
   d. Is compared to no contraception at all

22.2–22.4 Instructions: Match the mechanism of contraceptive action with the appropriate example(s).

22.2 Inhibiting the development and release of the egg _____

22.3 Impose a barrier between the sperm and egg _____

22.4 Alter the ability of the fertilized egg to implant and grow _____

   a. IUD
   b. Foam
   c. Oral contraceptive
   d. RU486
   e. Long-acting progesterone injection
   f. Diaphragm

22.5 Which of the following contraceptive method does *not* provide some measure of protection from sexually transmitted diseases?

   a. Male condom
   b. Diaphragm
   c. Spermicidal jelly
   d. Female condom
   e. IUCD

22.6 The most common method of contraception among women aged 20–24 in the United States is

   a. Spermicidal foam
   b. Male condom
   c. Long-acting hormone (rod or injection)
   d. Oral contraceptive
   e. Intrauterine device

22.7 The synthetic estrogen most frequently found in oral contraceptives is

   a. Ethinyl estradiol
   b. β-estradiol
   c. Mestranol
   d. Levonorgestrel
   e. Norethindrone

22.8 The hormone used in implantable contraceptive rods (Norplant) is

   a. Ethinyl estradiol
   b. β-estradiol
   c. Mestranol
   d. Levonorgestrel
   e. Norethindrone

22.9 Ethinyl estradiol is approximately _____ times as potent as the same weight of mestranol.

   a. 0.5
   b. 1.0
   c. 1.3
   d. 1.7
   e. 2.3

22.10 Which of the following progestins used in oral contraceptives has the *least* biologic potency?

   a. Norethindrone acetate
   b. Norgestrel
   c. Ethynodiol acetate
   d. Norethindrone
   e. Norethynodrel

22.11 Progesterone-only oral contraceptive agents are not widely used because they

   a. Cost more than mono-phasic oral contraceptives
   b. Cause breast tenderness
   c. Have a higher failure rate
   d. Raise serum HDL levels

22.12 Combination oral contraceptive pills mainly prevent pregnancy through which of the following mechanisms?

   a. Altering cervical mucous
   b. Inducing endometrial atrophy
   c. Causing elevated endometrial prostaglandin formation
   d. Suppressing FSH and LH release
   e. Altering tubal motility

22.13 The progestins used in most oral contraceptives tend to

   a. Increase the occurrence of acne
   b. Increase smooth muscle tone
   c. Decrease sebum production
   d. Decrease hair growth

Answers (22.1-22.13)

22.1 c	22.5 e	22.8 d	22.11 c
22.2 c, e	22.6 d	22.9 d	22.12 d
22.3 f	22.7 a	22.10 d	22.13 a
22.4 a, d			

22.14 Users of multiphasic (low-dose) oral contraceptives have a higher incidence of _____ than in the general population.

  a. Ovarian cancer
  b. Intermenstrual bleeding
  c. Ectopic pregnancy
  d. Anemia
  e. Dysmenorrhea

22.15 A 20-year-old G0 P0 moderately obese patient consults you about the use of oral contraceptives. Her menarche was at age 15 and her period comes every 30–45 days and lasts 2–4 days. If this patient were to use an oral contraceptive agent, she would be at greater risk for

  a. "Post-Pill amenorrhea"
  b. Endometrial cancer
  c. Ectopic pregnancy
  d. Acne

22.16 When taken concurrently, _____ will reduce the efficacy of oral contraceptives.

  a. Insulin
  b. Tricyclic antidepressants
  c. Oral penicillin
  d. Methyldopa
  e. Barbiturates

22.17 The most common side effect of injectable or implantable contraceptive steroids is

  a. Involuntary weight loss
  b. Dysmenorrhea
  c. Vaginal dryness
  d. Random vaginal bleeding

22.18 Which of the following is *not* an attribute of long-acting injectable and implantable progestins?

  a. Good compliance
  b. Patient-controlled reversibility
  c. Low failure rate
  d. Low incidence of major side effects

22.19 A couple wishes to use "natural family planning" for contraception. Her periods are regular, coming every 28 ±3 days. This patients's "fertile" period would be days

  a. 7–14
  b. 7–17
  c. 7–20
  d. 10–17
  e. 10–20

22.20–22.22 Instructions: A couple is using "natural family planning" for contraception. The chart shows the basal temperature graph made for the previous month. Using the chart, match the letter with the appropriate description.

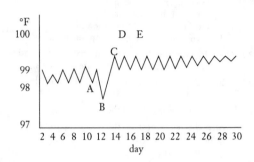

22.20 The time of ovulation _____

22.21 The time when unprotected intercourse may resume _____

22.22 The time when thin, "stretchy" cervical mucus would be found _____

22.23 Following unprotected intercourse, a high dose of oral estrogens may prevent pregnancy if they are given no later than

  a. 12 hr
  b. 24 hr
  c. 36 hr
  d. 72 hr
  e. 5 days

Answers (22.14-22.23)

22.14 b	22.17 d	22.20 b	22.22 c
22.15 a	22.18 b	22.21 e	22.23 d
22.16 c, e	22.19 c		

22.24–22.32 Instructions: Match the contraceptive method with its corresponding failure rate range (the estimated pregnancy rate).

22.24 Oral contraceptive _____

22.25 Implantable rod _____

22.26 Long-acting injectable progestin _____

22.27 IUD _____

22.28 Diaphragm _____

22.29 Condom _____

22.30 Spermicide _____

22.31 Rhythm (calendar) _____

22.32 Withdrawal _____

    a. <1%
    b. 1–2%
    c. 2–4%
    d. 5–15%
    e. 10–20%
    f. 15–30%
    g. 15–45%
    h. 20–25%

22.33 Which of the following are absolute contraindications to the use of oral contraceptives?

    a. Severe cardiovascular disease
    b. Obesity
    c. Vascular headaches
    d. Venous thrombosis
    e. History of obstructive jaundice of pregnancy
    f. Gallbladder disease
    g. Age greater than 35 years with smoking
    h. Current breast malignancy

22.34–22.40 Instructions: Match the symptom occurring in a patient taking an oral contraceptive with the appropriate action.

22.34 Diplopia _____

22.35 Hemoptysis _____

22.36 Hepatic mass _____

22.37 Slurring of speech _____

22.38 Severe headache _____

22.39 Chest/neck pain _____

22.40 Severe leg pain, tenderness _____

    a. Continue oral contraceptive but evaluate immediately
    b. Discontinue oral contraceptive and evaluate immediately, start nonhormal contraceptive method

22.41 Which of the following factors should be considered in the decision of which contraceptive method to use?

    a. Method failure rate
    b. Cost for the patient
    c. Partner satisfaction with method
    d. Patient satisfaction with method
    e. Availability

22.42 The failure of oral contraceptives usually is related to

    a. An inherent problem in the estrogen to progesterone ratio
    b. Interference by other medications that the patient is taking
    c. Missed doses of the oral contrasceptive
    d. Altered gastrointestinal absorption of the oral contraceptive due to hormonal influences

22.43 The estrogenic components of oral contraceptives preferentially inhibit

    a. FSH and are dose dependent
    b. FSH and are not dose dependent
    c. LH and are dose dependent
    d. LH and are not dose dependent

22.44 Oral contraceptives generally make cervical mucus

    a. Thicker
    b Thinner

22.45 The use of oral contraceptives offers some protection against

    a. Endometrial carcinoma
    b. Asthma
    c. Benign breast disease
    d. Ovarian carcinoma
    e. Ectopic pregnancy

22.46 Compared to low-dose oral contraceptives, high dose oral contraceptives have a _____ incidence of breakthrough bleeding.

    a. Higher
    b. Similar
    c. Lower

22.47 Which of the following are complications associated with oral contraceptive use?

    a. Venous thrombosis
    b. Stroke
    c. Myocardial infarction
    d. Cholestasis
    e. Pulmonary embolism

Answers (22.24–22.47)

22.24 b	22.30 f	22.36 b	22.42 c
22.25 a	22.31 g	22.37 b	22.43 a
22.26 a	22.32 h	22.38 a	22.44 a
22.27 c	22.33 a, d, e, g, h	22.39 b	22.45 a, c, d, e
22.28 e	22.34 b	22.40 b	22.46 c
22.29 d	22.35 b	22.41 all	22.47 all

22.48 Approximately what percent of patients will experience post-Pill amenorrhea after discontinuing oral contraceptives following long-term use?

    a. 1
    b. 3
    c. 5
    d. 7
    e. 9

22.49 Post-Pill amenorrhea is more likely to be experienced by

    a. Older women
    b. Younger women
    c. Smokers
    d. Nonsmokers
    e. Women with regular menses
    f. Women with irregular menses

22.50 What is the dosage of Depo-Provera that is given every 3 months for the purpose of contraception?

    a. 50 mg
    b. 100 mg
    c. 150 mg
    d. 200 mg
    e. 250 mg

22.51 Most women who discontinue Depo-Provera injections will not become fertile for _____ months.

    a. 1–2
    b. 2–3
    c. 3–4
    d. 4–5
    e. 5–6

22.52 Norplant is effective for _____ years after insertion.

    a. 1
    b. 2
    c. 3
    d. 4
    e. 5
    f. 6

22.53 Women using Norplant usually become amenorrheic.

    a. True
    b. False

22.54 Injectable and implantable progestin methods of contraception act by

    a. Suppressing ovulation
    b. Thickening the cervical mucus
    c. Thinning the cervical mucus
    d. Impeding sperm transport

22.55 Which of the following is *not* a positive attribute of barrier contraceptives?

    a. Need for good patient compliance
    b. Patient-controlled reversibility
    c. Low failure rate
    d. Low incidence of major side effects
    e. Low cost per month

22.56 In addition to the failure rate, which of the following is the *most* common problem associated with the use of condoms?

    a. Premature ejaculation
    b. Increased risk of vaginal yeast infection
    c. Contact dermatitis
    d. Urinary retention

22.57 When used for contraception, a diaphragm must be left in place following intercourse for a period of

    a. 30–60 min
    b. 2–3 hr
    c. 6–8 hr
    d. 12–18 hr
    e. 24 or more hrs

22.58 If a diaphragm is in place during the time following intercourse (the waiting time before diaphragm removal), what should be done before additional intercourse?

    a. Delay intercourse until the waiting time before diaphragm removal has expired
    b. Remove the diaphragm, reapply the contraceptive jelly, and restart the waiting time
    c. Insert additional jelly without disturbing the diaphragm and restart the waiting time
    d. Remove the diaphragm, reapply the contraceptive jelly, and remove the diaphragm at the end of the original waiting time
    e. Remove the diaphragm and use an alternate method of contraception

22.59 When correctly fitted and worn, a contraceptive diaphragm should

    a. Completely cover the posterior vaginal wall
    b. Have its apex in the posterior fornix
    c. Rest firmly against the anterior fourchette
    d. Sit 1–2 cm below the symphysis

22.60 Women who use diaphragms are _____ susceptible to urinary tract infections.

    a. Slightly more
    b. About as
    c. Slightly less

Answers (22.48-22.60)

22.48 b	22.52 f	22.55 a	22.58 c
22.49 b, f	22.53 b	22.56 c	22.59 b
22.50 c	22.54 a, b, d	22.57 c	22.60 a
22.51 d			

22.61 Following intercourse using a contraceptive foam, douching should be avoided for a period of at least

    a. 30–60 min
    b. 1–2 hr
    c. 4–6 hr
    d. 8–10 hr
    e. 12 or more hr

22.62 Spermicidal foams provide protection for

    a. A single act of intercourse.
    b. 1–3 hr
    c. 4–6 hr
    d. 10–12 hr
    e. up to 24 hr

22.63 The presence of a reservoir tip in a condom _____ the likelihood of breakage during use.

    a. Increases
    b. Does not affect
    c. Decreases

22.64 The vaginal sponge acted as a contraceptive primarily by

    a. Acting as a barrier
    b. Delivering spermicide
    c. Irritating the vaginal wall

22.65 Following unprotected intercourse, an intrauterine contraceptive device may prevent pregnancy if it is inserted within

    a. 12 hr
    b. 24 hr
    c. 36 hr
    d. 72 hr
    e. 5 days

22.66 The main contraceptive action of the intrauterine contraceptive device (IUCD) is to

    a. Inhibit ovulation
    b. Cause cervical mucus thickening
    c. Alter tubal motility
    d. Prevent implantation
    e. Cause heavy metal poisoning of passing sperm

22.67 Which of the following is *not* a frequent complication from the use of an intrauterine contraceptive device?

    a. Bloating
    b. Intermenstrual bleeding
    c. Dysmenorrhea
    d. Menorrhagia
    e. Increased risk of tubal infections

22.68 The spontaneous expulsion rate of intrauterine devices in the 1st year following insertion is

    a. 5%
    b. 10%
    c. 15%
    d. 20%
    e. 25%

22.69 Although IUDs may be inserted at any time in the menstrual cycle, many believe that insertion is best done

    a. At the time of ovulation
    b. In the time between the menstrual period and ovulation
    c. In the time between ovulation and the menstrual period
    d. At the time of the menstrual period

22.70 An effective postcoital antifertility method is

    a. Oral administration of diethyl stilbestrol
    b. Postcoital douche
    c. Immediate uterine curettage
    d. Carbonic anhydrase
    e. Hydroxyzine HCL

22.71 The two types of estrogen compounds commonly found in oral contraceptive preparations are

    a. Estrone and mestranol
    b. Ethinyl estradiol and mestranol
    c. Estradiol and estrone
    d. Estriol and mestranol

22.72 Which of the following oral contraceptive components has been implicated as the caustive agent of thromboembolism in women using oral contraceptives?

    a. Estrogen
    b. Progesterone

Answers (22.61-22.72)

22.61 d	22.64 b	22.67 a	22.70 a
22.62 a	22.65 e	22.68 b	22.71 b
22.63 c	22.66 d	22.69 d	22.72 a

Chapter 23 Final Questions (30 questions)

23.1   Sterilization ranks _____ in the United States among the methods used to control fertility.

  a. First
  b. Second
  c. Third
  d. Fourth

23.2   Roughly what proportion of married couples in the United States use sterilization for contraception?

  a. 1 in 8
  b. 1 in 5
  c. 1 in 3
  d. 1 in 2

23.3   Despite careful counseling, what percent of patients will request sterilization reversal?

  a. 1
  b. 3
  c. 5
  d. 8
  e. 12

23.4   Successful reversal of sterilization is possible in approximately what percent of cases?

  a. 5–10
  b. 20–30
  c. 40–60
  d. 70–80
  e. 90–95

23.5   Vasectomy accounts for approximately what percent of all sterilization procedures?

  a. 10–15
  b. 20–25
  c. 30–35
  d. 40–45
  e. 50–55

23.6   Antibodies against sperm are found in what proportion of men who have undergone vasectomy?

  a. 10–15%
  b. 20–25%
  c. 30–35%
  d. 40–45%
  e. 50–55%

23.7   When compared to female sterilization, which of the following is *not* an advantage of vasectomy?

  a. Lower incidence of postoperative depression
  b. Greater reversibility
  c. Lower cost
  d. Lower operative complication rate
  e. The possibility of routine postoperative verification

23.8   Which of the following are possible operative complications of vasectomy?

  a. Hematoma formation
  b. Wound infection
  c. Femoral nerve damage
  d. Continued bleeding of the operative site

23.9   The *most* common cause of pregnancy following a vasectomy is

  a. Recanalization
  b. Too short of a waiting period after surgery
  c. Ligation of the tunica albicans
  d. Operative hematoma formation

23.10   Sterilization after vasectomy usually is complete by

  a. 24–36 hr
  b. 3–5 days
  c. 2–3 weeks
  d. 4–6 weeks
  e. 8–10 weeks

23.11   Which of the following anesthetics is used for laparoscopic sterilization procedures?

  a. Local
  b. General
  c. Epidural
  d. Spinal

23.12   Which of the following female sterilization methods is *most* likely to result in future ectopic pregnancy?

  a. Hulka clip
  b. Falope ring
  c. Electrocautery
  d. Pomeroy tubal ligation
  e. Kroener fimbriectomy

23.13   Which of the following female sterilization methods is *most* likely to be successfully reversed?

  a. Hulka clip
  b. Falope ring
  c. Electrocautery
  d. Pomeroy tubal ligation
  e. Kroener fimbriectomy

23.14   Which of the following female sterilization methods is *most* likely to result in operative complications?

  a. Hulka clip
  b. Falope ring
  c. Electrocautery
  d. Pomeroy tubal ligation
  e. Kroener fimbriectomy

Answers (23.1-23.14)

23.1 d	23.5 c	23.9 b	23.12 c
23.2 c	23.6 e	23.10 d	23.13 a
23.3 a	23.7 a	23.11 all	23.14 c
23.4 c	23.8 a, b, d		

23.15 Which of the following female sterilization methods is most likely to result in postoperative pain, requiring strong analgesics?

    a. Hulka clip
    b. Falope ring
    c. Electrocautery
    d. Pomeroy tubal ligation
    e. Kroener fimbriectomy

23.16–23.21 Instructions: Match the tubal ligation technique with the appropriate description of the procedure.

23.16 Madlener _____

23.17 Pomeroy _____

23.18 Irving _____

23.19 Cook _____

23.20 Kroener _____

23.21 Aldridge _____

    a. Fimbriated end of tube excised
    b. Fimbriated end of tube buried in broad ligament
    c. Tube divided, proximal stump buried in uterine wall, distal stump buried in leaves of broad ligament
    d. Tube divided, proximal stump buried in round ligament, distal stump buried in leaves of broad ligament
    e. Tube elevated, base crushed in clamp, crushed area ligated with nonabsorbable suture
    f. Loop of tube from middle third of tube elevated, ligated with plain gut and excised

23.22 The Hulka clip has a _____ failure rate as compared to electrocautery.

    a. Higher
    b. Similar
    c. Lower

23.23 Which of the following is *not* required as part of vaginal tubal sterilization procedures?

    a. Specialized equipment
    b. Prophylactic antibiotics
    c. Restrictions on intercourse
    d. Restrictions on douching

23.24 The term "interval sterilization" refers to procedures

    a. In which a segment of the fallopian tube is removed
    b. That destroy a portion of the fallopian tube
    c. That are performed after the immediate postpartum period
    d. That are performed during the immediate postpartum period

23.25 Vasectomy is _____ tubal ligation.

    a. More easily reversed than
    b. As easily reversed as
    c. Less easily reversed than

23.26 A patient who has undergone tubal reversal after tubal ligation and becomes pregnant is presumed to have an ectopic pregnancy until the presence of intrauterine pregnancy is established.

    a. True
    b. False

23.27 Which of the following statements about surgical sterilization is *incorrect*?

    a. There is a less than 1% chance of pregnancy after female tubal sterilization
    b. The rate of permanent surgical sterilizations has steadily risen in recent years
    c. The number of men and women requesting surgical sterilization are roughly equal

23.28 Postoperative complications of vasectomy such as bleeding, hematoma formation, and local skin infection occur in about what percent of cases?

    a. <1
    b. 3–5
    c. 7–9
    d. 12–15

23.29 "Posttubal ligation syndrome" is described by some to encompass

    a. Menstrual dysfunction
    b. Dysmenorrhea
    c. Disruption of blood flow in the area of the fallopian tubes

23.30 Failure in the Pomeroy method of tubal ligation is approximately 1 in _____ procedures.

    a. 10
    b. 50
    c. 100
    d. 500
    e. 1000

Answers (23.15-23.30)

23.15 b	23.19 d	23.23 a	23.27 c
23.16 e	23.20 a	23.24 c	23.28 b
23.17 f	23.21 b	23.25 a	23.29 all
23.18 c	23.22 a	23.26 a	23.30 d

Chapter 24 Final Questions (36 questions)

24.1–24.2   Instructions: Match the type of dysmenorrhea with the appropriate precipitating condition(s).

24.1   Primary dysmenorrhea _____

24.2   Secondary dysmenorrhea _____

    a. Clinically identifiable cause
    b. Excess prostaglandins leading to painful muscle activity

24.3   The most common cause of dysmenorrhea in a 19-year-old is

    a. Anovulation
    b. Excess prostaglandin production
    c. Adenomyosis
    d. Endometriosis
    e. Pelvic congestion syndrome

24.4   The incidence of secondary dysmenorrhea _____ as a woman ages.

    a. Increases
    b. Remains the same
    c. Decreases

24.5   The agent thought to be responsible for causing primary dysmenorrhea is

    a. Estrogen
    b. Progesterone
    c. Prostaglandin E_2
    d. Prostaglandin $F_2\alpha$

24.6   Primary and secondary dysmenorrhea cause significant disability for approximately what percent of women?

    a. 1–2
    b. 5–8
    c. 10–15
    d. 20–25
    e. 30–35

24.7   Ischemia and stretching of tissues are postulated causes of pain associated with dysmenorrhea

    a. True
    b. False

24.8   Intrauterine resting pressure is _____ in primary dysmenorrhea.

    a. Decreased
    b. Unchanged
    c. Increased

24.9   During primary dysmenorrhea, intrauterine pressures may reach a maximum of

    a. 50 mm Hg
    b. 85 mm Hg
    c. 125 mm Hg
    d. 250 mm Hg
    e. 400 mm Hg

24.10   Dyspareunia is commonly associated with primary dysmenorrhea.

    a. True
    b. False

24.11–24.17   Instructions: Match the symptom associated with primary dysmenorrhea with the estimated incidence.

24.11   Pain _____

24.12   Nausea and emesis _____

24.13   Tiredness _____

24.14   Nervousness _____

24.15   Dizziness _____

24.16   Diarrhea _____

24.17   Headache _____

    a. 45%
    b. 60%
    c. 70%
    d. 85%
    e. 90%
    f. 100%

24.18   Which of the following is an action of prostaglandin $F_2\alpha$?

    a. Vasodilation
    b. Hyperemia
    c. Smooth muscle contraction
    d. Hypomotility of the intestines

24.19   In the uterus, the production of prostaglandins are most influenced by

    a. Estrogen
    b. Progesterone
    c. Epinephrine
    d. Acetylcholine
    e. Prolactin

Answers (24.1-24.19)

24.1 b	24.6 c	24.11 f	24.16 b
24.2 a	24.7 a	24.12 e	24.17 a
24.3 b	24.8 c	24.13 d	24.18 c
24.4 a	24.9 e	24.14 c	24.19 b
24.5 d	24.10 b	24.15 b	

24.20 A 43-year-old patient complains of increasing pelvic heaviness and cyclic lower abdominal pain that begins 1 day prior to her menstrual flow and lasts for 3 days. Periods are regular, but heavy with clots. She had a tubal ligation several years ago. Which of the following are possible diagnoses for this patient?

a. Primary dysmenorrhea
b. Adenomyosis
c. Uterine myomas
d. Endometriosis

24.21 A 23-year-old G0 P0 patient complains of increasing pelvic heaviness and cyclic lower abdominal pain that begins 1 day prior to her menstrual flow and lasts for 3 days. Periods are regular, but are heavy with clots. She has been attempting pregnancy for the past 3 years. Which of the following is not a likely diagnosis for this patient?

a. Primary dysmenorrhea
b. Adenomyosis
c. Uterine myomas
d. Endometriosis

24.22 A 23-year-old G0 P0 patient complains of increasing pelvic heaviness and cyclic lower abdominal pain that begins 1 day prior to her menstrual flow and lasts for 3 days. Periods are regular, but are heavy with clots. She has been attempting pregnancy for the past 3 years. Pelvic examination is normal except for painful nodules posterior to the cervix. Which of the following is the *most* likely diagnosis for this patient?

a. Primary dysmenorrhea
b. Adenomyosis
c. Uterine myomas
d. Endometriosis

24.23–24.24 Instructions: Use the following case history when answering questions 24.23 and 24.24: An 18-year-old G0 P0 patient complains of cyclic, sharp, crampy, lower abdominal pain that begins on the day of her menstrual flow and lasts for 3 days. Periods are regular, but are heavy, with clots. She has been attempting pregnancy for the past year. Pelvic examination is normal.

24.23 Which of the following is the *most* likely diagnosis for this patient? _____

a. Primary dysmenorrhea
b. Adenomyosis
c. Uterine myomas
d. Endometriosis

24.24 The *most* appropriate therapy for this patient would be

a. Low-dose, monophasic oral contraceptive pills
b. An acetaminophen/codeine combination
c. A nonsteroidal antiinflammatory agent
d. An injectable progestin contraceptive agent

24.25 An identifiable cause is found in what percent of patients who undergo diagnostic laparoscopy for pelvic pain?

a. 10–15
b. 30–40
c. about 50
d. 60–70
e. 90–95

24.26 Pain that continues between menstrual periods is consistent with

a. Primary dysmenorrhea
b. Secondary dysmenorrhea
c. Chronic pelvic pain

24.27 Extreme retroversion and retroflexion of the uterus can be causes of secondary dysmenorrhea.

a. True
b. False

24.28–24.31 Instructions: Match the symptom/finding with the possible diagnosis.

24.28 Heavy menstrual flow _____

24.29 Large, tender, symmetric uterus _____

24.30 Fever and chills _____

24.31 Infertility _____

a. Pelvic inflammatory disease
b. Leiomyoma uteri
c. Endometriosis
d. Adenomyosis uteri

24.32 Thickening in the adnexae is consistent with

a. Pelvic inflammatory disease
b. Leiomyoma uteri
c. Endometriosis
d. Adenomyosis uteri

24.33 The term "chronic pelvic pain" is applied to pain that has been present for

a. Three consecutive menstrual periods.
b. At least 6 months.
c. Three or more of a women's first six menstrual cycles
d. More than 21 days in a given month

24.34 Chronic pelvic pain may result from_____ etiologies.

a. Gynecologic
b. Nongynecologic

24.35 The goal of eliminating chronic pelvic pain is usually achieved.

a. True
b. False

24.36 Suppression of ovulation is often a useful diagnostic maneuver in the evaluation of chronic pelvic pain.

a. True
b. False

Answers (24.20-24.36)

24.20 all	24.25 d	24.29 b, d	24.33 b
24.21 b	24.26 b, c	24.30 d	24.34 a, b
24.22 d	24.27 a	24.31 a, b, c	24.35 b
24.23 a	24.28 b, d	24.32 a, c	24.36 a
24.24 c			

Chapter 25 Final Questions (28 questions)

25.1   Which of the following can be associated with pre-
        menstrual syndrome (PMS)?

        a. Physical symptoms
        b. Behavioral symptoms
        c. Emotional/mood changes

25.2   Which of the following statements about PMS is
        incorrect?

        a. PMS occurs in a regular, cyclical relationship to
           the luteal phase of the menstrual cycle
        b. The signs and symptoms can resemble certain
           psychiatric conditions
        c. There is a symptom-free period of at least 1
           week
        d. The signs and symptoms of PMS tend to in-
           crease in severity over time

25.3   What percent of women have some physical or
        emotional premenstrual symptoms?

        a. 30
        b. 50
        c. 70
        d. 90

25.4   PMS that is severe and debilitating occurs in what
        percent of women?

        a. 10
        b. 20
        c. 30
        d. 40

25.5   The signs and symptoms of PMS suggest that it is

        a. A single clinical entity.
        b. More than one clinical entity.

25.6   In making the diagnosis of PMS, the specific symp-
        toms are _____ the cyclic occurrence of the symp-
        toms.

        a. Less important than
        b. As important as
        c. More important than

25.7   PMS tends to be more common in women in which
        of the following age groups?

        a. 20–29
        b. 30–39
        c. 40–49
        d. 50–59
        e. 60–69

25.8   Of all the characteristics of symptoms of PMS, the
        _____ is most important.

        a. Severity
        b. Duration
        c. Cyclic occurrence
        d. Degree of disability
        e. Association with exogenous therapy

25.9   Which of the following physical symptoms are asso-
        ciated with PMS?

        a. Breast swelling and pain
        b. Headache
        c. Edema of the extremities
        d. Fatigue
        e. Tinnitus

25.10   Which of the following emotional symptoms are
        common in PMS?

        a. Anxiety
        b. Mania
        c. Irritability
        d. Euphoria
        e. Changes in libido

25.11–25.15   Instructions: Match the theoretical etiology
        of PMS with the appropriate supporting evidence.

25.11   Psychiatric basis _____

25.12   Endocrinologic basis _____

25.13   Dietary basis _____

25.14   Endorphin basis _____

25.15   Serotonin basis _____

        a. Occurrence of premenstrual hypoglycemic epi-
           sodes
        b. Production declines during the luteal phase
        c. Presence in luteal phase only
        d. Lower premenstrual levels than in comparable
           controlled patients, associated with depression
        e. Cyclic manifestation of underlying pathology

25.16   A strong argument for the endorphin basis of PMS
        comes from patients who report alleviation of symp-
        toms with

        a. Aspirin consumption
        b. Exercise
        c. Caffeine consumption
        d. Bedrest

25.17   The serotonin theory for PMS is based on the pres-
        ence of _____ levels of serotonin as compared with
        controls.

        a. Increased
        b. Unchanged
        c. Decreased

Answers (25.1-25.17)

25.1 all	25.6 a	25.10 a, c, e	25.14 b
25.2 d	25.7 b, c	25.11 e	25.15 d
25.3 c	25.8 c	25.12 c	25.16 b
25.4 a	25.9 a, b, d	25.13 a	25.17 c
25.5 b			

25.18 The most useful diagnostic tool with respect to PMS is

   a. Serial progesterone levels
   b. Serial blood glucose determinations
   c. A menstrual diary
   d. Cyclic vaginal wall cytology

25.19–25.23 Instructions: Match the type of PMS therapy with the appropriate description/example.

25.19 Diet _____

25.20 Exercise _____

25.21 Medication to induce anovulation _____

25.22 Diuretic _____

25.23 Anxiolytic _____

   a. Buspirone
   b. Spironolactone
   c. GnRH agonist
   d. Increased endorphins
   e. Decreased refined sugars and fats

25.24 Buspirone (BuSpar) has been found to have effect in PMS patients after approximately _____ weeks of therapy.

   a. 1
   b. 2
   c. 3
   d. 4
   e. 5

25.25 Which of the following dietary recommendations is *not* a component of PMS dietary therapy?

   a. Increased intake of fresh fruits and vegetables
   b. Decreased intake of refined sugars
   c. Intake of three substantial meals per day with no between meal snacking
   d. Decreased intake of salt
   e. Decreased intake of caffeine

25.26 Pyridoxine (vitamin B_6) therapy is a popular treatment for PMS, but has not been demonstrated to be helpful in rigorous scientific studies.

   a. True
   b. False

25.27 Which of the following may be useful in the treatment of PMS-associated mastodynia?

   a. Tetracycline
   b. Estrogen
   c. Bromocriptine
   d. Prostaglandin $F_2\alpha$

25.28 Although oral contraceptives are associated with anovulation, the side effects of these medications make them a poor choice for the treatment of PMS.

   a. True
   b. False

Answers (25.18-25.28)

25.18 c	25.21 c	25.24 b	25.27 c
25.19 e	25.22 b	25.25 c	25.28 b
25.20 d	25.23 a	25.26 b	

Chapter 26 Final Questions (31 questions)

26.1 What percent of couples are estimated to have sexual problems at some time during their relationship?

a. 20
b. 40
c. 60
d. 80
e. 100

26.2 During an individual's life, sexual identity

a. May change
b. Remains constant

26.3 The human sexual response is

a. Functionally volitional
b. Cycle dependent

26.4 The human sexual response is dependent upon

a. A physical and emotional system sufficiently functional to allow the sexual response
b. A sustained and sufficient sexual stimulation

26.5 The physiological components of the human sexual response are mediated by changes in

a. Hormone levels
b. Muscle tone (myotonic activity)
c. Blood flow (vasocongestion)

26.6 Sexual practices and attitudes may be classified as normal or abnormal based on standard psychological indices.

a. True
b. False

26.7–26.10 Instructions: Match the stages of the human sexual response according to Masters and Johnson with the appropriate description.

26.7 First stage _____

26.8 Second stage _____

26.9 Third stage _____

26.10 Fourth stage _____

a. Orgasmic phase
b. Plateau phase
c. Resolution phase
d. Excitement phase

26.11 The clinical and behavioral boundaries marking the different stages of the human sexual response are

a. Clear and well-defined
b. Unclear and ill-defined

26.12 The duration of the various phases of the human sexual response is _____ across individuals.

a. Variable
b. Constant

26.13 The orgasmic platform develops in the

a. Introitus
b. Vagina
c. Cervix
d. Uterus

26.14 Sexual flush, occurring in the face and anterior aspect of the thorax, is primarily mediated through

a. Myotonic activity
b. Vasocongestive activity

26.15 Introital muscle spasm inhibiting intercourse is termed

a. Lack of libido
b. Frigidity
c. Orgasmic dysfunction
d. Vaginismus
e. Dyspareunia

26.16–26.19 Instructions: Match the stage of the human sexual response according to Masters and Johnson with the corresponding description(s) of events occurring during the stage.

26.16 Excitement stage _____

26.17 Plateau stage _____

26.18 Orgasm stage _____

26.19 Resolution stage _____

a. Vagina begins to lubricate
b. Uterus contracts similar to labor
c. Orgasmic platform resolves
d. Uterus fully elevated
e. Expansion of vaginal barrel
f. Strong vaginal contractions of orgasmic platform
g. Uterus drops back into normal position
h. Clitoris increases in diameter

Answers (26.1-26.19)

26.1 b	26.6 b	26.11 b	26.16 a, h
26.2 b	26.7 d	26.12 a	26.17 d, e
26.3 a	26.8 b	26.13 b	26.18 b, f
26.4 a, b	26.9 a	26.14 b	26.19 c, g
26.5 b, c	26.10 c	26.15 d	

26.20 Which of the following is the initial determinant in the development of human sexuality?

  a. Distribution of the Y chromosome
  b. Learned behaviors from siblings and peers
  c. Learned behaviors from parents
  d. Endocrinologic development
  e. Mature adult evaluation of own character

26.21 Which of the following are required to initiate the human sexual response?

  a. Sustained sexual stimulation
  b. Sufficient sexual stimulation

26.22 The human sexual response is best considered as a continuum rather than as distinct, separate events.

  a. True
  b. False

26.23 Which of the following is *not* required of the physician in dealing with patient sexual issues?

  a. Exploring his or her own attitudes about the range of human sexual expression
  b. Exploring his or her own sexuality
  c. Accepting that the entire range of sexual expression is normal and nonpathological
  d. Attempting to address sexual issues in a supportive and nonjudgmental manner

26.24 Any sexual problem can be handled by the patient's primary physician.

  a. True
  b. False

26.25 Physician comfort with his or her own sexuality and/or with sexual issues is independent of the ability to appropriately and competently care for the sexual aspect of patient care.

  a. True
  b. False

26.26–26.29 Instructions: Match the components of the PLISSIT model for the treatment of sexual problems with the appropriate description(s).

26.26 P _____

26.27 LI _____

26.28 SS _____

26.29 IT _____

  a. Providing suggestions for action
  b. Referring to a specialist for intensive therapy
  c. Providing pertinent information
  d. Giving the patient permission to deal with sexual issues/problems

26.30 Sexual problems usually arise independent from medical problems and are best evaluated and treated separately.

  a. True
  b. False

26.31 Which of the following statements about the management of sexual problems is *incorrect*?

  a. In general, single disorders lasting less than 1 year in the context of a stable relationship, are more likely to be amenable to simple interventions.
  b. Sexual problems lasting longer than 1 year and/or with multiple dysfunctions are best referred to a sex therapist.
  c. Single sexual problems, even in the context of an unstable relationship, are best treated by the patient's primary physician.
  d. In general, sexual problems that are secondary and/or situational are more easily treated than those that are primary and constant.

Answers (26.20-26.31)

26.20 a	26.23 c	26.26 d	26.29 b
26.21 a, b	26.24 b	26.27 c	26.30 b
26.22 a	26.25 b	26.28 a	26.31 c

Chapter 27 Final Questions (72 questions)

27.1 Complaints of vulvar irritation account for approximately what percent of gynecologic office visits?

a. 3
b. 5
c. 10
d. 15
e. 25

27.2–27.13 Instructions: Match the statement with the condition with which it most closely associated.

27.2 A vaginal pH of 5.5 _____

27.3 A "fishy" odor after intercourse _____

27.4 Cervical petechia _____

27.5 Vaginal dryness _____

27.6 A yellow-green discharge _____

27.7 An intense itching _____

27.8 A thick, lumpy discharge _____

27.9 "Ground-glass" epithelial cells on microscopic examination _____

27.10 Motile protozoa on microscopic examination _____

27.11 Thin filaments found on microscopic examination _____

27.12 Few white blood cells and multiple, flat, polygonal cells with small nuclei on microscopic examination _____

27.13 Few white blood cells and multiple, rounded, parabasal epithelial cells on microscopic examination _____

a. Physiologic discharge
b. Bacterial vaginosis
c. Vaginal candidiasis
d. Vaginal trichomoniasis
e. Atrophic vaginitis

27.14 Which of the following is *not* characteristic of an infection that is the source of vulvar irritation?

a. Edema
b. Erythema
c. Skin ulceration
d. Vaginal discharge

27.15 Most of the liquid portion of physiologic vaginal secretions in a woman of reproductive age comes from

a. The cervix
b. Vaginal transudate
c. The Bartholin's glands
d. The Skene's glands

27.16 The creamy white portion of physiologic vaginal secretions in a woman of reproductive age comes from

a. Cervical mucus
b. Vaginal epithelium
c. The Bartholin's glands
d. Vaginal white blood cells

27.17 The average amount of vaginal secretion produced in 24 hr by a woman of reproductive age is approximately

a. 0.1 g
b. 0.5 g
c. 1.5 g
d. 3.0 g
e. 5.0 g

27.18 The normal pH of vaginal secretions found in women between menarche and menopause is

a. 3.5–4.5
b. 5.0–6.0
c. 6.5–7.5
d. 8.0–9.0

27.19 The normal pH of vaginal secretions found in women before menarche or after menopause (without hormonal replacement) is

a. 2.0–3.0
b. 3.5–5.5
c. 6.0–8.0
d. 9.0–11.0

27.20 The number of bacteria found in vaginal secretions a woman of reproductive age approximates

a. 10^2/mL
b. 10^3/mL
c. 10^6/mL
d. 10^9/mL

Answers (27.1-27.20)

27.1 c	27.6 d	27.11 c	27.16 b
27.2 b	27.7 c	27.12 a	27.17 c
27.3 b	27.8 c	27.13 e	27.18 a
27.4 d	27.9 b	27.14 d	27.19 c
27.5 e	27.10 d	27.15 a	27.20 d

27.21 The most common cause of persistently increased vaginal secretions is

    a. Sexual arousal
    b. Microbiologic infection
    c. Contact vulvitis
    d. Hormonal variation

27.22 The most common cause of increased vaginal discharge due to microbiological infection in the vagina is

    a. Candidiasis
    b. Trichomoniasis
    c. Bacterial vaginosis
    d. Human papilloma virus

27.23 In patients with the complaint of increased vaginal discharge, the diagnosis is established based on

    a. A description of the odor of the discharge
    b. Direct examination and microscopic examination of secretions
    c. The description of the symptoms reported by the patient
    d. The description of the color and texture of the discharge

27.24 Patients with bacterial vaginosis often complain of a foul odor after intercourse. This is a result of

    a. The alkaline pH of semen
    b. Colonization of the vagina by penile microorganisms
    c. Bacterial digestion of seminal proteins
    d. Liberation of prostaglandins from sperm

27.25 A "whiff test" is

    a. Mixing of vaginal secretions with 10% KOH to liberate amines
    b. Testing for odor in undiluted vaginal secretions from the apex of the vagina
    c. Mixing of vaginal secretions with normal saline to test dilution of odor
    d. Passing the speculum briefly under the nose to detect odor

27.26 "Clue cells" are

    a. Clumped white blood cells
    b. Immature vaginal epithelial cells
    c. Keratinized vaginal epithelial cells with adherent white blood cells
    d. Vaginal epithelial cells with adherent bacteria

27.27 Bacterial vaginosis is not thought to be sexually transmitted so that treatment of sexual partners is unnecessary.

    a. True
    b. False

27.28 *Trichomonas vaginalis* is a flagellate protozoan that can live in all of the following locations *except*

    a. Oral pharynx
    b. Vagina
    c. Male urethra
    d. Skene's ducts
    e. Female urethra

27.29 Approximately what percent of sexual partners of women with *Trichomonas* infections also have the infection?

    a. <10
    b. 20–30
    c. 40–50
    d. >60

27.30 Approximately what percent of women with *Trichomonas* infection of the vagina are symptomatic?

    a. 10
    b. 25
    c. 50
    d. 75
    e. 90

27.31 Which of the following is *not* characteristic of the appearance of *Trichomonas* organisms as seen through a microscope when vaginal secretions are suspended in saline?

    a. 3–5 flagella
    b. Fusiform shape
    c. Size about one-half that of a white blood cell
    d. Active movement

27.32 Characteristic petechia, or strawberry patches, are found in the upper vagina or on the cervix of patients with *Trichomonas vaginitis* in approximately what percent of cases?

    a. 10
    b. 30
    c. 50
    d. 70
    e. 90

27.33 The standard treatment for *Trichomonas* vaginal infection is

    a. Metronidazole 1 g p.o. in A.M. and P.M. for 1 day
    b. Metronidazole 250 mg p.o. q.d. for 14 days
    c. Clindamycin 1 g p.o. for one dose
    d. Ampicillin 500 mg p.o. q.i.d. for 10 days

Answers (27.21-27.33)

27.21 b	27.25 a	27.28 a	27.31 c
27.22 c	27.26 d	27.29 d	27.32 a
27.23 b	27.27 b	27.30 c	27.33 a
27.24 a			

27.34 The standard treatment for *Trichomonas vaginitis* will generally give a cure rate of

a. 100%
b. 90%
c. 80%
d. 70%
e. 60%

27.35 Because of the association of *Trichomonas vaginitis* with cervical dysplasia, the treatment of women with asymptomatic infections is mandatory.

a. True
b. False

27.36 It is estimated that up to _____ of patients with *Trichomonas vaginitis* will also have bacterial vaginosis.

a. 0%
b. 25%
c. 50%
d. 75%
e. 100%

27.37 When prescribing metronidazole for the treatment of *Trichomonas* infections, it is important to advise the patient to avoid alcohol intake because alcohol

a. Diminishes the gastric uptake of metronidazole
b. Induces metronidazole resistance in *Trichomonas*
c. Decreases tissue levels of metronidazole
d. May cause severe nausea and vomiting

27.38 The most common source of monilial infections of the vagina is from

a. Sexual contact with an infected partner
b. Airborne colonization
c. Contaminated clothing
d. Bath water retained in the vagina following bathing

27.39 Roughly 90% of vaginal "yeast" infections are caused by

a. *Candida albicans*
b. *Candida tropicalis*
c. *Candida glabrata*
d. *Torulopsis glabrata*

27.40 Which of the following is *not* thought to increase the risk of a vaginal "yeast" infection?

a. Use of oral contraceptives
b. Habitual use of panty liners
c. Obesity
d. Immunosuppression
e. Use of spermicidal foam

27.41 Approximately what percent of women with vaginal "yeast" infections are symptomatic?

a. 10
b. 25
c. 40
d. 60
e. 80

27.42 The normal pH of vaginal secretions found in women with vaginal "yeast" infections is

a. 4.0–4.5
b. 5.5–6.0
c. 6.5–7.0
d. 8.0–9.0

27.43 The most common presenting complaint in women with vaginal "yeast" infections is

a. Thick discharge
b. Vulvar burning
c. Dysuria
d. Intense itching

27.44 A 10% KOH solution is used for microscopic examination of vaginal secretions when a "yeast" infection is suspected because this solution

a. Renders *Candida albicans* noninfective
b. Causes lysis of white blood cells
c. Liberates amines from solution
d. Immobilizes *Trichomonas* organisms

27.45 Despite compliant therapy with an appropriate medication, the recurrence rate for vaginal yeast infections is

a. 5%
b. 10%
c. 25%
d. 40%
e. 60%

27.46 About 99% of "yeast infections" in the normal female are caused by *Candida albicans*.

a. True
b. False

27.47 The cottage cheese-like thick adherent vaginal discharge associated with *Candida* vaginitis is usually odorless.

a. True
b. False

Answers (27.34–27.47)

27.34 b	27.38 b	27.42 a	27.45 c
27.35 b	27.39 a	27.43 d	27.46 b
27.36 b	27.40 e	27.44 b	27.47 a
27.37 d	27.41 e		

27.48 The primary treatment of *Candida* vaginitis is

    a. Topical synthetic imidazoles
    b. Systemic synthetic imidazoles
    c. Topical cephalosporins
    d. Systemic cephalosporins

27.49 Treatment of the male partner _____ in reducing the rate of recurrences of vaginal "yeast" infections.

    a. Is effective
    b. Is not effective

27.50 Candidiasis is _____ occur in women with diabetes than in nondiabetic women.

    a. More likely to
    b. As likely to
    c. Less likely to

27.51–27.52 Instructions: Match the organism with the appropriate description.

27.51 *Pthirus pubis* (crab louse) _____

27.52 *Sarcoptes scabiei* (itch mite) _____

    a. Found exclusively in hairy areas of the body
    b. Acquired by close contact or infected bedding
    c. Treatment with γ-benzene hexachloride
    d. Itching on or about the mons suggestive of infection

27.53 The presence of "clue" cells is usually diagnostic of

    a. Tinea cruris
    b. Bacterial vaginosis
    c. Diabetic vulvitis
    d. Scabies

27.54–27.55 Instructions: Match the anatomical region with the statement(s) with which it is associated.

27.54 Vulva _____

27.55 Vagina _____

    a. Apocrine glands
    b. Sweat glands
    c. Stratified squamous epithelium
    d. Nonkeratinized epithelium
    e. Sebaceous glands
    f. Vulnerable to contact with external irritants
    g. Hair follicles

27.56 Because of the sensitivity of the vulvar skin, secondary allergic vulvitis almost always requires the use of hydrocortisone cream to achieve a satisfactory therapeutic resolution.

    a. True
    b. False

27.57 Vulvitis in the pediatric patient may be associated with

    a. Secondary allergic vulvitis
    b. Foreign body reaction
    c. Sexual abuse
    d. Pinworm infestation

27.58 In a patient with recurrent vulvar candida infection, what systemic disease should be considered as possibly coexistent?

    a. SLE
    b. Diabetes
    c. Syphilis
    d. Cushings' syndrome

27.59–27.62 Instructions: Match the dermatologic disease with the appropriate description(s).

27.59 Contact dermatitis _____

27.60 Psoriasis _____

27.61 Seborrheic dermatitis _____

27.62 Hidradenitis suppurative _____

    a. Pale to yellow-red edematous lesions covered with fine nonadherent scale
    b. Red, edematous skin surfaces, sometimes with vesicles and secondary infection
    c. Affects 1–3% of women and seems to have a familial pattern
    d. Deep painful scars and a foul discharge
    e. Treatment with local antibiotics and steroids is sometimes successful, but wide excision is often required
    f. Often refractory to simple fluorinated corticosteroids
    g. Treatment with Burrows solution, diluted 1 to 20 several times a day followed by drying
    h. Treatment with hydrocortisone
    i. Treatment involves removing offending substances or materials
    j. Treatment includes wet compresses

27.63 Any discharge from the vagina is abnormal and requires evaluation because of the high likelihood of infection or neoplasia.

    a. True
    b. False

27.64 What bacteria in the lower genital tract in normal women break down glycogen to lactic acid?

    a. *Gardnerella*
    b. *Streptococci*
    c. *Trichomonas*
    d. *Lactobacilli*

Answers (27.48–27.64)

27.48 a	27.53 b	27.57 all	27.61 a, h
27.49 b	27.54 a, b, c, e, f, g	27.58 b	27.62 d, e
27.50 a	27.55 c, d, f	27.59 b, g, h, i, j	27.63 b
27.51 all	27.56 b	27.60 c, f	27.64 d
27.52 b, c, d			

27.65 In the normal menstrual woman, most bacteria in the vagina are

   a. Aerobic
   b. Anaerobic

27.66 In bacterial vaginosis, the ratio of anaerobic to aerobic bacteria

   a. Increases
   b. Remains the same
   c. Decreases

27.67 Clumps of epithelial cells with numerous bacilli attached to their surface giving them indistinct borders and "ground glass" cytoplasm in appearance, is best associated with

   a. *Trichomonas vaginitis*
   b. *Candida* vaginitis
   c. bacterial vaginosis
   d. cervical dysplasia

27.68–27.71 Instructions: Match the condition with the associated characteristic vaginal discharge.

27.68 Physiologic vaginal secretion _____

27.69 Bacterial vaginosis _____

27.70 *Candida* vaginitis _____

27.71 *Trichomonas vaginitis* _____

   a. White, thick curdy discharge with a pH of 4–5
   b. Gray white thin discharge with a pH of 5–5.5
   c. Yellow white thin discharge with a pH of 3.5–4.5
   d. Yellow green, frothy discharge with a pH of 6–7

27.72 Prophylactic local vaginal therapy with an antifungal agent should be considered when systemic antibiotics (for example, ampicillin for a urinary tract infection) are prescribed.

   a. True
   b. False

Answers (27.65-27.72)

27.65 b	27.67 c	27.69 b	27.71 d
27.66 a	27.68 c	27.70 a	27.72 a

Chapter 28 Final Questions (101 questions)

28.1 For person-to-person transmission, the majority of sexually transmitted diseases require

    a. Exchange of body fluids
    b. Skin-to-skin contact
    c. Warm, dry environments
    d. Anaerobic conditions

28.2 Approximately what percentage of patients with a sexually transmitted disease (STD) have more than one STD?

    a. Less than 3
    b. 5–10
    c. 20–50
    d. 60–80
    e. 95–100

28.3 In approximately what percent of cases will a single sexual contact with a patient with an active herpes infection result in transmission of the infection?

    a. Less than 3%
    b. 5–10
    c. 20–50
    d. 60–80
    e. 95–100

28.4 The normal progression of symptoms in primary herpes infections is a prodromal phase followed by

    a. Ulcer, vesicle, crusting, resolution
    b. Ulcer, crusting, vesicle, resolution
    c. Crusting, vesicle, ulcer, resolution
    d. Vesicle, ulcer, crusting, resolution
    e. Vesicle, crusting, ulcer, resolution

28.5 What percent of genital herpes lesions are caused by the herpes simplex virus type II?

    a. 95
    b. 85
    c. 75
    d. 65
    e. 55

28.6 Generally, patients with herpes genitalis will be completely asymptomatic until the emergence of classic painful vesicular lesions.

    a. True
    b. False

28.7 Approximately what percent of patients with an initial herpes genitalis infection will require hospitalization for pain control or management of urinary complications?

    a. 10
    b. 20
    c. 30
    d. 40
    e. 50

28.8 Primary herpes genitalis infections are characterized by malaise, low grade fever, and inguinal adenopathy in about what percent of patients.

    a. 20
    b. 40
    c. 60
    d. 80

28.9 Viral cultures taken by swab from lesions _____ scrapings from vesicles stained by immunofluorescence techniques for detecting the presence of herpes viral particles.

    a. Are more sensitive than
    b. Are as sensitive as
    c. Are less sensitive than

28.10 Recurrent herpes genitalis lesions occur in approximately what percent of patients?

    a. 10
    b. 30
    c. 50
    d. 70

28.11 Recurrent herpes genitalis lesions are similar in character, _____ severity, and shorter in duration than primary genital lesions.

    a. Greater in
    b. Of the same
    c. Milder in

28.12 Oral acyclovir therapy (200 mg p.o. t.i.d.) is most often used in the treatment of

    a. Primary genital herpes infections
    b. Recurrent genital herpes infections

28.13 Vaginal delivery of a woman with vaginal herpetic lesions is associated with what percent infection in the newborn?

    a. 25
    b. 50
    c. 75
    d. 100

28.14 Neonatal herpes infection acquired at the time of delivery is associated with a mortality rate of approximately

    a. 100%
    b. 80%
    c. 60%
    d. 40%
    e. 20%

Answers (28.1-28.14)

28.1 a, b	28.5 b	28.9 a	28.12 b
28.2 c	28.6 b	28.10 b	28.13 b
28.3 d	28.7 a	28.11 c	28.14 b
28.4 d	28.8 b		

28.15 5% acyclovir cream applied to primary herpes vaginalis lesions for relief of symptoms is associated with _____ in the frequency of recurrence.

a. An increase
b. No change
c. A decrease

28.16 An 18-year-old patient presents with a 5-day history of very painful vulvar ulcers that began as small "blisters." She is now complaining of a low grade fever, headache, and meningismus. Large, painful vulvar and perineal ulcers and inguinal adenopathy are found on examination. The most likely diagnosis is

a. Disseminated gonococcal infection
b. Primary herpes vulvitis
c. Secondary syphilis
d. Lymphogranuloma venereum
e. Molluscum contagiosum

28.17 A 23-year-old G3 P2011 patient presents at term in early labor with an active herpes infection of the labia that has been present for the past 3 days. Membranes are intact. Contractions are regular at 3-min intervals and have been present for the last 3 hr. Her last term labor was 3 years ago and lasted 12 hr, ending in a vaginal delivery of a normal 7-lb infant. Which of the following is the best management of this patient?

a. Anticipate normal labor and delivery
b. Anticipate normal labor and delivery, plan acyclovir prophylaxis for the infant
c. Anticipate rapid labor and delivery but avoid episiotomy
d. Tocolysis and intravenous acyclovir (200 mg)
e. Immediate cesarean delivery

28.18 Which of the following is *not* caused by infection with *Chlamydia* species?

a. Cervicitis
b. Pelvic inflammatory disease
c. Lymphogranuloma venereum
d. Granuloma inguinale

28.19 Chlamydial infections are frequently associated with coinfections by

a. Herpes simplex
b. *N. gonorrhoeae*
c. Human papilloma virus
d. *Treponema pallidum*

28.20 Antibodies to *Chlamydia* are found in approximately what percent of sexually active women?

a. 1–5
b. 10–15
c. 20–40
d. 60–80
e. greater than 90

28.21 Which of the following statements concerning the laboratory diagnosis of *Chlamydia* infection is *not* correct?

a. *Chlamydia* cultures used to confirm the diagnosis require 48–72 hr for results.
b. The enzyme immunoassay (EIA) performed on cervical secretions has a 95% specificity.
c. The monoclonal fluorescent antibody test carried out on dry specimen is faster than the EIA, but has a 40–50% sensitivity and 50% specificity.

28.22 The outpatient treatment with doxycycline or erythromycin for suspected or confirmed *Chlamydia* infection is associated with a cure rate of

a. 95%
b. 80%
c. 65%
d. 50%

28.23 The partner of a patient with confirmed *Chlamydia* infection _____ receive treatment.

a. Should
b. Does not need to

28.24 A common sequela of infection by *Chlamydia trachomatis* is

a. Recurrent vulvar growths
b. Cyclic, migratory arthralgia
c. Involuntary infertility
d. Vaginismus

28.25 *Neisseria gonorrhoeae* is a

a. Gram-negative intracellular diplococcus
b. Gram-negative extracellular diplococcus
c. Gram-positive intracellular diplococcus
d. Gram-positive extracellular diplococcus

28.26 Infection of the pharynx is found in what percent of heterosexual women with confirmed *N. gonorrhoeae* infections?

a. 1–10
b. 10–20
c. 20–30
d. 30–40
e. 40–50

Answers (28.15-28.26)

28.15 b	28.18 d	28.21 c	28.24 c
28.16 b	28.19 b	28.22 a	28.25 a
28.17 e	28.20 c	28.23 a	28.26 b

28.27 For women, a single encounter with a partner infected with *Neisseria gonorrhoeae* is estimated to lead to infection in what percent of cases?

a. 20–30
b. 40–50
c. 60–70
d. 80–90
e. 100

28.28 Following initial infection by *N. gonorrhoeae*, symptoms first appear in

a. 1–2 days
b. 3–5 days
c. 1–2 weeks
d. 3–5 weeks

28.29 Anal infection with *Neisseria gonorrhoeae* is virtually always preceded by episodes of anal intercourse.

a. True
b. False

28.30 A 22-year-old G0 P0 patient has just been successfully treated for *N. gonorrhoeae* salpingitis and asks about her chances of infertility. Based on this single infection her chances of involuntary infertility are approximately

a. <1%
b. 3–5%
c. 8–10%
d. 15–20%

28.31 A 22-year-old G0 P0 patient has just been successfully treated for her third episode of *N. gonorrhoeae* salpingitis and asks about her chances of infertility. Based on these infections her chances of involuntary infertility are approximately

a. <10%
b. 20–25%
c. 40–50%
d. 70–80%

28.32 Lower genital tract infections by *N. gonorrhoeae* are usually characterized by

a. Malodorous, purulent vaginal or urethral discharge
b. Firm, painless vulvar ulcer
c. Inguinal adenopathy
d. Fever, malaise, and labial swelling bilaterally

28.33 The most frequent site of infection with gonorrhea in women is the

a. Bartholin's glands
b. Skene's glands
c. Cervix
d. Urethra
e. Rectal crypts

28.34 Which of the following are required to establish a diagnosis of pelvic inflammatory disease?

a. Cervical tenderness
b. Temperature greater than 38° C
c. Adnexal tenderness
d. Direct (abdominal) tenderness
e. WBC >10,000

28.35 Which of the following are criteria for the hospitalization of patients with pelvic inflammatory disease?

a. Coexisting pregnancy
b. Significant gastrointestinal symptoms
c. Patient less than 20 years of age
d. White blood count greater than 20,000
e. Tuboovarian abscess
f. Nulliparity

28.36 A temperature of at least _____ is a criterion for hospitalization for the treatment of PID.

a. 38° C
b. 38.5° C
c. 39° C
d. 39.5° C
e. 40° C

28.37 Patients with an IUD in place and the diagnosis of PID should be treated on an inpatient rather than outpatient basis.

a. True
b. False

28.38–28.42 Instructions: Match the incidence of the following diagnoses being confused with pelvic inflammatory disease.

28.38 Acute appendicitis _____

28.39 Endometriosis _____

28.40 Adhesions _____

28.41 Corpus luteum bleeding _____

28.42 Ectopic pregnancy _____

a. 7%
b. 11%
c. 12%
d. 17%
e. 25%

28.43 The initiation of treatment for presumed pelvic inflammatory disease (PID) is based on

a. Clinical suspicion
b. Cervical Gram stain
c. Anaerobic culture
d. White blood cell count less than 8,000
e. Rebound tenderness

Answers (28.27-28.43)

28.27 d	28.32 a	28.36 c	28.40 a
28.28 b	28.33 c	28.37 a	28.41 c
28.29 b	28.34 a, c, d	28.38 e	28.42 b
28.30 d	28.35 a, b, d, e, f	28.39 d	28.43 a
28.31 d			

28.44 Oral contraceptive use is associated with _____ incidence of pelvic inflammatory disease.

   a. An increased
   b. An unchanged
   c. A decreased

28.45 The development of cervical cancer is associated with

   a. *Chlamydia trachomatis* infections
   b. Herpes simplex type II infections
   c. Human papilloma virus infections
   d. *Herpes zoster* infections

28.46 In approximately what percent of cases will a single sexual contact with an individual with a human papilloma virus infection result in transmission of the infection?

   a. Less than 3
   b. 5–10
   c. 30–40
   d. 60–70
   e. 95–100

28.47 Lesions caused by human papilloma virus may be confused with those of

   a. Early herpes simplex type II infections
   b. Late lymphogranuloma venereum
   c. Granuloma inguinale
   d. Secondary syphilis

28.48 Human papilloma virus infection is associated with

   a. Condyloma lata
   b. Cyst formation
   c. *Trichomonas* or bacterial vaginosis
   d. Kissing lesions

28.49 Venereal warts caused by HPV are usually characterized by a narrower base and more "heaped-up" appearance, whereas a condyloma lata lesion has a more flattened top.

   a. True
   b. False

28.50 The human papilloma virus is found in approximately what percent of women?

   a. 2.5–4
   b. 6.5–7
   c. 8.5–10
   d   12–15

28.51 Which of the following modalities are used to treat simple condyloma acuminata?

   a. Podophyllin in tincture of Benzoin
   b. Trichloracetic acid
   c. 5-fluorouracil
   d. Acyclovir
   e. Penicillin

28.52 Condylomata acuminata are more resistant to therapy in patients who

   a. Are pregnant
   b. Are immunosuppressed
   c. Smoke
   d. Are overweight
   e. Are diabetic

28.53 Vaginal delivery of a patient with extensive condyloma acuminata of the vulva may result in

   a. Infant herpes encephalopathy
   b. Maternal hemorrhage
   c. Maternal febrile morbidity
   d. Infant laryngeal papillomas

28.54 Transplacental spread of *Treponema pallidum* can occur

   a. Only during the first trimester of pregnancy
   b. Only during the third trimester of pregnancy
   c. At any time during pregancy
   d. Only after rupture of the membranes

28.55 The chancre of primary syphilis will

   a. Spontaneously heal in 3–9 weeks
   b. Coalesce to form running sores
   c. Transform into raised fleshy growths that persist indefinitely
   d. Result in regional adenopathy and abscess formation within 2 weeks

28.56 Which of the following is characteristic of primary syphilis?

   a. Chancre appears 10–60 days after infection
   b. Chancre is often asymptomatic
   c. Serologic testing usually is positive
   d. Accompanying low-grade fever and anorexia are common

28.57 The most contagious stage of syphilis is

   a. Primary
   b. Secondary
   c. Tertiary
   d. Latent

28.58 The mucous patches of secondary syphilis will

   a. Spontaneously heal in 2–6 weeks
   b. Progress to coalesced running sores
   c. Progress to raised fleshy growths that persist indefinitely
   d. Progress with regional adenopathy and abscess formation

---

Answers (28.44-28.58)

28.44 c	28.48 c, d	28.52 a, b, c, e	28.56 a, b
28.45 c	28.49 a	28.53 d	28.57 b
28.46 d	28.50 a	28.54 c	28.58 a
28.47 d	28.51 a, b, c	28.55 a	

28.59–28.60 Instructions: Match the type of test for syphilis with the appropriate example(s).

28.59 Treponemal _____

28.60 Nontreponemal _____

    a. RPR
    b. FTA-ABS
    c. VDRL
    d. MHA-TP
    e. ART

28.61–28.64 Instructions: Match the test for syphilis with its approximate sensitivity in detecting primary syphilis.

28.61 VDRL _____

28.62 RPR _____

28.63 FTA-ABS _____

28.64 MHA-TP _____

    a. 45%
    b. 55%
    c. 65%
    d. 75%
    e. 85%

28.65 Which of the following serologic tests for syphilis has a sensitivity of approximately 100% for secondary syphilis?

    a. VDRL
    b. RPR
    c. FTA-ABS
    d. MHA-TP

28.66 Which of the following may be associated with a false-positive VDRL or RPR test?

    a. Gonorrhea
    b. Malaria
    c. Systemic lupus erythematosus
    d. Connective tissue disease
    e. Herpes virus infection

28.67 Which of the following are characteristic of secondary syphilis?

    a. Asymptomatic chancre that is often missed
    b. Highly infective mucous patches
    c. Low-grade fever, headache, malaise, sore throat, anorexia, and generalized lymphadenopathy
    d. Serologic testing for syphilis generally negative

28.68 Crippling damage to the central nervous system can occur in association with

    a. Primary syphilis
    b. Secondary syphilis
    c. Late (tertiary) syphilis

28.69 Without intervention, the risk of transmission of the HIV virus to a fetus is approximately

    a. 25%
    b. 50%
    c. 75%
    d. 100%

28.70 The diagnosis of HIV infection is established on the basis of

    a. Serum immunoassay
    b. Western blot testing
    c. CD_4 white blood cell counts
    d. Presence of clinical symptoms

28.71 Painless ulcerated vulvar lesions are characteristic of infections with

    a. Herpes simplex, type II
    b. *Chlamydia trachomatis*
    c. *Treponema pallidum*
    d. *Haemophilus ducreyi*

28.72 Which of the following conditions have an incubation period (from infection to clinical symptoms) of greater than 1 month?

    a. Genital herpes
    b. Condyloma acuminata
    c. Chancroid
    d. Lymphogranuloma venereum

28.73 Multiple vulvar vesicles are typical of which of the following infections?

    a. Genital herpes
    b. Condyloma acuminata
    c. Chancroid
    d. Lymphogranuloma venereum

28.74–28.79 Instructions: For genital lesions associated with the following sexually transmitted diseases, select whether the lesion is always/often or rarely/never accompanied by pain.

28.74 Herpes _____

28.75 Genital warts _____

28.76 Syphilis _____

28.77 Chancroid _____

28.78 Lymphogranuloma venereum _____

28.79 Granuloma inguinale _____

    a. Always/often
    b. Rarely/never

Answers (28.59-28.79)

28.59 b, d	28.65 all	28.70 b	28.75 b
28.60 a, c, e	28.66 b, c, d	28.71 c	28.76 b
28.61 d	28.67 b, c	28.72 b	28.77 a
28.62 e	28.68 a	28.73 a	28.78 b
28.63 e	28.69 b	28.74 a	28.79 b
28.64 d			

28.80–28.85 Instructions: Match the sexually transmitted disease with its incubation period.

28.80 Herpes _____

28.81 Genital warts _____

28.82 Syphilis _____

28.83 Chancroid _____

28.84 Lymphogranuloma venereum _____

28.85 Granuloma inguinale _____

    a. 1–8 months
    b. 2–6 days
    c. 8–12 weeks
    d. 1–4 weeks
    e. 10–60 days
    f. 3–7 day

28.86–28.90 Instructions: Match the sexually transmitted disease with the causative organism.

28.86 Genital wart _____

28.87 Syphilis _____

28.88 Chancroid _____

28.89 Lymphogranuloma venereum _____

28.90 Granuloma inguinale _____

    a. Human papilloma virus
    b. *Haemophilus ducreyi*
    c. *Calymmatobacterium granulomatis*
    e. *Chlamydia trachomatis*
    f. *Treponema pallidum*

28.91 Which of the following sexually transmitted diseases is generally *not* associated with lymphadenopathy?

    a. Herpes
    b. Genital warts
    c. Syphilis
    d. Chancroid
    e. Lymphogranuloma venereum
    f. Granuloma inguinale

28.92 Which of the following sexually transmitted diseases is associated with a purulent, hemorrhagic secretion?

    a. Herpes
    b. Genital warts
    c. Syphilis
    d. Chancroid
    e. Lymphogranuloma venereum
    f. Granuloma inguinale

28.93 Which of the following sexually transmitted diseases is characteristically associated with multiple vesicular lesions that often coalesce?

    a. Herpes
    b. Genital warts
    c. Syphilis
    d. Chancroid
    e. Lymphogranuloma venereum
    f. Granuloma inguinale

28.94 Mucopurulent cervicitis is more commonly associated with

    a. *Chlamydia trachomatis*
    b. *Neisseria gonorrhoeae*

28.95 Which of the following statements about acute cervicitis is *incorrect*?

    a. There is polymorphonuclear infiltration of the mucosa
    b. The presenting symptom is often leukorrhea
    c. It may be caused by acute *Neisseria gonorrhoeae* infection
    d. Treatment in the acute phase is surgical
    e. Patients may have associated acute salpingitis

28.96 What percent of normal women with *N. gonorrhoeae* cervicitis will develop acute pelvic inflammatory disease?

    a. 5
    b. 15
    c. 25
    d. 35
    e. 45

28.97 Indolent endometritis is more commonly associated with infection by

    a. *Neisseria gonorrhoeae*
    b. *Chlamydia trachomatis*

28.98–28.100 Instructions: Match the stage of lymphogranuloma venereum with the corresponding characteristic(s).

28.98 Primary lesions _____

28.99 Bubonic stage _____

28.100 Suppurative stage _____

    a. Regional lymphadenopathy
    b. Draining fistulas and lymphatic obstruction
    c. Papules or ulcers

28.101 Perihepatitis, the Fitz-Hugh-Curtis syndrome, is commonly associated with *Neisseria gonorrhoeae* infection but rarely with infection by *Chlamydia trachomatis*.

    a. True
    b. False

Answers (28.80–28.101)

28.80 f	28.86 a	28.92 d	28.97 b
28.81 a	28.87 f	28.93 a	28.98 c
28.82 e	28.88 b	28.94 a	28.99 a
28.83 b	28.89 e	28.95 d	28.100 b
28.84 d	28.90 c	28.96 b	28.101 b
28.85 c	28.91 b		

Chapter 29 Final Questions (41 questions)

29.1 Abortion is generally defined as termination of pregnancy prior to how many weeks of gestation?

a. 12 weeks
b. 15 weeks
c. 20 weeks
d. 25 weeks

29.2 Abortion is generally defined as a pregnancy loss where the fetus weighs less than _____ g?

a. 100
b. 200
c. 500
d. 1000

29.3 Approximately 80% of abortions occur by what gestational age?

a. 6 weeks
b. 8 weeks
c. 10 weeks
d. 12 weeks

29.4 What is the incidence of clinically recognized spontaneous abortion?

a. 5–10%
b. 15–25%
c. 30–40%
d. 50–60%

29.5 What is the most common chromosomal anomaly associated with early spontaneous abortion?

a. Trisomy
b. Monosomy
c. Triploidy
d. Tetraploidy

29.6 A 34-year-old patient reports that her first pregnancy ended in a chromosomally abnormal fetus at 10 weeks of gestation. Her risk of having another such event is

a. Increased compared to her first pregnancy
b. Decreased compared to her first pregnancy
c. The same as in her first pregnancy
d. Indeterminate

29.7 Which of the following are risk factors for spontaneous abortion?

a. Increasing maternal age
b. Increasing paternal age
c. Increasing parity
d. Increasing maternal weight

29.8 A spontaneous abortion at which of the following gestational ages is most likely to be chromosomally abnormal?

a. 6 weeks
b. 10 weeks
c. 14 weeks
d. 20 weeks

29.9 Which of the following is the least likely cause for a second trimester spontaneous abortion?

a. Abnormal placentation
b. Chromosomal abnormality
c. Maternal systemic disease
d. Uterine anomaly

29.10 Which of the following maternal infections has been associated with spontaneous abortion?

a. *Chlamydia trachomatis*
b. *Neisseria gonorrhoeae*
c. *Ureaplasma urealyticum*
d. Herpes zoster

29.11 How is luteal phase defect best diagnosed?

a. Timed serum progesterone
b. Timed endometrial biopsy
c. Timed serum estradiol
d. Timed serum luteinizing hormone
e. Hysterosalpingogram

29.12 Which of the following drugs is used to manage luteal phase defect?

a. Bromocriptine
b. Thyroxine
c. Estrogen
d. Clomiphene citrate

29.13 What is the effect on the rate of spontaneous abortion if the mother smokes more than one pack of cigarettes per day?

a. No effect on the rate
b. Twofold increase
c. Fourfold increase
d. Undetermined effect

29.14 Which location of leiomyomata is most associated with spontaneous abortion?

a. Subserosal
b. Submucosal
c. Intramural

Answers (29.1-29.14)

29.1 c	29.5 a	29.9 b	29.12 d
29.2 c	29.6 a	29.10 c	29.13 b
29.3 d	29.7 a, b, c	29.11 b	29.14 b
29.4 b	29.8 a		

29.15 Myomectomy is indicated only if it is determined that the leiomyomata were the cause of previous spontaneous abortion.

a. True
b. False

29.16 Pregnancies complicated by first trimester bleeding are at higher risk for which of the following?

a. Preeclampsia
b. Preterm delivery
c. Fetal macrosomia
d. Intrauterine infection

29.17 The combination of which two tests are most valuable in the evaluation of threatened abortion?

a. Ultrasound and CBC
b. hCG and CBC
c. Ultrasound and hCG

29.18 What is the lowest hCG level at which transabdominal ultrasound can identify an intact gestational sac?

a. 1500 mIU/mL
b. 2500 mIU/mL
c. 5000 mIU/mL
d. 7500 mIU/mL

29.19 What is the appropriate therapy for a missed abortion at 10 weeks of gestation?

a. Hysterotomy
b. Suction curettage
c. Administration of Methergine (methylergonovine maleate)
d. Dilatation and evacuation

29.20 Approximately what proportion of threatened abortions proceed to spontaneous abortion?

a. 10%
b. 25%
c. 50%
d. 75%

29.21 What is the appropriate time for placement of a McDonald cerclage?

a. Prior to pregnancy
b. Early in pregnancy, with minimal dilatation
c. Early in pregnancy, after dilation has reached 3 cm
d. After an abortion

29.22 Asherman's syndrome is best diagnosed by which of the following?

a. History
b. Physical examination
c. Hysteroscopy
d. Ultrasound

29.23 Which of the following are techniques for second trimester pregnancy termination?

a. Dilatation and evacuation
b. Prostaglandin vaginal suppository
c. Intraamniotic infusion of hypertonic saline
d. Suction curettage

29.24 Which of the following may characterize septic abortion?

a. Sepsis
b. Shock
c. Renal failure
d. Hemorrhage

29.25 Which of the following should be included in the management of septic abortion?

a. Intravenous fluids
b. Antibiotics
c. Evacuation of the uterus
d. Prostaglandins

29.26 Abortion is the termination of a pregnancy prior to viability, typically defined as _____ weeks from the first day of the last normal menstrual period.

a. 16
b. 18
c. 20
d. 22

29.27 Trisomy accounts for _____ of chromosomal abnormalities identified in early spontaneous abortion.

a. 20–30%
b. 30–40%
c. 40–50%
d. 50–60%
e. 60–70%

29.28 Recurrent abortion is defined as _____ consecutive abortions or a total of _____ spontaneous abortions.

a. 2, 2
b. 2, 3
c. 3, 2
d. 3, 3

29.29 Recurrent abortion is associated with a _____ chance that one parent is a symptomless carrier of a chromosomal abnormality.

a. 1%
b. 3%
c. 5%
d. 7%

Answers (29.15–29.29)

29.15 a	29.19 b	29.23 a, b, c	29.27 c
29.16 b	29.20 c	29.24 all	29.28 b
29.17 c	29.21 b	29.25 a, b, c	29.29 b
29.18 c	29.22 c	29.26 c	

29.30 Although septate uterus is associated with recurrent abortion, only about _____ of women with septate uteri have problems with fetal wastage.

 a. 5%
 b. 15%
 c. 25%
 d. 35%

29.31 The classic history of incompetent cervix is sudden symptomless expulsion of a normal sac and fetus.

 a. True
 b. False

29.32 When labor occurs with a cerclage in place, the laboring process is allowed to pull a cerclage suture through the effacing cervix so as to avoid precipitous labor.

 a. True
 b. False

29.33 Treatment of Asherman's syndrome involves lysis of the adhesions and treatment with

 a. Estrogen
 b. Progesterone
 c. Steroids
 d. Clomiphene citrate
 e. Oral contraceptives

29.34 The treatment of spontaneous first trimester abortion must include uterine curettage to ensure that all tissue is removed.

 a. True
 b. False

29.35 The differential diagnosis of threatened abortion includes

 a. Placental abruption
 b. Friable cervix
 c. Cervical laceration
 d. Polyp

29.36 The diagnosis of threatened abortion has no clinical implication when the pregnancy carries into the third trimester.

 a. True
 b. False

29.37 All causes of bleeding in the first trimester are classified as threatened abortion.

 a. True
 b. False

29.38 Women who smoke more than one package of cigarettes per day have a _____ increase in their rate of spontaneous abortion.

 a. Onefold
 b. Twofold
 c. Threefold
 d. Fourfold

29.39 Which of these medical conditions are associated with an increased risk of first trimester spontaneous abortion.

 a. Diabetes
 b. Luteal phase inadequacy
 c. Hypothyroidism
 d. Hyperthyroidism

29.40 Maternal infections associated with spontaneous abortion include

 a. *Listeria monocytogenes*
 b. *Candida albicans*
 c. *Mycoplasma hominis*
 d. *Ureaplasma urealyticum*

29.41 Second trimester abortions are less likely to be chromosomal and more likely to be due to maternal systemic disease, abnormal placentation, or other anatomic considerations than first trimester abortions.

 a. True
 b. False

Answers (29.30-29.41)

29.30 b	29.33 a	29.36 b	29.39 a, b, d
29.31 a	29.34 b	29.37 b	29.40 a, c, d
29.32 b	29.35 b, d	29.38 b	29.41 a

Chapter 30 Final Questions (49 questions)

30.1 About what percentage of patients with a prior ectopic pregnancy will have a subsequent full term birth?

    a. 30
    b. 50
    c. 70
    d. 90

30.2 Currently, the ratio of ectopic:intrauterine pregnancies in the United States is about 1:

    a. 25
    b. 65
    c. 125
    d. 275

30.3 Which of the following causes the greatest increase in the risk of ectopic pregnancy?

    a. Use of oral contraceptives
    b. Intrauterine device contraceptive use
    c. Previous elective abortion
    d. Previous ectopic pregnancy

30.4 At what gestational age do tubal ectopic pregnancies usually present clinical symptoms?

    a. 2 weeks
    b. 4 weeks
    c. 6 weeks
    d. 8 weeks
    e. Varies with location

30.5 Ectopic pregnancy should be suspected in women who present with which of the following?

    a. Acute pelvic pain
    b. Lower abdominal pain
    c. Vaginal bleeding
    d. Acute nausea and vomiting
    e. Amenorrhea

30.6 Which of the following physical findings is potentially compatible with the diagnosis of ectopic pregnancy?

    a. Abdominal tenderness
    b. Adnexal mass
    c. Uterine enlargement
    d. Normal blood pressure

30.7 What is the etiology for vaginal bleeding in cases of ectopic pregnancy?

    a. Coagulopathy
    b. Sloughing of decidua
    c. Bleeding from the tube
    d. Progesterone excess

30.8 If no villi are observed on uterine curettage, which of the following diagnoses are ruled out?

    a. Combined pregnancy
    b. Heterotropic pregnancy
    c. Tubal pregnancy
    d. None of the above diagnoses are ruled out

30.9 The great majority of ectopic pregnancies implant in the

    a. Ovary
    b. Cervix
    c. Peritoneal cavity
    d. Fallopian tube

30.10 Of those ectopic pregnancies that implant in the fallopian tube, about 80% implant in the

    a. Isthmus
    b. Fimbriae
    c. Ampulla

30.11 Which of the following laboratory and radiologic findings are consistent with the diagnosis of ectopic pregnancy?

    a. Empty uterine cavity on ultrasound
    b. A white blood count of 16,500
    c. A hematocrit of 37%
    d. Serum progesterone of 25 ng/mL

30.12 A culdocentesis that obtains 3 cc of straw-colored fluid would be considered

    a. Negative
    b. Positive
    c. Nondiagnostic
    d. Unsatisfactory

30.13 A pregnancy in which of the following implantation sites is *likely* to reach term?

    a. Abdomen
    b. Ovary
    c. Cervix
    d. Fallopian tube
    e. None of the above implantation sites is likely to reach term

30.14 A heterotopic pregnancy is defined as

    a. An ectopic pregnancy outside the fallopian tube
    b. Twin ectopic pregnancy in the same site
    c. Coexistent intrauterine and ectopic pregnancies
    d. Ectopic pregnancy in two different sites outside the uterus

Answers (30.1-30.14)

30.1 b	30.5 a, b, c, e	30.9 d	30.12 a
30.2 b	30.6 all	30.10 c	30.13 e
30.3 d	30.7 b	30.11 all	30.14 c
30.4 e	30.8 d		

30.15 Which of the following is *not* one of Spiegelberg's criteria for ovarian pregnancy?

    a. An intact fallopian tube
    b. Ovary in the normal position
    c. Ovarian tissue in the wall of the gestational sac
    d. A fallopian tube connected to the uterus by the ovarian ligament

30.16 Methotrexate is classified as an

    a. Antibiotic
    b. Alkylating agent
    c. Antiviral
    d. Folinic acid antagonist

30.17 Which of the following is not useful in the diagnosis of an ectopic pregnancy?

    a. Arias-Stella reaction on histologic examination
    b. Gestational sac visualized on ultrasound examination of the fallopian tube
    c. Empty uterus on ultrasound accompanied by hCG level of 8500 mlU/mL
    d. Laparoscopic visualization of 3-cm mass in the fallopian tube

30.18 The incidence of tubal ectopic pregnancy has been steadily rising in the United States, primarily because of an increased

    a. Use of oral contraceptives
    b. Incidence of elective abortion
    c. Incidence of pelvic inflammatory disease
    d. Delay in the onset of sexual activity in couples

30.19 The mortality associated with ectopic pregnancy has decreased from 3.5 maternal deaths per 1000 cases of ectopic pregnancy to less than 1 case per 1000 cases of ectopic pregnancy, primarily because of

    a. Earlier detection of ectopic pregnancy
    b. Greater availability of blood
    c. Modern intensive care technology to combat shock and blood loss
    d. The increased use of sophisticated laparoscopic surgical techniques

30.20 Fewer than _____ of women who have had an ectopic pregnancy subsequently are successful in having a live full term birth.

    a. One-quarter
    b. One-half
    c. Three-quarters

30.21 Which of the following is the most significant risk factor for ectopic pregnancy.

    a. Oral contraceptive use
    b. IUD use
    c. Salpingitis
    d. Abnormal Pap smear

30.22 Women 35–44 years of age have a _____ increase in the rate of ectopic pregnancy as compared with women 15–23 years of age.

    a. Twofold
    b. Threefold
    c. Fourfold
    d. Fivefold

30.23 Over one-half of all ectopic pregnancies occur in women who have had _____ or more pregnancies.

    a. 2
    b. 3
    c. 4
    d. 5

30.24 Sterilization increases the risk of ectopic pregnancy.

    a. True
    b. False

30.25 The classic symptom triad of abdominal pain, amenorrhea, and vaginal bleeding is noted in virtually all cases of ectopic pregnancy.

    a. True
    b. False

30.26 The pain of tubal ectopic pregnancy is on the side of the ectopic pregnancy in virtually all cases.

    a. True
    b. False

30.27 Tubal ectopic pregnancy is more likely to be symptomatic if located in the _____ portion of the fallopian tube.

    a. Proximal
    b. Distal

30.28 Hemoperitoneum associated with ruptured ectopic pregnancy may result in irritation of the diaphragm and referred pain to the

    a. Flank
    b. Shoulder
    c. Mid-chest
    d. Arm

Answers (30.15-30.28)

30.15 d	30.19 a	30.23 b	30.26 b
30.16 d	30.20 b	30.24 b	30.27 a
30.17 a	30.21 c	30.25 b	30.28 b
30.18 c	30.22 b		

30.29   Syncope is reported in about _____ patients with ruptured tubal ectopic pregnancies and hemoperitoneum.

    a. one-third of
    b. two-thirds of
    c. all

30.30   The pain of tubal ectopic pregnancy is virtually always constant and unilateral.

    a. True
    b. False

30.31   Nowadays, about _____ of patients with tubal ectopic pregnancy present with hypovolemic shock.

    a. 5%
    b. 15%
    c. 25%
    d. 35%

30.32   Patients with a fever *and* the symptoms of ectopic pregnancy are usually found to have pelvic inflammatory disease or appendicitis rather than ectopic pregnancy.

    a. True
    b. False

30.33   The absence of a tender adnexal mass on pelvic examination essentially rules out ectopic pregnancy as a diagnosis after 6 weeks of amenorrhea.

    a. True
    b. False

30.34   Urinary pregnancy tests in common use are positive in _____ of ectopic pregnancy.

    a. 90%
    b. 80%
    c. 70%
    d. 60%

30.35   Failure of a quantitative β-hCG level to increase by at least _____ in 48 hr indicates the pregnancy is not growing and increases the suspicion of ectopic pregnancy.

    a. 90%
    b. 75%
    c. 66%
    d. 50%

30.36   A rise of a quantitative β-hCG level of 32% in 48 hr is diagnostic of a tubal ectopic pregnancy.

    a. True
    b. False

30.37   Transabdominal pelvic ultrasonography should be able to identify an intrauterine pregnancy by the time the serum β-hCG level reaches 6000 mIU/mL.

    a. True
    b. False

30.38   Transvaginal pelvic ultrasonography should be able to identify an intrauterine pregnancy by the time the serum β-hCG level reaches at least _____ mIU/mL.

    a. 500
    b. 1500
    c. 2500
    d. 3500

30.39   In a patient with symptoms consistent with ectopic pregnany, a white blood cell count of greater than 20,000 WBC/dL may be more consistent with infection than ectopic pregnancy.

    a. True
    b. False

30.40   As a clinical cut-off, a serum progesterone of _____ ng/mL or less indicates a nonviable pregnancy.

    a. 1
    b. 5
    c. 10
    d. 15

30.41   What percent of all abnormal pregnancies, ectopic or intrauterine, are associated with serum progesterone levels of greater than 25 ng/mL?

    a. 0.5
    b. 2.5
    c. 4.5
    d. 6.5
    e. 7.5

30.42   The identification of an intrauterine gestation in a patient with symptoms consistent with ectopic pregnancy rules out the diagnosis of ectopic pregnancy.

    a. True
    b. False

30.43   The Arias-Stella reaction is diagnostic of ectopic pregnancy.

    a. True
    b. False

Answers (30.29-30.43)

30.29 a	30.33 b	30.37 a	30.41 b
30.30 b	30.34 a	30.38 b	30.42 b
30.31 a	30.35 c	30.39 a	30.43 b
30.32 b	30.36 b	30.40 b	

30.44 A positive culdocentesis is diagnostic of ectopic pregnancy.

a. True
b. False

30.45 Because of the small amount of gestational tissue involved in most tubal ectopic pregnancies, the administration of Rh immune globulin (Rho-GAM) is not required after surgical treatment.

a. True
b. False

30.46 Combined pregnancy (simultaneous intrauterine and extrauterine gestations) occurs in about 1 in _____ pregnancies.

a. 10,000
b. 20,000
c. 30,000
d. 40,000

30.47 Survival of the intrauterine twin of a combined pregnancy is resported in about one in _____ cases.

a. Two
b. Three
c. Four
d. Five

30.48 Spiegelberg's criteria for ovarian pregnancy include

a. Fallopian tube intact
b. Fallopian tube separate from ovary
c. Fallopian tube free of gestational tissue
d. Ovary in normal positon
e. Ovarian tissue in wall of gestational sac

30.49 Rubin's criteria for cervical pregnancy include

a. Cervical glands opposite placental attachment
b. Chorionic villi in cervical canal
c. Chorionic villi in corpus uteri
d. Internal cervical os closed, external cervical os open or closed

Answers (30.44-30.49)

30.44 b
30.45 b
30.46 c
30.47 b
30.48 all
30.49 a, b, d

Chapter 31 Final Questions (59 questions)

31.1   Which of the following may be symptoms of pelvic relaxation?

   a. Pelvic pressure
   b. Dyspareunia
   c. Stress incontinence (urinary)
   d. Intermittent diarrhea

31.2   The approximate percent of women who will at some point in their lifes have loss of urine during coughing, laughing, or other stress is

   a. 5
   b. 20
   c. 50
   d. 70
   e. 90

31.3   Approximately what percent of women suffer significant, recurrent urinary incontenence in the presence of increased intraabdominal pressure?

   a. <5
   b. 10–15
   c. 20–25
   d. 30–35
   e. 40–45

31.4   Pelvic support is provided by which of the following structures?

   a. Pelvic floor muscles
   b. Fascia
   c. Ligaments

31.5   In a patient with enterocele there is a descent or herniation of the

   a. Uterus
   b. Peritoneal cavity through the vagina
   c. Bladder
   d. Urethra
   e. Rectum

31.6–31.9   Instructions: Match the clinical situation with the appropriate definition.

31.6   A 45-year-old patient complains of frequent loss of urine when she coughs, laughs, or strains. The volume lost is small, but it occurs frequently. She does not report any dysuria. _____

31.7   A 45-year-old diabetic patient presents complaining of frequent loss of urine. The volume lost is small, but it occurs almost continuously. She does not report any sense of fullness, urgency, or dysuria. She voids frequently but in small amounts. She does not ever feel "full" but also never has the sense that she has completely emptied her bladder. _____

31.8   A 22-year-old patient presents complaining of occasional loss of urine. The volume lost is large when it occurs. She reports a sense of intense fullness and urgency just before the urine is lost. She voids infrequently but in large amounts. She does not ever feel that she "gets enough warning" to get to the bathroom. _____

31.9   A 22-year-old patient presents complaining of occasional loss of urine. The volume lost is large when it occurs. She reports the loss occurs primarily when she changes position (e.g., rising from a chair) or when she is around running water. _____

   a. Stress incontinence
   b. Urgency incontinence
   c. Overflow incontinence
   d. Behavioral incontinence
   e. Enuresis

31.10   A symptomatic rectocele is often characterized by

   a. Loss of urine during stress
   b. Urinary retention
   c. Intermittent diarrhea
   d. Difficulty passing stools

31.11   A cystocele may best be demonstrated clinically by means of

   a. Supine Valsalva maneuver
   b. Use of a Sims speculum to retract the anterior vaginal wall
   c. Gentle traction on the cervix
   d. Observing posterior rotation of the anterior vaginal wall in response to change in position

Answers (31.1-31.11)

31.1 a, b, c	31.4 a, b, c	31.7 c	31.10 d
31.2 c	31.5 b	31.8 b	31.11 a
31.3 b	31.6 a	31.9 b	

31.12 A patient who needs to press on the back of her vagina with her fingers to facilitate having a bowel movement is most likely to have a(n)

 a. Rectocele
 b. Cystocele
 c. Urethral prolapse (urethrocele)
 d. Enterocele

31.13 A patient who loses urine when she coughs or sneezes is most likely to have a(n)

 a. Rectocele
 b. Cystocele
 c. Urethral prolapse (urethrocele)
 d. Enterocele

31.14 Small bowel herniation is found in

 a. Rectocele
 b. Cystocele
 c. Urethral prolapse (urethrocele)
 d. Enterocele

31.15 Which of the following is lined with peritoneum, making it a true hernia?

 a. Rectocele
 b. Cystocele
 c. Urethral prolapse (urethrocele)
 d. Enterocele

31.16 Which of the following is *not* a manifestation of pelvic relaxation?

 a. Uterine prolapse
 b. Procidentia
 c. Vaginal vault prolapse
 d. Uterine retroversion

31.17 A cough causes genuine stress incontinence when the bladder pressure _____ urethral pressure.

 a. Is less than
 b. Is the same as
 c. Is greater than

31.18 Which of the following conditions are associated with urinary incontinence?

 a. Bladder atony
 b. Bladder spasm
 c. Psychosis
 d. Fistulous tract

31.19–31.21 Instructions: Match the clinical situation with the type of prolapse.

31.19 The structure (e.g., the cervix) is noted to descend to the upper third of the vagina _____

31.20 The structure is noted to descend to the vaginal introitus _____

31.21 The structure is noted to descend to outside the vaginal opening _____

 a. First-degree prolapse
 b. Second-degree prolapse
 c. Third-degree prolapse
 d. Procidentia

31.22 A "Q-tip test" is used to evaluate

 a. The presence of residual urine
 b. Supports for the posterior vaginal wall
 c. Cervical descent down the vaginal canal
 d. Urethral mobility
 e. Urethral sensitivity

31.23 When performing a "Q-tip test," incontinence is generally associated with upward rotation of

 a. Less than 5 degrees
 b. 10 degrees
 c. 20 degrees
 d. 30 degrees

31.24 The key anatomic abnormality in stress incontenence is

 a. A urethrovesical angle less than 90 degrees
 b. The urethra prolapsing at times of increased intraabdominal pressure
 c. The pressure of bladder herniation
 d. The urethra dropping outside the influence of intraabdominal pressure while the bladder remains within

31.25 Which of the following may result from the vaginal mucosa prolapsing beyond the introitus?

 a. Bleeding
 b. Ulceration
 c. Infection

31.26 How is pelvic relaxation best demonstrated?

 a. With the patient at rest, supine
 b. With the patient at rest, upright
 c. With the patient straining
 d. With the patient under anesthesia

Answers (31.12-31.26)

31.12 a	31.16 d	31.20 b	31.24 d
31.13 c	31.17 c	31.21 c	31.25 all
31.14 d	31.18 all	31.22 d	31.26 c
31.15 d	31.19 a	31.23 d	

31.27   While a speculum is retracting the posterior vaginal wall, a 51-year-old patient is asked to strain down. There is a bulge from the anterior vaginal wall. This is most likely a

a. Rectocele
b. Cystocele
c. Enterocele
d. Vaginal vault prolapse

31.28   Which of the following is often associated with procidentia?

a. Fecal incontinence
b. Constipation
c. Ureteral obstruction
d. Bladder atony

31.29–31.31   Instructions: Match the drug used to treat incontinence with its appropriate category.

31.29   Anticholinergic _____

31.30   Musculotropic _____

31.31   Antidepressant _____

a. Oxybutynin chloride (Ditropan)
b. Metaproterenol sulfate (Alupent)
c. Flavoxate hydrochloride (Urispas)
d. Diazepam (Valium)
e. Imipramine hydrochloride (Tofranil)

31.32   Which of the following is the *least* effective treatment for urgency incontinence?

a. Biofeedback
b. Surgery
c. Bladder training
d. Medical therapy

31.33   Bladder training programs have which of the following goals?

a. Increasing the amount of time between voiding
b. Decreasing the duration of urine flow
c. Decreasing bladder volume
d. Increasing midstream urine flow

31.34   The purpose of Kegel exercises is to

a. Strengthen pelvic floor muscles
b. Improve bladder capacity and control
c. Tighten uterine ligaments
d. Increase bladder awareness

31.35   Kegel exercises may be useful in patients with

a. Second degree prolapse of the uterus
b. Symptomatic rectoceles
c. Mild stress incontinence
d. Dyspareunia

31.36   The main function of pessaries is to

a. Obstruct the urethra
b. Provide mechanical support
c. Focus intraabdominal pressure toward the introitus
d. Decrease bladder capacity

31.37–31.40   Instructions: Match the procedure with the pelvic defect it is designed to correct.

31.37   Hysterectomy _____

31.38   Colpocleisis _____

31.39   Posterior colporrhapy _____

31.40   Paravaginal repair _____

a. Vaginal vault prolapse
b. Stress incontinence
c. Uterine prolapse
d. Rectocele

31.41–31.44   Instructions: Match the statement with the surgical procedure for that best relates to it.

31.41   Does not require an abdominal incision _____

31.42   Obliterates the vaginal canal _____

31.43   Provides a sling for the vagina _____

31.44   Decreases the possibility of future enterocele formation _____

a. Marshall-Marchetti-Krantz
b. Burch
c. Pereyra
d. LeFort
e. Moskowitz

31.45   The first step in the treatment of a vesicovaginal fistula first noted 4 days after an abdominal hysterectomy is

a. Catheter drainage of the bladder
b. Insertion of a vaginal pessary
c. Surgical dissection of the fistulous tract
d. Irradiation to create scarring

31.46   Approximately what percent of women will suffer a urinary tract infection during their lifetime?

a. Less than 5
b. 10–15
c. 20–25
d. 30–35
e. 40–45

Answers (31.27-31.46)

31.27 b	31.32 b	31.37 c	31.42 d
31.28 c	31.33 a	31.38 a	31.43 c
31.29 a	31.34 a	31.39 d	31.44 e
31.30 c	31.35 c	31.40 b	31.45 a
31.31 e	31.36 b	31.41 d	31.46 b

31.47 The relative prevalence of urinary tract infections in men and women (M:F) is

  a. 10:1
  b. 5:1
  c. 1:1
  d. 1:5
  e. 1:10

31.48 In women, most urinary tract infections occur through

  a. Hematogenous seeding
  b. Lymphatic spread
  c. Ascending urethral contamination
  d. Retained urine

31.49 Which of the following increase the risk of bladder infection in women as compared to men

  a. Relatively shorter urethra in women
  b. Estrogen effects
  c. Sexual activity
  d. Trauma
  e. Proximity of rectal organisms

31.50 Asymptomatic bacteria is found in approximately what percent of postmenopausal women?

  a. Less than 5
  b. 10–15
  c. 20–25
  d. 30–35
  e. 40–45

31.51 Most first urinary tract infections in women are caused by

  a. β-streptococcus
  b. *Proteus mirabilis*
  c. *E. coli*
  d. *Clostridium perfringens*

31.52 Irritation of the trigone (trigonitis) causes which of the following symptoms?

  a. Frequency
  b. Urgency
  c. Nocturia
  d. Dysuria

31.53 A single drop of uncentrifuged urine is examined under the microscope and two white blood cells per high power field are found. The likelihood that this patient has bladder infection is

  a. 15%
  b. 30%
  c. 50%
  d. 70%
  e. 90%

31.54 The culture of a urine sample is reported to show greater than 100,000 colonies of "mixed flora." This is indicative of

  a. Infection of the proximal urethra
  b. Trigonitis
  c. Upper urinary tract infection
  d. Contaminated specimen

31.55 In a symptomatic patient, which of the following is indicative of lower urinary tract infection?

  a. 10,000 colonies of *E. coli*
  b. 10,000 colonies of *Staphylococcus aureus*
  c. >100,000 colonies of mixed flora
  d. 1,000 colonies of *Bacteroides* sp.

31.56 When treating an uncomplicated first episode of lower urinary tract infection, which of the following is most likely to precipitate a concomitant vaginal yeast infection?

  a. Ascorbic acid
  b. Phenazopyridine hydrochloride (Pyridium)
  c. Nitrofurantoin (Macrodantin)
  d. Ampicillin

31.57 Which is the *least* likely finding in patients with simple cystitis?

  a. Frequency
  b. Dysuria
  c. Fever
  d. Suprapubic tenderness

31.58 Which of the following provides urinary analgesia?

  a. Ascorbic acid
  b. Phenazopyridine hydrochloride (Pyridium)
  c. Nitrofurantoin (Macrodantin)
  d. Ampicillin

31.59 In the region where the urethra joins the bladder, the urethra is surrounded by circular smooth muscle fibers called

  a. The pubovesicocervical neck
  b. The external sphincter
  c. Retzius' angle
  d. The internal sphincter

Answers (31.47-31.59)

31.47 e	31.51 c	31.54 d	31.57 c
31.48 c	31.52 a, b, c	31.55 a	31.58 b
31.49 a, c, d, e	31.53 e	31.56 d	31.59 d
31.50 b			

Chapter 32 Final Questions (37 questions)

32.1 Which of the following symptoms is *not* associated with endometriosis?

a. Infertility
b. Dysmenorrhea
c. Incontinence
d. Dyspareunia
e. Chronic pelvic pain

32.2 The diagnosis of endometriosis is suspected on the basis of

a. Culture and sensitivity
b. Histology
c. Typical history
d. Pelvic examination
e. Family history

32.3 Which of the following is thought to be associated with an increased risk of endometriosis?

a. Early menopause
b. Multiparity
c. First degree relative with endometriosis
d. Middle to upper income socioeconomic status

32.4 Sampson's theory of the development of endometriosis is based on the occurrence of

a. Retrograde menstruation
b. Multipotent celomic cells
c. Vascular and lymphatic dissemination
d. A viral DNA vector

32.5 The occurrence of distant implants of endometriosis (such as in the pleural cavity or kidney) supports the theory of endometriosis development based on

a. Retrograde menstruation
b. Multipotent celomic cells
c. Vascular and lymphatic dissemination
d. A viral DNA vector

32.6 The most common site in which endometriosis is found is the

a. Posterior cul-de-sac
b. Uterosacral ligaments
c. Ovary
d. Fallopian tube

32.7 Which of the following findings at the time of laparoscopy is *not* consistent with a diagnosis of mild endometriosis?

a. 1-mm vascular hemorrhagic area in the posterior cul-de-sac
b. Multiple rust-colored spots on peritoneal surfaces, 1–2 mm in diameter
c. Small puckered white lesions on the uterosacral ligaments
d. Small, firm, yellow nodules on the anterior surface of the uterus

32.8 What percent of women with endometriosis have ovarian involvement?

a. 10
b. 20
c. 40
d. 60
e. 90

32.9 The term *endometrioma* refers to

a. An isolated collection of endometriosis involving an ovary and creating a tumor
b. Any endometrial implant greater than 5 cm
c. Endometrial tissue found deep within the wall of the uterus
d. Endometrial implants that are symptomatic

32.10 The histologic diagnosis of endometriosis requires the presence of which of the following?

a. Glands
b. Stroma
c. Decidual reaction
d. Hemosiderin-laden macrophages

32.11 In what percent of cases will the clinical diagnosis of endometriosis *not* be supported by histological findings?

a. 5
b. 15
c. 30
d. 50

32.12 The presence of endometrial glands and stroma within the wall of the uterus is termed

a. Endometriosis
b. Adenomyosis
c. Endometrial hyperplasia
d. Endometrioma

32.13 It is estimated that approximately _____ of women with adenomyosis are asymptomatic.

a. 5%
b. 15%
c. 40%
d. 60%
e. 85%

32.14 Which of the following symptoms is *not* consistent with a clinical diagnosis of endometriosis?

a. Cyclic pelvic pain
b. "Deep thrust" dyspareunia
c. Vaginal bleeding between periods
d. Intermittent fevers
e. Painful bowel movements

Answers (32.1–32.14)

32.1 c	32.5 c	32.9 a	32.12 b
32.2 c, d	32.6 c	32.10 a, b, d	32.13 c
32.3 c	32.7 d	32.11 c	32.14 d
32.4 a	32.8 d		

32.15 The most common cause for infertility in patients with endometriosis is

a. Pelvic scarring
b. Persistent anovulation
c. Elevated levels of FSH
d. Increased macrophage activity

32.16 What is the estimated overall incidence of endometriosis in women in the general population?

a. 0.1%
b. 1%
c. 10%
d. 20%
e. 35%

32.17 The prevalence of endometriosis in infertile women is approximately

a. 5%
b. 10–15%
c. 20–25%
d. 35–40%
e. 60–65%

32.18 In which age group is endometriosis most likey to be diagnosed?

a. Prepubertal (less than 12 years of age)
b. Adolescent (13–17 years)
c. 20–35 years
d. Perimenopausal (45–52 years)
e. Postmenopausal (63–68 years)

32.19 Vaginal bleeding between periods occurs in approximately what proportion of women with endometriosis?

a. less than 5%
b. 10–15%
c. 20–25%
d. 30–35%
e. 40–45%

32.20 The dysmenorrhea associated with endometriosis is

a. Not necessarily proportional to the extent of the disease
b. Due to a fixed, retroverted uterus
c. A result of uterosacral involvment
d. Worse in patients who are infertile

32.21 A typical finding on pelvic examination of patients with adenomyosis is

a. Retroversion of the uterus
b. Reduced mobility of the uterus
c. Adnexal thickening
d. Nodularity of the cul-de-sac
e. Firm, symmetrical enlargement of the uterus

32.22 Which of the following physical findings is consistent with a clinical diagnosis of endometriosis?

a. Retroversion of the uterus
b. Reduced mobility of the uterus
c. Adnexal thickening
d. Nodularity of the cul-de-sac
e. Firm, symmetrical enlargement of the uterus

32.23 According to the American Fertility Society classification of endometriosis, a patient with complete obliteration of the cul-de-sac by adhesions has

a. Minimal disease
b. Mild disease
c. Moderate disease
d. Severe disease

32.24 According to the American Fertility Society classification of endometriosis, a patient with extensive ovarian adhesions enclosing two-thirds of both ovaries but no other signs of disease has

a. Minimal disease
b. Mild disease
c. Moderate disease
d. Severe disease

32.25 Infertility in the presence of minimal endometriosis is due to

a. Adhesions
b. Tubal obstruction
c. Autoantibodies
d. Prostaglandin overproduction
e. Unknown causes

32.26 What type of abnormal bleeding is *not* associated with endometriosis?

a. Menorrhagia
b. Anovulatory bleeding
c. Premenstrual staining

32.27 A 25-year-old patient is found to have minimal endometriosis at the time of laparoscopy for infertility. Appropriate treatment for this patient is

a. Administration of oral contraceptives.
b. Administration of a GnRH agonist.
c. Laser surgery
d. Expectant management

Answers (32.15-32.27)

32.15 a	32.19 d	32.22 a, b, c, d	32.25 e
32.16 b	32.20 a	32.23 d	32.26 a
32.17 d	32.21 e	32.24 c	32.27 d
32.18 c			

32.28   In a patient that has undergone total abdominal hysterectomy and bilateral salpingo-oophorectomy for endometriosis, estrogen-replacement therapy should be

   a. Begun immediately
   b. Begun after follow-up laparoscopy 1 year later
   c. Begun only after 5 symptom free years
   d. Avoided indefinitely

32.29   Continuous administration of combination oral contraceptives is effective in treating endometriosis because they

   a. Lower FSH and LH levels
   b. Induce anovulation
   c. Reduce endometrial prostaglandin production
   d. Induce a decidual reaction in the endometrial implants

32.30   Medical therapy for endometriosis can be expected to accomplish which of the following?

   a. Improvement of dyspareunia
   b. Reduction of adhesions
   c. Reduction of cyclic pain
   d. Reduced menstrual flow

32.31   Conservative surgical therapy for moderate endometriosis is associated with a pregnancy rate of approximately

   a. Less than 10%
   b. 20%
   c. 40%
   d. 60%
   e. 80%

32.32–32.34   Instructions: Match the drug(s) used to treat endometriosis with the appropriate description.

32.32   Induces "pseudopregnancy" _____

32.33   Side effects include hot flushes and alterations of lipoprotein metabolisms _____

32.34   Suppresses FSH and LH _____

   a. Oral contraceptives
   b. Danazol (17 α-ethinyl testosterone derivative)
   c. GnRH agonist
   d. Medroxyprogesterone acetate

32.35   GnRH agonists act by

   a. Suppression of endometrial responsiveness
   b. Down-regulation of the pituitary gland
   c. Hyperstimulation of the ovary
   d. Stimulation of the metabolism of progesterone

32.36   Definitive surgical therapy for endometriosis includes

   a. Total abdominal hysterectomy
   b. Bilateral salpingo-oophorectomy
   c. Lysis of adhesions
   d. Removal of endometriotic implants

32.37   The diagnosis of endometriosis is confirmed on the basis of

   a. Culture and sensitivity
   b. Histology
   c. Typical history
   d. Pelvic examination
   e. Family history

Answers (32.28-32.37)

32.28 a	32.31 d	32.34 b, c	32.36 all
32.29 d	32.32 a	32.35 b	32.37 b
32.30 a, c, d	32.33 b		

Chapter 33 Final Questions (33 questions)

33.1   What percent of women and children in the United States are victims of sexual assault?

a. Less than 1
b. 5
c. 15
d. More than 25

33.2   Because of the stigmata associated with sexual assault, it is estimated that only 1 in _____ victims seeks help of any kind.

a. 2
b. 4
c. 6
d. 8
e. 10

33.3   Which of the following are direct responsibilities of the health care team related to victims of sexual assault?

a. Care for the victim's emotional needs
b. Assistance to authorities in identifying the perpetrator
c. Collection of forensic specimens
d. Evaluation and treatment of the victim's medical condition

33.4   The most serious emotional problem faced by the sexual assault victim is

a. Gender identity conflict
b. Fear of infection
c. Loss of control
d. Uncontrolled anger

33.5   Threatened or actual violence is always an integral part of sexual assault.

a. True
b. False

33.6–33.8   Instructions: Match the stage of the rape trauma syndrome with the statements that best describe it.

33.6   Acute phase _____

33.7   Middle phase _____

33.8   Late phase _____

a. Unrealistic plans to avoid further sexual assault
b. Readjustment
c. Rationalization that the victim should or could have prevented the assault
d. Begins with the assault
e. May not be fully manifested until time of initial disclosure
f. May be associated with cognitive dysfunction
g. Safety and regaining control are the victims main emotional needs during this time
h. Reorganization
i. Retreat to routine activities
j. Emotionally volatile time
k. May be associated with drastic changes in lifestyle, friends, and work

33.9   To retreat to routine activities during the acute phase of the rape trauma syndrome is often misinterpreted by health care team members and police as evidence that a sexual assault did not actually occur.

a. True
b. False

33.10   The rape trauma syndrome

a. Is reproducible in all victims
b. Has a predictable onset
c. Is involuntary in nature
d. Typically is of short duration

33.11   The presence or absence of retreat to routine activities is directly related to the severity of a victim's assault experience.

a. True
b. False

33.12   The inability of a patient to think clearly after an assault is

a. A manifestation of an underlying psychosis
b. Usually perceived by the health care team but not by the victim
c. Involuntary in nature
d. Relatively rare in occurrence

Answers (33.1-33.12)

33.1 d	33.4 c	33.7 a, b, c	33.10 c
33.2 e	33.5 a	33.8 h, k	33.11 b
33.3 a, c, d	33.6 d, e, f, g, i, j	33.9 a	33.12 c

33.13   Counseling and support are indicated during which phase of the rape trauma syndrome?

a. Acute
b. Readjustment
c. Reorganization

33.15   The initial care of the sexual assault victim should include

a. The provision of a safe environment
b. The treatment of serious or life-threatening trauma
c. The avoidance of discussion of the details of the assault
d. Gentle encouragement to work with the police

33.16   If a victim is hitchhiking at night and is assaulted, she should be reassured that such activity was not inappropriate and was not the cause of her being assaulted.

a. True
b. False

33.17   Minor trauma is seen in approximately what percent of sexual assault victims?

a. 1
b. 10
c. 25
d. 50

33.18   Victims of sexual assault characteristically perceive themselves as guilty and responsible for their assault, regardless of the situation.

a. True
b. False

33.19   Which of the following statements about the physical examination of a sexual assault victim is *correct*?

a. A general complete physical examination is beneficial but not required if it is felt that it would be too traumatic for the patient
b. Forensic specimens should be collected and cultures sent to test for sexually transmitted disease
c. Forensic specimens should be kept in the health professional's possession or control until turned over to an appropriate representative of the police laboratory
d. Genital and rectal evaluations are mandatory in the evaluation of a sexual assault victim

33.20   Antibiotic prophylaxis for sexually transmitted disease should be offered to all adult and child victims of sexual assault.

a. True
b. False

33.21   Which of the following is included in routine laboratory tests in cases of sexual assault?

a. Complete blood count
b. Liver function tests
c. Renal function tests
d. Hepatitis screen

33.22   An immediate posttreatment telephone evaluation of the sexual assault victim, usually within 24–48 hr, is needed to

a. Provide emotional support
b. Confirm further appointments for therapy and counseling
c. Confirm billing and financial arrangements
d. Identify physical and emotional problems that have arisen after initial care

33.23   If diethylstilbestrol (DES) is used as a postcoital contraceptive method following sexual assault, it should be combined with an antiemetic such as compazine (prochlorperazine).

a. True
b. False

33.24   If a female victim of sexual assault of menstrual age is using an effective method of contraception, a pregnancy test is not required as part of the sexual assault evaluation.

a. True
b. False

33.25   Which of the following antibiotics is appropriate to administer prophylactically following sexual assault?

a. Penicillin
b. Doxycycline
c. Cephalexin
d. Ciprofloxin

Answers (33.13-33.25)

33.13 all	33.17 c	33.20 b	33.23 a
33.15 a, b, d	33.18 a	33.21 d	33.24 b
33.16 b	33.19 b, c, d	33.22 a, b, d	33.25 b

33.26 Under what circumstances should ceftriaxone (Rocephin) be offered victims of sexual assault?

a. For all patients where the culture is positive for *N. gonorrhoeae*
b. If the patient is penicillin allergic
c. When the prevalence rate of antibiotic resistant strains of *N. gonorrhoeae* exceeds 1%
d. If the victim is pregnant

33.27 What is the appropriate dose of diethylstilbesterol (DES) for postcoital contraception?

a. 2 tablets b.i.d. × 3 days
b. 2 tablets q.d. × 3 days
c. 2 tablets b.i.d. × 5 days
d. 2 tablets q.d. × 5 days

33.28 Which of the following statements about child sexual victimization is correct?

a. Victimization is most commonly by parents, family members, or family friends
b. Rape by a stranger is relatively uncommon in children
c. It is best to interview child victims apart from parents and other family members
d. The use of anatomically correct dolls is a useful routine adjunct to history taking in young children as it will offset the lack of communication children are often able to provide

33.29 Because the physical examination of a small child is often difficult, routine sedation should be given prior to attempting examination.

a. True
b. False

33.30 The high prevalence of sexually transmitted diseases requires the routine prophylactic antibiotic therapy of child victims of sexual assault.

a. True
b. False

33.31 Suspected child sexual abuse must be reported to the police, but is reported to child welfare authorities only with the permission of the parents.

a. True
b. False

33.32 It is the responsibility of the _____ to determine if a child may safely return home after evaluation of sexual assault or if the risk of ongoing abuse requires foster home placement or hospitalization.

a. Health care team
b. Department of Social Work
c. Police
d. State's attorney

33.33 A child who displays a knowledge of sexual matters, anatomy, or function beyond that is expected for her years should be evaluated for the possibility of sexual abuse.

a. True
b. False

Answers (33.26-33.33)

33.26 c	33.28 all	33.30 b	33.32 a
33.27 a	33.29 b	33.31 b	33.33 a

Chapter 34 Final Questions (50 question)

34.1 At what average age is a regular, predictable reproductive cycle established in women?

    a. 11 years
    b. 13 years
    c. 15 years
    d. 18 years

34.2 At what average age does the female reproductive cycle become inefficient?

    a. 30 years
    b. 35 years
    c. 40 years
    d. 45 years

34.3 A woman's optimal reproductive time occupies _____ years?

    a. 10
    b. 15
    c. 20
    d. 30

34.4 On average, how many times a year will a healthy, nonpregnant woman ovulate?

    a. 6–8 times
    b. 10–12 times
    c. 13–14 times
    d. 16–18 times

34.5 What is the average length of the female reproductive cycle for a healthy woman in her mid-20s?

    a. 26 days
    b. 28 days
    c. 30 days
    d. 32 days

34.6 What is the name of the pulse generator that secretes gonadotropin-releasing hormone (GnRH)?

    a. Arcuate nucleus of the anterior hypothalamus
    b. Anterior lobe of the pituitary gland
    c. Posterior lobe of the pituitary gland
    d. Third ventricle

34.7 What is the route of flow of GnRH from the hypothalamus to the anterior pituitary gland?

    a. Through the cerebrospinal fluid
    b. Through the lymphatic system
    c. Through the pituitary portal venous plexus

34.8 What is the pulse frequency of hypothalamic GnRH secretion?

    a. Every 50–60 min
    b. Every 70–90 min
    c. Every 100–120 min
    d. Greater than 140 min

34.9 Given a woman with the inability to secrete GnRH (Kallmann syndrome), at what pulse frequency should an external GnRH pump be set?

    a. Every 50–60 min
    b. Every 70–90 min
    c. Every 100–120 min
    d. Greater than 140 min

34.10 Which of the following is a gonadotropic hormone that stimulates the granulosa cells of the primary ovarian follicle?

    a. Luteinizing hormone (LH)
    b. Follicle-stimulating hormone (FSH)
    c. Thyroid-stimulating hormone (TSH)
    d. Melanocyte-stimulating hormone (MSH)

34.11 Which of the following is a gonadotropic hormone that triggers ovulation?

    a. Luteinizing hormone (LH)
    b. Follicle-stimulating hormone (FSH)
    c. Thyroid-stimulating hormone (TSH)
    d. Melanocyte-stimulating hormone (MSH)

34.12 What is the result if any pituitary hormone becomes tonically elevated?

    a. Menorrhagia
    b. Hyperstimulation of the ovary
    c. Chronic anovulation
    d. Hirsuitism

34.13 Which of the following is the principal sex steroid hormone secreted by the granulosa cells of the ovarian follicle?

    a. Estriol
    b. Androstenedione
    c. Estrone
    d. 17β-estradiol

34.14 Which is the principal sex steroid hormone secreted by the theca lutein cells?

    a. Estradiol
    b. Testosterone
    c. Progesterone
    d. Estriol

34.15 Which of the following is secreted by the theca lutein cells during the follicular phase of the cycle and acts as a precursor for granulosa cell sythesis of sex steroid hormone?

    a. Androgens
    b. Prostaglandins
    c. Estrogens
    d. Endorphins

Answers (34.1-34.15)

34.1 c	34.5 b	34.9 b	34.13 d
34.2 d	34.6 a	34.10 b	34.14 c
34.3 d	34.7 c	34.11 a	34.15 a
34.4 c	34.8 b	34.12 c	

34.16   The oocyte in the primordial follicle is arrested in what stage?

   a.   Prophase of meiosis
   b.   Metaphase of meiosis
   c.   Prophase of mitosis
   d.   Metaphase of mitosis

34.17   What is required in order to stimulate the arrested oocyte to complete maturation?

   a.   Critical levels of FSH
   b.   The LH surge
   c.   An FSH:LH ratio of 3:1
   d.   A critical level of estradiol

34.18   Which of the following stimulates the pregranulosa cells of the primordial follicle to become granulosa cells?

   a.   LH
   b.   FSH
   c.   GnRH
   d.   Progesterone

34.19   What endocrine event initiates the onset of menstruation?

   a.   LH surge
   b.   Estradiol peak
   c.   Involution of the corpus luteum with decline in plasma progesterone
   d.   An FSH:LH ratio of 3:1

34.20   What is the average volume of blood lost each menstrual cycle?

   a.   10–25 mL
   b.   30–50 mL
   c.   70–90 mL
   d.   120–150 mL

34.21   Where do the prostaglandins that initiate uterine contractions during menstruation originate?

   a.   Ovary
   b.   Endocervix
   c.   Uterine musculature
   d.   Endometrium

34.22   Name the clinical condition associated with intrinsic symptomatic uterine contractions during menstruation.

   a.   Primary dysmenorrhea
   b.   Secondary dysmenorrhea
   c.   Dyspareunia
   d.   Dyschezia

34.23   What is the preferred form of medical treatment for women who suffer from primary dysmenorrhea?

   a.   β-blockers
   b.   Calcium channel blockers
   c.   Prostaglandin synthetase inhibitors
   d.   Narcotics

34.24   When during the female reproductive cycle does the pituitary gland begin to secrete FSH to initiate a new cycle?

   a.   Just before ovulation
   b.   Just after ovulation
   c.   24–48 hr prior to the onset of menstruation
   d.   24–48 hr after the onset of menstruation

34.25   What is the feedback relationship between FSH and 17β-estradiol?

   a.   Positive
   b.   Negative

34.26   What is the feedback relationship between 17β-estradiol and LH?

   a.   Positive
   b.   Negative

34.27–34.28   Instructions: Match the ratio of FSH:LH with the appropriate phase of the menstrual cycle.

34.27   Early follicular phase _____

34.28   Late follicular phase _____

   a.   <1
   b.   0
   c.   >1

34.29   What is the consequence of an androgen:estrogen ratio of >1 in a follicle undergoing stimulation?

   a.   Multiple gestation
   b.   Atretic follicle
   c.   Chromosomal abnormalities
   d.   Spontaneous abortion

34.30   What is the presumed chemical mechanism for extrusion of the oocyte from the follicle at the time of ovulation?

   a.   Metabolism of endorphins
   b.   Release of progesterone
   c.   Synthesis of prostaglandins
   d.   Liberation of intrafollicular prostaglandins

34.31   What is the consequence if prostaglandin synthetase inhibitors are administered at the expected time of ovulation?

   a.   The oocyte may be retained in the follicle
   b.   Mittelschmerz is intensified
   c.   Progesterone synthesis is enhanced
   d.   The corpus luteum is ruptured

Answers (34.16-34.31)

34.16 a	34.20 b	34.24 c	34.28 a
34.17 b	34.21 d	34.25 b	34.29 b
34.18 b	34.22 a	34.26 a	34.30 d
34.19 c	34.23 c	34.27 c	34.31 a

34.32 What term is given to the pain associated with ovulation?

a. Premenstrual syndrome
b. Dysmenorrhea
c. Dyspareunia
d. Mittelschmerz

34.33 What method can be used to follow follicular maturation during a reproductive cycle?

a. Transabdominal ultrasound
b. Transvaginal ultrasound
c. Serial hCG levels
d. Serum prolactin levels

34.34 Which steroid hormone facilitates preparation of the endometrium for implantation of the blastocyst following fertilization?

a. Estradiol
b. Estriol
c. Estrone
d. Progesterone
e. Testosterone

34.35 The clinical term for insufficient progesterone production by the corpus luteum is

a. Secondary dysmenorrhea
b. Primary dysmenorrhea
c. Inadequate luteal phase
d. Premenstrual syndrome
e. Spontaneous abortion

34.36 Which hormone is necessary to sustain the life of the corpus luteum beyond 14 days?

a. Progesterone
b. Human chorionic gonadotropin (hCG)
c. Estradiol
d. Human chorionic somatomammotropin (hCS)

34.37 What is the functional life of the corpus luteum during a normal intraterine pregnancy?

a. 1–2 weeks
b. 3–5 weeks
c. 6–7 weeks
d. 8–10 weeks

34.38 At about what age will a woman begin to notice changes in her reproductive cycle associated with perimenopause?

a. 30–32 years
b. 34–36 years
c. 38–42 years
d. 45–48 years

34.39 What is the first evidence of diminished reproductive efficiency in a woman?

a. A change in the length of the reproductive cycle
b. Hot flushes
c. Vaginal atrophy
d. Premenstrual mood changes

34.40 The clinical condition when the few remaining ovarian follicles are resistant to stimulation by FSH is called

a. Polycystic ovarian disease
b. Menopause
c. Kallman syndrome
d. Premenstrual syndrome

34.41 Recording the basal body temperature is an inexpensive, dynamic (recorded on a daily basis) technique for evaluating the female reproductive cycle.

a. True
b. False

34.42 Which steroid hormone affects the hypothalamic thermoregulatory center?

a. Etsradiol
b. Estriol
c. Estrone
d. Progesterone
e. Testosterone

34.43 Which of the following are clinical manifestations of progesterone secretion?

a. Breast fullness
b. Abdominal bloating
c. Fluid retention
d. Mood changes
e. Uterine bleeding

34.44 Which hormone is associated with the development of a secretory endometrium?

a. Estradiol
b. Estriol
c. Estrone
d. Progesterone
e. Testosterone

34.45 What procedure is used for endometrial dating, to diagnose inadequate luteal phase?

a. Transvaginal ultrasound
b. Hysteroscopy
c. Endometrial biopsy
d. Hysterosalpingogram

34.46 What is the primary reproductive function of the endocervix?

a. To act as a barrier to infection
b. To store spermatozoa for release at the time of ovulation
c. To maintain normal menstrual flow
d. To provide vaginal lubrication

Answers (34.32-34.46)

34.32 d	34.36 b	34.40 b	34.44 d
34.33 b	34.37 c	34.41 a	34.45 c
34.34 d	34.38 c	34.42 d	34.46 b
34.35 c	34.39 a	34.43 a, b, c, d	

34.47 The ductal elements of the breasts (nipples, areolae, and ducts) respond primarily to which hormone?

a. Estradiol
b. Estriol
c. Estrone
d. Progesterone
e. Testosterone

34.48 The acinar elements of the breasts (milk-producing glands) respond primarily to which hormone?

a. Estradiol
b. Estriol
c. Estrone
d. Progesterone
e. Testosterone

34.49 What is the common condition manifested by breast tenderness, mood changes, fluid retention, abdominal bloating, and weight gain?

a. Primary dysmenorrhea
b. Secondary dysmenorrhea
c. Premenstrual syndrome
d. Perimenopause

34.50 Which hormone is associated with the development of a proliferative endometrium?

a. Estradiol
b. Estriol
c. Estrone
d. Progesterone
e. Testosterone

Answers (32.47-32.50)

34.47 a   34.48 d   34.49 c   34.50 a

Chapter 35 Final Questions (35 questions)

35.1   The developmental events at puberty follow an un-predictable pattern.

   a. True
   b. False

35.2   What is known about the endocrine events surrounding the onset of secondary sexual maturation?

   a. A critical level of prolactin is necessary
   b. A critical LH:FSH ratio is necessary
   c. A critical level of dihydrotestosterone is necessary
   d. The critical endocrine event is unknown

35.3   At what age is the hypothalamic-pituitary axis first known to function?

   a. 6 weeks of gestation
   b. 10 weeks of gestation
   c. 15 weeks of gestation
   d. 28 weeks of gestation

35.4   What is the first known endocrine event associated with secondary sexual maturation?

   a. Secretion of dehydroepiandrosterone by the adrenal glands
   b. Ovarian hormone secretion
   c. Pituitary development
   d. Hypothalamus down-regulation

35.5   What is the usual length of time from the first physical signs of secondary sexual maturation until the time that sexual maturation is complete?

   a. 1 year
   b. 2 years
   c. 3 years
   d. 4 years
   e. 5 years

35.6   What is the expected sequence of secondary sexual development in girls?

   a. Adrenarche, growth spurt, thelarche, menarche, ovulation
   b. Menarche, growth spurt, thelarche, adrenarche, ovulation
   c. Growth spurt, menarche, adrenarche, thelarche, ovulation
   d. Thelarche, adrenarche, growth spurt, menarche, ovulation

35.7   Which of the following is a critical element required for timely secondary sexual maturation?

   a. Body fat level
   b. Amount of sleep
   c. Serum prolactin level
   d. Amount of light exposure

35.8   What is the baseline percentage of body fat needed to sustain female reproductive function?

   a. 6
   b. 12
   c. 24
   d. 30

35.9   What would be the earliest sign of delayed puberty in girls?

   a. Failure of growth spurt by age 10
   b. Failure of menarche by age 12
   c. Failure of breast budding by age 13
   d. Failure of ovulation by age 17

35.10 What is the normal interval between adrenarche and thelarche, when adrenarche occurs first?

   a. 4–5 months
   b. 6–9 months
   c. 12–15 months
   d. 24 months

35.11 Which of the following is not a cause of premature ovarian failure in adolescent girls?

   a. Turner syndrome (45X karyotype)
   b. X chromosome long arm deletion
   c. Mature teratoma
   d. Alkylating chemotherapy

35.12 Which of the following is a common cause of inadequate gonadotropin-releasing hormone (GnRH)?

   a. Marijuana use
   b. Inadequate body fat
   c. Environmental radiation exposure
   d. Constitutional delayed puberty

35.13 What is the most common genital tract cause of primary amenorrhea?

   a. Congenital absence of the uterus
   b. Imperforate hymen
   c. Asherman's syndrome
   d. Premature ovarian failure

35.14 Which of the following is a method for the treatment of vaginal agenesis?

   a. Vaginoplasty
   b. Vulvectomy
   c. Pressure dilatation of the vaginal space

35.15 What is the simple, definitive treatment for imperforate hymen?

   a. Hymenectomy
   b. Hymenotomy
   c. Vaginal reconstruction
   d. Administration of a GnRH agonist

Answers (35.1-35.15)

35.1 b	35.5 d	35.9 c	35.13 b
35.2 d	35.6 d	35.10 b	35.14 a, c
35.3 b	35.7 a, b, d	35.11 c	35.15 b
35.4 a	35.8 c	35.12 a, b, c	

35.16 What is the definitive chemical evidence of ovarian failure?

   a. Depressed estradiol
   b. Elevated prolactin
   c. Elevated follicle-stimulating hormone (FSH)
   d. Depressed testosterone

35.17 Genetic information that regulates the rate of ovarian follicular atresia is located on

   a. The short arm of the X chromosome
   b. The long arm of the X chromosome
   c. Chromosome 21
   d. Chromosome 18

35.18 Genetic information that determines height and somatic characteristics is located on

   a. The short arm of the X chromosome
   b. The long arm of the X chromosome
   c. Chromosome 21
   d. Chromosome 18

35.19 Which of the following will result from the deletion of part of the long arm of the X chromosome in a female?

   a. She will have premature ovarian failure
   b. She may have normal secondary maturation
   c. She may be able to become pregnant
   d. She will be of short stature

35.20 In girls with premature ovarian failure, which of the following hormones must be replaced?

   a. Prolactin
   b. Progesterone
   c. 17β-estradiol
   d. Testosterone

35.21 What is the risk of administering excessive 17β-estradiol (or other estrogens) in girls with pubertal failure?

   a. Endometrial cancer
   b. Short stature
   c. Hirsuitism
   d. Vaginal adenosis

35.22 What is the risk of delaying administration of 17β-estradiol in girls with pubertal failure?

   a. Short stature
   b. Mental retardation
   c. Osteoporosis
   d. Clinical depression

35.23 Alteration of the GnRH pulse frequency in adolescent girls will result in

   a. Ovarian hyperstimulation
   b. Ovarian atrophy
   c. Ovarian neoplasm
   d. No pituitary stimulation of the ovary

35.24 What condition is associated with olfactory tract hypoplasia and failure of GnRH secretion?

   a. Turner syndrome
   b. Cushing syndrome
   c. Kallmann syndrome
   d. Swyer syndrome

35.25 What condition is associated with failure to establish secondary sexual development, a webbed neck, and short stature?

   a. Turner syndrome
   b. Cushing syndrome
   c. Kallmann syndrome
   d. Swyer syndrome

35.26 How can Kallmann syndrome be recognized on clinical evaluation?

   a. Serum estradiol levels
   b. Visual field evaluation
   c. Serum FSH
   d. Olfactory challenge

35.27 How would a patient with Kallmann syndrome be treated to help her conceive?

   a. Artificial insemination
   b. Pulsatile administration of GnRH
   c. Administration of clomiphene citrate
   d. Administration of sequential estrogen and progesterone

35.28 What would be evidence of marijuana use in adolescents leading to incomplete puberty?

   a. Elevated estradiol
   b. Elevated testosterone
   c. Suppressed gonadotropins (FSH and LH)
   d. Suppressed prolactin

35.29 What is the prognosis for adolescent girls who have delayed puberty or secondary amenorrhea due to participation in competitive athletics?

   a. Increased incidence of congenital anomalies in offspring
   b. Infertility can be anticipated
   c. Normal secondary sexual development can be anticipated
   d. Normal reproductive capacity can be anticipated
   e. Early menopause can be anticipated

35.30 A woman with uterine and vaginal agenesis can produce her own genetic child through

   a. Sequential administration of estrogen and progesterone
   b. Pelvic reconstructive surgery
   c. In vitro fertilization and pregnancy carried by a surrogate

Answers (35.16-35.30)

35.16 c	35.20 c	35.24 c	35.28 c
35.17 b	35.21 b	35.25 a	35.29 c, d
35.18 a	35.22 c	35.26 d	35.30 c
35.19 a, b, c	35.23 d	35.27 b	

35.31 What is the criterion for precocious puberty in girls?

a. Growth spurt before 8 years
b. Growth spurt before 10 years
c. Breast development before 8 years
d. Growth spurt before 10 years

35.32 Isosexual precocious puberty is defined as

a. Premature sexual maturation following the normal sequence
b. Premature sexual maturation following an abnormal sequence
c. Sexual maturation on time but following an abnormal sequence
d. Sexual maturation on time but following a prolonged sequence

35.33 What is the most common cause of inappropriate hormone secretion leading to precocious puberty in girls?

a. Cushing syndrome
b. Addison syndrome
c. Adrenal hyperplasia, 21-hydroxylase type
d. Adrenal hyperplasia, 11-hydroxylase type

35.34 What is the treatment of choice for children with isosexual precocious puberty?

a. Steroids
b. Estrogen alone
c. Gonadotropin-releasing hormone agonist
d. Oral contraceptives

35.35 What is the primary physical consequence of isosexual precocious puberty?

a. Increased adult height
b. Short stature
c. Excess addition of weight
d. Excess weight loss

Answers (35.31-35.35)

35.31 c   35.33 a   35.34 c   35.35 b
35.32 a

Chapter 36 Final Questions (31 questions)

36.1 At what average chronologic age is a regular, predictable reproductive cycle established?

a. 9 years
b. 11 years
c. 13 years
d. 15 years

36.2–36.4 Instructions: Match the term with its definition.

36.2 Primary amenorrhea _____

36.3 Secondary amenorrhea _____

36.4 Dysfunctional uterine bleeding _____

a. Failure ever to menstruate
b. Irregular menstruation without anatomic lesions of the uterus
c. Failure to menstruate within 6 months of a previous menstrual cycle
d. Failure to menstruate due to obstruction of outflow

36.5 Which of the following do amenorrhea and dysfunctional uterine bleeding have in common?

a. Association with endometriosis
b. Anovulation
c. Levels of testosterone

36.6 What is the most common cause of amenorrhea?

a. Ovarian failure
b. Cervical stenosis
c. Pregnancy
d. Vaginal agenesis

36.7 What is the most common cause of pathologic amenorrhea?

a. Outflow obstruction
b. Disruption of the hypothalamic-pituitary axis
c. Asherman syndrome
d. Kallmann syndrome

36.8 In a woman presenting with a complaint of amenorrhea, the first evaluation that should be taken is to rule out pregnancy.

a. True
b. False

36.9 Disruption of the pulsatile secretion of gonadotropin-releasing hormone (GnRH) interferes with the secretion of

a. Follicle-stimulating hormone (FSH)
b. Luteinizing hormone (LH)
c. Catecholamines
d. Prolactin

36.10 Which of the following affects GnRH release?

a. Blood glucose level
b. Catecholamines
c. Estrogen
d. Progesterone

36.11 Which of the following is a functional cause of hypothalamic-pituitary amenorrhea?

a. Weight loss
b. Disrupted light-dark cycle
c. Chronic anxiety
d. Excessive exercise

36.12 Which of the following is associated with drug-induced hypothalamic-pituitary amenorrhea?

a. Codeine
b. Tetracycline
c. Tranquilizers
d. Nonsteroidal antiinflammatory drugs

36.13 Which of the following tests can help differentiate hypothalamic-pituitary amenorrhea from ovarian failure?

a. Measurement of FSH levels
b. Measurement of serum estradiol
c. Pregnancy test
d. Measurement of prolactin

36.14 Which of the following are immediate symptoms of estrogen deficiency in women with ovarian failure?

a. Hot flushes
b. Sleep disturbances
c. Mood changes
d. Vaginal dryness

36.15 What is the most common cause of secondary amenorrhea that results from anatomical abnormalities of the genital outflow tract?

a. Cervical stenosis
b. Vaginal septum
c. Asherman syndrome
d. Intact hymen
e. Labial adhesions

36.16 What is the typical cause of the endometrial scarring that characterizes Asherman syndrome?

a. Infection
b. Previous dilatation and curettage
c. Previous IUD use
d. Previous hysterosalpingogram

Answers (36.1-36.16)

36.1 c	36.5 b	36.9 a, b	36.13 a, d
36.2 a	36.6 c	36.10 b, c, d	36.14 a, b, c
36.3 c	36.7 b	36.11 a, c, d	36.15 c
36.4 b	36.8 a	36.12 c	36.16 b

36.17   What is the method of treating scarring of the uterine cavity?

    a. Estrogen alone
    b. Lysis of intrauterine adhesions alone
    c. Lysis of intrauterine adhesions and estrogen
    d. Sequential estrogen and progesterone

36.18   The first principle of treatment of hypothalamic-pituitary amenorrhea is to establish the etiology.

    a. True
    b. False

36.19   What is the definition of dysfunctional uterine bleeding?

    a. Any irregular bleeding
    b. Irregular bleeding with pain
    c. Irregular bleeding causing functional disability
    d. Irregular bleeding in the absence of anatomical lesions

36.20   What is the endocrine environment that leads to dysfunctional uterine bleeding?

    a. Falling prolactin
    b. Chronic progesterone effect
    c. Chronic estrus
    d. Fluctuating testosterone

36.21   Dysfunctional uterine bleeding is always frequent and heavy.

    a. True
    b. False

36.22   What causes irregular bleeding in women with dysfunctional uterine bleeding?

    a. Subclinical infection
    b. Progesterone withdrawal
    c. Noncyclical stimulation of endometrial polyps
    d. Endometrium outgrows its blood supply

36.23   What is the medical treatment of choice for immediate treatment of dysfunctional uterine bleeding?

    a. Daily oral contraceptives
    b. Progestin for 10 days
    c. Progesterone in oil for 1 month

36.24   What is the medical treatment of choice for chronic treatment of dysfunctional uterine bleeding?

    a. Daily oral contraceptives
    b. Progestin for 10 days
    c. Progesterone in oil for 1 month

36.25   What is the surgical treatment of choice for dysfunctional uterine bleeding that cannot be controlled with medical therapy?

    a. Hysterectomy
    b. Myomectomy
    c. Dilatation and curettage
    d. Hysteroscopy

36.26   Which of the following conditions may result in dysfunctional uterine bleeding?

    a. Adrenal hyperplasia
    b. Hypertension
    c. Obesity
    d. Polycystic ovarian disease

36.27   Dysfunctional uterine bleeding can occur in association with ovulation.

    a. True
    b. False

36.28   In luteal phase defect, there is insufficient _____ produced to maintain the endometrium.

    a. Estrogen
    b. Progesterone
    c. Prolactin
    d. FSH

36.29   Which of the following anatomical conditions can cause irregular bleeding?

    a. Endometrial adenocarcinoma
    b. Cervical carcinoma
    c. Endometrial polyps
    d. Uterine leiomyomata

36.30   In addition to history and physical examination, which of the following help differentiate anatomical causes of abnormal uterine bleeding from dysfunctional uterine bleeding?

    a. Endometrial biopsy
    b. Basal body temperature chart
    c. Daily FSH levels
    d. Daily prolactin levels

36.31   Which of the following are risks from untreated dysfunctional uterine bleeding?

    a. Endometrial carcinoma
    b. Adenomyosis
    c. Endometrial hyperplasia
    d. Blood loss causing anemia

Answers (36.17–36.31)

36.17 c	36.21 b	36.25 c	36.29 all
36.18 a	36.22 d	36.26 a, c, d	36.30 a, b
36.19 d	36.23 b	36.27 a	36.31 a, c, d
36.20 c	36.24 a	36.28 b	

Chapter 37 Final Questions (57 questions)

37.1 The climacteric is defined as the

a. Time of the last menstrual flow
b. Beginning of menopause
c. The transition from the reproductive to the nonreproductive years
d. The last five regular menstrual cycles

37.2 The mean age of menopause is about

a. 40 years
b. 45 years
c. 50 years
d. 55 years
e. 60 years

37.3 Approximately what percent of women will experience menopause prior to the age of 45?

a. 5
b. 15
c. 25
d. 35
e. 45

37.4 Ovarian function ceases by age 55 years in what percent of women?

a. 80
b. 85
c. 90
d. 95
e. 99

37.5 Between infancy and the time of menopause, the number of oocytes in the ovary

a. Steadily rises
b. Rises and then falls
c. Steadily falls

37.6 Approximately how many oocytes will a woman ovulate during her reproductive years?

a. 100
b. 200
c. 300
d. 400
e. 500

37.7 At the time of puberty, a woman has about _____ oocytes.

a. 4,000
b. 40,000
c. 400,000
d. 4 million

37.8 The major hormonal product of the postmenopausal ovary is

a. Luteinizing hormone
b. 17β-estradiol
c. Testosterone

37.9 As a women approaches menopause, the remaining oocytes become increasingly _____ to follicle stimulating hormone.

a. Resistant
b. Sensitive

37.10–37.12 Instructions: Match a woman's age with the average number of times that she will ovulate during a year.

37.10 25 years old _____

37.11 40 years old _____

37.12 45 years old _____

a. 13–14 times per year
b. 11–12 times per year
c. 3–4 times per year

37.13 The withdrawal of _____ is responsible for the vasomotor symptoms of the menopause.

a. Estrogen
b. Progesterone
c. Prolactin
d. Oxytocin
e. Testosterone

37.14 With aging, the change in the overall length of menstrual cycle is a function of variations in the

a. Follicular phase
b. Luteal phase

37.15 The 5–10-year period prior to menopause is called the

a. Climacteric
b. Perimenopause

37.16 Which of the following is generally the first physical manifestation of ovarian failure?

a. Sleep disturbance
b. Vaginal dryness
c. Hot flushes
d. Mood changes
e. Skin thickening

37.17 The plasma concentration of FSH begins to increase

a. Several years before menopause
b. At the time of menopause
c. Several years after menopause

Answers (37.1-37.17)

37.1 c	37.6 d	37.10 a	37.14 a
37.2 c	37.7 c	37.11 b	37.15 b
37.3 c	37.8 c	37.12 c	37.16 c
37.4 d	37.9 a	37.13 a	37.17 a
37.5 c			

37.18–37.21 Instructions: Match the life stage with the corresponding FSH level that would be expected in a normal physiologic state.

37.18 Childhood _____

37.19 Prime reproductive years _____

37.20 Perimenopause _____

37.21 Menopause _____

   a. Greater than 30 mIU/mL
   b. 14 to 24 mIU/mL
   c. 6 to 10 mIU/mL
   d. Less than 4 mIU/mL

37.22 Which of the following statements about hot flushes is *incorrect*?

   a. Over 95% of perimenopausal and menopausal women experiences hot flushes (vasomotor instability)
   b. As a woman approaches menopause, the frequency and intensity of hot flushes increases
   c. Hot flushes may be associated with disabling diaphoresis
   d. If a menopausal woman does not receive estrogen-replacement therapy, hot flushes will continue indefinitely

37.23 Hot flushes are the result of _____ 17β-estradiol secretion by the ovarian follicles.

   a. Increased
   b. Decreased

37.24 What is the effect of decreasing estrogen on the sleep cycle?

   a. Latent phase shortened, sleep period shortened
   b. Latent phase shortened, sleep period lengthened
   c. Latent phase lengthened, sleep period shortened
   d. Latent phase lengthened, sleep period lengthened

37.25 Which of the following statements about vaginal atrophy associated with menopause is *incorrect*?

   a. The vaginal epithelium becomes thin
   b. Vaginal but not cervical secretions diminish in quantity
   c. Many patients experience diminished sexual pleasure and dyspareunia
   d. Vaginal tissue is more likely to become infected by local flora, resulting in atrophic vaginitis

37.26 Which of the following is an estrogen-dependent tissue?

   a. Ovary
   b. Vaginal mucosa
   c. Endocervix
   d. Endometrium
   e. Myometrium

37.27 Which of the following is an effect of estrogen deficiency on paravaginal tissue?

   a. Bladder and rectal prolapse
   b. Uterine retroversion
   c. Dysuria and urinary frequency
   d. Vaginal vault prolapse

37.28 In a postmenopausal woman, symptomatic pelvic relaxation cannot be improved by the administration of estrogens.

   a. True
   b. False

37.29 Which of the following is *not* a consequence of estrogen deficiency?

   a. Acne
   b. Thinning of the skin
   c. Brittle nails
   d. Synchronous hair shedding

37.30 What is the mechanism responsible for increased facial hair in menopausal women?

   a. Increased testosterone production
   b. Increased dihydrotestosterone production
   c. Increased DHEAS production
   d. Reduction in sex hormone–binding globulin

37.31 What is the expected rate of bone loss in perimenopausal women?

   a. 0.1%/year
   b. 0.5%/year
   c. 1%/year
   d. 5%/year

37.32 What is the expected rate of bone loss in postmenopausal women?

   a. 0.1–0.2%/year
   b. 0.5%/year
   c. 1–2%/year
   d. 5%/year

37.33 If a woman begins estrogen-replacement therapy prior to or at the time of menopause, bone density is maintained at the premenopausal levels.

   a. True
   b. False

37.34 Calcium supplementation in a postmenopausal woman appears to be just as effective as estrogen-replacement therapy with respect to osteoporosis.

   a. True
   b. False

Answers (37.18–37.34)

37.18 d	37.23 b	37.27 a, c	37.31 b
37.19 c	37.24 c	37.28 b	37.32 c
37.20 b	37.25 b	37.29 a	37.33 a
37.21 a	37.26 b, c, d, e	37.30 d	37.34 b
37.22 d			

37.35 Which of the following is *not* a risk factor for osteo-porosis?

    a. Reduced height for weight
    b. Family history of osteoporosis
    c. Late menopause
    d. Low calcium intake
    e. Cigarette smoking
    f. Nulliparity
    g. High alcohol intake
    h. High caffeine intake

37.36 The decrease in estrogen associated with menopause _____ total cholesterol.

    a. Increases
    b. Does not affect
    c. Decreases

37.37 The decrease in estrogen associated with menopause _____ high-density lipoprotein.

    a. Increases
    b. Does not affect
    c. Decreases

37.38 The administration of exogenous estrogens to per-imenopausal and postmenopausal women promotes normalization of the cardiovascular lipid profile.

    a. True
    b. False

37.39 Estrogen-replacement therapy reduces cholesterol levels equally in smokers and nonsmokers.

    a. True
    b. False

37.40 Premature ovarian failure is defined as menopause that occurs prior to the age of

    a. 32
    b. 37
    c. 42
    d. 47

37.41 In Savage syndrome, the number of ovarian follicles is _____ as compared to normal women.

    a. Increased
    b. Unchanged
    c. Reduced

37.42 Cigarette smoking has what effect on the timing of menopause?

    a. Smokers experience menopause 3–5 years earlier than nonsmokers
    b. Smokers experience menopause at about the same time as nonsmokers
    c. Smokers experience menopause 3–5 years later than nonsmokers

37.43–37.48 Instructions: Match the type of estrogen with the corresponding example(s).

37.43 Conjugated estrogens _____

37.44 Ethinyl estradiol _____

37.45 17β-estradiol _____

37.46 Piperazine estrone sulfate _____

37.47 Estropipate _____

    a. Dienestrol cream
    b. Estratest
    c. Estraderm transdermal patch
    d. Premarin
    e. Ogen
    f. Estratab
    g. Estrace

37.48 Which of the following common estrogen prepara-tions used in the treatment of postmenopausal pa-tients also contains testosterone?

    a. Premarin
    b. Estratab
    c. Estrace
    d. Estratest
    e. Ogen

37.49–37.50 Instructions: Match the type of progestin used in the treatment of menopausal patients with the corresponding common progestin preparation.

37.49 Medroxyprogesterone _____

37.50 Norethindrone acetate _____

    a. Depo-Provera
    b. Aygestin
    c. Norlutate
    d. Provera

37.51 Hot flushes occur more often and with greater se-verity in women with premature ovarian failure as compared to women undergoing menopause at the normal time.

    a. True
    b. False

37.52 Which of the following may be responsible for pre-mature menopause?

    a. Chromosomal abnormalities
    b. Follicle resistance to FSH/LH
    c. Production of autoantibodies
    d. Alkylating cancer chemotherapy

37.53 Simple hysterectomy is not routinely associated with an alteration in the normal time of ovarian failure (menopause).

    a. True
    b. False

Answers (37.35-37.53)

37.35 c	37.40 c	37.45 c	37.50 b, c
37.36 a	37.41 b	37.46 e	37.51 b
37.37 c	37.42 a	37.47 e	37.52 all
37.38 a	37.43 d	37.48 d	37.53 b
37.39 b	37.44 none	37.49 a, d	

37.54   Individuals who smoke

    a.   Do not respond as well as nonsmokers to estrogen-replacement therapy

    b.   Do not respond as well as nonsmokers to estrogen replacement-therapy only if they also drink alcohol

    c.   Respond equally well as nonsmokers to estrogen-replacement therapy

    d.   Respond better than nonsmokers to estrogen-replacement therapy

37.55   Women with a history of thromboembolic disease

    a.   Should not receive estrogen-replacement therapy

    b.   May receive oral or injectable estrogen-replacement therapy

    c.   May be candidates to receive transdermal estrogen-replacement therapy

37.56   Which of the following is a known risk of unopposed estrogen-replacement therapy?

    a.   Endometrial hyperplasia

    b.   Leiomyoma uteri

    c.   Endocervical adenocarcinoma

    d.   Squamous cell carcinoma of the cervix

37.57   Women with a history of carcinoma limited to the endometrium and myometrium should never receive estrogen-replacement therapy because of the risk of recurrence of the carcinoma in metastatic sites.

    a.   True

    b.   False

Answers (37.54-37.57)

37.54 a   37.55 c   37.56 a   37.57 b

Chapter 38 Final Questions (56 questions)

38.1 Approximately _____ of normal couples would conceive within 1 year.

    a. 55%
    b. 65%
    c. 75%
    d. 85%
    e. 95%

38.2 Infertility affects _____ of reproductive age couples in the United States.

    a. 1%
    b. 5%
    c. 10%
    d. 15%
    e. 25%

38.3 Infertility is defined as a couple's failure to conceive following _____ year(s) of unprotected sexual intercourse.

    a. 0.5
    b. 1
    c. 2
    d. 3
    e. 4

38.4 What percent of couples with a clinical diagnosis of infertility may expect to have a child with appropriate specific diagnosis and treatment?

    a. 55
    b. 65
    c. 75
    d. 85
    e. 95

38.5 Although there is considerable emotional burden during the initial phase of the evaluation of the infertile couple, this usually resolves spontaneously with specific diagnosis as the patients then understand the problem and do not feel guilty or unduly stressed.

    a. True
    b. False

38.6 Anovulation, anatomical defects of the female genital tract, and abnormal spermatogenesis together account for what percent of reproductive dysfunction?

    a. 65
    b. 75
    c. 85
    d. 95

38.7 Which of the following is *not* part of the initial evaluation of the infertile couple?

    a. Basal body temperature recording
    b. Hysterosalpingogram
    c. Semen analysis
    d. Diagnostic laparoscopy

38.8 The characteristic biphasic temperature shift associated with ovulation occurs in what percent of ovulating women?

    a. 60
    b. 70
    c. 80
    d. 90
    e. 99

38.9 About _____ days after ovulation, the basal temperature drops and menstruation begins within 24–36 hr.

    a. 11–12
    b. 13–14
    c. 15–16
    d. 17–18

38.10 A temperature elevation of longer than _____ days suggests pregnancy.

    a. 12
    b. 14
    c. 16
    d. 18
    e. 20

38.11 The _____ part of an ejaculate contains the greatest density of sperm.

    a. First
    b. Middle
    c. Last

38.12 Semen analysis should be performed no longer than _____ hr after the specimen is collected.

    a. 1
    b. 2
    c. 4
    d. 6
    e. 10

Answers (38.1–38.12)

38.1 d	38.4 d	38.7 d	38.10 c
38.2 d	38.5 b	38.8 d	38.11 a
38.3 b	38.6 d	38.9 b	38.12 b

38.13–38.16 Instructions: Match the cause of infertility with the tests which may be used for their evaluation.

38.13 Anovulation _____

38.14 Anatomic disorder _____

38.15 Abnormal spermatogenesis _____

38.16 Immunologic disorder _____

    a. Postcoital test
    b. Diagnostic laparoscopy
    c. Hysteroscopy
    d. Serum progesterone
    e. Basal body temperature
    f. Endometrial biopsy
    g. Hysterosalpingogram
    h. Urinary ovulation detection kit
    i. Semen analysis
    j. Antisperm antibodies

38.17 A sperm count of between 5 and 20 million per milliliter would be defined as

    a. Infertile
    b. Subfertile
    c. Fertile

38.18 A normal semen analysis is characterized by less than _____ abnormal sperm forms.

    a. 10%
    b. 15%
    c. 20%
    d. 25%
    e. 30%

38.19 A normal semen analysis is characterized by a minimum of _____ motile sperm

    a. 40%
    b. 50%
    c. 60%
    d. 70%
    e. 80%

38.20 A normal semen analysis excludes a male cause for infertility in what percent of cases?

    a. 50
    b. 60
    c. 70
    d. 80
    e. 90

38.21 A normal semen analysis is characterized with respect to viscosity by full liquification within

    a. 30 min
    b. 60 min
    c. 90 min
    d. 120 min

38.22 A hysterosalpingogram has a diagnostic accuracy of approximately _____ for detecting anatomic abnormalities of the genital tract.

    a. 30%
    b. 50%
    c. 70%
    d. 90%

38.23 The menstrual cycle of a healthy young woman between ages 18 and 36 is characterized by

    a. Ovulation 13–14 times per year
    b. Ovulation occurring on the 14th day
    c. Menstruation beginning on the 28th day
    d. Menstruation lasting approximately 5 days

38.24–38.25 Instructions: Match the phase of the ovulatory menstrual cycle with the appropriate descriptive statements.

38.24 Follicular phase _____

38.25 Luteal phase _____

    a. Acinar elements of the breast alter to produce rounding of the lateral quadrants
    b. Increased production of clear, watery endocervical mucus
    c. Proliferation of the endometrium
    d. Predominant hormone, 17β-estradiol
    e. Increased turgor of the ductal elements of the breast
    f. Predominant hormone, progesterone
    g. Conversion of cervical mucus to sticky mucoid nature
    h. Conversion of endometrium to secretory pattern

38.26 Following ovulation, the basal body temperature increases by approximately

    a. 0.2°F
    b. 0.4°F
    c. 0.6°F
    d. 0.8°F
    e. 1.0°F

38.27 Which of the following cyclic changes is presumptive evidence of ovulation?

    a. Fullness and heaviness of the breasts
    b. Increased vaginal secretions
    c. Abdominal bloating
    d. Minor peripheral edema with a slight increase in body weight
    e. Occasional episodes of depression

Answers (38.13-38.27)

38.13 d, e, f, h	38.17 b	38.21 b	38.25 a, f, g, h
38.14 b, c, g	38.18 d	38.22 c	38.26 c
38.15 a, i	38.19 c	38.23 all	38.27 a, c, d, e
38.16 a, j	38.20 e	38.24 b, c, d, e	

38.28 The measurement of serum progesterone is a much more sensitive and specific test for ovulation than the basal body temperature curve.

a. True
b. False

38.29 Ovulation-detection kits measure changes in urinary LH and are, therefore, specific for confirming ovulation.

a. True
b. False

38.30–38.31 Instructions: Match the abnormal sperm level with the appropriate causes.

38.30 No sperm (azoospermia) _____

38.31 Few sperm (oligospermia) _____

a. Varicocele
b. Kleinfelter syndrome
c. Exogenous factors, including heat
d. Endocrinopathies, including androgen receptor defects
e. Leydig cell failure

38.32 Abnormal sperm morphology can be caused by which of the following?

a. Varicocele
b. Infection
c. Immunologic factors, including antisperm antibodies
d. Stress

38.33 Capacitation of sperm occurs in the

a. Fallopian tube
b. Endometrial cavity
c. Endocervix
d. Vagina

38.34–38.37 Instructions: Match the possible cause of infertility with the appropriate evaluation(s).

38.34 Anovulation _____

38.35 Anatomic disorder _____

38.36 Abnormal spermatogenesis _____

38.37 Immunologic disorder _____

a. Endometrial biopsy
b. Postcoital test
c. Hysterosalpingogram
d. Serum progesterone
e. Antisperm antibodies

38.38 Which of the following statements about hysterosalpingograms is *correct*?

a. The test should be performed between the 7th and 11th day of the menstrual cycle
b. The endometrial cavity should appear smooth and symmetrical if there are no abnormalities
c. The distal third of the fallopian tubes should be slender, approximating the diameter of a pencil lead
d. Fimbrial fold should appear as linear radiolucencies along the longitudinal access of the tube

38.39 Hysterosalpingograms performed during the menses produce the risk of iatrogenic retrograde menstruation.

a. True
b. False

38.40 A hysterosalpingogram that shows radiographic crescents throughout the pelvis, caused by dye spilling from the fallopian tubes, is considered

a. Normal
b. Abnormal

38.41 Diagnostic laparoscopy provides information about the external surfaces of the pelvic organs, while hysterosalpingography provides information about the internal surfaces of the same organs.

a. True
b. False

38.42 The sperm generation time is approximately

a. 33 days
b. 53 days
c. 73 days
d. 93 days
e. 113 days

38.43 The success of treatment for oligospermia is observable within 1 month.

a. True
b. False

38.44 Sperm production occurs at a temperature of approximately _____ below body temperature.

a. 1°F
b. 2°F
c. 3°F
d. 4°F
e. 5°F

Answers (38.28-38.44)

38.28 b	38.33 c	38.37 b, e	38.41 a
38.29 b	38.34 a, d	38.38 a, b, d	38.42 c
38.30 a, b, c, e	38.35 c	38.39 a	38.43 b
38.31 a, c, d	38.36 b	38.40 a	38.44 a
38.32 a, b, d			

38.45 Which of the following can result in decreased sperm production resulting from thermal shock?

a. Spending excessive time in hot tubs or hot baths
b. Sitting on the testicles for long periods of time with poor heat dispersion
c. Wearing tight clothing
d. Living in a climate where the temperature exceeds 90°F for long periods

38.46 Men with poor sperm production as a result of hormonal abnormalities usually respond well to the induction of spermatogenesis with drugs such as clomiphene citrate.

a. True
b. False

38.47 If antisperm antibodies exist in the male, timed intrauterine insemination of washed sperm is often effective in producing pregnancy.

a. True
b. False

38.48 Which of the following statements about the postcoital (Sims-Huhner) test is *correct*?

a. Test best done during late follicular phase
b. Test best done with intercourse approximately 8 hr before the test
c. Normal result is 3–4 motile sperm per high power field in cervical mucus
d. Test provides information about coitus, ejaculation, sperm pickup, and sperm storage within the endocervical canal

38.49 If the woman produces antisperm antibodies, the sperm will be _____ in the cervical mucus.

a. Agglutinated
b. Immobilized

38.50 Which of the following statements about the use of clomiphene citrate is *correct*?

a. Clomiphene citrate acts by stimulating estrogen production and binding
b. Clomiphene citrate should be given in combination with progesterone
c. Clomiphene citrate administration results in an increase in FSH release from the pituitary
d. Dosage with clomiphene citrate must not exceed 50 mg per day

38.51 Significant risks of treatment of anovulation with menotropins include

a. Ovarian hyperstimulation
b. Multiple gestation
c. Fetal wastage
d. Hirsutism

38.52 The success rate of the induction of spermatogenosis by the administration of clomiphene citrate is generally less than

a. 5%
b. 10%
c. 15%
d. 20%
e. 25%

38.53 The expected successful outcome from *in vitro* fertilization in properly selected couples is approximately _____ per cycle.

a. 13–17%
b. 18–22%
c. 23–27%
d. 28–32%
e. 33–37%

38.54 How many days after the completion of therapy with clomiphene citrate do presumptive signs of ovulation occur?

a. 1–3
b. 4–6
c. 7–11
d. 12–14
e. 15–17

38.55 "Spinnbarkheit" is a term that means

a. Mucus secretion of the cervix
b. Thinning of the cervical mucus
c. Threading of cervical mucus
d. Crystallization of the cervical mucus

38.56 Luteal phase failure as a cause of infertility is treated by

a. Thyroid hormone
b. Estrogens and progestins combined
c. Progesterone alone
d. Pergonal

Answers (38.45-38.56)

38.45 a, b, c	38.48 a, b, d	38.51 a, b, c	38.54 c
38.46 b	38.49 b	38.52 d	38.55 c
38.47 b	38.50 c	38.53 b	38.56 c

Chapter 39 Final Questions (54 questions)

39.1 Which of the following is a common cause of hirsutism and virilization?

   a. Hilus cell tumor
   b. Polycystic ovarian disorder
   c. Congenital adrenal hyperplasia
   d. Sertoli-Leydig tumor
   e. Exogenous testosterone administration

39.2 Hirsutism and virilization are characterized as

   a. Estrogen excess disorders
   b. Androgen excess disorders
   c. Progesterone excess disorders
   d. Prolactin excess disorders

39.3 Which of the following is *not* a major role of androgens in female reproductive function?

   a. Precursors for estrogen biosynthesis
   b. Stimulate and maintain sexual hair growth
   c. Precursors for progesterone biosynthesis
   d. Influences the female libido

39.4 The treatment for androgen excess disorders is directed at

   a. Suppressing the source of androgen excess
   b. Stimulating hormones that produce feminization to compensate for androgen action
   c. Blocking androgen action at receptor sites

39.5–39.7 Instructions: Match the site with the normal percent of dehydroepiandrosterone (DHEA) production that occurs at the site.

39.5 Adrenal glands _____

39.6 Ovary _____

39.7 Extraglandular _____

   a. 0
   b. 10
   c. 25
   d. 50
   e. 90

39.8–39.10 Instructions: Match the site with the normal percent of testosterone production that occurs at the site.

39.8 Adrenal glands _____

39.9 Ovary _____

39.10 Extraglandular _____

   a. 0
   b. 10
   c. 25
   d. 50
   e. 90

39.11 What histologic structure is characteristic of the hilus cell tumor?

   a. Signet cell
   b. Clue cell
   c. Reinke crystalloid
   d. Donovan body

39.12–39.13 Instructions: Match the potential androgen excess disorder with the statement that best describe it.

39.12 Hirsutism _____

39.13 Virilization _____

   a. Increased circulating testosterone
   b. Temporal balding
   c. Often associated with acne
   d. Terminal hair on lower abdomen
   e. Remodeling of the limb-shoulder girdle

39.14 Which is the first event usually associated with virilization?

   a. Involution of the breasts
   b. Deepening of the voice
   c. Enlargement of the clitoris
   d. Temporal balding

39.15 Which of the following hormones are routinely measured in the evaluation of a woman with hirsutism and virilization?

   a. Dehydroepiandrosterone sulfate (DHEAS)
   b. Androstenedione (A)
   c. Estrone
   d. Testosterone (T)

39.16 In adipose tissue there is extraglandular production of testosterone from

   a. Dehydroepiandrosterone
   b. Androstenedione
   c. Estrone
   d. Estriol

39.17 In the hair follicles, dihydrotestosterone is produced by the local action of 5α-reductase on

   a. Dehydroepiandrosterone
   b. Testosterone
   c. Estrone
   d. Prolactin

39.18 Deficiencies of 21-hydroxylase and 11β-hydroxylase results in an accumulation of

   a. Dehydroepiandrosterone
   b. Estrone
   c. Testosterone
   d. Androstenedione

Answers (39.1-39.18)

39.1 b, c	39.6 b	39.11 c	39.15 a, b, d
39.2 b	39.7 a	39.12 c, d	39.16 b
39.3 c	39.8 c	39.13 a, b, e	39.17 b
39.4 a, c	39.9 c	39.14 c	39.18 a, c, d
39.5 e	39.10 d		

39.19 When a woman becomes obese, the conversion of androstenedione to testosterone in adipocytes

a. Increases
b. Is unchanged
c. Decreases

39.20 What percent of testosterone is not bound to sex hormone-binding globulin?

a. 1–3
b. 5–7
c. 10–15
d. 20–25

39.21 The measurement of total testosterone is a good surrogate measure for the fraction of free testosterone

a. True
b. False

39.22 Greater estrogen production is associated with _____ free testosterone.

a. More
b. The same amount of
c. Less

39.23 The hepatic production of sex hormone-binding globulin (SHBG) is stimulated by

a. Testosterone
b. Dihydrotestosterone
c. Estrogen
d. ACTH

39.24 The most common cause of hirsutism in women associated with androgen excess is

a. Luteinizing hormone excess
b. Genetic predisposition
c. Obesity
d. Polycystic ovarian disease

39.25 Which of the following is *not* a characteristic symptom of polycystic ovarian disease?

a. Oligomenorrhea
b. Amenorrhea
c. Anovulation
d. Acne
e. Virilization

39.26 The results of hormonal studies in women with polycystic ovarian disease are characterized by which of the following?

a. Increased LH:FSH ratio
b. Estradiol in greater concentration than estrone
c. Androstenedione at the upper limits of normal or increased
d. Testosterone at the upper limits of normal or slightly increased

39.27 Which of the following is *not* a result of the oral contraceptive treatment of polycystic ovarian disease?

a. Suppressed LH production
b. Decreased production of androstenedione
c. Decreased production of testosterone
d. Increased ovarian contribution to total androgen pool
e. Decreased incidence of endometrial hyperplasia

39.28 Which of the following statements about the pathophysiology of polycystic ovarian disease is correct?

a. LH stimulates the theca lutein cells to increase androstenedione production
b. Androstenedione is converted to estrone within fat cells
c. Estrone has a weak positive-feedback action or stimulates the pituitary secretion of LH
d. With increasing obesity there is a decreased conversion of androstenedione
e. With a rise in androstenedione, there is increased testosterone production

39.29 Once polycystic ovarian disease is established in an obese woman, weight reduction is rarely associated with a return to ovulation, even after administration of clomiphene citrate.

a. True
b. False

39.30 Which of the following medical therapies for the treatment of polycystic ovarian disease is *not* appropriate for a woman who wishes to conceive?

a. Oral contraceptive therapy with "mini-pills"
b. Medroxyprogesterone (Provera)
c. Medroxyprogesterone (Provera) plus clomiphene citrate

39.31 Thickening of the skin on the back of the neck, under the breasts, and in the intertriginous zones of the thighs in patients with polycystic ovarian disease is called

a. Vitiligo
b. Psoriasis
c. Acanthosis nigricans
d. Acne

39.32 Virilization associated with polycystic ovarian disease is seen in a disorder known as

a. Hyperthecosis
b. Androgen insensitivity syndrome
c. Hyperandrogenic syndrome
d. Acanthosis nigricans

39.33 Like polycystic ovarian disease, hyperthecosis is amenable to therapy with oral contraceptives or cyclic progestins.

a. True
b. False

Answers (39.19-39.33)

39.19 a	39.23 c	39.27 d	39.31 c
39.20 a	39.24 d	39.28 a, c, d, e	39.32 a
39.21 b	39.25 e	39.29 b	39.33 b
39.22 c	39.26 a, c, d	39.30 a	

39.34 Sertoli-Leydig cell tumors are characterized by which of the following?

a. Secrete testosterone
b. Common form of ovarian tumor
c. Occur usually in women between the ages of 50 and 60
d. Usually unilateral

39.35 Which of the following is *not* true of women with Sertoli-Leydig cell tumors?

a. There is a rapid onset of acne
b. Hirsutism occurs in approximately 75% of patients
c. Amenorrhea occurs in 95% of patients
d. Virilization occurs in most patients

39.36 In patients with Sertoli-Leydig cell tumors, hirsutism usually precedes breast atrophy.

a. True
b. False

39.37 Patients with Sertoli-Leydig cell tumors have which of the following laboratory findings?

a. Suppression of FSH
b. Suppression of LH
c. High plasma androstenedione levels
d. Elevation of testosterone levels

39.38 Which of the following statements about patients who have had surgical removal of a unilateral Sertoli-Leydig cell tumor is *incorrect*?

a. Ovulatory cycles return spontaneously in most patients
b. Further progression of hirsutism is arrested in most patients
c. Clitoral enlargement will usually revert to its pretreatment dimensions
d. The 10-year survival rate approximates 90–95%

39.39–39.41 Instructions: Match the uncommon virilizing-masculinizing ovarian tumor with the appropriate description(s).

39.39 Gynandroblastoma _____
39.40 Lipid (lipoid) cell tumors _____
39.41 Hilus cell tumors _____

a. Overgrowth of mature hilus cells or from the ovarian mesenchyme
b. Small ovarian tumors containing sheets of round, clear, pale-staining cells
c. Granulosa cell and arrhenoblastoma components
d. Contain Reinke crystalloids
e. Elevated 17-ketosteroids in many cases
f. Small, unilateral, and benign

39.42 Which ovarian tumor is associated with clinical masculinization, endometrial hyperplasia, and irregular uterine bleeding?

a. Lipoid cell tumors
b. Hilus cell tumors
c. Gynandroblastoma tumors
d. Sertoli-Leydig cell tumors

39.43–39.44 Instructions: Match types of congenital adrenal hyperplasia with the appropriate descriptions.

39.43 21–hydroxylase deficiency _____
39.44 11β–hydroxylase deficiency _____

a. Diagnosis made by measuring increased dehydroepiandrosterone sulfate and androstenedione in plasma
b. Increased plasma dehydroepiandrosterone sulfate, increased androstenedione, and normal and slightly increased testosterone
c. Increased plasma desoxycorticosterone
d. Associated with mild hypertension and mild hirsutism
e. Severe form associated with female infant virilization
f. History of pubic hair growth occurring prior to the onset of breast development may be a clinical clue to this disorder

39.45 Which of the following statements about the medical treatment of adrenal hyperplasia with prednisone is *incorrect*?

a. Facial acne usually clears promptly
b. Ovulation is usually restored
c. New terminal hair growth ensues
d. Hirsutism resolves quickly

39.46 Androgen-associated adrenal adenomas are associated with

a. Hirsutism
b. Acne
c. Amenorrhea
d. Virilization

39.47 Women with constitutional hirsutism are characterized by

a. Greater activity of 5α-reductase
b. Responsiveness to treatment with spironolactone, which blocks androgen receptor action
c. Regular ovulation and normal hormone levels
d. Severe acne

39.48 Danazol may be associated with which of the following effects?

a. Hirsutism
b. Deepening of the voice
c. Clitoral enlargement
d. Acne

Answers (39.34-39.48)

39.34 a, d	39.38 c	39.42 all	39.46 all
39.35 c	39.39 c	39.43 a, b, e, f	39.47 a, b, c
39.36 b	39.40 b	39.44 c, d	39.48 a, b, d
39.37 a, b, d	39.41 a, d	39.45 d	

39.49–39.50   Instructions: Match the type of hair with the appropriate descriptions.

39.49   Terminal hair _____

39.50   Vellus hair _____

    a. Coarse, kinky, dark
    b. Soft, downy, light in color
    c. Not under the influence of androgens
    d. Under the metabolic influence of androgens

39.51   The cause of androgen excess may often be established solely on clinical evidence without specific laboratory testing.

    a. True
    b. False

39.52   The finding of terminal hair on the lower back usually implies that a woman has had androgen excess of some variety for a long duration of time.

    a. True
    b. False

39.53   The more potent metabolite of testosterone that is produced in genital skin and hair follicles is

    a. Dehydroepiandrosterone
    b. Dihydrotestosterone
    c. Androstenedione

39.54   The essential role of androgens within the ovarian follicle is to serve as a precursor for estrogens.

    a. True
    b. False

Answers (39.49-39.54)

39.49 a, d
39.50 b, c

39.51 b
39.52 a

39.53 b

39.54 a

Chapter 40 Final Questions (44 questions)

40.1   The treatment plan for a gynecologic carcinoma is determined exclusively by the type and stage of the carcinoma.

a.   True
b.   False

40.2   Cells are especially vulnerable to anticancer therapies during the _____ portion of the cell cycle.

a.   Dividing
b.   Resting

40.3–40.7   Instructions: Match the phase of the cell cycle with the major event occurring during the phase.

40.3 G_0 _____

40.4 G_1 _____

40.5 G_2 _____

40.6   S _____

40.7   M _____

a.   Synthesis of RNA and protein in preparation for DNA synthesis
b.   DNA synthesis
c.   Additional RNA, protein, and specialized DNA synthesis
d.   Cell division occurs
e.   Resting phase

40.8   Anticancer therapies specifically designed to effect cells engaged in synthetic activities are least effective during which stage of the cell cycle?

a. G_0
b. G_1
c. G_2
d.   S

40.9   The growth fraction is the number of cells in a tumor that are not in the

a. G_0 phase
b.   S phase.
c. G_1 phase
d. G_2 phase

40.10   As a tumor enlarges in size, the growth fraction

a.   Increases
b.   Decreases
c.   Remains the same

40.11   Cytoreductive debulking surgery can result in G_0 cells _____ the cell cycle.

a.   Leaving
b.   Entering

40.12   Cyctoreductive debulking surgery is often associated with a decreased vulnerability to chemotherapy and radiation therapy.

a.   True
b.   False

40.13–40.16   Instructions: Match the class of antineoplastic drug with its major characteristic/action(s).

40.13   Alkylating agents _____

40.14   Antitumor antibiotics _____

40.15   Antimetabolites _____

40.16   Plant alkaloids _____

a.   Affects assembly of microtubles
b.   Structural analogs of normal molecules for necessary for cell function
c.   Intercalates between DNA base pairs
d.   Inhibits DNA directed RNA synthesis
e.   Interferes with base pairs, producing cross links, causing single and double strand breaks

40.17–40.20   Instructions: Match the class of antineoplastic drug with the phase of the cell cycle in which the drugs are most active.

40.17   Alkylating agents _____

40.18   Antitumor antibiotics _____

40.19   Antimetabolites _____

40.20   Plant alkaloids _____

a. G_1
b.   S
c. G_2
d.   M
e.   phase nonspecific

40.21   Suppression of blood cell formation is a known side effect of the

a.   Alkylating agents
b.   Antitumor antibiotics
c.   Antimetabolites
d.   Plant alkaloids

40.22   The phase of the cell cycle that is the most variable in length is

a. G_1
b.   S
c. G_2
d.   M

Answers (40.1–40.22)

40.1 b	40.7 d	40.13 e	40.18 e
40.2 a	40.8 a	40.14 c, d	40.19 b
40.3 e	40.9 a	40.15 b	40.20 d
40.4 a	40.10 b	40.16 a	40.21 all
40.5 c	40.11 b	40.17 a, b	40.22 a
40.6 b	40.12 b		

40.23–40.26 Instructions: Match the class of antineoplastic drug with examples of drugs from that class.

40.23 Alkylating agents _____

40.24 Antitumor antibiotics _____

40.25 Antimetabolites _____

40.26 Plant alkaloids _____

a. Busulfan (Myleran)
b. Chlorambucil (Leukeran)
c. Bleomycin (Blenoxane)
d. Actinomycin D
e. Methotrexate
f. 6-mercaptopurine
g. 5-fluorouracil
h. Hydroxyurea
i. Mitoxantrone
j. Nitrogen mustard
k. Cyclophosphamide
l. Doxorubicin
m. Melphalan
n. Hexamethylmelamine
o. Vinblastine
p. Vincristine
q. *Cis*-diammine-dichloroplatimum

40.27 Impaired renal function is most often associated with the use of which antineoplastic drug?

a. Methotrexate
b. Cisplatin
c. Busulfan
d. Hydroxyurea

40.28 Antineoplastic drugs are toxic because they act on normal as well as cancer cells.

a. True
b. False

40.29 In order for antineoplastic drugs to be used in combination, they must first fulfill which of the following criteria?

a. They must be effective when used singularly
b. They must have different mechanisms of action
c. They must be additive in action
d. They must not lead to drug resistance

40.30–40.32 Instructions: Match the type of interaction between antineoplastic drugs with the appropriate definition.

40.30 Additive _____

40.31 Antagonistic _____

40.32 Synergistic _____

a. Improved antitumor activity or decreased toxicity compared to each agent alone
b. Enhanced antitumor activity equal to the sum of each of the individual agents
c. Less antitumor activity that each individual agent

40.33–40.35 Instructions: Match the type of chemotherapy regimen with its definition and therapeutic goal.

40.33 Adjuvant chemotherapy _____

40.34 Induction chemotherapy _____

40.35 Maintenance chemotherapy _____

a. A short course of combination chemotherapy given in high doses for the purpose of eliminating residual cancer cells
b. Long-term and low-dose therapy designed to keep a patient in remission by inhibiting the growth of remaining cancer cells
c. Combination chemotherapy in high doses with a purpose of causing remission

40.36 Like chemotherapy, radiation therapy kills cells according to first-order kinetics.

a. True
b. False

40.37 A single large focused dose of radiation is more likely to be effective in destroying a tumor than fractionated small doses.

a. True
b. False

40.38 Cells are more vulnerable to radiation in the _____ of oxygen.

a. Presence
b. Absence

40.39 Local irradiation of tumor cells is termed

a. Teletherapy
b. Brachytherapy

40.40 The use of encapsulated sources of ironizing radiation is best associated with

a. Teletherapy
b. Brachytherapy

Answers (40.23-40.40)

40.23 a, b, j, k, m, n	40.28 a	40.33 a	40.37 b
40.24 c, d, i, l	40.29 a, b, c	40.34 c	40.38 a
40.25 e, f, g, h	40.30 b	40.35 b	40.39 b
40.26 o, p	40.31 c	40.36 a	40.40 b
40.27	40.32 a		

40.41 One Gray equals _____ rad.

    a. 1
    b. 10
    c. 100
    d. 1000

40.42 One Gray is defined as one joule per

    a. kilogram
    b. meter squared
    c. meter
    d. rad

40.43 Tamoxifen acts as a competitive inhibitor of

    a. Progesterone binding
    b. Estrogen binding
    c. Prolactin binding
    d. FSH binding

40.44 Cytoreductive debulking surgery often makes gynecologic malignancies more susceptible to adjuvant therapy.

    a. True
    b. False

Answers (40.41-40.44)

40.41 c   40.42 a   40.43 b   40.44 a

Chapter 41 Final Questions (46 questions)

41.1–41.4   Instructions: Match the common vulvar dermatoses with the appropriate statements about their
identification.

41.1   Lichen simplex chronicus (LSC) _____

41.2   Lichen planus _____

41.3   Psoriasis _____

41.4   Seborrheic dermatitis _____

a. Usually a desquamative lesion of the vagina;
occasionally it will develop on the vulva near the
inner aspects of the labia minora and vulvar
vestibule

b. Lesions of pale to red to yellow-pink and may be
covered by an oily appearing, scaly crust

c. Lesions are typically sightly raised, round, or
ovoid patches with a silver scale appearance atop
an erythematous base

d. Areas of whitish lacy bands of keratosis near reddish ulcerated-like lesions

e. Diffusely reddened areas with occasional hyperplastic or hyperpigmented plaques of red to reddish brown on the skin of the labia majora, labia
minora, and perineal body

41.5–41.8   Instructions: Match the common vulvar derma-
tosis with its treatment.

41.5   Lichen simplex chronicus _____

41.6   Lichen planus _____

41.7   Psoriasis _____

41.8   Seborrheic dermatitis _____

a. Empiric treatment includes antipruritic to inhibit nighttime itching and topical steroid
creams

b. Treatment with topical steroid preparations, but
with hyperkeratosis stronger fluorinated steroid
preparations may be used

c. Treatment includes topical cold tar preparations,
followed by exposure to ultraviolet light

d. Treatment includes use of Burrow's solution
soaks followed by topical corticosteroid lotions
or creams

41.9   Which of the following statements about vulvar vestibulitis is *incorrect*?

a. Vulvar vestibulitis involves the vestibular glands
located just inside the vaginal introitus near the
hymeneal ring, most commonly the posterolateral
vestibular glands in the 4 and 8 o'clock positions

b. Most commonly, patients report a progressive
worsening of the condition over 3 to 4 months

c. Light touch of a moistened cotton tip applicator
to the proper anatomic areas will duplicate the
pain of complaint

d. The affected areas are often evident as small,
reddened, patchy areas

e. Treatment with hydrocortisone ointments and
topical xylocaine jelly is uniformly successful

41.10   New onset insertional dyspareunia is especially associated with

a. Chronic cervicitis

b. Vulvar dysplasia

c. Vestibulitis

d. Bartholin's abscess

41.11–41.15   Instructions: Match the benign vulvar lesion
with the appropriate descriptive statement.

41.11   Inclusion cyst _____

41.12   Hydrocele _____

41.13   Fibroma _____

41.14   Hidradenoma _____

41.15   Nevi _____

a. Rising from fibrous tissue, usually small although occasionally may reach large proportions

b. Cyst of the canal of Nuck

c. Inflammatory blockage of gland ducts causes
small smooth nodular masses containing cheesy
material

d. Arises from the sweat glands of the vulva

e. Must be distinguished from a common malignant lesion that may occur on the external
genitalia

f. Almost always benign and found on the inner
surface of the labia majora

Answers (41.1–41.15)

41.1 e	41.5 a	41.9 e	41.13 a
41.2 a, d	41.6 b	41.10 c	41.14 d, f
41.3 c	41.7 c	41.11 c	41.15 e
41.4 b	41.8 d	41.12 b	

41.16 Which of the following lesions is *not* generally treated by simple excision, especially if symptomatic?

   a. Inclusion cyst
   b. Hydrocele
   c. Fibroma
   d. Hidradenoma
   e. Nevi

41.17 Which of the following conditions may be associated with high urinary oxalic acid concentrations?

   a. Hidradenoma
   b. Seborrheic dermatitis
   c. Lichen simplex chronicus
   d. Vestibulitis
   e. Psoriasis

41.18 Lichen sclerosis and hyperplastic dystrophy without atypia carry an estimated _____ risk of the development of vulvar carcinoma.

   a. 0–1%
   b. 2–3%
   c. 4–5%
   d. 6–7%
   e. 8–9%

41.19 Which of the following is *not* characteristic of squamous cell hyperplasia without atypia?

   a. Hyperkeratosis
   b. Acanthosis
   c. Abundant mitotic figures

41.20 The treatment of mixed dystrophy, i.e., lichen sclerosis admixed with areas of hyperplastic dystrophy, is

   a. Corticosteroid cream alone
   b. Testosterone appropionate cream alone
   c. Corticosteroid cream for 2–3 weeks, then topical testosterone appropionate
   d. Topical testosterone appropionate for 2–3 weeks, then corticosteroid cream
   e. Laser ablation

41.21–41.22 Instructions: Match the chronic vulvar disease with the appropriate statement(s) about its identification and clinical course.

41.21 Hyperplastic dystrophy _____

41.22 Lichen sclerosis _____

   a. Lesion is unlikely to totally resolve, requiring intermittent treatment for an indefinite period
   b. Lesion usually resolves completely within 6 months of therapy
   c. Vulva is characteristically diffusely involved with very thin whitish epithelium, often termed "onion skinned" epithelium
   d. Obviously hyperkeratotic skin with secondary excoriation

41.23–41.26 Instructions: Match the vulvar lesion with the appropriate statement(s) about its identification and progression.

41.23 Vulvar interepithelial neoplasia I and II (VIN I and VIN II) _____

41.24 Vulvar intraepithelial neoplasia III (VIN III, carcinoma in situ) _____

41.25 Paget's disease _____

41.26 Melanoma _____

   a. May be associated with carcinoma of the skin
   b. Associated with a higher incidence of underlying internal carcinoma, particularly colon and breast
   c. HPV changes occasionally seen in these lesions
   d. Full-thickness loss of maturation
   e. Raised gross lesions
   f. High predilection for progression to severe intraepithelial lesions and eventually carcinoma
   g. Associated with vulvar pruritus and chronic irritation
   h. Raised, irritated, pruritic pigmented lesion

41.27 If VIN III is identified, biopsy is made

   a. At a single site, in the center of the lesion
   b. At multiple sites in the lesion(s)

41.28 Vulvar carcinoma accounts for approximately what percent of all gynecologic malignances?

   a. 4
   b. 8
   c. 12
   d. 20

41.29 What percent of vulvar carcinomas are of the squamous cell type?

   a. 60
   b. 70
   c. 80
   d. 90

41.30 Extended VIN I and VIN II lesions are best treated by

   a. Cryocautery
   b. Electrodessication
   c. Laser cautery, using local anesthetic
   d. Laser ablation, using general anesthetic

41.31 The most common presenting complaint in cases of vulvar carcinoma is

   a. An exophytic ulcerative lesion on a labium majus
   b. Vulvar pruritis
   c. Dysuria
   d. Dyspareunia

Answers (41.16–41.31)

41.16 e	41.20 c	41.24 d, e, g	41.28 a
41.17 d	41.21 b, d	41.25 a, b	41.29 d
41.18 b	41.22 a, c	41.26 h	41.30 d
41.19 c	41.23 c, e, f, g	41.27 a	41.31 b

41.32 Which of the following statements concerning squamous cell carcinoma of the vulva is *correct*?

  a. The disease remains localized in most incidences for a relatively long period of time
  b. Spread is usually predictable along the regional lymph nodes
  c. Lesions greater than 2 cm in diameter and 0.5 cm in depth have an increased incidence of nodal metastasis
  d. Lesions rising in the anterior third of the vulva may spread directly to the deep pelvic nodes

41.33 The overall incidence of lymph node metastasis in squamous cell carcinoma of the vulva is approximately

  a. 10%
  b. 20%
  c. 30%
  d. 40%

41.34 Because of the high incidence of regional lymph node metastasis and the usual delay in diagnosis, vulvectomy of the radical nature with bilateral node dissection is mandatory for full evaluation and treatment in patients with vulvar carcinoma.

  a. True
  b. False

41.35 The primary factor affecting of 5-year survival in vulvar carcinoma is the presence of inguinal or femoral lymph node metastasis.

  a. True
  b. False

41.36 Which of the following statements about carcinoma of the Bartholin's gland is *incorrect*?

  a. Arises either from the squamous epithelium of the ducts or the glandular epithelium of the greater vestibular glands
  b. Most common in the fifth decade or later
  c. Treatment is radical vulvectomy and bilateral lymphectomy with radiation therapy, in most cases
  d. The 5-year overall survival rate is 85–95%

41.37–41.38 Instructions: Match the benign vaginal mass with the appropriate description(s).

41.37 Gartner duct cyst _____

41.38 Inclusion cyst _____

  a. Arise from vestigial remnants of the wolffian or mesonephric system
  b. Arise from imperfect alignment of childbirth lacerations or episiotomy
  c. Lined with stratfied squamous epithelium, and filled with "cheesy" material
  d. Are found along outer aspect of vaginal canal
  e. Should be excised if symptomatic

41.39 Vaginal carcinoma in situ is a rare gynecologic condition, but somewhat more common in patients

  a. With preexisting lower genital tract neoplasia
  b. Who have undergone hysterectomy for cervical carcinoma in situ
  c. Who have undergone radiation therapy for other gynecologic malignancy
  d. Who have been exposed to DES in utero

41.40 Invasive vaginal cancer accounts for about what percent of gynecologic malignancies?

  a. 1–2
  b. 3–4
  c. 5–6
  d. 7–8
  e. 9–10

41.41 Which of the following statements about sarcoma botryoides is *incorrect*?

  a. Presents as a mass of polyps protruding from the introitus of very young girls and infants
  b. Arises from the undifferentiated mesenchyme of the lamina propria of the anterior vaginal wall
  c. Often associated with a bloody discharge
  d. Treated in almost all cases by radical pelvic exenteration

---

Answers (41.32-41.41)

41.32 all	41.35 a	41.38 b, c, e	41.40 a
41.33 c	41.36 d	41.39 a, b, c	41.41 d
41.34 b	41.37 a, d, e		

41.42 Screening for the recognition of potential malignancy of the cervix is best accomplished by

    a. Self-investigation of the vagina
    b. Papanicolau (Pap) smear
    c. Cervical canal curettage
    d. Aspiration of endocervical mucus
    e. Posterior fornix aspiration

41.43 Diethylstilbestrol administered to the pregnant
mother is associated with which condition?

    a. Clear-cell adenocarcinoma of the vagina
    b. Endometrial carcinoma
    c. Hidradenosis
    d. Carcinoma in situ of the vagina
    e. Embryonal rhabdomyosarcoma

41.44 The recommended procedure for the evaluation of a
chronic vulvar ulcer is

    a. Darkfield examination
    b. Biopsy
    c. Pap smear
    d. Culture of lesion
    e. Lymphangiography

41.45 The most common cause of the delay in diagnosing
vulva carcinoma is the

    a. Unreliability of a Pap smear of vulva
    b. Equivocal histology of early lesions
    c. Failure to biopsy lesions
    d. Lack of visibility of most lesions

41.46 The most common malignant tumor of the vagina is

    a. Adenocarcinoma
    b. Squamous cell carcinoma
    c. Sarcoma botryoides
    d. Melanoma
    e. Paget's disease

Answers (41.42–41.46)

41.42 b	41.44 b	41.45 c	41.46 b
41.43 a			

Chapter 42 Final Questions (73 questions)

42.1 In most series, what percent of Pap smears are abnormal?

    a. 1–10
    b. 11–20
    c. 21–30
    d. greater than 30

42.2 Which of the following risk factors associated with cervical neoplasia is considered by most to be of special importance.

    a. Early intercourse
    b. Multiple sexual partners
    c. Early childbearing
    d. Low socioeconomic status
    e. Previous venereal infection
    f. Altered immune status
    g. Cigarette smoking
    h. Intrauterine DES exposure
    i. All contraceptive use
    j. Male factors, "high-risk" sex partner

42.3 Which of the following statements best describes cervical "erosion?"

    a. Cervical tissue exposed to trichomonas vaginalis
    b. Exocervical tissue undergoing squamous metaplasia
    c. Normal endocervical tissue that has "moved" to the cervical surface
    d. Endocervical tissue undergoing squamous metaplasia
    e. Endocervical tissue associated with mechanical abrasion

42.4 The transformation zone develops

    a. Prior to puberty
    b. During puberty and adolescence
    c. At the time of menopause

42.5 In the menopausal years, the squamocolumnar junction "moves"

    a. Into the endocervical canal
    b. Just outside the external os
    c. Onto the cervical surface

42.6 What percent of squamous intraepithelial neoplasia occurs within the transformation zone?

    a. 55
    b. 65
    c. 75
    d. 85
    e. 95

42.7 Which of the following statements about human papilloma virus is *correct*?

    a. The human papilloma virus is the single, direct cervical carcinogen
    b. The human papilloma virus may serve as a cofactor in the abnormal maturation and division of epithelial cells
    c. The great majority of women who harbor the human papilloma virus have accompanying cervical intraepithelial neoplasia

42.8 Which of the following types of human papilloma virus is associated with a particularly high risk of squamous intraepithelial neoplasia?

    a. 16
    b. 18
    c. 21
    d. 30
    e. 31

42.9 The current recommendation of the American College of Obstetricians and Gynecologists with respect to Pap smear screening is to obtain the first Pap smear at the time a woman becomes sexually active or reaches the age of

    a. 14
    b. 16
    c. 18
    d. 20

42.10 According to the recommendations of the American College of Obstetricians and Gynecologists, Pap smears should be obtained

    a. yearly
    b. every 2 years
    c. every 3 years
    d. at no set interval

42.11–42.15 Instructions: Match the Pap smear class system classification with the appropriate description.

42.11 Class 1 _____
42.12 Class 2 _____
42.13 Class 3 _____
42.14 Class 4 _____
42.15 Class 5 _____

    a. CIS
    b. Severe dysplasia
    c. Moderate dysplasia
    d. Mild dysplasia
    e. Inflammation
    f. Normal
    g. Squamous cell CA

Answers (42.1-42.15)

42.1 a	42.5 a	42.9 c	42.13 c, d
42.2 a, b, f, g, j	42.6 e	42.10 a	42.14 a, b
42.3 c	42.7 b	42.11 f	42.15 g
42.4 b	42.8 a, b, e	42.12 e	

42.16–42.19 Instructions: Match the Bethesda system of Pap smear classification with the appropriate descriptions.

42.16 Within normal limits _____

42.17 Low grade SIL _____

42.18 High grade SIL _____

42.19 Squamous cell cancer _____

  a. CIS
  b. Severe dysplasia
  c. Moderate dysplasia
  d. Mild dysplasia
  e. Inflammation
  f. Normal
  g. Squamous cell CA

42.20 Carcinoma in situ of the cervix becomes classified as invasive cervical cancer when the dysplastic cells traverse the

  a. Transformation zone
  b. Squamocolumnar junction
  c. Basement membrane
  d. Endocervical canal
  e. Canal of Nuck

42.21 Of all cases of mild dysplasia of the cervix, what percent will spontaneously regress?

  a. 5
  b. 25
  c. 45
  d. 65
  e. 85

42.22 Of all cases of mild dysplasia of the cervix, what percent will progress to worsening disease?

  a. 5
  b. 10
  c. 15
  d. 20
  e. 25

42.23–42.26 Instructions: Match the Bethesda system classifications of cervical cytology with the appropriate follow-up.

42.23 Atypical squamous cells of undetermined significance (ASCUS) _____

42.24 Low-grade squamous intraepithelial lesions (LSIL) _____

42.25 High-grade squamous intraepithelial (HSIL) _____

42.26 Atypical glandular cells of undetermined significance (AGUS) _____

  a. Repeat Pap every 4–6 months for 2 years until there are three consecutive negative smears; if second abnormal Pap, colposcopy should be considered
  b. Colposcopy with endocervical curettage and directed biopsies as indicated
  c. If Pap report is qualified by severe inflammation, any specific infection should be treated and the Pap repeated in 2–3 months
  d. In postmenopausal patient, repeat Pap smear following course of vaginal estrogen therapy; if still abnormal, colposcopy should be considered
  e. Options including repeat Pap with endocervical brush, endometrial biopsy, and/or cone biopsy

42.27 A colposcopic examination is defined as satisfactory when

  a. The entire squamocolumnar junction is visualized
  b. The entire external cervical os is visualized
  c. The entire internal cervical os is visualized
  d. The entire vesicouterine reflection is visualized
  e. The entire erosive zone is visualized

42.28 Which of the following is an indication for conization of the cervix?

  a. Unsatisfactory colposcopy
  b. Atypical squamous cells of undetermined significance
  c. Positive endocervical curettage
  d. Two-step discrepancy between Pap smear and cervical biopsy results
  e. Atypical glandular cells of undetermined significance

42.29 Acetic acid solution is used to wash the cervix prior to colposcopy, functioning as a

  a. Stain
  b. Emulsifyer
  c. Desiccant
  d. Antiseptic

Answers (42.16-42.29)

42.16 e, f	42.20 c	42.24 a, b	42.27 a
42.17 d	42.21 d	42.25 b	42.28 a, c, d
42.18 a, b, c	42.22 c	42.26 e	42.29 c
42.19 g	42.23 a, c, d		

42.30 Biopsies based on the findings of colposcopy should come from at least three of the four quadrants of the cervix in order to ensure adequate evaluation of any cervical abnormalities.

a. True
b. False

42.31 The endocervical curettage will be positive for dysplasia in what percent of women with a dysplastic Pap smear?

a. Less than 5
b. 5–10
c. 11–15
d. 16–20
e. 21–25

42.32 Approximately what percent of colposcopically directed biopsies and endocervical curettages will demonstrate a significant discrepancy between the screening Pap smear and the histologic data.

a. 1
b. 5
c. 10
d. 15
e. 20

42.33 A colposcopy may be considered satisfactory if the entire limits of some lesions are not totally visualized as long as the entire squamocolumnat junction is visualized entirely.

a. True
b. False

42.34 Which of the following is required for a conization specimen to be considered satisfactory?

a. The specimen encompasses the entire cervix
b. The specimen encompasses the entire squamocolumnar junction
c. The specimen encompasses the entire extent of identified lesions
d. The specimen encompasses a portion of the endocervical canal

42.35 If a conization specimen does not encompass the margins of the disease, repeat conization is always required.

a. True
b. False

42.36 Which of the following techniques is *not* commonly used for conization of the cervix?

a. Scalpel and scissors
b. Heated electric wire
c. Super-cooled electric wire
d. Laser

42.37 Which of the following is a risk factor for women undergoing conization of the cervix who desire future childbearing?

a. Incompetent cervical os
b. Abnormal cervical contours impeding coitus
c. Reduced cervical capacity to facilitate sperm transport due to loss of mucus secreting endocervical glands
d. Loss of uterus secondary to hysterectomy associated with hemorrhage

42.38 A major problem with the loop electro excisional procedure (LEEP) for conization is damage to the pathology specimen at the margins of excision, which interferes with pathologic diagnosis.

a. True
b. False

42.39–42.42 Instructions: Match the methods of treatment of cervical intraepithelial neoplasia with the appropriate descriptions.

42.39 Cryocautery _____

42.40 Laser therapy _____

42.41 Cervical conization _____

42.42 Excisional biopsy _____

a. May be considered for the treatment of specific focal areas of abnormality
b. May involve the use of a hot wire loop
c. May involve the use of "mushroom-tip" stainless-steel probe, super-cooled with circulating liquid nitrogen or carbon dioxide
d. Permits precise control of depth of ablation
e. Popular method for the treatment of low-grade CIN
f. Procedure is routinely considered both therapeutic and diagnostic
g. Procedure associated postoperatively with profuse watery discharge admixed with necrotic cellular debris
h. May be used for the treatment of high-grade intraepithelial lesions

42.43 Patients who have been treated for cervical intraepithelial neoplasia need to be followed by Pap smears at approximately 3-month intervals for 1 year. If these Pap smears are all normal, they may routinely be returned to a yearly Pap smear schedule.

a. True
b. False

Answers (42.30-42.43)

42.30 b	42.34 b, c, d	42.38 b	42.41 b, f, h
42.31 b	42.35 b	42.39 a, c, e, g	42.42 a
42.32 c	42.36 c	42.40 a, d, h	42.43 b
42.33 b	42.37 a, c, d		

42.44 The average age at diagnosis of invasive cervical carcinoma is approximately

a. 20 years
b. 30 years
c. 40 years
d. 50 years
e. 60 years

42.45 Advanced cervical intraepithelial neoplasia is thought to precede the occurrence of invasive cervical carcinoma by an average of

a. 1 year
b. 5 years
c. 10 years
d. 15 years
e. 20 years

42.46 What percentage of cervical cancer is of the squamous cell variety?

a. 45
b. 55
c. 65
d. 75
e. 85
f. 95

42.47 Approximately what percentage of cervical carcinoma is adenocarcinomas arising from the cervical glands?

a. 5
b. 15
c. 25
d. 35
e. 45
e. 55

42.48 Clear-cell carcinoma of the cervix is associated with intrauterine exposure to

a. Progesterone
b. Estrone
c. Dehydroepinandrosterone
d. Diethylstilbesterol
e. Cigarette smoke

42.49–49.52 Instructions: Match the stage of cervical carcinoma with the approximate 5-year survival.

42.49 Stage 1 _____
42.50 Stage II-A _____
42.51 Stage III-A _____
42.52 Stage IV _____

a. 5
b. 14
c. 25
d. 45
e. 64
f. 83
g. 91

42.53 Which of the following symptoms is *not* a classical finding or historical presentation for cervical cancer.

a. Postcoital bleeding
b. Pain
c. Abnormal uterine bleeding

42.54 If there is a visible lesion on the cervix, Pap smear will virtually always be an accurate method of evaluation.

a. True
b. False

Answers (42.44-42.54)

42.44 d	42.47 b	42.50 f	42.53 b
42.45 c	42.48 d	42.51 d	42.54 b
42.46 e	42.49 g	42.52 b	

42.55–42.63 Instructions: Match the clinical staging of carcinoma of the cervix (FIGO) with the appropriate description(s).

42.55 Stage I AI _____

42.56 Stage I AII _____

42.57 Stage IB _____

42.58 Stage IIA _____

42.59 Stage IIB _____

42.60 Stage IIIA _____

42.61 Stage IIIB _____

42.62 Stage IVA _____

42.63 Stage IVB _____

a. Carcinoma involves the lower third of the vagina, but there is no extension to the pelvic wall
b. Carcinoma extends beyond the cervix but not to the pelvic wall, there is no obvious parametrial involvement
c. All cases of Stage I cancer not included in other classifications or divisions
d. Minimal evidence stromal invasion on microscopic examination
e. Microscopic lesion(s) no more than 5 mm in depth measured from base of epithelial surface or glandular surface from which it originates, and horizontal spread not to exceed 7 mm
f. Carcinoma extends beyond cervix with obvious parametrial involvement
g. Carcinoma is extended to pelvic side wall
h. Carcinoma has spread to adjacent pelvic organs
i. Carcinoma has spread to distant organs

42.64 All patients with cervical carcinoma with hydronephrosis or a nonfunctioning kidney should be included in at least stage

a. I
b. II
c. III
d. IV

42.65 When there is a gross cervical lesion of the cervix, colposcopic evaluation is mandatory prior to biopsy.

a. True
b. False

42.66 Cervical carcinoma spreads through

a. Lymphatic metastasis
b. Direct extension
c. Both
d. Neither

42.67 In general, surgical therapy for cervical carcinoma is indicated for most patients with

a. Stage I
b. Stage II
c. Stage III
d. Stage IV

42.68 If a patient undergoes radical surgery for cervical carcinoma, the ovaries must be removed because of the additional risk to the patient caused by the continued cyclic estrogen production.

a. True
b. False

42.69 Which of the following is a complication noted after radiation therapy for cervical carcinoma?

a. Radiation cystitis
b. Radiation proctitis
c. Dyspareunia
d. Fistulae

42.70 Radiation therapy for cervical carcinoma is generally reserved for patients with stage IB or IIA disease who are poor surgical candidates and for all patients with more advanced disease.

a. True
b. False

42.71 A 31-year-old female with three living children and a tubal ligation has a Pap smear reported as HGSIL. There are no macroscopic lesions. The management should involve which of the following?

a. Hysterectomy
b. Radiotherapy
c. Local chemotherapy
d. Colposcopically directed cervical biopsies
e. Systemic chemotherapy

42.72 The primary lymph nodes involved in spread of cervical carcinoma is (are):

a. Paracervical and obturator
b. Sacral and inguinal
c. Common iliac and aortic
d. Perineal
e. Femoral

42.73 Metastatic cervical carcinoma can cause

a. Hydronephrosis
b. Paraplegia
c. Hematemesis

Answers (42.55–42.73)

42.55 d	42.60 a	42.65 b	42.70 a
42.56 e	42.61 g	42.66 c	42.71 d
42.57 c	42.62 h	42.67 a	42.72 a
42.58 b	42.63 i	42.68 b	42.73 all
42.59 f	42.64 c	42.69 all	

Chapter 43 Final Questions (42 questions)

43.1 Which of the following statements about leiomyoma uteri is *incorrect*?

a. An estimated 70% of American women have these benign tumors

b. The majority of women with leiomyoma do not require hysterectomy

c. Leiomyoma is an indication in approximately one-third of hysterectomies performed

d. Histologically these are benign tumors with localized proliferation of smooth muscle cells surrounded by a pseudocapsule

e. Leiomyoma are hormonally responsive to estrogen and progesterone

43.2 Which of the following are common symptoms or clinical manifestations of uterine fibroids?

a. Pain

b. Pressure

c. Anemia

d. Bleeding

e. Constipation

43.3 Leiomyosarcoma occur in what percent of leiomyoma?

a. 0.1–1.0

b. 2.1–3.0

c. 4.1–5.0

d. 6.1–7.0

e. 8.1–9.0

43.4 Which of the following statements about leiomyosarcoma is *correct*?

a. Leiomyosarcoma form from degeneration of a normal fibroid

b. This malignancy is more common in patients below the age of 40

c. Patients typically present with a rapidly enlarging uterine mass, unusual vaginal discharge and pelvic pain

d. The tumor consists of a cell types found only in the uterus

43.5–43.7 Instructions: Match the type of benign uterine myoma with the appropriate description(s):

43.5 Intravenous leiomyomatosis _____

43.6 Benign metastasizing leiomyoma _____

43.7 Leiomyomatosis peritonealis disseminata _____

a. Thought to be somewhat estrogen dependent

b. Has been reported in cardiac, pulmonary, and lymphatic nodules

c. Has been found in pelvic veins and the vena cava

d. Implants on peritoneal surfaces

43.8 Postmenopausal patients who present with rapidly enlarging uterine masses should be considered at high risk for

a. Uterine leiomyoma

b. Uterine leiomyosarcoma

c. Intravenous leiomyomatosis

d. Benign metastasizing leiomyoma

e. Leiomyomatosis peritonealis disseminata

43.9 The most common change occurring in myomas in pregnancy is

a. Red degeneration

b. Calcification

c. Liquefaction

d. Hyalinization

e. Parasitic growth

43.10 Red degeneration of uterine leiomyoma refers to

a. Hyalinization of the smooth muscle elements

b. Calcification of the smooth muscle stroma

c. Hemorrhagic changes in the myometrium associated with rapid growth

43.11 Menorrhagia associated with uterine leiomyoma is characterized by increased

a. Amount of menstrual flow only

b. Duration of menstrual flow only

c. Amount and duration of menstrual flow

d. Amount and frequency of menstrual flow

e. Frequency of menstrual flow

43.12 Menorrhagia associated with uterine leiomyoma is defined as a menstrual blood loss of greater than

a. 40 mL

b. 80 mL

c. 120 mL

d. 160 mL

e. 200 mL

43.13 Which of the following is a possible mechanism to explain the increased bleeding associated with the uterine fibroids.

a. Alteration of normal myometrial contractual function in the small artery and the arteriolar blood supply underlying the endometrium

b. Inability of the overlying endometrium to respond to the normal estrogen-progesterone menstrual phases

c. Pressure necrosis of the overlying endometrial bed exposing vascular surfaces that bleed excessively with endometrial sloughing

d. Increased proliferation of small blood vessels under hormonal stimulation

Answers (43.1-43.13)

43.1 a	43.5 a, c	43.8 b	43.11 c
43.2 a, b, d	43.6 a, b	43.9 a	43.12 b
43.3 a	43.7 a, d	43.10 c	43.13 a, b, c
43.4 c			

43.14   The most common type of leiomyoma associated
        with abnormal uterine bleeding is

        a. Subserosal
        b. Intramural
        c. Submucous

43.15   The occurrence of an isolated submucous fibroid
        is common and a major cause of fibroid-associated
        menorrhagia and anemia.

        a. True
        b. False

43.16   Which of the following is a uncommon clinical
        complication of large uterine leiomyoma.

        a. Hydroureter
        b. Hydronephrosis
        c. CVA tenderness

43.17   Which of the following statements about the physi-
        cal examination and physical diagnosis of uterine
        fibroids is *incorrect*?

        a. There is characteristic presence of a large mid-
            line mobile mass with an irregular contour
        b. The mass usually has a "hard-feel" or solid
            quality
        c. Subserosal pedunculated myomas are easily dis-
            tinguishable from solid adnexal masses
        d. Uterine fibroids are usually appreciable on ab-
            dominal examination when they are greater than
            14–16 weeks equivalent gestational size

43.18   Which of the following has the highest cost-benefit
        for imaging uterine myomas?

        a. Magnetic resonance imaging
        b. Computerized axial tomography
        c. Ultrasound

43.19   Which of the following statements about the ultra-
        sound evaluation of presumed uterine leiomyoma is
        correct?

        a. Ultrasound is commonly used for confirmation
            of uterine myomas
        b. Ultrasound can usually demonstrate hypoecho-
            genicity amid otherwise normal myometrial
            patterns
        c. Ultrasound can usually resolve the presence of a
            distorted endometrial stripe
        d. Ultrasound cannot usually distinguish a myoma
            from a solid adnexal mass

43.20   Present data suggest that _____ of patients under-
        going hysteroscopic removal of submucous leiomy-
        oma will require additional therapy within 10 years.

        a. 10%
        b. 20%
        c. 30%
        d. 40%
        e. 50%

43.21   Pedunculated uterine leiomyoma may occasionally
        be removed at the time of dilatation and curettage
        or hysteroscopy, ameliorating symptoms such as
        menorrhagia.

        a. True
        b. False

43.22   Which of the following statements about the treat-
        ment of patients with uterine fibroids is *correct*?

        a. The majority of patients with uterine leiomyoma
            do not require surgical treatment
        b. Assessment of uterine growth requires regular
            CT scans
        c. Uterine bleeding may be minimized by intermit-
            tent progestin supplementation, if significant en-
            dometrial cavity distortion is not present
        d. Myomectomy may be warranted in young pa-
            tients whose fertility is being compromised by
            intracavitary distortion

43.23   Which of the following statements about the use of
        gonadotropin-releasing hormone agonists (GnRH
        analogs) is *incorrect*?

        a. They may be used as temporary treatment (3–6
            months) prior to surgery
        b. They may be used for relatively long-term ther-
            apy (12–36 months) to bring about major reduc-
            tion in large tumor size
        c. Treatment is often associated with reduction in
            uterine masses by as much as 40–60%
        d. Treatment will not permanently reduce the size
            of myomas as withdrawal of the medication
            commonly results in growth of the myomas

43.24   Which of the following statements about pregnancy
        associated with leiomyoma uteri is correct?

        a. The overall course of pregnancy is usually unre-
            markable
        b. There is usually a normal labor and delivery
        c. Myomas typically shrink during pregnancy
        d. Pregnancy is sometimes associated with red or
            carneous degeneration of myomas

43.25   Vaginal births after myomectomy is absolutely con-
        traindicated because of the risk of uterine rupture
        along the myomectomy incision line.

        a. True
        b. False

43.26   Soft tissue dystocia is quite common in association
        with uterine leiomyoma.

        a. True
        b. False

Answers (43.14–43.26)

43.14 c	43.18 c	43.21 a	43.24 a, b, d
43.15 b	43.19 a, b, c	43.22 a, c, d	43.25 b
43.16 all	43.20 b	43.23 b	43.26 b
43.17 c			

43.27 Adenomyosis is found in coexistence with leiomyoma in about what percent of hysterectomy specimens?

    a. 10
    b. 20
    c. 30
    d. 40
    e. 50

43.28 The standard treatment for adenomyosis of the uterus is

    a. Hormone therapy with estrogens
    b. Therapy of GnRH agonists
    c. "Watchful waiting"
    d. Hysterectomy

43.29 Leiomyosarcoma accounts for approximately what percent of cancers involving the body of the uterus?

    a. 1
    b. 3
    c. 6
    d. 9
    e. 12

43.30 The virulence of uterine sarcomas are directly related to

    a. Number of mitotic figures
    b. Degree of cellular proliferation
    c. Association with leiomyoma
    d. Fundal position

43.31 The overall 5-year survival rate for patients with leiomyosarcoma is approximately

    a. 30%
    b. 50%
    c. 70%
    d. 90%

43.32 Like adenocarcinoma of the endometrium, uterine sarcomas are extremely sensitive to progestin therapy.

    a. True
    b. False

43.33 Dilatation and curettage has a 95% success rate in the diagnosis of uterine leiomyosarcoma.

    a. True
    b. False

43.34 Indications and actions prior to myomectomy for infertility patients should include

    a. The presence of leiomyoma of sufficient size or location to be a probable factor in infertility
    b. The absence of a more likely explanation for the failure to conceive
    c. Evidence of normal ovarian function
    d. Evidence of normal fallopian tube function

43.35 Which of the following criteria is required for hysterectomy for leiomyoma?

    a. The presence of asymptomatic leiomyoma of such a size that they are palpable abdominally and of concern to the patient
    b. The presence of uterine bleeding that is uncomfortable for the patient, but without anemia
    c. The presence of acute or severe pelvic discomfort caused by myoma

43.36 Which of the following are relative contraindications to hysterectomy as treatment for leiomyoma?

    a. Acute onset anemia
    b. Possible extension into the broad ligament
    c. Desire to maintain fertility
    d. Asymptomatic leiomyoma of size less than 12 weeks gestation

43.37 Which of the following actions is *not* necessary prior to hysterectomy for leiomyoma uteri?

    a. Confirmation of the absence of cervical malignancy
    b. Elimination of anovulation or other sources of abnormal bleeding
    c. Confirmation of the absence of endometrial malignancy by endometrial biopsy in all patients over the age of 25
    d. Assessment of surgical risk from anemia and the need for presurgical treatment
    e. Consideration of psychological risk associated with hysterectomy

43.38 Which of the following statements about leiomyomas is *not* correct?

    a. Sarcomatous changes are frequent
    b. They are the most common benign tumors in women
    c. They are often asymptomatic and are commonly diagnosed on routine pelvic examination
    d. Regression after menopause is common
    e. Etiologic factors may include estrogenic stimulation

Answers (43.27–43.38)

43.27 c	43.30 a, b	43.33 b	43.36 c, d
43.28 d	43.31 b	43.34 all	43.37 c
43.29 b	43.32 b	43.35 a, c	43.38 a

43.39 Which of the following is *not* a sign or symptom of uterine myomata?

a. Bladder irritability with urinary frequency
b. Heavy periods
c. Amenorrhea
d. Pressure on the rectum with pain on defecation
e. A palpable pelvic mass

43.40 Adenomyosis is characterized by

a. Invasion of the myometrium with benign endometrial cells
b. Infiltration of the myometrium with lymphocytes secondary to endometritis
c. Invasion of the myometrium with endometrial adenocarcinoma
d. Invasion of pelvic tissues with endometrial adenocarcinoma
e. Invasion of the myometrium with squamous cell carcinoma of the cervix

43.41 Uterine sarcomas may originate from all of the following tissues *except*

a. Blood vessels
b. Uterine fibroids (myomata)
c. Endometrium
d. Nerve fibers
e. Myometrium

43.42 The most common malignant nonepithelial tumor of the uterus is

a. Leiomyosarcoma
b. Hemangiopericytoma
c. Fibrosarcoma
d. Endometrial sarcoma
e. Mixed mesodermal tumor

Answers (43.39–43.42)

43.39 c   43.40 a   43.41 d   43.42 a

Chapter 44 Final Questions (55 questions)

44.1 Endometrial carcinoma is the most common genital tract malignancy.

    a. True
    b. False

44.2 Approximately what proportion of patients with invasive endometrial carcinoma are diagnosed in the postmenopausal years?

    a. One-quarter
    b. One-half
    c. Three-quarters
    d. All

44.3 The risk factors for the development of endometrial carcinoma include clinical factors associated with a _____ environment.

    a. Progesterone-rich
    b. Estrogen-rich
    c. Prolactin-rich
    d. Prostaglandin-rich
    e. Testosterone-rich

44.4 Endometrial hyperplasia and endometrial carcinoma are overgrowths of the endometrium in response to

    a. Glandular or ovarian estrogen production
    b. Peripheral conversion of androstenedione to estrone to estrogen
    c. Exogenous estrogen sources
    d. Progesterone production by the endometrium
    e. Testosterone production by the ovary

44.5 Conversion of androstenedione to estrogen occurs mainly in

    a. Peripheral tissue stroma
    b. Peripheral muscular tissue
    c. Peripheral fat tissue
    d. Centers of bone marrow activity

44.6 Endometrial hyperplasia is defined as abnormal proliferation of

    a. Both glandular and stromal elements, with altered histologic architecture
    b. Only glandular elements, with altered histologic architecture
    c. Only stromal elements, with altered histologic architecture
    d. Both glandular and stromal elements, with normal histologic architecture

44.7–44.9 Instructions: Match the traditional histologic classifications of endometrial hyperplasia with the appropriate International Society of Gynecologic Pathologist Classification.

44.7 Cystic hyperplasia _____

44.8 Adenomatous hyperplasia _____

44.9 Atypical adenomatous hyperplasia _____

    a. Complex hyperplasia
    b. Atypical hyperplasia
    c. Simple hyperplasia
    d. Adenomatous hyperplasia without cytologic atypia
    e. Adenomatous hyperplasia with cytologic atypia

44.10 If no clinical intervention occurs, which of the following histologic variations of endometrial hyperplasia will uniformly become endometrial carcinoma?

    a. Cystic glandular hyperplasia
    b. Adenomatous hyperplasia
    c. Atypical adenomatous hyperplasia
    d. None of the above

44.11 Which of the following patient groups is *not* at special risk for endometrial hyperplasia?

    a. Patients only exposed to exogenous estrogen
    b. Patients who have a history of regular ovulation and associated regular estrogen stimulation
    c. Obese postmenopausal women
    d. Women with menopause at greater than 55 years of age

Answers (44.1-44.11)

44.1 a	44.4 a, b, c	44.7 c	44.10 d
44.2 c	44.5 c	44.8 a, d	44.11 b
44.3 b	44.6 a	44.9 b, e	

44.12–44.14   Instructions: Match the type of endometrial hyperplasia with the appropriate statement(s) about its morphology.

44.12   Cystic endometrial hyperplasia (simple hyperplasia) _____

44.13   Adenomatous hyperplasia (complex hyperplasia) _____

44.14   Atypical adenomatous hyperplasia (atypical hyperplasia with cytologic atypia) _____

    a. Significant numbers of glandular elements exhibiting cytologic atypia
    b. Increased gland: stroma ratio giving a "crowded" or "back to back" appearance
    c. Simple tubules are noted with marked variation in size from small to enlarged, cystic dilated glands
    d. "Carcinoma in situ of the endometrium"
    e. A significant amount of disordered maturation
    f. Abnormal proliferation of primarily glandular elements without proliferation of stromal elements
    g. Both glandular and stromal elements proliferate excessively

44.15   Which of the following has an approximately 20–30% risk for malignant transformation?

    a. Cystic endometrial hyperplasia
    b. Adenomatous hyperplasia
    c. Atypical adenomatous hyperplasia

44.16   Special consideration should be given to endometrial sampling in patients over the age of _____ who present with abnormal uterine bleeding.

    a. 30
    b. 35
    c. 40
    d. 45
    e. 50

44.17   The endometrial biopsy of a healthy, thin postmenopausal woman not on estrogen-replacement therapy and without medical problems, is reported as "insufficient tissue for diagnosis." What should be the follow-up testing for this patient?

    a. D&C
    b. Hysteroscopic evaluation
    c. No follow-up testing needed

44.18   The main disadvantage of the "office endometrial biopsy" technique is the

    a. Patient discomfort
    b. Cost
    c. Need for cervical dilation and instrumentation to perform this procedure
    d. Small part of the endometrial surface sampled

44.19–44.22   Instructions: Match the type of endometrial hyperplasia with the appropriate medical therapy

44.19   Simple endometrial hyperplasia _____
44.20   Atypical adenomatous hyperplasia _____
44.21   Cystic endometrial hyperplasia _____
44.22   Adenomatous endometrial hyperplasia _____

    a. Cyclic oral medroxyprogesterone (Provera)
    b. High-dose intramuscular depomedroxyprogesterone acetate (Depo-Provera)
    c. Continuous oral megestrol acetate (Megase)

44.23   Atypical adenomatous hyperplasia in a postmenopausal women is best treated

    a. Medically
    b. Surgically

44.24   Patients with endometrial polyps most commonly present with

    a. Abrupt onset pelvic pain
    b. Abnormal bleeding
    c. Abnormal vaginal discharge
    d. Pelvic pressure

44.25   About what percent of endometrial polyps show malignant change?

    a. 5
    b. 10
    c. 20
    d. 30
    e. 40

44.26   Polyps in postmenopausal women are _____ to be associated with endometrial carcinoma than those in menstrual age women.

    a. More likely
    b. As likely
    c. Less likely

44.27   Endometrial polyps are most commonly associated with women who have had surgery of the uterine corpus with the disruption of the endometrium, decidua, and myometrium.

    a. True
    b. False

44.28   Approximately what percent of postmenopausal women with bleeding have uterine malignancy?

    a. 5–15
    b. 15–25
    c. 30–40
    d. 50–60

Answers (44.12-44.28)

44.12 c, g	44.17 c	44.21 a	44.25 a
44.13 b, f	44.18 d	44.22 a	44.26 a
44.14 a, d, e	44.19 a	44.23 b	44.27 b
44.15 c	44.20 b, c	44.24 b	44.28 b
44.16 b			

44.29 Approximately what percent of patients with endometrial carcinoma are postmenopausal?

    a. 45
    b. 55
    c. 65
    d. 75
    e. 85

44.30 Approximately what percent of women with endometrial carcinoma are menstrual aged?

    a. less than 5
    b. 5–10
    c. 15–20
    d. 25–30
    e. 35–40

44.31–44.40 Instructions: Match the FIGO surgical staging of endometrial carcinoma with the appropriate descriptions about spread.

44.31 Stage IA _____

44.32 Stage IB _____

44.33 Stage IC _____

44.34 Stage IIA _____

44.35 Stage IIB _____

44.36 Stage IIIA _____

44.37 Stage IIIB _____

44.38 Stage IIIC _____

44.39 Stage IVA _____

44.40 Stage IVB _____

    a. Vaginal metastases
    b. Cervical stromal invasion
    c. Endocervical glandular involvement only
    d. Invasion to more than one half of the myometrium
    e. Tumor invades serosa, adnexa, or both and/or positive peritoneal cytology
    f. Metastases to pelvic and/or periaortic lymph nodes
    g. Tumor invades bladder, bowel mucosa, or both
    h. Invasion to less than one-half of the myometrium
    i. Tumor limited to the endometrium
    j. Distant metastases including intraabdominal and/or inguinal lymph nodes

44.41 The term *adenoacanthoma* refers to the situation where the squamous element of the tumor comprises more than _____ of the histologic picture?

    a. 5%
    b. 10%
    c. 15%
    d. 20%
    e. 25%

44.42 The diagnosis of endometrial carcinoma is most frequently made by

    a. Pap smear
    b. Endometrial sampling
    c. Laparoscopy

44.43 Hematogenous spread occurs _____ in endometrial carcinoma than in cervical or ovarian carcinoma.

    a. More frequently
    b. As frequently
    c. Less frequently

44.44 Papillary serous adenocarcinoma tends to be _____ in abdominal pelvic spread than the more common adenocarcinoma of the endometrium.

    a. More aggressive
    b. As aggressive
    c. Less aggressive

44.45 The most important prognostic factor for endometrial carcinoma is

    a. The depth of invasion of the myometrium
    b. The cytologic grade
    c. Patient age at time of diagnosis

44.46 The FIGO guidelines for cervical staging of endometrial carcinoma suggests the need for sampling of the periaortic and pelvic lymph nodes when indicated, especially when the depth of invasion of the myometrium is more than

    a. One-third of the myometrial thickness
    b. Two-thirds of the myometrial thickness
    c. The total myometrial thickness

44.47–44.49 Instructions: Match the grading using the International Federation of Gynecology and Obstetrics System for endometrial carcinoma the best description of tumor type.

44.47 G1 _____

44.48 G2 _____

44.49 G3 _____

    a. Predominantly solid or entire undifferentiated carcinoma
    b. Mildly differentiated adenomatous carcinoma with partly solid areas
    c. High differentiated adenomatous carcinoma

Answers (44.29-44.49)

44.29 d	44.35 b	44.40 j	44.45 b
44.30 b	44.36 e	44.41 b	44.46 a
44.31 i	44.37 a	44.42 b	44.47 c
44.32 h	44.38 f	44.43 a	44.48 b
44.33 d	44.39 g	44.44 a	44.49 a
44.34 c			

44.50 The 5-year survival rate for grade 1 tumors of the endometrium is approximately

  a. 95%
  b. 85%
  c. 75%
  d. 65%
  e. 55%

44.51 What is the incidence of vaginal apex recurrence when simple hysterectomy is used for the treatment of endometrial carcinoma?

  a. less than 5%
  b. 5–10%
  c. 15–20%
  d. 25–30%

44.52 The primary surgical treatment of endometrial carcinoma is

  a. Total abdominal hysterectomy alone
  b. Total abdominal hysterectomy with bilateral salpingo-oophorectomy
  c. Vaginal hysterectomy
  d. Radical hysterectomy
  e. Pelvic exenteration

44.53 The first line of treatment for recurrent endometrial carcinoma is

  a. Debulking surgery
  b. Hormonal therapy, usually progestins
  c. Radiation therapy
  d. Chemotherapy

44.54 The use of estrogen replacement therapy in patients previously treated for endometrial carcinoma is absolutely contraindicated.

  a. True
  b. False

44.55 Endometrial carcinoma is often associated with

  a. Chronic pelvic inflammatory disease
  b. Feminizing ovarian neoplasms
  c. Endometriosis
  d. Mesonephroma

Answers (44.50-44.55)

44.50 a	44.52 b	44.54 b	44.55 b
44.51 b	44.53 b		

Chapter 45 Final Questions (74 questions)

45.1–45.4   Instructions: Match the ovarian neoplasm from each tissue type with the appropriate specific example(s).

45.1   From celomic epithelium (epithelial) _____

45.2   From gonadal stroma _____

45.3   From germ cells _____

45.4   Miscellaneous cell line sources _____

   a. Sertoli-Leydig cell tumor
   b. Teratoma
   c. Lymphoma
   d. Brenner tumor
   e. Endometrioid
   f. Granulosa theca
   g. Metastatic tumor from colon, breast, and endometrium
   h. Dysgerminoma
   i. Choriocarcinoma
   j. Sarcoma
   k. Serous epithelial tumor
   l. Mucinous tumor
   m. Lipid cell fibroma
   n. Endodermal sinus tumor

45.5–45.7   Instructions: Match the histologic classification of common epithelial tumors of the ovary with the appropriate specific example(s).

45.5   Serous tumors _____

45.6   Mucinous tumors _____

45.7   Endometrioid tumors _____

   a. Mucinous, cystadenoma
   b. Serous cystadenomas with low malignant potential
   c. Mucinous cystadenocarcinoma
   d. Serous cystadenomas
   e. Endometrioid benign cysts
   f. Adenocarcinoma
   g. Serous cystadenocarcinoma
   h. Endometrioid tumors of low malignant potential
   i. Mucinous cystadenoma of low malignant potential

45.8–45.11   Instructions: Match the FIGO staging for primary carcinoma of the ovary with the degree of tumor spread.

45.8   Stage 1 _____

45.9   Stage 2 _____

45.10   Stage 3 _____

45.11   Stage 4 _____

   a. Growth involving one or both ovaries with pelvic extension
   b. Tumor involving one or both ovaries with peritoneal implants outside the pelvis and/or positive retroperitoneal or inguinal nodes
   c. Growth limited to the ovaries
   d. Growth involving one or both ovaries with distant metastasis

45.12   Which of the following is *not* contained within the adnexae?

   a. Fallopian tubes
   b. Appendix
   c. Ovaries
   d. Upper portion of the broad ligament
   e. Mesosalpinx

45.13   Which structure of the GU system may mimic a solid adnexal mass?

   a. Bladder
   b. Kidney
   c. Ureter
   d. Urethra
   e. Renal pelvis

45.14   In which age group of women is it abnormal for the ovaries to be palpable?

   a. Premenarchal
   b. Reproductive
   c. Postmenopausal

45.15   In the postmenopausal patient, palpable ovarian enlargement is _____ to be the result of a malignancy than in reproductive age patients.

   a. More likely
   b. As likely
   c. Less likely

Answers (45.1-45.15)

45.1 d, e, k, l	45.5 b, d, g	45.9 a	45.13 b
45.2 a, f, m	45.6 a, c, i	45.10 b	45.14 a, c
45.3 b, h, i, n	45.7 e, f, h	45.11 d	45.15 a
45.4 c, g, j	45.8 c	45.12 b	

45.16   The use of oral contraceptives makes the ovaries
        _____ to be palpable.

        a. More likely
        b. As likely
        c. Less likely

45.17   A small, unilocular ovarian mass in a patient within
        3 years of natural menopause is managed by

        a. Surgical removal of the mass
        b. Observation through serial transvaginal ultra-
            sound examinations

45.18   Functional ovarian cysts are

        a. Neoplasms
        b. Anatomic variations
        c. Malignant tumors

45.19   Which of the following statements about ovarian
        follicular cysts is *incorrect*?

        a. They arise from the failure of an ovarian follicle
            to rupture
        b. They are associated with a shortening of the fol-
            licular phase
        c. Cysts are lined with normal granulosa cells
        d. Cysts are filled with estrogen-rich fluid

45.20   The rupture of a follicular cyst usually results in an
        acute abdomen requiring surgical evaluation

        a. True
        b. False

45.21   Alterations in the menstrual cycle associated with
        follicular cysts are due to

        a. Failed subsequent ovulation
        b. Stimulation by the large amount of estradiol pro-
            duced by the granulosa cells within the follicle
        c. Large concentrations of progesterone produced
            by the ovary in response to cyst growth

45.22   Follicular cysts usually are followed for _____
        weeks with or without accompanying oral contra-
        ceptive treatment, before consideration of surgical
        evaluation.

        a. 2–4
        b. 6–8
        c. 10–12
        d. 14–16

45.23   A patient not using oral contraceptives, with regular
        periods, presents with acute pain late in the luteal
        phase. Her pregnancy test is negative. This clinical
        picture is most consistent with

        a. Serous cystadenoma
        b. Mucinous cystadenoma
        c. Corpus hemorrhagicum
        d. Dermoid cyst
        e. Follicular cyst

45.24   Corpus luteum cysts are often associated with a de-
        lay in menstruation for 1–2 weeks and dull lower
        quadrant pain. Which of the following must be mea-
        sured prior to the consideration of conservative
        management of this situation?

        a. Progesterone
        b. Estrogen
        c. Estradiol
        d. β-hCG
        e. FSH

45.25–45.27   Instructions: Match the site of origin with the
        resulting ovarian neoplasm.

45.25   From coelomic epithelium _____

45.26   From gonadal stroma _____

45.27   From germ cells _____

        a. Teratoma
        b. Granulosa-theca
        c. Serous
        d. Mucinous
        e. Choriocarcinoma

45.28   Approximately what percent of serous cystadenomas
        are benign?

        a. 20
        b. 30
        c. 40
        d. 50
        e. 60
        f. 70

45.29–45.32   Instructions: Match the epithelial tumor of
        the ovary with its corresponding characteristics

45.29   Serous cystadenoma _____

45.30   Mucinous cystadenoma _____

45.31   Endometrioid tumor _____

45.32   Brenner cell tumor _____

        a. Potentially the largest type of cystic tumor
        b. The most common epithelial cell neoplasm
        c. Bilateral about 15% of the time
        d. Bilateral 5% of the time
        e. Most common in perimenopausal and postmen-
            opausal women
        f. Large amount of stroma and fibrotic tissue sur-
            rounds the epithelial cells
        g. Cyst lined by well-differentiated endometrial-
            like glandular tissue

Answers (45.16–45.32)

45.16 c   45.21 a, b   45.25 c, d   45.29 b, c, e
45.17 b   45.22 b   45.26 b   45.30 a, d
45.18 a, b   45.23 c   45.27 a, e   45.31 g
45.19 b   45.24 d   45.28 f   45.32 f
45.20 b

45.33 Because of the risk of malignancy, the treatment of serous cystadenoma is removal of the associated adnexa at a minimum.

a. True
b. False

45.34 Hyperthyroidism is associated with what ovarian neoplasm?

a. Mucinous cystadenoma
b. Serous cystadenoma
c. Stroma ovarii
d. Benign cystic teratoma

45.35 Which of the following is *not* characteristic of benign cystic teratomas?

a. They contain derivates from all of the embryonic germ layers.
b. The most common elements are mesodermal in origin
c. 10–20% are bilateral
d. Diagnosis can be confirmed on ultrasound
e. They often are felt anterior to the broad ligament on physical examination

45.36–45.38 Instructions: Match the stromal cell tumor of the ovary with its characteristics.

45.36 Granulosa-theca cell tumor _____

45.37 Sertoli-Leydig cell tumor _____

45.38 Ovarian fibroma _____

a. Produces hormones
b. May contribute to precocious puberty
c. Produces androgenic components
d. Produces estrogenic components
e. May contribute to hirsutism or virilizing symptoms
f. May result in feminization
g. May be associated with ascites

45.39 Benign ovarian neoplasms are _____ malignant tumors of the ovary in all age groups.

a. More common than
b. As common as
c. Less common than

45.40 A woman's risk of developing ovarian cancer during her lifetime is approximately

a. 1%
b. 3%
c. 5%
d. 7%
e. 9%

45.41 Ovarian cancer presents more commonly in which decades of life?

a. 3rd
b. 4th
c. 5th
d. 6th
e. 7th

45.42 Approximately what percent of patients with ovarian cancer have metastatic disease at the time of diagnosis?

a. 20
b. 30
c. 40
d. 50
e. 60

45.43 Which ovarian tumor has the highest malignant potential?

a. Cystadenofibroma
b. Brenner tumor
c. Mucinous cystadenoma
d. Serous cystadenoma
e. Dermoid

45.44 Which of the following have been associated with developing ovarian cancer?

a. Use of hormone replacement therapy
b. Low parity
c. Delayed childbearing
d. Familial predisposition

45.45 Malignant ovarian epithelial cell tumors spread primarily by

a. Direct extension within the peritoneal cavity
b. Lymphatic dissemination
c. Hematogenous dissemination

45.46 Serum tumor markers are useful in the diagnosis and clinical follow-up of epithelial cell neoplasms of the ovary.

a. True
b. False

45.47 The combination of benign ovarian fibroma and ascites and right unilateral hydrothorax is termed

a. Sertoli-Leydig syndrome
b. Familial cancer syndrome
c. Meigs syndrome
d. Hydrotubae profluens

Answers (45.33-45.47)

45.33 b	45.37 a, c, e	45.41 c, d	45.45 a
45.34 c	45.38 g	45.42 e	45.46 b
45.35 b	45.39 a	45.43 d	45.47 c
45.36 a, b, d, f	45.40 a	45.44 b, c, d	

45.48   What percent of all ovarian malignancies are of the epithelial cell type?

    a. 90
    b. 70
    c. 50
    d. 30

45.49–45.51   Instructions: Match the epithelial cell ovarian carcinoma with the appropriate descriptions.

45.49   Malignant epithelial serous tumors _____

45.50   Malignant mucinous epithelial tumors _____

45.51   Malignant endometrioid tumors _____

    a. Associated with pseudomyxomatous peritonei
    b. Most common malignant epithelial cell tumors
    c. 10–15% bilateral
    d. 30% bilateral
    e. Typically multiloculated
    f. Contain histologic features similar to endometrial carcinoma
    g. May be associated with widespread peritoneal extensions

45.52   The most common ovarian cancer in women under the age of 20 is

    a. Malignant serous cystadenocarcinoma
    b. Malignant mucinous cystadenocarcinoma
    c. Clear cell carcinoma
    d. Germ cell tumor

45.53   The primary surgical approach involved in the surgical treatment of ovarian carcinoma is

    a. Total abdominal hysterectomy
    b. Cytoreductive surgery or "tumor debulking"
    c. Radical hysterectomy
    d. Laparoscopically assisted vaginal hysterectomy

45.54   Which of the following statements about dysgerminomas is *correct*?

    a. They are most commonly bilateral
    b. They are more likely than epithelial cell tumors to spread via lymphatic channels
    c. The tumors are radiosensitive
    d. The 5-year survival rate for patients with small, unilateral tumors is approximately 50%

45.55   Which of the following statements about treatment of dysgerminomas is *correct*?

    a. If tumor size is less than 10 cm and there is no evidence of extraovarian spread, treatment may include only the removal of the affected ovary
    b. Pelvic and periaortic nodes must be assessed at the time of surgery
    c. There should be postoperative irradiation to the abdomen and pelvis
    d. Chemotherapy usually is reserved for primary treatment failures

45.56–45.57   Instructions: Match the gonadal stromal cell tumor with its appropriate characteristics.

45.56   Granulosa cell tumor _____

45.57   Sertoli-Leydig cell tumor _____

    a. Secretes testosterone
    b. Secretes estrogen
    c. May result in endometrial hyperplasia
    d. Occur in patients of all ages
    e. More common in older patients

45.58   Tumors that are metastatic to the ovary from other sites are

    a. Krukenberg tumors
    b. Malignant mesodermal sarcomas
    c. Fibrosarcomas

45.59   The least common of these carcinomas of the female genital tract is

    a. Carcinoma of the fallopian tube
    b. Bartholin gland carcinoma
    c. Vulvar carcinoma
    d. Leiomyosarcoma

45.60   Which of the following statements about fallopian tube carcinoma is *incorrect*?

    a. The most common primary fallopian tube carcinomas are adenosquamous carcinoma and sarcoma
    b. Primary fallopian tube carcinoma is associated with a profuse serosanguineous discharge, hydrotubae profluens
    c. Overall 5-year survival rate for primary fallopian tube carcinoma is 35–45%
    d. Carcinoma metastatic to the fallopian tube is more common than primary fallopian tube carcinoma

---

Answers (45.48-45.60)

45.48 a	45.52 d	45.55 a, b, d	45.58 a
45.49 b, d, e	45.53 b	45.56 b, c, d	45.59 a
45.50 a, c, g	45.54 b, c	45.57 a, e	45.60 a
45.51 f			

45.61 A pathognomonic sign of tubal carcinoma is

a. Secondary amenorrhea coupled with intermittent pelvic pain
b. A pelvic mass
c. Profuse serosanguineous vaginal discharge
d. Colicky abdominal pain

45.62 Which of the following is appropriate when clinically palpable ovarian enlargement is detected in a
postmenopausal woman?

a. Take a Pap smear and review in 6 weeks
b. Treat with parenteral progestins
c. X-ray to evaluate osteoporosis and collect urine
for 24-hr total estrogen excretion
d. Take a Pap smear and review in 6 months
e. Take a sonogram of pelvis and consider surgical
evaluation

45.63 Which of the following is *not* a complication of
functional ovarian cysts (follicular or luteal)?

a. Hemorrhage into the cyst
b. Rupture with hemoperitoneum
c. Rupture with brief acute pelvic pain
d. Pseudomyxoma peritonei
e. Torsion

45.64 Granulosa theca cell ovarian tumors are seen most
frequently

a. Before puberty
b. In the childbearing years
c. Postmenopausal

45.65 Abnormal uterine bleeding due to an ovarian neoplasm is secondary to

a. Pressure
b. Increased vascularity
c. Metastasis
d. Biological activity of the hormones produced

45.66 Which ovarian tumor has the highest malignant potential?

a. Cystadenofibroma
b. Brenner tumor
c. Mucinous cystadenoma
d. Serous cystadenoma
e. Dermoid

45.67 Physiological enlargement of the ovaries can be due
to

a. Follicle cysts
b. Corpus luteum cysts
c. Theca lutein cysts

45.68 The most common masculinizing ovarian tumor is

a. Arrhenoblastoma
b. Gynandroblastoma
c. Adrenal rest tumor
d. Leydig cell tumor

45.69 Arrhenoblastomas are usually

a. Unilateral
b. Bilateral

45.70 The hormone responsible for the findings in arrhenoblastoma is

a. Androstedione
b. Androsterone
c. Testosterone
d. Estriol

45.71 Dermoids are more commonly

a. Unilateral
b. Bilateral

45.72 Brenner tumors are usually

a. Unilateral
b. Bilateral

45.73 The treatment of Brenner tumors of the ovary is

a. Simple excision
b. Excision and exploration of the other ovary
c. Excision and hysterectomy

45.74 The presence of a signet-ring cell type in ovarian
tumors is usually indicative of

a. Hilus cell tumors
b. Adrenal rest tumors
c. Brenner tumors
d. Krukenberg tumors
e. Serous adenoma

Answers (45.61–45.74)

45.61 c	45.65 d	45.69 a	45.72 a
45.62 e	45.66 d	45.70 c	45.73 a
45.63 d	45.67 all	45.71 a	45.74 d
45.64 c	45.68 a		

Chapter 46 Final Questions (24 questions)

46.1   About _____ of patients with gestational trophoblastic disease will develop persistent or malignant
disease.

   a. 10%
   b. 20%
   c. 30%
   d. 40%
   e. 60%

46.2   The incidence of gestational trophoblastic disease in
the United States is approximately 1 in pregnancies.

   a. 500
   b. 1000
   c. 1500
   d. 2000
   e. 2500
   f. 3000

46.3   Genetically, complete moles are of

   a. Paternal origin only
   b. Maternal origin only
   c. Mixed paternal and maternal origin

46.4   Approximately what percent of molar pregnancies
are of the complete mole type?

   a. 50
   b. 60
   c. 70
   d. 80
   e. 90

46.5–46.6 Instructions: Match the type of molar pregnancy with its appropriate characteristics.

46.5   Complete molar pregnancy _____

46.6   Incomplete molar pregnancy _____

   a. Karyotype commonly 69, XXY
   b. Karyotype commonly 46, XX
   c. Fetal membranes absent
   d. Chromosomally abnormal fetus present
   e. Proliferations of the syncytotrophoblast
   f. Proliferation from the cytotrophoblast
   g. All villi edematous

46.7   The potential for malignant transformation in a
complete mole is _____ in a partial mole.

   a. Greater than
   b. The same as
   c. Less than

46.8   Abnormal bleeding during a complete molar pregnancy most commonly occurs early in the _____
trimester.

   a. First
   b. Second
   c. Third

46.9   A discrepancy between the uterine size and the gestational age is seen in approximately what percent of
patients with complete molar pregnancy?

   a. 30
   b. 50
   c. 70
   d. 90

46.10   Patients with molar pregnancy may present with
which of the following signs and symptoms?

   a. Pregnancy-induced hypertension
   b. Severe nausea
   c. Bradycardia
   d. Visual disturbances

46.11   A molar pregnancy is confirmed through

   a. Serial measurement of hCG levels
   b. Use of ultrasound imaging
   c. Bimanual pelvic examination

46.12   Patients with partial molar pregnancy typically present at _____ patients with complete molar pregnancy.

   a. An earlier gestational age than
   b. The same gestational age as
   c. A later gestational age than

46.13   Theca lutein cysts accompany molar pregnancy in
almost all cases.

   a. True
   b. False

46.14   The determination of hCG titers associated with
molar pregnancy is used to

   a. Classify the risk category for the tumor
   b. Serve as a tumor marker in follow-up of therapy
   c. Ascertain whether the pregnancy is a partial or
       complete mole

46.15   Which of the following is not characteristic of high
risk gestational trophoblastic disease?

   a. Uterus greater than 16-week size
   b. Presence of a large theca lutein cyst
   c. Marked trophoblastic proliferation and/or ana-
       plasia
   d. Hyperthyroidism
   e. 46-XX karyotype

46.16   The basic treatment of molar pregnancy is

   a. Evacuation of the uterine contents
   b. Abdominal hysterectomy
   c. Abdominal hysterectomy with bilateral salpingo-
       oophorectomy
   d. Radiation therapy
   e. Chemotherapy

Answers (46.1–46.16)

46.1	a	46.5	b, c, e, g	46.9	c	46.13	b
46.2	d	46.6	a, d, f	46.10	a, b, d	46.14	a, b
46.3	a	46.7	a	46.11	b	46.15	e
46.4	e	46.8	b	46.12	c	46.16	a

46.17 Because of the abnormal genetic karyotype of molar pregnancies, RhoGAM administration following molar evacuation is not required.

    a. True
    b. False

46.18 In the follow-up of a molar pregnancy, serum hCG levels should be obtained monthly for _____ months, after obtaining the first normal level following the evacuation.

    a. 6
    b. 12
    c. 18
    d. 24

46.19 Choriocarcinoma occurs in about one-third of patients with gestational trophoblastic disease.

    a. True
    b. False

46.20 Which of the following is an indication for chemotherapy in trophoblastic disease?

    a. Histologic diagnosis of choriocarcinoma
    b. Evidence of metastatic disease
    c. Plateaued or rising hCG titers after evacuation
    d. β-hCG titer that has not returned to normal after 12 weeks postevacuation
    e. Increased β-hCG titer after a normal level has been obtained, exclusive of a normal pregnancy

46.21 The treatment of a patient with a hydatidiform mole may include all of the following *except*

    a. Periodic assays of serum β-hCG
    b. Periodic clinical examinations for the detection of malignant changes
    c. Radiotherapy
    d. Prophylactic chemotherapy
    e. Evacuation of the uterus

46.22 Eclampsia in the first trimester is most frequently due to

    a. Abruptio placenta
    b. Acute glomerulonephritis
    c. Molar degeneration
    d. Pregnancy-induced hypertension
    e. Berry aneurysm

46.23 A serious complication of choriocarcinoma is

    a. Intestinal obstruction
    b. Uterine perforation and massive bleeding
    c. Sudden unexpected death

46.24 An antecedent term pregnancy is associated with a _____ prognosis in malignant gestational trophoblastic disease.

    a. Good
    b. Poor

Answers (46.17–46.24)

46.17 b	46.19 b	46.21 c	46.23 b
46.18 b	46.20 all	46.22 c	46.24 b

Chapter 47 Final Questions (22 questions)

47.1   A 32-year-old patient has delivered at 25 weeks of gestation, 3 days after premature rupture of the membranes. She has discussed the circumstances with her obstetrician and requests that no attempts at resuscitation should be done. At delivery there are rare gasping breathing movements. The pediatrician demands that intubation be done. The individual with the clearest primary responsibility for this decision is the

a.   Mother
b.   Pediatrician
c.   Obsetrician
d.   Hospital attorney

47.2   Which of the following is *not* among the main domains of ethical concern in medical care?

a.   Justice issues
b.   Patient preference issues
c.   Legal issues
d.   Medical indications or benefit issues
e.   Quality of life issues

47.3   Quality of life issues primarily concern the

a.   Physician's estimate of outcome
b.   Patient's experience of outcome
c.   Population-based evaluation of outcome
d.   Patient's choice of outcome

47.4   Respect for patient wishes (autonomy) requires that there be assessment of the

a.   Patient's ability to consider information in their framework
b.   Severity of the illness and the potential success of the proposed therapy
c.   Impact of the patient's choice on family
d.   Cost of the proposed treatment

47.5   A 62-year-old woman with newly diagnosed stage III ovarian cancer refuses chemotherapy. She wants to "go home to die." The next step in evaluating this patient is to

a.   Assess the patient's comprehension, evidence of depression
b.   Accept patient wishes and discharge from hospital
c.   Call hospital attorney to assess risk of malpractice
d.   Call the family for a conference

47.6   A 90-year-old woman is found to have a 20-cm pelvic/abdominal mass. Her Ca125 is 90. Your recommendation for care should be based in the ethical area of

a.   Beneficence/nonmaleficence
b.   Statutory law
c.   Autonomy
d.   Justice
e.   Quality of life
f.   Conflict of interest
g.   Futility
h.   Surrogate decision making
i.   Advance directives

47.7   A 33-year-old physician sees a 21-year-old pregnant primigravid woman in the emergency room for a UTI. She discovers the patient is going to give the child up for adoption and gives the patient her lawyer's phone number. She states she has been looking for a child to adopt and goes over all the advantages she can offer the child. Her actions fall into the ethical area of

a.   Beneficence/nonmaleficence
b.   Statutory law
c.   Autonomy
d.   Justice
e.   Quality of life
f.   Conflict of interest
g.   Futility
h.   Surrogate decision making
i.   Advance directives

47.8   A 60-year-old woman is admitted semicomatose with fever and a white blood count of 1000, 10 days after chemotherapy for breast cancer. She has an advance directive on record and her husband accompanies her. The decision to treat is made based on the ethical area of

a.   Beneficence/nonmaleficence
b.   Statutory law
c.   Autonomy
d.   Justice
e.   Quality of life
f.   Conflict of interest
g.   Futility
h.   Surrogate decision making
i.   Advance directives

Answers (47.1-47.8)

47.1 a	47.3 b	47.5 a	47.7 f
47.2 c	47.4 a, b, c	47.6 a	47.8 h

47.9   A 28-year-old with metastatic breast cancer wants to try a bone marrow transplant-supported treatment. Her insurance company refuses. The ethical area involved is

   a. Beneficence/nonmaleficence
   b. Statutory law
   c. Autonomy
   d. Justice
   e. Quality of life
   f. Conflict of interest
   g. Futility
   h. Surrogate decision making
   i. Advance directives

47.10–47.13   Instructions: Match the area of concern with the corresponding illustrative questions.

47.10   Medical indication _____
47.11   Patient preference _____
47.12   Quality of life _____
47.13   Contextual issues _____

   a. What does the patient want?
   b. What are the needs of society?
   c. What impact will the proposed treatment or lack of it have on the patient's life?
   d. What is the best treatment? Best alternatives?

47.14–47.17   Instructions: Match the ethical concern with the corresponding ethical principle.

47.14   Medical indication _____
47.15   Patient preference _____
47.16   Quality of life _____
47.17   Contextual issues _____

   a. Beneficence
   b. Nonmaleficence
   c. Autonomy
   d. Justice

47.18–47.21   Instructions: Match the ethical principle with the appropriate definition.

47.18   Beneficence _____
47.19   Nonmaleficence _____
47.20   Autonomy _____
47.21   Justice _____

   a. The patient should be given what is "due"
   b. There should be respect for the patient's right to self-determination
   c. There is a duty not to inflict harm or injury
   d. There is a duty to promote the good of the patient

47.22   Ethically, the physician-patient relationship is paramount to the physician-fetus relationship.

   a. True
   b. False

Answers (47.9-47.22)

47.9 d	47.13 b	47.17 d	47.20 b
47.10 d	47.14 a	47.18 d	47.21 a
47.11 a	47.15 c	47.19 c	47.22 a
47.12 c	47.16 b		

APGO OBJECTIVES INDEX

This index is different from the usual Subject Index. It is designed to help the reader study a topic designated in one of the educational objectives of the Association of Professors of Gynecology and Obstetrics (APGO).

The objectives are listed on the left. On the right are the pages in the book where there are major discussions of the topic.

Unit 1 : Approach to the Patient

Unit 2 : Obstetrics

SECTION A : NORMAL OBSTETRICS

SECTION B : ABNORMAL OBSTETRICS

INDEX

Page numbers followed by "f" denote figures; those followed by "t" denote tables.